Antimicrobial Resistance

INFECTIOUS DISEASE AND THERAPY

Series Editor

Burke A. Cunha

Winthrop-University Hospital Mineola and
State University of New York School of Medicine
Stony Brook, New York

Antimicrobial Resistance
Problem Pathogens and Clinical Countermeasures

Edited by

Robert C. Owens, Jr.
Maine Medical Center
Portland, Maine, USA

Ebbing Lautenbach
University of Pennsylvania
Philadelphia, Pennsylvania, USA

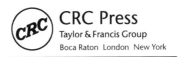

CRC Press
Taylor & Francis Group
Boca Raton London New York

CRC Press is an imprint of the
Taylor & Francis Group, an **informa** business

CRC Press
Taylor & Francis Group
6000 Broken Sound Parkway NW, Suite 300
Boca Raton, FL 33487-2742

First issued in paperback 2019

ISBN 13: 978-0-367-45278-0 (pbk)
ISBN 13: 978-0-8247-2941-7 (hbk)

Library of Congress Cataloging-in-Publication Data

Antimicrobial resistance: problem pathogens and clinical countermeasures / edited by Robert C. Owens Jr., Ebbing Lautenbach.
  p. ; cm. – (Infectious disease and therapy ; v. 48)
  Includes bibliographical references and index.
  ISBN-13: 978-0-8247-2941-7 (hb : alk. paper)
  ISBN-10: 0-8247-2941-2 (hb : alk. paper)
1. Drug resistance in microorganisms. I. Owens, Robert C. Jr. II. Lautenbach, Ebbing. III. Series.
  [DNLM: 1. Drug Resistance, Microbial. W1 IN406HMN v.48 2007/QW 45 A6313 2007] QR177.A588 2007
  616.9'041–dc22

2007024842

Visit the Taylor & Francis Web site at
http://www.taylorandfrancis.com

and the CRC Press Web site at
http://www.crcpress.com

This is for my dear wife, Christy,
and our children, Aleksandr and Ekaterina,
who have inspired me in every way and through every day.

—RCO, Jr.

To my parents, John and Monika,
for a lifetime of encouragement, guidance, and love.

—EL

Foreword

Few would argue with the fact that the discovery and subsequent clinical application of antimicrobial agents represents one of the crowning achievements of medical science in the twentieth century. This is clearly reflected in the fact that the names of many of the pioneers in antimicrobial chemotherapy, including Paul Ehrlich, Gerhard Domagk, Alexander Fleming, Howard Florie, Edward P. Abraham, Ernst Boris Chain, and Selman Waxman, were all awarded Nobel Prizes for their scientific achievements. The initial reaction of the medical and lay communities alike was one of optimism that the problems of bacterial infections throughout the world would clearly be solved by antibiotic therapy. As recently as the 1970s, statements were made by prominent scientists suggesting that bacterial infections were no longer a problem worthy of concern. Nothing, of course, could have been further from the truth. The microbial world shows remarkable adaptivity, and nowhere is this more evident than in the ability of bacteria to develop resistance to all antimicrobial agents that have thus far been discovered. Shortly after the turn of the century, ethyl hydrocupreine (optochin) was tried for the treatment of pneumococcal pneumonia. Although the initial trial was terminated because of drug toxicity, the emergence of resistance to optochin during therapy was also noted—probably the first documentation of the emergence of resistance to an antimicrobial agent by pathogenic bacteria in humans. The enzyme beta-lactamase was described by Abraham and Chain in 1939, before the first clinical use of penicillin. Nonetheless, once this enzyme surfaced in *Staphylococcus aureus*, it was responsible for the rapid world-wide emergence of resistance to penicillin in this important pathogen. This scenario has been repeated over and over as new antimicrobials have entered the therapeutic armamentarium.

Most of the clinically useful antimicrobial agents (with some notable exceptions like the sulfonamides and oxazolidinones) are natural products. It is not surprising, knowing this, that genes encoding resistance to these antimicrobials are found in nature as well. Indeed, many of these genes come from the antibiotic-producing microbes themselves, where they are useful to prevent the organisms from committing microbiological suicide. It was originally hoped that resistance to synthetic molecules would be less likely to develop since they did not necessarily have distributions in the natural habitats of bacteria and other microorganisms. However, as already mentioned, microorganisms are remarkably resourceful and have succeeded in developing resistance by various mechanisms to the sulfonamides and even the oxazolidinones. It was hoped that resistance to the latter class of compounds would be particularly difficult to achieve by bacteria since there are multiple copies of the target 23S ribosomal RNA in many important Gram-positive bacterial pathogens. While this has slowed the development of resistance to the oxazolidinones among staphylococci, for example, it has not prevented it. Moreover, recent descriptions of a plasmid-mediated enzyme that methylates a common target for chloramphenicol, the lincosamides, the oxazolidinones, the pleuromutilins, and streptogramins, has been described. If further dissemination of this occurs, it will cause problems for all five classes of these antimicrobials!

Over the years, it has become clear that it is the selective pressure exerted by the clinical and other use of antimicrobial agents that leads to the emergence and persistence of resistant organisms in a given environment. Antimicrobials are used for the prophylaxis and treatment of infections in humans and animals. They are also used as agricultural growth-promotants. They are widely used in aquaculture and have industrial uses as broad as the management of bacterial causes of fruit and vegetable blights to the prevention of barnacle formation on military and commercial ships.

Clinicians play an important role in contributing to the selective pressure that leads to resistance. Nonetheless, the use of antimicrobials for veterinary, agricultural, aquacultural, and other commercial applications dwarfs the clinical use of antibiotics in humans. Indeed, the tonnage of antimicrobials used in growth-promotion and therapeutic use in farm animals in the United States is more than four times the amount used therapeutically in humans. The prophylactic and therapeutic use of antimicrobials by health professionals, especially in the confines of the hospital and the intensive care unit, has a dramatic impact on antimicrobial resistance in these areas, and it is therefore appropriate that this book is directed primarily at practicing physicians, pharmacists, microbiologists, hospital epidemiologists, and hospital administrators. Its subtitle, *Problem Pathogens and Clinical Countermeasures*, sums up the editors' intention to hone in on the problematic commonplace organisms and to provide opportunities to intervene and begin addressing the magnitude of antimicrobial resistance. Unless the tide of antimicrobial resistance is stemmed quickly, we face the real possibility of a world once more full of untreatable bacteria and other microorganisms.

Antimicrobial Resistance: *Problem Pathogens and Clinical Countermeasures* is filled with chapters written by renowned experts in their respective fields who provide real insight into this problem. The value of surveillance in establishing appropriate areas for intervention is covered nicely. Excellent chapters on problem bacterial pathogens provide insight into the issues that confront the clinician trying to choose appropriate antimicrobial therapy for organisms as diverse as methicillin-resistant staphylococci, vancomycin-resistant enterococci, extended spectrum beta-lactamase producing enterobacteriaceae, *Pseudomonas aeruginosa*, and *Acinetobacter species*. The emerging area of antifungal resistance is also addressed. In addition, the importance of properly evaluating studies of resistant organisms (versus their susceptible counterparts) is addressed so the reader can effectively evaluate this growing body of literature, and is but one area that differentiates this book from others addressing antimicrobial resistance. Not content to describe and define the problem of resistance, the editors have concluded with a series of chapters defining potential methods to deal with antimicrobial resistance. These include discussions of the importance of appropriate initial therapy, de-escalation therapy, pharmacodynamic dose optimization, including the role of prolonged infusions of beta-lactams, infection control controversies, the burgeoning topic of antimicrobial stewardship, and the role of computers in this and other processes to limit the spread of resistant organisms, short course antibiotic therapy, and the role of combination therapy. Taken in aggregate, the chapters in this book provide a fresh and very valuable look at the problems posed by antimicrobial resistance as we enter the twenty-first century! These are issues that are of critical importance to research scientists, physicians, allied health care professionals, administrators, and patients alike. Unless we deal effectively with the problem as outlined by this detailed book, its title will be more prophetically written "Antimicrobial Armageddon"!

Robert C. Moellering, Jr., M.D.
Shields Warren-Mallinckrodt Professor of Medical Research
Harvard Medical School
Department of Medicine
Beth Israel Deaconess Medical Center
Boston, Massachusetts, U.S.A.

Preface

With more than two million infections occurring in the United States alone each year, and a substantial proportion of them being caused by antimicrobial resistant organisms, interventions are desperately needed. Antimicrobial resistance has the potential to impact everyone. In fact, antimicrobials are the only category of drugs that have "societal" consequences. In other words, antihypertensives or lipid lowering agents only impact the person receiving these drugs. With antimicrobials, in contrast, an individual can receive these drugs, develop resistance to them, and then pass along the newly created resistant organism to individuals that have never been exposed to the antimicrobial(s) administered. This so-called "societal" impact of antimicrobials can be seen with not only traditional antibiotics used to treat bacteria and fungal pathogens (both of which this book will focus on), but also antivirals used to treat human immunodeficiency virus, influenza A, avian flu virus, and anti-tuberculosis agents to treat tuberculosis. The latter examples have received considerable press attention due to the fact that multiple antiviral-resistant human immunodeficiency virus strains can be transmitted to an individual who is treatment naïve, with the same being true for extrapulmonary tuberculosis , or extensively drug-resistant tuberculosis. The examples of highly resistant human immunodeficiency virus and extrapulmonary tuberculosis portray the societal consequences well to the general public because of the therapeutic challenges they create and the poor associated outcomes. For bacteria and fungi, there does not yet seem to be a public eruption about bacteria and fungi that are resistant to multiple drugs and are in part responsible for numerous deaths in the developed world each day.

Sometimes these resistant organisms occur as a consequence of treatment that has been suboptimally selected, dosed, and/or given for an appropriate duration (usually too long). However, a significant proportion of resistance is created in patients who are receiving antimicrobial therapy that is *not* optimized in terms of its selection, dose, and duration, and/or the adherence to the regimen by the patient is poor or non-existent. In the spirit that this book, *Antimicrobial Resistance: Problem Pathogens and Clinical Countermeasures*, was developed, our intentions were to focus on the more common pathogens that are causing significant disease and pathogens that have also developed multiple drug resistance, and, perhaps most importantly, to discuss interventions to minimize the development, spread, and impact of antimicrobial resistance.

This book is divided into three sections. The first section tackles several background subjects germane to antimicrobial resistance, including the subject of measuring the cost of resistance from the healthcare and clinician's perspective. The intention of this is to enable administrators, clinician administrators, as well as clinicians themselves to understand the direct and indirect costs of antimicrobial resistance. It is in the hope that, as more administrators understand (and more clinicians are able to speak to) these issues, more progress will be made in the investment of programs designed to prevent infection and use antimicrobials more judiciously in the healthcare setting. Other chapters in this section deal with quantifying escalating resistance rates through national and international surveillance projects, their limitations, and ultimately quantifying and benchmarking resistance at the local level through the use of modified antibiograms. A chapter is also dedicated to tackling the troubling issues surrounding why we have seen a seventy five percent reduction in new antimicrobials for human use over the last two decades. What is driving this reduction in antimicrobial development? Why are large pharmaceutical companies who have brought more than ninety percent of our current antimicrobial arsenal to the market leaving anti-infective development? Finally, a chapter is included that addresses the types of methodologies used by investigators to understand the impact of antimicrobial resistance compared with infections caused by antimicrobial-susceptible organisms. This section is designed to help the reader understand the general methodologies currently in use, when to use certain methodologies, and the strengths and limitations of each.

The next section deals with clinically important pathogens ranging from community- to healthcare-associated bacteria, as well as the troubling developments in *Clostridium difficile* and fungi. The topic of *Staphlyococcus aureus* is covered nicely, addressing both community-acquired methicillin-resistant staphylococci as well as healthcare-associated methicillin-resistant staphylococci in terms of both virulence characteristics and treatment. *Streptococcus pneumoniae*, the leading community-acquired pathogen is discussed, as are enterococci. In addition, the most common and refractory healthcare-associated pathogens are discussed, including *Pseudomonas aeruginosa* and *Acinetobacter spp.* The chapters are designed to give the clinician a general overview of the organism, including resistance mechanisms and recent trends as well as potential treatment options. In the case of *C. difficile*, this chapter focuses on a novel aspect of resistance, that is, resistance to certain antimicrobials has lead to an increased risk of developing *C. difficile*-infection. Recent and historical data are reviewed in an effort to simplify this complex association between antimicrobial use and risk for *C. difficile*-infection. Furthermore, an up-to-date *C. difficile* treatment algorithm is proposed that has been in clinical use since the time of the BI/NAP1/027 outbreak strain. A chapter on emerging beta-lactamases was developed, in part, due to the overwhelming changes that have occurred with this sophisticated mechanism of resistance. Within this chapter, a variety of organisms are discussed as well as the types of beta-lactamases they are most associated with.

The final section is one that may separate it from traditional books on antimicrobial resistance. The intention is to discuss clinically relevant options to minimize the development of resistance, ranging from a nicely written chapter overviewing infection control interventions, to a chapter discussing the merits and practical implementation issues related to antimicrobial stewardship programs. Some components of antimicrobial stewardship programs require their own chapter. These include the a review of antimicrobial de-escalation/streamlining, use of computer assisted technology to optimize antimicrobial use, employing shorter courses of therapy when appropriate, and using guidelines to drive appropriate antimicrobial use, as examples.

This book has an appeal to all who are involved in the ordering and oversight of antimicrobial agents or are responsible for antimicrobial policy or guideline creation in both community and healthcare practice venues. Also, with the advancing era of computerization and physician order entry, this book provides an ideal perspective on the use of computerized decision support to optimize the use of antimicrobials.

Robert C. Owens, Jr.
Ebbing Lautenbach

Contents

Contributors

Cybele L. Abad   Department of Medicine, University of Wisconsin Medical School, Madison, Wisconsin, U.S.A.

Nicole Akar   Center for Tuberculosis Research, Johns Hopkins University School of Medicine, Baltimore, Maryland, U.S.A.

Sujata M. Bhavnani   Institute for Clinical Pharmacodynamics, Ordway Research Institute, Inc., Albany, New York, U.S.A.

William R. Bishai   Center for Tuberculosis Research, Johns Hopkins University School of Medicine, Baltimore, Maryland, U.S.A.

Bernard C. Camins   Division of Infectious Diseases, Washington University School of Medicine, Saint Louis, Missouri, U.S.A.

Donald E. Craven   Department of Infectious Diseases, Lahey Clinic Medical Center, Burlington, Massachusetts and Tufts University School of Medicine, Boston, Massachusetts, U.S.A.

Kathleen Steger Craven   Consultant in Infectious Diseases and Public Health, Wellesley, Massachusetts, U.S.A.

George L. Drusano   Ordway Research Institute and New York State Department of Health, Albany, New York, U.S.A.

Thomas M. File   Northeastern Ohio Universities College of Medicine, Rootstown, Ohio and Summa Health System, Akron, Ohio, U.S.A.

Victoria J. Fraser   Division of Infectious Diseases, Washington University School of Medicine, Saint Louis, Missouri, U.S.A.

Marion S. Helfand   Infectious Diseases Section and Research Division, Louis Stokes Cleveland Department of Veterans Affairs Medical Center and the Case Western Reserve School of Medicine, Cleveland, Ohio, U.S.A.

James M. Hollands   Department of Pharmacy, Barnes-Jewish Hospital, Saint Louis, Missouri, U.S.A.

George A. Jacoby   Department of Infectious Diseases, Lahey Clinic Medical Center, Burlington, Massachusetts and Harvard Medical School, Boston, Massachusetts, U.S.A.

Sanjay K. Jain   Department of Pediatrics and Center for Tuberculosis Research, Johns Hopkins University School of Medicine, Baltimore, Maryland, U.S.A.

Marin H. Kollef   Pulmonary and Critical Care Division, Washington University School of Medicine, Saint Louis, Missouri, U.S.A.

Ebbing Lautenbach   Center for Clinical Epidemiology and Biostatistics, University of Pennsylvania, Philadelphia, Pennsylvania, U.S.A.

Ingi Lee   Division of Infectious Diseases, Hospital of the University of Pennsylvania, Philadelphia, Pennsylvania, U.S.A.

Peter K. Linden   Department of Critical Care Medicine, University of Pittsburgh Medical Center, Pittsburgh, Pennsylvania, U.S.A.

Thomas P. Lodise   Albany College of Pharmacy, Albany, New York, U.S.A.

Karen Lolans   Chicago Infectious Disease Research Institute, Chicago, Illinois, U.S.A.

Ben M. Lomaestro   Albany Medical Center Hospital, Albany, New York, U.S.A.

Lisa L. Maragakis   Department of Medicine, Division of Infectious Diseases, and Department of Hospital Epidemiology and Infection Control, Johns Hopkins Medical Institutions, Baltimore, Maryland, U.S.A.

Peggy S. McKinnon   Department of Pharmacy, Barnes-Jewish Hospital, Saint Louis, Missouri, U.S.A.

Daniel P. McQuillen   Department of Infectious Diseases, Lahey Clinic Medical Center, Burlington, Massachusetts and Tufts University School of Medicine, Boston, Massachusetts, U.S.A.

Sharon B. Meropol   Center for Clinical Epidemiology and Biostatistics, Penn Center for Education and Research on Therapeutics, and Department of Biostatistics and Epidemiology, University of Pennsylvania School of Medicine, Philadelphia, Pennsylvania, U.S.A.

Joshua P. Metlay   Center for Clinical Epidemiology and Biostatistics, Penn Center for Education and Research on Therapeutics, Department of Biostatistics and Epidemiology, and Division of General Internal Medicine, Department of Medicine, University of Pennsylvania School of Medicine, and Veterans Administration National Center, Philadelphia, Pennsylvania, U.S.A.

Scott T. Micek   Department of Pharmacy, Barnes-Jewish Hospital, Saint Louis, Missouri, U.S.A.

Pamela A. Moise   Department of Pharmacy Practice, Thomas J. Long School of Pharmacy and Health Sciences, University of the Pacific, Stockton, California, U.S.A.

Jonathan B. Olson   TheraDoc, Incorporated, Salt Lake City, Utah, U.S.A.

Winnie W. Ooi   Department of Infectious Diseases, Lahey Clinic Medical Center, Burlington, Massachusetts and Tufts University School of Medicine, Boston, Massachusetts, U.S.A.

Robert C. Owens, Jr.   Department of Clinical Pharmacy Services, Division of Infectious Diseases, Maine Medical Center, Portland, Maine and the Department of Medicine, University of Vermont, College of Medicine, Burlington, Vermont, U.S.A.

Trish M. Perl   Department of Medicine, Division of Infectious Diseases, and Department of Hospital Epidemiology and Infection Control, Johns Hopkins Medical Institutions, Baltimore, Maryland, U.S.A.

Stanley L. Pestotnik   TheraDoc, Incorporated, Salt Lake City, Utah, U.S.A.

John P. Quinn   Chicago Infectious Disease Research Institute, John. H. Stroger Jr. Hospital of Cook County, and Rush University Medical Center, Chicago, Illinois, U.S.A.

Efren L. Rael   Department of Medicine, Lahey Clinic Medical Center, Burlington, Massachusetts, U.S.A.

Louis B. Rice   Louis Stokes Cleveland Department of Veterans Affairs Medical Center and the Case Western Reserve School of Medicine, Cleveland, Ohio, U.S.A.

Rebecca R. Roberts Department of Emergency Medicine, John H. Stroger Jr. Hospital of Cook County, Chicago, Illinois, U.S.A.

Nasia Safdar Department of Medicine, University of Wisconsin Medical School, Madison, Wisconsin, U.S.A.

George Sakoulas Department of Medicine, Division of Infectious Diseases, New York Medical College, Valhalla, New York, U.S.A.

R. Douglas Scott II Division of Healthcare Quality Promotion, National Center for Infectious Diseases, Centers for Disease Control and Prevention, Atlanta, Georgia, U.S.A.

Glenn S. Tillotson Replidyne, Inc., Milford, Connecticut, U.S.A.

August J. Valenti Department of Hospital Epidemiology and Infection Prevention, Division of Infectious Diseases, Maine Medical Center, Portland, Maine and Department of Medicine, College of Medicine, University of Vermont, Burlington, Vermont, U.S.A.

Maria Virginia Villegas CIDEIM, International Center for Medical Research and Training, Cali, Columbia

Mark H. Wilcox Consultant, Clinical Director of Microbiology, Pathology Lead Infection Control Doctor, Leeds Teaching Hospitals NHS Trust, and Professor of Medical Microbiology, University of Leeds, Leeds, West Yorkshire, U.K.

Theoklis Zaoutis Department of Pediatrics and Epidemiology, University of Pennsylvania School of Medicine, and Division of Infectious Diseases, The Children's Hospital of Philadelphia, Philadelphia, Pennsylvania, U.S.A.

1 The Attributable Costs of Resistant Infections in Hospital Settings: Economic Theory and Application

R. Douglas Scott II

Division of Healthcare Quality Promotion, National Center for Infectious Diseases,
Centers for Disease Control and Prevention, Atlanta, Georgia, U.S.A.

Rebecca R. Roberts

Department of Emergency Medicine, John H. Stroger Jr. Hospital of
Cook County, Chicago, Illinois, U.S.A.

INTRODUCTION

The emergence of antibiotic resistance in healthcare settings and the community continues to prompt greater policy efforts from public health organizations. In 2001, the World Health Organization issued its global strategy to contain the spread of antimicrobial resistance (AR) (1). In the United States, the coordinated efforts of various agencies of the federal government were published in "A Public Health Action Plan to Combat Antimicrobial Resistance" by the Interagency Task Force on Antimicrobial Resistance (2). The Centers for Disease Control and Prevention (CDC) has initiated two education campaigns to reduce AR in healthcare settings and in the community. The Campaign to Prevent Antimicrobial Resistance in Healthcare Settings promotes AR prevention in hospitals and long-term care facilities, whereas the Get Smart: Know When Antibiotics Work Campaign is designed to affect provider prescription and patient consumption behavior to promote greater adherence to appropriate prescribing guidelines (3).

While the epidemiologic evidence on AR continues to show that the prevalence of resistant hospital-associated infections (HAI) is increasing (4), quantifying the health and economic impact of AR in hospital settings has been elusive. In addition to causing adverse patient outcomes and treatment dilemmas for physicians, infections with microorganisms resistant to conventional antimicrobial drug therapy present difficult problems for hospital management. Such infections complicate patient treatment, often driving the use of broad-spectrum (and usually more expensive) drugs (5). Just as important, many resistant infections are acquired within healthcare settings and thus are an important patient safety issue (6).

Accurately estimating the economic costs to hospitals and society has proven challenging because of difficulties in both developing standard economic methods to accurately measure the excess or attributable costs of resistant infections and understanding the epidemiology of drug resistance. This is highlighted by various estimates of the aggregate annual economic cost of AR in the United States (published between 1989 and 1995), which ranged from $4 billion to $5 billion to $100 million to $30 billion (7,8). This disparity illustrates how different assumptions and economic perspectives in an analytic framework can influence the final results. A recent systematic review on the economic benefits from infection control programs aimed at hospital-associated methicillin-resistant *Staphylococcus aureus* (MRSA) concluded that there was a lack of well-conducted economic evaluations on this subject (9).

This chapter reviews the methods of measuring the direct excess or attributable hospital patient cost resulting from acquiring an antimicrobial resistant organism from the cost perspective of the hospital. As many resistant infections are associated with hospital stays, hospitals absorb much of the direct medical cost of their treatment. Although the direct attributable medical cost due to resistant infections comprises only a small portion of the potential cost to society, economic analysis conducted from the perspective of hospital administrators is most likely to encourage hospitals to make the financial investment in improved infection control programs and interventions in order to reduce overall hospital costs. Therefore, our emphasis is limited to measuring the potential patient costs that are a result of acquiring an infection during a hospital stay, and does not consider other issues such as economic evaluations of infection control interventions where the program and/or the social costs must be measured as well (10).

First, we present a brief overview of important general economic concepts and how they relate to AR, including a discussion of market failure, the opportunity cost of resistance infections that are hospital acquired, and the role of relative price comparisons. The second section discusses the divergence of perspectives on healthcare costs resulting from the imperfect nature of markets for healthcare and how perspectives on cost vary when considering AR. The elements of the cost of drug resistance consistent with the narrow cost perspective of hospital administrators is distinguished from the cost of resistance to society. The third section focuses on the epidemiologic models used to measure the attributable costs of drug-resistant HAI from the cost perspective of hospitals, and considers both the choice of (*i*) surrogates used to represent hospital costs, and (*ii*) measures used to adjust for the confounding impact of the severity of underlying patient illness on cost estimates. Finally, the chapter concludes with some recommendations to improve the quality of the economic information that can be provided by hospital-based observational studies and their use in economic evaluations of AR in hospitals.

OVERVIEW OF ECONOMIC THEORY

Everyone has heard of the "market." Another term for market is "resource allocation mechanism." Design of resource allocation mechanisms for allocating scarce resources across unlimited consumer demands is a key function of economic theory. There are three main issues at work in the design of markets. First, suppliers will want an allocation mechanism that promotes efficiency—getting the greatest output of goods or services from the resources used in production. Commonly, product suppliers who sell products to the consumer are called "firms." Second, consumers will want a mechanism that provides the goods and services they want. And finally, the mechanism must be able to efficiently distribute the products among those who want them.

Next, it is worthwhile to understand what is meant by the perfectly competitive market. Characteristics of a perfectly competitive market include: (*i*) no barriers to the movement of suppliers or firms into or out of the market; (*ii*) many buyers and sellers where no single seller or consumer can influence the exchange of goods among participants—the opposite of a monopoly; (*iii*) a homogeneous or standardized product that pıoducers cannot alter to collect a higher price; (*iv*) all market participants have perfect knowledge of market conditions such as product quality, price, and availability; (*v*) a fully defined and stable system of property rights in which ownership of all products and productive resources is assigned (11).

This perfectly competitive market provides a social environment in which producers and consumers can freely interact and the traditional supply and demand curves are operational. As the price of a product declines, consumers will want to buy more of it. Conversely, as the price of a product increases, firms will try to produce more of it. With free interaction in the perfectly competitive market an equilibrium price will emerge that matches the amount of product consumers want to buy with the amount of product that firms want to produce. If the price is higher than this equilibrium price, excess product will accumulate in warehouses, unsold. If the price is lower, demand will cause shortages and the price will rise. This is the equilibrium price (Fig. 1).

Why is the concept of the perfectly competitive market such an important model of resource allocation in modern economic theory? The predominant reason is that perfectly competitive markets generate values or "prices" that reflect the scarcity of physical resources used in the production of the goods and services for

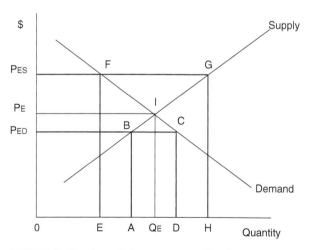

FIGURE 1 Supply and demand curves. X axis represents quantity of a good purchased and quantity of a good supplied. Y axis represents price of a good in dollars. The demand curve is downward sloping (as prices fall, consumers will buy more of the goods), while the supply curve is upward sloping (as prices rise, producers will supply more of the goods). At price level P_E, the two curves intersect and the market clears (the quantity demanded by consumers is equal to the quantity supplied by producers at Q_E). At price level P_{ES}, producers will supply a greater quantity of the goods than consumers will purchase (the excess supply is equal to the line segment EH on the quantity axis, and the valuation of the excess supply is represented by the rectangle EFGH). At price level P_{ED}, consumers will demand a greater quantity of the goods than suppliers will produce (the excess demand is equal to the line segment AS on the quantity axis, and the valuation of the exceess demand is represented by the rectangle ABCD). *Source*: Adapted from Ref. 25.

members of society. The essence of economic theory is about decision making (either by government, business, households, or individuals) when scarce resources cannot be stretched to accommodate all the possible wants and desires of society. A decision to make a particular purchase, or invest in a particular project, implies that the resources used to fulfill this decision will not be available for other alternative uses. A concept in economic theory that reflects this tradeoff is opportunity cost. In economics, the real social cost associated with using a resource is not the financial or accounting cost associated with the resource, but the foregone value or benefit of the resource if employed in its *next best alternative use* (12).

For example, the financial decision to turn a children's daycare center into a parking lot includes the cost of demolition, parking lot construction, and the loss of the childcare center's revenue. This loss is frequently measured in money, such as the annual profit the center netted. The opportunity cost of this decision would also include the lost benefits to society of having a daycare center that contributed to the long run development of children and/or allowed a parent to enter the workforce. The latter foregone benefits are not easily determined. If resources used in this context could be allocated through a perfectly competitive market, the value of these societal benefits would be processed by market participants, and the prices of these resources determined in the market would more closely represent their true opportunity costs.

Market Failure and Opportunity Costs

The markets for healthcare goods and services do not fit the perfect competitive model for several reasons. (*i*) There is not free entry of firms into and out of the market. This is especially true of hospital care. Very few groups could decide to set up and operate a new hospital. Conversely, existing hospitals are often kept open as a service to the community, even when doing poorly financially. (*ii*) Pharmaceutical patents are a clear example of how a single firm can influence the market, especially with extended antimicrobial patent durations (13). (*iii*) Hospitals provide different types and quantities of vast numbers of medical services, and pharmaceutical companies provide unique products, again high-lighting the deviation from the conditions of a perfect market. (*iv*) On a patient level, healthcare outcomes and cost are not predictable; and insured patients are not directly responsible for payment of services rendered. It is also difficult for patients and third-party payers to assess the quality of the services rendered. Even among physicians, opinions vary on best treatment practices and outcome values. (*v*) Property rights are well defined, with at least one possible exception, which we discuss below. (*vi*) In healthcare, there are often limited satisfactory substitute products in the market, especially among antimicrobials. Medical terminology has many references to this fact such as "treatment of choice," "standards of care," or "best practices." The presence of health insurance and third party payers removes some of the direct decision making from the consumer and physician. The result is that the "price" paid is often only indirectly related to the decision to seek or render a particular medical service. Under these circumstances, prices that come from such "imperfect" markets will not accurately reflect the true opportunity costs of resources used in healthcare.

This shortcoming becomes evident when valuing the resources used for hospital care. An important consideration in the measure of hospital cost is making the distinction between "costs" or expenditures the hospital makes for goods and services, and what the hospital "charges" for providing care (14,15). The current reimbursement system leads to distortions such as cost shifting, where the hospital raises charges above those that would accurately reflect costs so that payers with more generous reimbursement schedules are, in effect, subsidizing less generous payers as well as patients whose care is uncompensated. Thus, hospital charges will often overestimate the actual cost of resources consumed (16–18). Similarly, cost shifting may occur within the hospital when some services are reimbursed at a higher rate or percentage of cost than others.

The failure of market prices to represent opportunity cost is particularly true for the consumption of antimicrobials. Unfettered use of antimicrobials has a downside. An important attribute of antimicrobials is that over time, current use decreases future effectiveness as organisms develop resistance to the drug. On one hand, antimicrobials are given to promote an individual patient's health, but the decision to provide antimicrobial treatment to one patient can affect the future efficacy and quality of treatments to others (19–21). In the broader societal view, this feature of antimicrobial drug use places these agents within a class of economic goods called common property resources. The characteristic that distinguishes common property resources from other goods and services is that an individual consumption of such a good can affect the consumption of the resource by others, without their permission. In economics, this phenomenon is called an externality (21–23). An example of a common property resource in basic economics is a fishery (24). Individual commercial fishermen seek to maximize their profit by attempting to catch as many fish as their boats will hold. However, the operation of one boat catching as many fish as possible causes a reduction in the stock of fish. This increases the cost of fishing for all fishermen and an increase in the average cost for harvested fish. The result is overfishing, that in the long run could lead to the biologic collapse of the fish population, which ultimately is detrimental to all users of the fishery. An economic model for this problem (developed by Gordon in 1954) predicted most fishermen would be forced to quit fishing because of high harvest costs before this level of biologic collapse takes place (24). The problem of common property resource externalities stems from violating the last condition for a perfectly competitive market: a fully defined system of property rights. Because the resource belongs to no one particular individual or group, the resource is held "in common." No user of the resource must pay anyone to get access to the fishery and harvest fish. Without prices to provide feedback concerning the long-term economic value (or opportunity cost) of maintaining a sustainable fish population, the market fails to be perfectly competitive. In cases of market failure such as this, the resource allocation mechanism designed for common property resources is usually a modified market mechanism with rights to use the resource held within a government agency or some collective organization made up of users (25). These bodies oversee the use of regulations, taxes, and/or subsidies to act as surrogates for market prices to reflect the value of a sustainable resource.

A similar situation can occur when an individual clinician decides to administer antimicrobial treatment to an infected patient without consideration of the impact on future users of the drug. Such use for one patient may increase the cost or reduce the effectiveness of care for other patients without their permission. At present, there is no broadly applicable formal regulatory mechanism in place for antimicrobial therapy that provide feedback about the future effectiveness of antimicrobials based on current use. However, hospitals, government health agencies, and organizations of healthcare professions are developing and advocating appropriate-use guidelines and even antimicrobial management programs (26). Time will tell if these types of institutional arrangements, based on voluntary associations or local controls, will be capable of responding to the challenges that the emerging pattern of resistance places on national and global public health.

Opportunity Costs and Relative Prices

The practical implication of this discussion is that measuring opportunity costs for economic evaluations of AR is problematic and requires the use of surrogate information. Once the surrogate information is obtained, how can opportunity cost of patient resources in these studies be represented? Opportunity costs can be represented using comparisons of relative prices (11). A primary implication of the role of prices in resource allocation is that prices relative to each other are important when considering changes in the demand and supply for goods and services (27). Using national trade policy as an example, a nation's decision to import or export a commodity can be assessed by comparing the price of a domestically produced commodity to its price in the international market. A cheaper domestic price indicates that the opportunity costs of producing domestically are cheaper relative to the costs of production in other countries. In this instance, it is in the country's best economic interest, to export the commodity.

Opportunity costs associated with drug resistant HAIs are usually expressed in terms of alternative uses within the hospital. Given that much of the cost structure for a U.S. hospital is fixed (costs associated with resources that must be in place before a patient is admitted), these fixed resources cannot be easily re-employed to some other use within a short time frame (10,28). Studies of attributable costs of resistant HAIs usually make comparisons involving the three clinical situations ("states") related to resistance: (*i*) patient costs with no infection, (*ii*) patient costs with a susceptible HAI (infections due to organisms that can be treated by the usual antimicrobials), and (*iii*) patient costs with resistant infections. One of the earliest assessments of the economic impact of drug resistance in hospitals estimated that the cost of infection when nosocomial pathogens are antibiotic resistant is double the cost of infection when these organisms are antibiotic susceptible (29). Combining this relative price ratio and information from the Study on the Efficacy of Nosocomial Infection Control (SENIC) project, the U.S. Office of Technology Assessment (OTA) estimated the nationwide hospital cost associated with six different resistant nosocomial pathogens to be $1.3 billion annually (in 1992 dollars) (30).

Studies of HAIs have also used attributable length of hospital stay and patient mortality as outcomes (31–35). Recognizing that much of the cost of HAIs will be borne by the hospitals, these outcomes do not directly translate into the dollar costs that hospitals must cover (36–38). Assessing the economic impact of drug-resistant hospital pathogens in terms of dollar costs provides the type of evidence hospitals need to make investment decisions for infection control (39).

In concluding this section, the most important consequence of market failure and the allocation of antimicrobial effectiveness is the divergence of perspectives on the cost of AR. When ownership of a good or resource is fully specified, the resource owner is the only individual who accrues any benefits or costs that the resource will produce. This provides the resource owner the incentive to make the best possible use of the resource, which in turn benefits society. The level of prices determined in the marketplace will incorporate all economic factors and reflect the true opportunity cost of the resources used to produce goods and services. This is not the case of antimicrobial drugs when future and current consumers obtain a different value or effectiveness from the product. Given this failure, traditional tools of market analysis (which relies on having prices observed in markets) will not provide all the relevant costs that can be associated with drug resistance. How these various economic perspectives diverge is considered next.

ANALYTIC PERSPECTIVES ON THE COSTS OF RESISTANT INFECTIONS

What are the implications for conducting cost studies of resistant infections in hospitals? There are three important decisions an analyst must make when beginning any economic evaluation: choosing an analytic perspective, determining the relevant costs, and deciding how to measure cost (40). Because of the heterogeneous nature of the healthcare market, the economic impact of changes in the allocation of resources will be viewed differently by the various market participants. The costs and benefits of an expensive new healthcare intervention to mitigate AR may be received differently by physicians, patients, healthcare facilities, drug industry firms, third party payers, and society. The perspective that is chosen for the study will determine which costs and benefits should be included in the analysis. If the analytic perspective chosen is from the hospital administration point of view, the primary economic impact stems from the direct medical costs of additional patient care resulting from infection. Alternatively, a broader societal perspective would consider other costs such as pain, suffering and the loss of working productivity due to delayed recovery from the infection. This section discusses the various cost perspectives related to AR (Table 1) (20).

Physicians

Physicians' main concerns are the individual patients and their motivation to eliminate disease in patients (Table 1). The economic consequences of resistant infections are related to ineffective treatment leading to the patient's continued illness or death. From the clinician's perspective, it is a grave concern if the

TABLE 1 Different Perspectives of Economic Impact of Antimicrobial Resistance

	Medical	Patient	Healthcare business	Drug industry	Public ("society")
Focus	Individual	Individual	Care group	Potential clients	Population
Outcome	Absence of disease	Absence of disease	Reduce cost of care	Product sales	Maximize health
Time frame	Short	Short	Short	Short, long	Long
Motivation	Professionalism	Personal well-being	Profit	Profit	Social good
Approach	Treatment	Treatment	Cost containment	Develop new drugs, maintain life of old drugs	Reduce forces leading to resistance

Source: From Cordell RE, Solomon SE, Scott RD, and McGowan JE, unpublished data, 2000.

available supply of antimicrobials becomes "ineffective." The economic impact of diminishing effectiveness of a given drug or group of drugs depends on the availability of other drugs that could be substituted to treat a given type of infection.

Patients

Infected patients have a perspective on cost similar to that of physicians, because the patient's focus is on successful treatment. Patients are motivated by their desire to obtain improved health. The direct costs to patients of resistant infection include the extra cost of drugs and health services that resulted from the infection. These are paid directly out of pocket or indirectly through insurance premiums. From this perspective, costs of resistant infections should include not only the added costs of treatment but also the costs associated with morbidity, mortality, pain, suffering, and time lost from work due to delayed recovery.

Healthcare Businesses

In the United States, a large share of the financial resources of the health system, and their allocation, are controlled by hospital administrators, financial managers, insurance companies, and government agencies at the local, state, and federal level, with less control by healthcare providers. Here, the perspective on the costs of resistant infections and their economic impact comes from a focus on treating patients (customers) who are part of a well-defined population being served, but doing so to maximize financial returns or minimize costs to boards of directors, or shareholders. Resistance becomes a problem when reduced drug effectiveness causes patient-care cost to rise as additional resources such as alternative drugs, personnel time, supplies, space, and equipment are required for patient care. To minimize this cost, health system administrators often attempt to monitor or control drug effectiveness through pharmacy and therapeutics committees, drug utilization reviews, and formularies.

From this perspective, a resistant infection in settings outside the population served by a particular healthcare organization becomes of interest only when it affects its client population or care group. Healthcare businesses, particularly hospitals, may provide the easiest setting for measuring the economic impact of resistant infections on their costs. The economic impact is limited to the costs of specific antimicrobial drugs and the extra costs of care in specific patient groups. These costs can be calculated for a specific healthcare organization and used to assess the value of programs to preserve the effectiveness of available drugs.

Even among healthcare businesses, cost perspectives may diverge. Third-party payers such as health insurance companies are interested in having health-care services delivered in a cost-effective manner to minimize reimbursements to providers. Reimbursement policies that allow hospitals to pass along added treatment expenses from resistant HAIs could act as a financial disincentive for hospitals to invest in improved infection control programs, because the hospital does not absorb these costs.

Drug Industry Firms

Pharmaceutical firms operate similarly to healthcare businesses in that they seek to generate profits. They produce a variety of antimicrobial compounds and vaccines used to treat or prevent infectious diseases for potential clients. Clients can be direct users, such as patients, or indirect users, such as healthcare systems and government health agencies. Firms look to high product sales as the desired outcome, usually in the short-term. However, firms must also take a longer view and consider the impact of resistance as a potential for the introduction and sale of new products. This requires a two-pronged strategy. First, the firm wishes to extend the effective life of its current drug line against infecting organisms. Second, the pattern of resistance may make competitors' products obsolete, providing the firm with a new marketing opportunity for an existing product of its own that may have in the past been more expensive, less safe, or less effective than the now-obsolete drug.

Public or Societal View

The societal perspective is concerned with the well-being of members of society, which may be expressed in terms of populations in cities, states, countries, or even the entire world. The goal of this perspective is to promote health for the entire defined population, usually over a long time horizon. For this reason, antimicrobials are a scarce resource that must be managed wisely to prevent and treat infectious diseases. Appropriate use of antimicrobials might lead to an eventual, but acceptable, decrease in effectiveness, whereas overuse or misuse would lead to an inappropriate or unacceptable loss of effectiveness. If the treatment of one patient leads to decreased effectiveness in treatment for the next patient using the same drug, society is adversely affected.

The Appropriate Perspective?

The economic costs and benefits of programs to preserve antimicrobial effectiveness must be interpreted in the context of the differing points of view illustrated above. In any single study, it is essential to keep the same perspective consistently throughout. The business viewpoint might place a positive value on the loss of effectiveness of a competitor's cheap antimicrobial if it leads to increased use of that same manufacturer's more expensive agent. The physician's viewpoint might consider the loss of effectiveness of the cheaper drug of little consequence as long as other effective drugs are available and there is no clinical or economic impact in using a different drug.

Another example of varying perspectives is the use of policies and formularies to control the provider's choice of antimicrobial agents. This step may make great sense to hospital and healthcare administrators if it is likely to produce more efficient use of resources. However, these measures might be seen as having no positive value to clinicians who are willing to use any and all resources to cure their current patients.

Antimicrobial drugs could potentially be managed collectively with a market-based resource allocation mechanism, which can distribute the current supply of antimicrobials between current and future users. However, the detrimental effect of current use on long-term effectiveness has not been quantified for most situations (41). This makes it difficult to design a resource allocation mechanism that can distribute antimicrobial value from a social perspective.

Table 2 illustrates the variety of cost factors that are important to the differing perspectives when conducting an economic analysis of HAIs that are susceptible or resistant to antimicrobials (20). When comparing the costs of

TABLE 2   Elements of the Economic Impact of HAIs by Perspective Affected

Element	Measurement[a]	Perspective affected
Mortality	Costs associated with treatment failure (R) (S)	Physician, patient, HCB
Morbidity	Costs associated with pain, suffering, inconvenience (R) (S)	Physician, patient
Care cost	Charges for care (R) (S)	Patient
Care time	Time devoted to care (R) (S)	Physician, HCB
	Length of process (R) (S)[b]	Patient, society
Diagnosis costs	Costs for diagnosis (R) (S)	HCB
Treatment costs	Costs for drugs, etc (R) (S) (additional drugs and treatments, more expensive drugs, etc.)	HCB
Diminished marketability	Market for drug use (R) (S)	Drug Industry
New markets	Market for new drug (S) (R) (replace current market leader; replace inexpensive drug with more expensive drug; provide new product)	Drug Industry
Impact on non-treated	Increased resistance (R) (S)	Society

[a](R)=extent in patients infected with resistant organism; (S)=extent in patients infected with susceptible organism.
[b]Costs associated with lack of usual function during infection, including for patient loss of work, quality of life, etc. (includes both inpatient and outpatient components); for society, reduction of useful function in workforce.
Abbreviations: HAI, healthcare-associated infection; HCB, healthcare business.

resistant infections to susceptible infections, the added cost for each factor is shown along with its impact on the various perspectives. The example in Table 2, the direct medical costs for diagnostic procedures, such as laboratory, radiology, bronchoscopy, the cost for additional or more expensive antimicrobial drugs, and the increased length of hospital stay, are primarily of concern to healthcare institutions when these costs cannot be passed on to third-party payers or patients. Patients also experience indirect costs due to lost income from missed workdays, travel costs associated with frequent hospital or doctor visits, and possible declines in quality of life. Businesses experience productivity losses when patients are ill with resistant infections. The drug industry may also experience indirect costs due to diminishing marketability of their drugs as they lose effectiveness.

Studies of the economic impact of resistance have not included measurement of the full range of these variables. Most studies on HAIs have conducted their economic analysis from the cost perspective of hospital administrators or third-party payers and frequently substitute hospital charges for costs. From this perspective, the additional direct costs of diagnosis and treatment of a resistant pathogen are measured to determine the magnitude of the potential per-patient cost savings that could result from reducing the incidence of resistant infections.

The SENIC project, conducted during the late 1970s to early 1980s, showed that hospitals employing infection control surveillance and other preventive interventions had lower rates of HAIs (42). In order to further justify investment in surveillance programs, researchers conducted economic studies of the cost-effectiveness of infection control programs and the cost savings they could generate from the perspective of both the hospital and society at large. The analytic approaches used to examine the overall economic impact of antibiotic susceptible HAIs in hospital settings were later used to assess the economic impact of resistant infections. Because most of the work was done from the hospital perspective, the remainder of this discussion focuses specifically on the economic studies of resistant infections from that point of view.

EPIDEMIOLOGIC MODELS OF THE ATTRIBUTABLE COST OF RESISTANT INFECTIONS FROM THE HOSPITAL PERSPECTIVE

The most common analytic approach for measuring the attributable costs of resistant infections in hospitals has been to conduct an observational epidemiologic study (24). This approach was routinely used in studies of the attributable cost of antimicrobial-drug susceptible HAIs and was adopted by researchers to measure the attributable cost of drug resistant HAIs when these became more prominent. Two groups of patients matched for similar characteristics but different infection status (usually susceptible vs. resistant infection) and are followed to see if the patient cost outcome differs between the groups. To better understand the epidemiologic studies used to analyze cost outcomes in hospitals, we need to address the use of severity of illness (SOI) indexes to control for the confounding caused by the high cost of underlying disease severity that is frequently associated with and preceding susceptible and resistant HAIs, and the use of various cost measures for hospital resources.

Focusing on susceptible HAIs, Haley (43) provided a summary of the observational study designs and cost measurement issues that may be considered when estimating the cost savings to a hospital from infection control programs and interventions. Two study designs have been used to assess the cost savings achieved by infection control programs: the concurrent method and the comparative method. The concurrent method involves following each case of infection on a daily basis and itemizing all resources consumed (labor, supplies, equipment) to treat the infection. Costs associated with each resource are then combined with the volume of resources used to estimate the total costs attributable to the infection. Such studies usually employ an appropriateness evaluation protocol to determine whether a particular service, procedure, or day in the hospital was attributable to the infection or the pre-existing condition of hospitalization (44).

Most comparative studies, although sometimes erroneously referred to as case-control studies, have used a cohort or case-cohort approach. Exposed subjects are defined as those with an identified HAI, while a comparison group is selected from patients who do not have an HAI. Common outcome variables include some measure of cost, length of hospital stay, or mortality. A true case-control study would involve assigning subjects to groups on the basis of their having or not having a particular outcome—in this instance, a high cost of care—and then looking for risk factors, such as having a resistant HAI, that are positively associated with the high cost of care.

In studies of the overall excess cost of HAIs, it was recognized that patients acquiring an HAI have a greater severity of underlying disease upon admission to the hospital than patients who did not become infected (43,45–48). This introduced an upward bias in cost measures because the group who became infected were already more costly than those less sick who also had lower rates of infection. Investigators frequently match subjects with and without resistant infections on other factors, such as age, diagnosis, or SOI in an attempt to improve the comparability of the two groups.

These same issues hold true for measuring the excess costs for resistant infections as well (20,38). Controlling for the confounding effects of severity of underlying disease both in patients with susceptible HAIs and in those with resistant HAIs has been a particularly difficult analytic issue to overcome in epidemiologic studies of AR. A number of recommendations have been advanced on the best way to adjust for differences in patient characteristics and severity of disease in studies of HAIs. Haley (43) recommended that researchers use multiple matching criteria, by selecting one or more control patients for every infected patient, in order to obtain a group of control subjects that would have "the same expected length of hospital stay and hospital costs" as infected patients would have had if they had not developed an infection. He further suggested the use of diagnosis-related groups (DRGs) as the best measure to predict patient length of stay and total hospital costs. Alternatively, Gross et al. (49) advocated using the number of comorbidities as a measure to control for severity of disease. Harris et al. (50) suggested that using SOI indexes that possess standardized scores would promote the comparison of results from different studies. Standardized scores that have been used include the Acute Physiology and Chronic Health Evaluation (APACHE) system, the Charlson index, and the McCabe-Jackson scale (51–53). Other indexes specific to a patient diagnosis, like the Zawacki score for burn victims, have also been used (54).

The Measurement of Cost

Recognizing the limitations of using charges as a surrogate for costs, Haley (43) offered several methods to overcome the problem of this substitution. One approach involves adjusting charges by the overall hospital cost-to-charge ratio to get an improved surrogate measure of cost. A modification would be to determine the cost-to-charge ratio for each service department and then sum all subtotals for each department in which the patient received services. This eliminates the distortion in costs introduced by cost shifting between departments. Another approach would be to use micro-costing or cost accounting data, which are usually available from hospital expenditure reports or hospital accounting departments. These costs are the actual hospital expenditures on all resources hospitals consume in order to provide health services (28,55). Of the various approaches, micro-costing provides the most accurate measure of direct costs from the hospital perspective. Although difficult to obtain, they would most likely prove more credible to administrators interested in the study results (38).

When choosing between methods, it is important to consider the issue of statistical power. Medical cost data are highly skewed, and the standard deviations are typically large relative to the group means. The implication is that studies with small- to medium-sized samples will be underpowered or fail to reject the null hypothesis or fail to detect a cost difference when one truly exists. Indeed, most of the studies reviewed below lack statistical power, and thus findings of no difference in costs for resistant infections must be viewed with caution.

Overview of Studies on the Economic Impact of
Resistant Infections in Hospitals

The perspective having been determined, the key considerations from economic theory are: (*i*) prices are ordinal and are used to rank whether different states or conditions result in a high level of economic well-being; (*ii*) measures of hospital costs should reflect the opportunity cost of resources used in hospital services as closely as possible; and (*iii*) at baseline, noninfected patients selected to be controls must be equally as ill as infected patients in order to address the potential confounding from underlying severity of disease. Without comparable controls, the economic resources consumed will always be different between the two groups. Table 3 summarizes recent studies examining the hospital costs associated with resistant pathogens, reported in U.S. dollars. The papers were selected to illustrate the various approaches for measuring opportunity costs, controlling for underlying SOI, and comparing important patient groups. The results summarize cost comparisons between groups of patients with the infection states of: no infection, susceptible infection, and resistant infection. The table allows the reader to compare the variables used to control for the confounding associated with SOI, and the methods used to measure cost.

The evidence from the selected studies presents a varied picture of the magnitude of the attributable cost of resistant HAIs, the use of SOI measures, and the surrogates used for patient costs. With the exception of studies by Rubin et al. (56) and Engemann et al. (57), most of the studies do not compare costs across patients in all possible infection states: those without infection, those with a susceptible infection, and those with a resistant infection. Rubin et al. found that methicillin-sensitive *S. aureus* (MSSA) infection results in a $27,700, or 108%, increase in the direct medical costs in infected versus noninfected nonobstetrical patients (mean cost of $13,263). MRSA infection increased costs by 137% over the mean cost for noninfected patients. The increase in average cost when comparing MSSA-infected ($27,700) to MRSA-infected patients ($31,400) was approximately 13%.

The Engemann paper provides an example of the differences between cost comparisons using crude, unadjusted cost data and cost data adjusted for confounding variables including SOI. While the focus of the paper was on identifying the attributable cost differences between MSSA surgical-site infection (SSI) patients and MRSA SSI patients, the data presented in the paper allowed for separate crude cost comparisons between noninfected surgical patients with those acquiring MSSA and those acquiring MRSA infections. Although relative costs were not reported in the paper, these were calculated for both the mean and median cost. The presence of MSSA resulted in a 79% increase over the unadjusted mean cost of treating noninfected surgical patients. MRSA SSI patients had a 244% increase over that same mean cost and a 214% increase over median cost of the MSSA SSI cases. After adjustment for cost confounders, the adjusted mean cost for MRSA was only 19% greater than MSSA infections—a much smaller impact than indicated from the unadjusted cost comparison.

The remaining papers on MRSA compared two of the three states of infection using a variety of total and attributable cost estimators. Chaix et al. (58) compared intensive care unit (ICU) patients with MRSA infection to ICU patients with no HAI, but did not include MSSA. They estimated the mean attributable cost due to resistance to be $9275 relative to similar noninfected control cases; a 44% increase. Abramson et al. reported attributable cost increases due to *S. aureus* of $9661 for susceptible cases and $27,083 for resistant cases (59). Comparing patients with MRSA bloodstream infections (BSIs) to patients with MSSA BSIs, Roughman et al. (60) reported an average attributable direct cost of $24,552 above the cost for those with MSSA infection; a 95% increase. Welch et al. (61) reported a mean total cost of $23,075 for MRSA, which was 18% greater than in patients who acquired MSSA infections. Reed et al. (62) found a mean attributable cost for MRSA of $7273; a 52% increase, over costs for hemodialysis-dependent end-stage

(*text continues on p.17*)

TABLE 3 Studies on the Direct Medical Cost of Resistant Nosocomial Infections

Ref.	Design (n)	Study setting	Type of (resistant) infection	Site of infection	Total noninfected patient costs	Measure of cost for sensitive infections	Increase in relative cost of sensitive infections over noninfected patient costs	Measure of cost for resistant infections	Increase in relative cost of resistance over noninfected patient costs	Increase in relative cost of resistance over sensitive infection costs	Cost data	SOI controls
56	RC and modeling (1,351,362 including 6,300 NIs)	All New York State nonobstetrical discharges	Noninfected vs. MSSA; noninfected vs. MRSA	Pneumonia, bacteremia, endocarditis, SSI, osteomyelitis, septic arthritis	$13,263 (mean)	$27,700 (mean total costs)	2.08[a]	$31,400 (mean total costs)	2.37[a]	1.13[a]	Hospital charges; medicare physician fees; wholesale drug prices	None
57	PC, retrospective cost data, and modeling (479)	U.S. teaching TCH	Noninfected vs. MSSA; noninfected vs. MRSA; MSSA vs. MRSA	SSIs	$29,455 (median) $34,395 (mean)	$23,336 (unadjusted median attributable costs)[a] $38,770 (unadjusted mean attributable costs)[a]	1.79 (median unadjusted)[a] 2.13 (mean unadjusted)[a]	$62,908 (unadjusted median attributable costs)[a] $84,020 (unadjusted mean attributable costs)[a] $13,901 (mean attributable costs after model adjustment)[c]	3.14 (median unadjusted)[a] 3.44 (mean unadjusted)[a]	1.75 (unadjusted median)[a] 1.62 (unadjusted mean)[a] 1.19 (mean adjusted)[c]	Hospital charges	NNIS risk index; ASA score; duration of surgery; wound class
58	Matched retrospective case-control; modeling (54)[b]	ICU in French hospital	Noninfected vs. MRSA	Bacteremia, catheter-related, lower respiratory tract, UTI	$20,950 (mean)	NA	NA	$9,275 (mean attributable cost)	1.44[a]	NA	Hospital costs	McCabe-Jackson; SAPS II
59	Prospective matched nested case-control study (38)[b]	U.S. University TCH	MSSA vs. MRSA	Primary BSI	NA	$9,661 (median attributable cost)	NA	$27,083 (median attributable cost)	NA	NA	Hospital costs	Comorbidities; primary and secondary diagnosis
61	Retrospective case-control; matched (296)[b]	U.S. multi-center hospitals	MSSA vs. MRSA	All patients with MRSA or MSSA bacteremia	NA	$19,487 (total MSSA patient costs)	NA	$23,075 (total MRSA patient costs)	NA	1.18[a]	Hospital charges adjusted to costs	DRG; ICD-9 codes

#	Study (n)	Setting	Comparison	Infection sites							
62	Prospectively identified cohort (143)	U.S. university TCH	MSSA vs. MRSA	Bacteremia in patients with ESRD	NA	$13,978 (mean total costs for initial hospitalization)	NA	$21,251 (mean total costs for initial hospitalization)	NA	1.52[a]	Hospital costs	APACHE II
63	RC (353)	U.S. teaching TCH	MSSA vs. MRSA	Bacteremia	NA	$11,668 (mean total cost)	NA	$21,577 (mean total cost)	NA	1.85	Hospital costs	APACHE II
64	RC (348)	U.S. university TCH	MSSA vs. MRSA	Bacteremia	NA	$19,212 (mean total cost)	NA	$26,424 (mean total cost) $6,916 (attributable costs after model adjustment)	NA	1.36 (based on adjusted costs)	Hospital charges adjusted to costs	McCabe-Jackson; number of comorbidities
65	Matched RC (62)	U.S. teaching TCH ICU	Noninfected vs. susceptible and resistant Acinetobacter baumannii	Sputum, wound	$49,708 for noninfected patient matched on primary diagnosis	NA	NA	$206,648 (includes cases with susceptible infections)	4.14[a]	NA	Hospital charges	APACHE II
66	Case-control study (68)[b]	U.S. teaching TCH burn unit	Multi-drug resistant A. baumannii	Wound, respiratory, blood, urine, other sites	$102,983 for noninfected patient matched on TBSA	NA	NA	$201,558	1.96[a]	NA	Hospital charges adjusted to costs	TBSA; Zawacki score
67	Matched case-control (99)[b]	U.S. teaching TCH	ESBL-producing Escherichia coli or Klebsiella Pnuemoniae	UTI, wound, catheter, blood, respiratory, abdominal	NA	$22,231 (median total costs)	NA	$66,590 (unadjusted median total costs)	NA	3.0 (un-adjusted)[a] 1.71 (model adjusted)	Hospital charges	APACHE II
68	Nested matched cohort (477)	U.S. teaching TCH	Cephalosporin sensitive vs. resistant Enterobacter	BSI, respiratory tract, UTI, wound, effusion	NA	$40,406 (median total costs) $57,606 (mean total costs)	NA	$79,323 (unadjusted median total costs) $29,379 (model adjusted attributable costs above costs of susceptible infections)	NA	1.96[a] (un-adjusted)[a] 1.51 (model adjusted)	Hospital charges	McCabe-Jackson
69	Matched case-control (72)	U.S. hospital level 1 trauma center	VSE vs. VRE	Urinary, skin, IV catheter, intraabdominal	NA	$16,692 (mean total VSE patient costs)	NA	$38,226 (mean total VRE patient costs)	NA	2.29[a]	NA	APACHE II

(Continued)

TABLE 3 Studies on the Direct Medical Cost of Resistant Nosocomial Infections (*Continued*)

Ref. Design (n)	Study setting	Type of (resistant) infection	Site of infection	Total noninfected patient costs	Measure of cost for sensitive infections	Increase in relative cost of sensitive infections over noninfected patient costs	Measure of cost for resistant infections	Increase in relative cost of resistance over noninfected patient costs	Increase in relative cost of resistance over sensitive infection costs	Cost data	SOI controls
70 Matched case-control (34)	U.S. teaching TCH	VSE vs. VRE	Bacteremia in liver transplant patients	NA	$91,833 (mean total VSE patient costs)	NA	$190,728 (mean total VRE patient costs)	NA	2.08[a]	Hospital charges adjusted to costs	None
60 Matched RC (190)	U.S. hospital adult ICU unit	MSSA vs. MRSA; VSE vs. VRE	BSIs	NA	$25,888 (mean total MSSA costs) $34,469 (mean total VSE costs)	NA	$50,440 (mean total MRSA costs) $60,798 (mean total VRE costs)	NA	1.95 (MSSA vs. MRSA) 1.76 (VSE vs. VRE)	NA	None
71 Matched RC (51)	U.S. teaching TCH	VSE vs. VRE	Bacteremia	NA	$56,707 (mean total costs)	NA	$83,897 (mean total costs)	NA	1.32	Hospital costs	SOI index for bacteremia patients
72 Matched RC (277)	U.S. TCH hospital	Noninfected vs. VRE	VRE bacteremia	$46,699 (mean)	NA	NA	$81,208 (risk adjusted estimate for total cost)	1.74[a]	NA	Hospital charges	APR-DRG complexity index

[a]Increase in relative costs have been estimated when not directly reported. Relative costs based on crude costs comparisons of infection states using the following formulas:

Increase in relative cost of patients with sensitive infection over noninfected patient costs = total patient cost of sensitive infections/total cost of noninfected patients

Increase in relative cost of patients with resistant infection over noninfected patient costs = total patient costs of resistant infection/total patient costs of noninfected patient

Increase in relative cost of patients with resistant infection over patients with sensitive infection = total patient cost with resistant infections/total patient costs with sensitive infections

[b]Authors report as case-control studies when the design is actually a matched retrospective cohort study.

[c]Paper presents information that allows for both crude cost comparison and cost comparisons after model adjustment.

Abbreviations: APACHE II, Acute Physiology, Age, Chronic Health Evaluation II; APR-DRG, all patient refined-diagnosis related group; ASA, America Society of Anesthesiologist Score; BSI, blood stream infection; DRG, diagnosis related group; ESBL, extended-spectrum beta-lactamase; ESRD, hemodialysis-dependent end-stage renal disease; ICD-9, International Classification of Disease, version 9; ICU, intensive care unit; IV, intervenous catheter; MRSA, methicillin-resistant *S. aureus*; MSSA, methicillin-susceptible *S. aureus*; NA, not measured in study; NI, nosocomial infection; NNIS, National Nosocomial Surveillance risk index; NR, estimate measured but not reported; PC, prospective cohort; RC, retrospective cohort; SAPS II, Simplified Acute Physiology Score II; SOI, severity of illness; SSI, surgical site infection; TBSA, total body surface area; TCH, tertiary-care hospital; UTI, urinary tract infection; VRE, vancomycin-resistant *enterococcus*; VSE, vancomycin-susceptible *enterococcus*.

renal disease patients with MSSA infections. For MRSA bacteremia, Lodise and McKinnon (63), and Cosgrove et al. (64) found that MRSA increased patient costs by 85% and 36%, respectively, over infections with MSSA (comparisons to noninfected patients were not made in either paper).

For the remaining pathogens, resistant *Acinetobacter baumannii* infections have resulted in cost increases of 96% and 314% over costs of control group patients with no infection (65,66). Extended-spectrum beta-lactamase (ESBL)-producing *Escherichia coli* and *Klebsiella pnuemoniae* infections resulted in a 71% increase in cost compared to patients with susceptible infection (67). Infections with cephalosporin-resistant *Enterobacter* caused an excess cost increase of 51% compared to the costs for control group patients with susceptible infections (68). For studies on vancomycin-resistant *enteroccocus* (VRE), McKinnon et al. (69), Linden et al. (70), Roughmann et al. (60), and Stosor et al. (71) found that the costs associated with VRE were 129%, 108%, 76%, and 32% greater, respectively, than costs for control group patients with vancomycin-susceptible *enteroccocus.* Song et al. (72) found that costs for patients with VRE bacteremia were 66% higher than those for noninfected control patients.

As presented above, the published evidence has been difficult to synthesize because of the differences in infection type, treatment location, patient type, and comparisons made. It should also be apparent that this literature does not provide enough evidence on the opportunity costs of resistant infections and their impact on hospital resources. However, all studies have been consistent in demonstrating a significant increase in costs for patients with antimicrobial susceptible HAIs and an even greater cost in those who acquire antimicrobial resistant infections. With the exception of the studies by Rubin et al. (56) and Welch et al. (61), these studies were conducted at single centers, so the results could be influenced by a variety of localized patient management practices, particularly empiric therapy regimens and the transfer of infected patients between acute care hospitals and long-term care facilities. In hospitals where drugs active against resistant strains are used as empiric therapy, the cost differential may be less between patients infected with resistant strains compared with those with susceptible strains. Single-center studies should provide detailed information on antimicrobial regimens to facilitate comparisons. Making inferences at the regional or national level based on single-center findings is probably inappropriate. Much larger multi-center studies are needed to control for differences in hospital practices.

As shown in Table 3, several different types of SOI measures have been used to control for confounding in these economic studies. The underlying theory is that more severely ill patients will require more hospital services and so incur higher costs. Among these measures are the APACHE II and III, Charlson, McCabe-Jackson scores, the Simplified Acute Physiology Score (SAPS) II, the All Patient Refined Diagnosis Related Group (APR-DRG), an SOI index developed for bacteremia patients, as well as simply counting the number of comorbidities listed (51–53,73–75). The APACHE II, APACHE III, and SAPS II are primarily physiologic indexes that were designed to predict death upon admission to an ICU, whereas the Charlson index was originally developed to predict death in breast cancer patients over one year and is based on the number and type of pre-existing comorbidities. The McCabe-Jackson score is a prospective and subjective measure of the likelihood of death based on observations of an attending physician on patient hospital admission. The APR-DRG complexity index is an extension to the DRG codes to reflect patient SOI. The diversity of measures used in various studies demonstrates there is no consensus on which SOI indexes are the most appropriate controls for observational comparisons of resistant infection costs. These scoring indexes are not good predictors of the risk of developing HAIs in ICU populations (76). They are instead used to control for cost confounding. Many of the standardized SOI indexes were developed for other uses and have not been evaluated as control measures in the study of resistant infections (77). This is a fruitful area for future research.

A narrow majority of studies used actual hospital costs or charges adjusted by cost-to-charge ratios; others used unadjusted hospital charges. As unadjusted hospital charges often overstate the actual cost of resistant infections, the upward bias in these estimates may be substantial. Published cost-to-charge ratios for the United States range from just over 50% to 80% (78). These ratios are readily available and when cost accounting is not possible, should be used to adjust hospital charges to more closely approximate the opportunity cost of resistant infections.

Implications for Future Studies on Attributable Cost of Resistant Infections

Measuring the absolute attributable cost is useful for determining the potential cost savings associated with interventions that reduce resistant infections within a given healthcare setting. In addition, it is important to measure the relative cost of HAIs, both susceptible and resistant, because they indicate the magnitude of these costs to society. Comparison studies are needed to evaluate the cost differences between the three states of infection status for specific hospital populations. The attributable costs of the different infection states should be examined within the same research study so that the matching criteria, control variables such as SOI indexes, and cost measures are internally consistent. Within this framework, hypothesis testing on the significance of the attributable cost differences can be performed, the existence of differences can be verified, and the relative costs can be estimated. As a single, large, multi-site may not be currently feasible, use of standardized comparison methods and variables will allow synthesis of cost results from a number of reports from single-hospital studies.

Similarly, the use of SOI indexes should be evaluated to determine if attributable cost results are sensitive to the severity measures used as either matching criteria or controls in multivariate models. As noted earlier, clinical SOI indices have not been good predictors of the risk of HAI occuring during a hospital stay; a simple tally of the number of comorbidities present appears to be an equally reliable predictor (79). A recent study has shown that the APACHE III index is statistically correlated with patient cost (39). In models with patient cost as a dependent variable, this index was used to control for the increased costs associated with the baseline underlying disease, independent of the occurrence of infection. More studies are needed to understand how SOI indexes can be used in cost models so that they can be compared and examined for the different effects they may have on cost study results.

The advent of electronic surveillance to help curb the incidence of resistant infection can potentially influence how comparison studies of resistant infections are done (80). As electronic medical records become more common, studies of resistant HAIs will be much cheaper to conduct in terms of research and data collection costs. This will allow the use of larger data sets that could greatly increase the robustness of the analyses. SOI indices constructed from electronic patient data may prove to be the best measures for use in future comparison studies.

Further Considerations

Can retrospective cohort studies be successfully expanded to make comparisons of results for the three infection states feasible? There are other measurement issues to be addressed in cohort studies. A workshop held at Emory University on methodological issues concerning cost measurement of resistant infections in hospitals (38) resulted in a number of recommendations for such studies including:

- Increase study populations by using multi-center study populations because the lack of statistical power in single-center studies with small sample sizes limits the use of statistical controls for SOI as well as the ability to make generalizations to larger populations.
- Develop standardized definitions of resistance, because several microorganisms of clinical importance lack well-defined criteria to be categorized as resistant.
- Assess cost of infection longitudinally, as attributable costs may still accrue after the patient is discharged from the hospital.

Although cohort studies can measure the attributable costs of resistant infections, the reporting of results needs to be consistent and complete. The difficulty and associated research cost in conducting these studies increases when the three infection states are compared and matched. Because many cohort studies employ the strategy of matching, many patients who do not fit the matching criteria are excluded from the study population. A matching strategy may exclude patients with excess cost that should be measured, particularly if an intervention is hospital-wide.

In order to develop cost estimates to be used to evaluate a hospital-wide intervention to reduce infection rates, an alternative analytic approach to concurrent and comparison studies was employed by Roberts et al. (39). This study measured the attributable costs of HAIs in a random sample of hospitalized adult medical patients. The patients in this study were grouped into three categories: (*i*) no infection; (*ii*) confirmed infection, based on modified National Nosocomial Infection Surveillance (NNIS) definitions; and (*iii*) suspected infection representing patients who met most but not all of the NNIS definitions. The cost-confounding effects of underlying disease were controlled for using APACHE III score and ICU admission in a linear regression model. Estimates from the model showed that the attributable cost due to confirmed HAI was over $15,000 and over $6800 for suspected infection. This strategy is currently being used at the same hospital in another study sized to capture a sufficient number of patients to measure costs due to resistant infections.

Another area for future research is the measurement of cost related to the increasing use of alternative antimicrobials for empiric therapy (5,81–83). Patients are often given empiric therapy before an infecting organism has been identified. As the prevalence of resistant infection increases in a given hospital or geographic area, physicians are more likely to use broad-spectrum and expensive drugs for everyone than would have been used if resistance were less prevalent in the population. These excess costs, which include side effects or complications resulting from the alternative treatment, have rarely been measured but potentially could exceed the costs of treatment failure (5). Howard estimated that this substitution effect in the United States amounted to approximately $20 million (during 1980–1996) for the treatment of otitis media in outpatient settings (83). These costs may not be relevant from the perspective of the hospital, but may be very relevant to third-party payers and society.

Another important measurement issue is the endogenous relationship between hospital length of stay and the risk of acquiring an HAI (84). Patients experiencing longer hospitals stays have higher cost, but also a greater chance of acquiring a nosocomial infection. Conversely, patients acquiring an HAI tend to require longer hospital stays and, therefore, higher cost. This implies that an endogenous problem exists between cost and infection. A two-stage modeling process that includes a model of the probability of acquiring infection (stage 1) and a model of patient cost (stage 2) can test the statistical significance of this endogenous relationship and correct the model estimates to account for this bias.

CONCLUSIONS

Recent studies of the attributable cost of resistant nosocomial infections from the hospital perspective have indicated that hospitals can realize cost savings by reducing the incidence of resistant nosocomial infections. The attributable cost studies published in the medical literature are mostly retrospective cohort studies in which cost becomes the outcome variable. The economic evidence presented tends to ignore the relative costs of the various states of infection and to compare just two of the three possible states of infection. The limited evidence indicates that MRSA infections tend to increase costs anywhere from 137% to 244% over noninfected control patients, with no control for underlying SOI. However, the single study making this same comparison with adjusted results estimated a cost increase of only 44%. For comparison of MSSA versus MRSA patient groups, the cost increase ranges from 13% to 95% (including both unadjusted and adjusted cost results). Similar cost disparities were also evident for both VRE and resistant *Acinetobacter baumannii*. The wide disparity in estimates may be partly the result of the differing research strategies regarding the use of SOI measures as controls, the type of information used to represent hospital cost, the site of infection (surgical vs. bloodstream), and the size of the study sample. Although reporting the absolute dollar costs associated with resistance is important for conducting a cost-effectiveness or cost-benefit analysis of a particular intervention, reporting the cost differences as relative proportions between different infections will provide the evidence that can be used to estimate the economic burden of disease from the hospital perspective.

Cohort studies face challenges in controlling the confounding influence of the severity of the underlying disease and finding appropriate measures to represent opportunity costs of resources. More research is needed to evaluate various SOI measures that have been used as controls to see if attributable cost estimates change based on the measures used. Opportunity costs of hospital resources are best reflected in the micro-costing data of hospital expenditures, but such data are difficult to collect. At a minimum, when hospital charges are used as surrogates for cost, they must be adjusted by cost-to-charge ratios to remove the upward bias present in charges due to cost shifting. Implementing the above recommendations can improve the quality of economic information, but places informational burdens on reasearches.

REFERENCES

1. World Health Organization. Global Strategy for the Containment of Antimicrobial Resistance: Executive Summary. (Accessed at http://www.who.int/drugresistance/guidance/en/index.html)
2. Centers for Disease Control and Prevention. A Public Health Action Plan to Combat Antimicrobial Resistance. Part 1: Domestic Issues. (Accessed at http://www.cdc.gov/drugresistance/actionplan/html/index.htm)
3. Centers for Disease Control and Prevention. Antibiotic/Antimicrobial Resistance. (Accessed at http://www.cdc.gov/drugresistance/)
4. Muto CA. Why are antibiotic-resistant nosocomial infections spiraling out of control? Infect Control Hosp Epidemiol 2005; 26:10–12.
5. Howard DH, Scott RD II, Packard R, Jones D. The global impact of drug resistance. Clin Infect Dis 2003; 36(Suppl. 1):S4–10.
6. Kohn LT, Corrigan JM, Donaldson MS, eds. To Err Is Human: Building a Safer Health System. Washington, DC: National Academy Press, 2000.
7. Jones D. Antimicrobial drug resistance: issues and options. Workshop report. Washington, DC: National Academy Press, 1998.
8. Phelps DE. Bug/Drug resistance. Med Care 1989; 27:194–203.
9. Loveday HP, Pellowe CM, Jones SRLJ, Pratt RJ. A systematic review of the evidence for interventions for the prevention and control of methicillin-resistant *Staphylococcus aureus* (1996–2004): report to the Joint MRSA Working Party (Subgroup A). J Hosp Infect 2006; 635:S45–70.
10. Graves N. Economics and preventing hospital-acquired infection. Emerg Infect Dis 2004; 10:561–6.
11. Mankiw NG. Principles of Economics. Orlando: The Dryden Press, 1998.
12. Baumol WJ, Blinder AS. Microeconomics. 9th ed. Belmont: South-Western College Publishing, 2004.
13. Horowitz JB, Hoehring HB. How property rights and patents affect antibiotic resistance. Health Econ 2004; 13:575–83.
14. Finkler SA. The distinction between cost and charges. Ann Intern Med 1982; 96: 102–9.
15. Haddix AC, Schaffer PA. In: Haddix AC, Teutsch SM, Shaffer PA, Dunet DO, eds. Cost-effectiveness Analysis. New York: Oxford University Press, 1996.
16. Dranove D. Pricing by non-profit institutions: the case of hospital cost shifting. J Health Econ 1988; 7:47–57.
17. Dor A, Farley DE. Payment source and the cost of hospital care: evidence from a multiproduct cost function with multiple payers. J Health Econ 1996; 15:1–21.
18. Tompkins CP, Altman SH, Eilat E. The precarious pricing system for hospital services. Health Aff 2006; 25:45–56.
19. McGowan JE Jr. Antimicrobial resistance in hospital organisms and its relation to antibiotic use. Rev Infect Dis 1983; 5:1033–48.
20. McGowan JE Jr. Economic impact of antimicrobial resistance. Emerg Infect Dis 2001; 7:286–92.
21. Tisdell C. Exploitation of techniques that decline in effectiveness. Public Finance 1982; 3:428–37.
22. Coast J, Smith RD, Millar MR. Superbugs: should antimicrobial resistance be included as a cost in economic evaluation? Health Econ 1996; 5:217–26.
23. Coast J, Smith RD, Millar MR. An economic perspective on policy to reduce antimicrobial resistance. Soc Sci Med 1998; 46:29–38.
24. Gordon HS. Economic theory of a common property resource: the fishery. J Political Econ 1954; 62:124–42.

25. Scott RD II, Solomon SL, McGowan JE Jr. Applying economic principles to health care. Emerg Infect Dis 2001; 282–5.
26. Shlaes DM, Gerding DN, John JF Jr, et al. Society for Healthcare Epidemiology of America and Infectious Diseases Society of America Joint Committee on the prevention of antimicrobial resistance: guidelines for the prevention of antimicrobial resistance in hospitals. Clin Infect Dis 1997; 25:584–99.
27. Varian HR. Microeconomic Analysis. 3rd ed. New York: WW Norton, 1992.
28. Roberts RR, Frutos PW, Ciavarella GC, et al. Distribution of fixed vs variable costs of hospital care. JAMA 1999; 281:644–9.
29. Holmberg SD, Solomon SL, Blake PA. Health and economic impacts of antimicrobial resistance. Rev Infect Dis 1987; 9:1065–78.
30. U.S. Congress, Office of Technology Assessment. Impacts of Antibiotic Resistant Bacteria. OTA-H-629. Washington, DC: US Government Printing Office, 1995.
31. Haley RW, Crossley KB, Von Allmen SD, McGowen JE Jr. Extra Charges and prolongation of stay attributable to nosocomial infections: a prospective interhospital comparison. Am J Med 1981; 70:51–8.
32. Schulgen G, Kropec A, Kappstein I, Daschner F, Schmacher M. Estimation of extra hospital stay attributable to nosocomial infections: heterogeneity and timing of events. J Clin Epidemiol 2000; 53:409–17.
33. Edmond MB, Ober JF, Weinbaum DL, Wenzel RP. Vancomycin-resistant enterococcal bacteremia; natural history and attributable mortality. Clin Infect Dis 1996; 23:1234–9.
34. Harbarth S, Rutschmann O, Sudre P, Pittet D. Impact of methicillin resistance on the outcome of patients with bacteremia caused by *Staphylococcus aureus*. Arch Intern Med 1998; 158:182–9.
35. Lodise TP, McKinnon PS, Tam VH, Rybak MJ. Clincial outcomes for patients with bacteremia caused by vancomycin-resistant enterococcccus in a level 1 trauma center. Clin Infect Dis 2002; 34:922–9.
36. Farber BF. Reimbursement for nosocomial infections under the prospective payment plan: the future or decline of infection control? Infect Control 1984; 5:425–6.
37. Haley RW, White JW, Culver DH, Hughes JM. The financial incentive for hospitals to prevent nosocomial infections under the prospective payment system: an empirical determination from a nationally representative sample. JAMA 1987; 257:1611–4.
38. Howard D, Cordell R, McGowan JE, Packard RM, Scott RD II, Solomon SL. Measuring the economics of antimicrobial resistance in hospital settings: summary of the Centers for Disease Control and Prevention—Emory workshop. Clin Infect Dis 2001; 33:1573–8.
39. Roberts RR, Scott RD II, Cordell R, et al. The use of economic modeling to determine the hospital costs associated with nosocomial infections. Clin Infect Dis 2003; 36: 1424–32.
40. Farnham PG, Haddix AC. Study Design. In: Haddix AC, Teutsch SM, Shaffer PA, Dunet DO, eds. Prevention Effectiveness: a Guide to Decision Analysis and Economic Evaluation. 2nd ed. New York: Oxford University Press, 2003.
41. Zanetti G, Platt R. Cost-effectiveness of vancomycin use versus cefazolin for perioperative antibiotic prophylaxis in coronary artery bypass graft surgery (abstract). Am J Infect Control 2000; 28:79.
42. Haley RW, Culver DH, White JW, et al. The efficacy of infection surveillance and control programs in preventing nosocomial infections in US hospitals. Am J Epidemiol 1985; 121:182–205.
43. Haley RW. Measuring the costs of nosocomial infections: methods for estimating economic burden on the hospital. Am J Med 1991; 91(Suppl. 3B):32S–38S.
44. Wakefield DS, Pfaller MA, Hammons GT, Massanari RM. Use of the appropriateness evaluation protocol for estimating the incremental cost associated with nosocomial infections. Med Care 1987; 25:481–8.
45. Haley RW, Schaberg DR, Von Allmen SD, McGowan JE. Estimating the extra charges and prolongation of hospitalization due to nosocomial infections: a comparison of methods. J Infect Dis 1980; 141:248–57.

46. Freeman J, McGowan JE Jr. Methological issues in hospital epidemiology: III. Investigating the modifying effects of time and severity of underlying illness on estimates of cost of nosocomial infection. Rev Infect Dis 1984; 6:285–300.

47. Rello J. Impact of nosocomial infections on outcomes: myths and evidence. Infect Control Hosp Epidemiol 1999; 20:392–94.

48. Paladino JA, Sunderlin JL, Price CS, Schentag JT. Economic consequences of antimicrobial resistance. Surg Infect 2002; 3:259–67.

49. Gross PA, DeMauro PJ, Van Antwerpen C, Wallenstein S, Chiang S. Number of co-morbidities as a predictor of nosocomial infection acquisition. Infect Control Hosp Epidemiol 1988; 9:497–500.

50. Harris AD, Karchmer TB, Carmeli Y, Samore MH. Methodological principles of case-control studies that analyzed risk factors for antibiotic resistance: a systematic review. Clin Infect Dis 2001; 32:1055–61.

51. Knaus WA, Wagner DP, Draper EA, et al. The APACHE III prognostic system: risk prediction of hospital mortality for critically ill hospitalized adults. Chest 1991; 100:1619–36.

52. Charleson ME, Pompei P, Ales KL, MacKenzie CR. A new method of classifying prognostic comorbidity in longitudinal studies: development and validation. J Chronic Dis 1987; 40:373–83.

53. McCabe WR, Jackson GG. Gram-negative bacteremia. I. Etiology and ecology. Arch Intern Med 1962; 110:847–53.

54. Zawacke BE, Azen SP, Imbus SH, Chang YT. Multifactorial probit analysis of mortality in burn patients. Ann Surg 1979; 189:1–5.

55. Stone PW, Gupta A, Loughrey M, et al. Attributable costs and length of stay of an extended-spectrum beta-lactamase-producing *Klebsiella pneumoniae* outbreak in a neonatal intensive care unit. Infect Control Hosp Epidemiol 2003; 24:601–6.

56. Rubin RJ, Harrington CA, Poon A, Dietrich K, Greene J, Moiduddin A. The economic impact of *Staphylococcus aureus* Infection in New York hospitals. Emerg Infect Dis 1999; 5:9–17.

57. Engemann JJ, Carmeli Y, Cosgrove SE, et al. Adverse clinical and economic outcomes attributable to methicillin resistance among patients with *Staphylococcus aureus* surgical site infection. Clin Infect Dis 2003; 36:592–8.

58. Chaix C, Durand-Zaleski I, Corinne A, Alberti C, Brun-Buisson C. Control of endemic methicillin-resistant *Staphylococcus aureus*: a cost-benefit analysis in an intensive care unit. JAMA 1999; 282:1745–51.

59. Abramson MA, Sexton JS. Nosocomial methicillin-resistant and methicillin-susceptible *Staphylococcus aureus* primary bacteremia: at what costs. Infect Control Hosp Epidemiol 1999; 20:408–11.

60. Roughmann M, Bradham D, South B, Fridkin S, Perl T. The clinical and economic impact of antimicrobial drug resistance on nosocomial bloodstream infections (abstr). Infect Control Hosp Epidemiol 2000; 21:97.

61. Welch KE, Goff DA, Fish N, Sierawski SJ, Paladino JA. A multi-center economic analysis of bacteremia caused by methicillin-resistant *Staphylococcus aureus*. (abstr) presented at the 39th International Conference of Antimicrobial Agents and Chemotherapy, Sept. 26–29, 1999.

62. Reed SD, Friedman JY, Engeman JJ, et al. Cost and outcomes among *hemodialysis*-dependent patients with methicillin-resistant or methicillin-susceptible *Staphylococcus aureus* bacteremia. Infect Control Hosp Epidemiol 2005; 26:175–83.

63. Lodise TP, McKinnon. Clinical and economic impact of methicillin resistance in patients with *Staphylococcus aureus* bacteremia. Diagn Microbiol Infect Dis 2005; 52:113–22.

64. Cosgrove SE, Youlin Q, Kaye KS, Harbarth S, Karchmer AW, Carmeli Y. The impact of methicillin resistance in *Staphylococcus aureus* bacteremia on patient outcomes: mortality, length of stay, and hospital charges. Infect Control Hosp Epidemiol 2005; 26:166–74.

65. Weingarten CM, Rybak MJ, Jahns BE, Stevenson JG, Brown WJ, Levine DP. Evaluation of *Acinetobactoer baumannii* infection and colonization, and antimicrobial treatment patterns in an urban teaching hospital. Pharmacotherapy 1999; 19:1080–5.

66. Wilson SJ, Knipe CJ, Zieger MJ, et al. Direct costs of multidrug-resistant *Acinetobactoer baumannii* in the burn unit of a public teaching hospital. Am J Infect Control 2004; 32:342–4.
67. Lautenbach E, Patel JB, Bilker WB, Edelstein PH, Fishman NO. Extended-spectrum β-lactamase-producing *Escherichia coli* and *Klebsiella pneumoniae*: risk factors for infection and impact of resistance on outcomes. Clin Infect Dis 2001; 32:1162–71.
68. Cosgrove SE, Kaye KS, Eliopoulous GM, Carmeli Y. Health and economic outcomes of the emergence of third-generation cephalosporin resistance in *Enterobacter* species. Arch Intern Med 2002; 162:185–90.
69. McKinnon PS, Tam VH, Kwa AL, Rybak MJ. An economic analysis of bacteremia caused by vancomycin resistant *Enterococcus* in patients admitted to a level-1 trauma center. Abstract presented at the 40th International Conference of Antimicrobial Agents and Chemotherapy, Chicago, IL; Sept. 17–20, 2000.
70. Linden P, Paladino J, Saul M, Stoffer D. The economic impact of bacteremia due to vancomycin-resistant *Enterococcus faecium*: a case control study. Abstract presented at the 38th International Conference of Antimicrobial Agents and Chemotherapy, San Diego, CA; Sept.24–27, 1998.
71. Stosor V, Peterson LR, Postelnick, Noskin GA. *Enterococcus faecium* bacteremia: does vancomycin resistance make a difference? Arch Inter Med 1998; 158:522–7.
72. Song X, Srinivasan A, Perl T. Effect of nosocomial vancomycin-resistant enterococcal bacteremia on mortality, length of stay, and costs. Infect Control Hosp Epidemiol 2003; 24:251–6.
73. Le Gall JR, Lomeshow S, Saulnier F. A new Simplified Acute Physiology Score (SAPS II) based on a European/North American multicenter study. JAMA 1993; 270:2957–63.
74. Saulnier F. All Patient Refined-Diagonosis Related Groups Definitions Manual, version 15.0. St. Paul, MN: 3M Health Information Systems; 1998.
75. Chow JW, Fine MJ, Shlaes DM, et al. *Enterobacter* bacteremia: clinical features and emergence of antibiotic resistance during therapy. Ann Intern Med 1991; 155:585–90.
76. Keita-Perse O, Gaynes RP. Severity of illness scoring systems to adjust nosocomial infection rates: a review and commentary. Am J Infect Control 1996; 24:429–34.
77. Harris AD, Karchmer TB, Carmeli Y, Samore MB. Methodological principles of case-control studies that analyze risk factors for antibiotic resistance: a systematic review. Clin Inf Dis 2001; 32:1055–61.
78. Haddix AC, Teutsch SM, Shaffer PA. Prevention Effectiveness: A Guide to Decision Analysis and Economic Evaluation. 2nd ed. New York: Oxford University Press, 2003.
79. Gross PA, Stein MR, van Antwerpen C, et al. Comparison of severity of illness indicators in an intensive care unit. Arch Intern Med 1991; 151:2201–5.
80. Wisnieski MF, Kieszkowski P, Zagorski BM, Trick WE, Sommers M, Weinstein RA. Development of a clinical data warehouse for hospital infection control. J Am Med Inform Assoc 2003; 10:454–62.
81. Phillips M, Phillips-Howard P. Economic implications of resistance to antimalaria drugs. Pharmacoeconomics 1996; 10:225–38.
82. Howard DH, Rask KJ. The impact of resistance on antibiotic demand in patients with ear infections. In: Laxminarayan R, Brown G, eds. The Economics of Resistance. Washington, DC: Resources for the Future, 2003.
83. Howard DH. Resistance-induced antibiotic substitution. Health Econ 2004; 13:585–95.
84. Graves N, Weinhold D, Roberts JA. Correcting for bias when estimating the cost of hospital acquired infections; an analysis of lower respiratory tract infections in non-surgical patients. Unpublished paper. June 2002.

2

Benchmarking: Its Utility in the Fight Against Antibacterial Resistance

Sujata M. Bhavnani
Institute for Clinical Pharmacodynamics, Ordway Research Institute, Inc., Albany, New York, U.S.A.

Glenn S. Tillotson
Replidyne, Inc., Milford, Connecticut, U.S.A.

INTRODUCTION

Antibacterial resistance is a burgeoning and global problem, involving multiple species of bacteria and most antibacterial agents. Although antibacterial resistance rates for both Gram-negative and Gram-positive pathogens continue to rise, increases in the resistance rates of Gram-negative bacilli to many commonly used broad spectrum agents, especially in intensive care units, is particularly ominous. While awareness of antibacterial resistance is increasing among medical practitioners, the public is likewise becoming increasingly cognizant of pathogens such as multi-drug resistant *Streptococcus pneumoniae* (MDRSP) and methicillin-resistant *Staphylococcus aureus* (MRSA), the latter of which has become the focus of sports news as athletes increasingly acquire MRSA infections. For example, Toronto Blue Jays outfielder Alex Rios was sidelined for over a month in the summer of 2006 due to a drug-resistant staphylococcal infection arising from an otherwise trivial injury. Traditionally seen as a hospital problem, data from large surveillance programs demonstrate that these resistant pathogens are now originating in the community rather than in the hospital setting (1).

Various strategies have been developed to stem or even reduce this emerging threat, one of which is "benchmarking." In this context, benchmarking typically involves a process of pooling clinical and laboratory data from multiple institutions to identify "benchmarks" against which individual institutions can measure the effectiveness of their own antimicrobial management programs. The utility of benchmarking techniques in the fight against antibacterial resistance, including the incorporation of valuable data from large surveillance systems, is reviewed here.

BENCHMARKING AND INFECTIOUS DISEASES

Benchmarking refers to a continuous process of measuring the products, services, or practices of an institution against those of its peer groups or leaders in the field (external benchmarking), or against its own past performance (internal benchmarking). Ideally, benchmarking involves an ongoing and self-reflective process of establishing preliminary procedures and target goals, periodically reviewing performance, and instituting appropriate modifications to each part of the process as needed. The principles of benchmarking, originally cited by Deming (2), have been successfully applied to various industries including healthcare. Benchmarking in institutional settings, such as hospitals and long-term care facilities, and even in the outpatient setting, has proven to be of value in identifying potential problem areas in healthcare delivery and in aiding the establishment of appropriate and attainable target goals (3–6). In the last decade, the benefits of benchmarking have been increasingly recognized, and the practice of benchmarking has become important to the hospital accreditation process. Hospitals are assessed by whether or not their systems and databases support benchmarking, and by whether or not institutions are actively participating in an ongoing benchmarking process with other institutions (7).

Using national data sources, standards of practice have been compared to patient outcomes. In an effort to compare rates of urinary tract infections in home care, Woomer and colleagues (3) described a collaborative approach in which six home care agencies developed standards to define and monitor urinary tract infections. Narong et al. (4), using data from the National Nosocomial Infection Surveillance (NNIS) System as a reference, benchmarked rates of surgical site infections in patients undergoing major operations in a university hospital setting. Benchmarking has also been used to reveal the positive impact of a change in practice. For example, Bissell (5) described the experience of the Latter Day Saints Hospital in Salt Lake City. Through the use of internal and retrospective data, the beneficial impact on patient outcomes of computerized decision-support was demonstrated, based both on laboratory and clinical data. Similarly, but on a large scale, after collecting and benchmarking data on vancomycin use and the prevalence of vancomycin-resistant enterococci (VRE) in 50 intensive care units (ICUs) among 20 U.S. NNIS hospitals participating in Project Intensive Care Antimicrobial Resistance Epidemiology (Project ICARE), Fridkin et al. assessed whether or not such comparative information led to quality improvement (6). These authors reported that specific and targeted changes in practices, arising from the benchmarking process, were associated with both decreases in vancomycin use and prevalence of VRE in the ICU.

In addition to Project ICARE, other programs have collected antibacterial use and resistance data in hospitals for the purposes of benchmarking and evaluating the relationship between antibacterial use and resistance. Perhaps the longest running program of this nature is the Benchmarking Program (8–12), which has been building a database of U.S. hospitals since 1993. Participants complete an annual survey to report hospital demographic information such as number of beds, occupancy rates, number of inpatient days and case mix index, and annual inpatient expenditures, including cost/gram for many individual antimicrobial agents. Hospital antibiograms, which describe annual rates of resistance for various microorganisms of interest, are also provided. Lastly, each participant provides information regarding the types of antibiotic management activities performed at their institution, including whether or not antibiotic formularies are enforced (and if so, how), what types and choices for therapeutic substitution are used, and whether programs such as streamlining broad-spectrum to narrow-spectrum antibiotics exist (11). In addition to receiving an annual report that allows for comparison of the above-described measures and characteristics to peer hospitals of similar size and type, these data have also allowed for the exploration of certain relationships including the impact on treatment cost of certain antimicrobial stewardship practices such as intravenous-to-oral therapy (IV-to-PO) switching programs (8) and the relationship between use of certain antibacterial agents and susceptibility of microorganisms of interest to those same agents (13).

While many hospitals have embraced benchmarking or similar continuous quality improvement (CQI) tools in an effort to manage antibacterial resistance, studies have mainly been focused in specific units or specialty areas. The more general collection of susceptibility data for community-originated bacterial strains, the comparison of their emergence relative to antibacterial usage, and the impact of changes in medical practice designed to address this issue, have not been undertaken consistently by institutions. Furthermore, even if a hospital routinely collected such data, finding appropriate comparative data with which they might benchmark their efforts has been a challenge. To this end, data from surveillance systems represent an important and under-utilized resource that institutions can use to benchmark their rates of antibacterial resistance.

OVERVIEW OF EXISTING ANTIMICROBIAL SURVEILLANCE SYSTEMS

In the context of antibacterial resistance, the term surveillance refers to a process of systematic and ongoing data collection, analysis, and reporting in order to characterize temporal trends in the occurrence and distribution of susceptibility and resistance to antibacterial agents. As described by the World Health Organization (WHO), the establishment of "effective, epidemiologically sound surveillance of antimicrobial resistance among common pathogens in the community, hospitals, and other healthcare facilities" is a fundamental public health priority in the effort to confront antimicrobial drug-resistant organisms (14). Consequences of nonsystematic and discontinuous surveillance of antibacterial resistance include the following: the inability to establish meaningful baseline trends, low sensitivity in detecting new resistance threats, and inadequate information to provide the basis to identify populations at risk or interventions required. Data from large surveillance systems provide the opportunity to address these issues.

Over the last decade, many surveillance systems have been established to evaluate changing patterns of antibacterial susceptibility. A summary of various national and international antimicrobial surveillance programs, past and present, including those that have received support from industry (15–22), is provided in Table 1. Surveillance studies sponsored by industry are crucial for supporting the registration of new agents. These data are important for pharmacokinetic-pharmacodynamic (PK-PD) analyses to support dose selection and derive susceptibility breakpoints, as well as for providing global and regional susceptibility information for product labeling. Additionally, such data provide a basis to differentiate new agents from those already marketed. Ongoing surveillance data may also be used to demonstrate the validity of original data provided at the time of registration, to assist in predictions about future resistance trends, and to support marketing and life cycle management (23). In addition to industry-based objectives, data from such systems are very useful guides for formulary decisions, prescribing empiric therapy, and creating programs to contain antimicrobial resistance (24).

One important though inevitable limitation of such industry-sponsored surveillance programs is their sometimes narrow focus or testing bias (e.g., it is unlikely that generically-available drugs would be widely tested). Testing and reporting is typically limited to the investigational or approved agent of interest and those comparators of direct marketing relevance for certain pathogens. In addition, factors associated with decreased susceptibility within a particular

TABLE 1 A Summary of Various National and International Antimicrobial Surveillance Programs

Study	Acronym	Funding/sponsor	Start date	Notes	References
Industry-supported program					
Alexander Project		GlaxoSmithKline	1992	Inactive	15
Meropenem Yearly Susceptibility Test Information Collection	MYSTIC	AstraZeneca	1997	Global	16
SENTRY Antimicrobial Surveillance Program	SENTRY	Multiple	1997	Global, 6 continents	17
The Surveillance Network	TSN	Eurofins Medinet	1998	United States	18
Prospective Resistant Organism Tracking and Epidemiology for the Ketolide Telithromycin	PROTEKT	Sanofi-Aventis	1999	United States and Europe	19
LIBRA Surveillance Program	LIBRA	Bayer	2000	Compilation of fluoroquinolone studies	20
Academia/government-driven programs					
European Antimicrobial Resistance Surveillance System	EARSS	European Commission	1998	European Union only	See reports on website
European Surveillance of Antibiotic Resistance	ESAR	European Commission	1998	European Union only	See reports on website
Active Bacterial Core Surveillance Program	ABCs	U.S. CDC	1995	United States only	21
Antimicrobial Resistance Information Bank	AR InfoBank	World Health organization	1999	Global	See website
Intensive Care Antimicrobial Resistance Evaluation	ICARE	Pharmaceutical companies under auspices of CDC	1996	Surveillance of ICUs across the United States	22
British Society for Antimicrobial Chemotherapy Resistance Surveillance Project	BSAC	Multiple pharmaceutical companies	1999	Ireland and United Kingdom	See website

Abbreviations: CDC, Centers for Disease Control and Prevention; ICU, intensive care unit.
Source: Adapted from Ref. 31.

institution or geographical regions are often not characterized. This latter limitation could be overcome by broadening the nature of data collection. For example, information about the strategies used to contain the emergence of resistance in a hospital setting could be collected, the results of which could be used by hospitals for benchmarking.

As a result of the recent decline of antibacterial drug development and the increasing number of off-patent agents, fewer large pharmaceutical companies are involved in supporting large-scale surveillance studies. Also, those companies that are developing antibacterial agents are generally more selective about the studies performed and/or often have insufficient resources to support these large and expensive programs. In this climate, programs such as the SENTRY Antimicrobial Resistance Program (17), which represents a long-standing program that originally received funding from one sponsor (Bristol-Myers Squibb) and which now receives funding from a number of pharmaceutical companies, is an example of an effective paradigm for a broad-based surveillance program that ensures longevity of data collection.

In addition to funding programs such as SENTRY (17), the Meropenem Yearly Susceptibility Test Information Collection (MYSTIC) (16), and The Surveillance Network® (TSN®) (18), pharmaceutical companies also support large coordinated surveillance efforts, which pool and compare data in order to detect early patterns of antimicrobial resistance. Recognizing the value of joint surveillance collaborations to provide the broadest set of data to policymakers and researchers, the Alliance for the Prudent Use of Antibiotics, a nonprofit organization, established the Global Advisory for Antibiotic Resistance Data (GAARD) (25) in 1999 for the purposes of collaboration among large international surveillance programs, and the Centers for Disease Control and Prevention (CDC), the WHO, and the WHO Collaborating Centre for Surveillance of Antimicrobial Resistance, which serve in advisory roles. GAARD studies have been based on data from Astra-Zeneca International (supporting the MYSTIC surveillance project), Bayer AG (TARGETed), Bristol-Myers Squibb Company (SENTRY), GlaxoSmithKline (Alexander Project), and Ortho-McNeil Pharmaceuticals (TRUST) (26).

In one such study, which pooled data from the MYSTIC and SENTRY Antimicrobial Surveillance Programs, two large international datasets allowed for the exploration of temporal, geographic, and demographic trends in *Escherichia coli* resistance to various agents from 1997 to 2001. These analyses served to demonstrate the elevated rates of nonsusceptibility in certain regions compared to others (e.g., compared to the rates seen in North America, higher rates of nonsusceptibility were evident in Latin America, southern Europe, and the western Pacific) and the differences in nonsusceptibility in cohorts of interest including older versus younger patients and patients in the intensive care unit. Although the finding of greater nonsusceptibility of isolates among patients in the intensive care unit was not unexpected, confidence in the reliability and validity of such findings is perhaps greater when identified in two separate programs. Thus, the potential benefit of GAARD projects that represent pooled analyses of data gathered from multiple sources, are the following: (*i*) increased statistical power to detect outcomes of interest and to evaluate risk factors associated with emergence of antimicrobial resistance and spread; (*ii*) greater geographic and demographic representation and time span for bacterial isolates collected as compared to those isolates collected from a single system with limited resources; and (*iii*) ability to cross-validate findings from similar data sources (27).

Along with such industry-sponsored programs, a growing number of academia- or government-sponsored programs have been established. The bedrock of such programs has been the utilization of data from routine susceptibility testing of clinical isolates. Such data banks are frequently very accessible and inexpensive and allow for the potential to benchmark rates of antimicrobial resistance against peer hospitals of similar size, type, and even patient population. Despite these benefits, limitations of pooling data from routine susceptibility testing have been identified (28) and include the following: (*i*) poor standardization of methodology and interpretative criteria; (*ii*) many laboratories test a small number of agents and they do not all test the same compounds; (*iii*) so-called "second-line" agents are only tested against isolates known to be resistant to first-line drugs; and (*iv*) isolates are often not fully identified but rather "pooled," allowing for major resistance development to be potentially missed.

In an effort to address these limitations and to harmonize antimicrobial resistance surveillance in Europe, the European Antimicrobial Resistance Surveillance System (EARSS), a network of European laboratories in 31 countries coordinated by Rijksinstituut voor de Volksgezondheid en Milieu (RIVM) and the National Institute of Public Health and the Environment of the Netherlands, was established. This surveillance system, which is funded by the European Commission's Directorate-General Health and Consumer Protection, was created in an effort to monitor antibacterial resistance using data based on comparable sampling polices, testing systems, and adopted breakpoints. Through EARSS, susceptibility test results for invasive isolates and background information about patients are reported (29).

Although systems such as EARSS allow for cost-effective monitoring and benchmarking of national antibacterial resistance trends based on a large sample with wide geographic representation, the data collected and evaluated are often only qualitative [i.e., data for isolates indicate whether they are susceptible, intermediate, or resistant to the antibacterial tested, but the actual minimum inhibitory concentration (MIC) value is not provided]. In addition, data are collected from a wide variety of laboratory systems, and thus are subject to sampling bias. One example of such bias that may contribute to differences in rates of antibacterial resistance among European countries is the differing practices for requesting blood cultures. As described by Bronzwaer et al. (30), clinicians in northern European countries may request blood cultures more frequently than those from southern European countries, who typically only request blood cultures in the case of empiric treatment failure. Higher rates of antibacterial resistance in the latter countries may be due in part to this sampling bias. Thus, while potentially valuable, data from modestly-funded academia- or government-sponsored surveillance programs also suffer from some important limitations.

Using a consensus process involving a large group of experts from across Europe, antimicrobial resistance surveillance was recently addressed by the European Society of Clinical Microbiology and Infectious Diseases (ESCMID) Study Group for Antimicrobial Resistance Surveillance (ESGARS) (24). One of the key issues identified by this group was the need for high quality surveillance data on which to base decisions. It was also recognized that different types of surveillance studies should fulfill different requirements. Accordingly, individualized consideration with regard to data collection and reporting, the anticipated use of the data, and the necessity for networking to disseminate the data will be required. Another important concept identified centers on the need for relevant indicators for antimicrobial resistance data based on the use of adequate denominators and stratifying variables such as infection type (community- vs. hospital-based infections), patient location, and severity of illness. Also, data from such systems would be infinitely more valuable if clinical outcomes of patients with infections arising from the isolates collected were to be captured (31,32).

Although data from different states in the United States are not pooled in a large coordinated effort as previously described for Europe (29), the Division of Healthcare Quality Promotion at the CDC has worked collaboratively with the Rollins School of Public Health of Emory University through Project ICARE to establish the relationship between antimicrobial use and resistance. Data from this program have been used to aid healthcare professionals in understanding and controlling antimicrobial resistance in the healthcare system. Unlike other resistance surveillance systems, Project ICARE focuses on a narrow list of problem pathogens, such as staphylococci with decreased sensitivity to vancomycin, daptomycin, and linezolid, and Gram-negative organisms that are resistant to fluoroquinolones, extended-spectrum cephalosporins, and carbapenems. Currently, emphasis is placed upon the molecular characterization and typing of isolates, new methods for detecting antimicrobial resistance in the diagnostic laboratory, and educational efforts to improve laboratory testing and reporting (33).

CHALLENGES IN MEASURING ANTIBACTERIAL RESISTANCE

Although valuable, longitudinal data collected through large national and international surveillance programs is not without complications, some of which may hamper efforts to utilize the data for benchmarking purposes. Chief among these are regional differences in susceptibility breakpoints, inappropriately set susceptibility breakpoints, and changes in susceptibility breakpoints over time.

Susceptibility breakpoints vary from one region of the world to another. There are often valid reasons for this variation. For instance, the dose and dosing interval in different countries can vary markedly. In North America, most fluoroquinolones are typically dosed 250 to 750 mg one to two times daily, while in Japan these drugs are typically dosed 100 to 200 mg two to three times daily. This difference in dosing would suggest a higher North American susceptibility breakpoint compared to that in Japan. Such regional differences in susceptibility breakpoints can affect comparisons between countries.

Inappropriately set susceptibility breakpoints also pose a challenge to resistance benchmarking efforts. Historically, most susceptibility breakpoints have been epidemiological. That is, they are set to discriminate between the "wild type" subpopulation and those with one or more resistance determinants. For instance, macrolide susceptibility breakpoints for *S. pneumoniae* were set in such a manner. Figure 1 shows the clarithromycin MIC distribution for *S. pneumoniae* (34). Three subpopulations can be discerned, which are differentiated by the presence or absence of *mef*(A) and *erm*(B) resistance determinants. Clarithromycin's pneumococcal susceptibility breakpoints separate three subpopulations with ≤0.25 mg/L considered susceptible and ≥1 mg/L resistant. The problem with epidemiologically set susceptibility breakpoints is that they often do not predict clinical failure, but rather the presence or absence of a factor that results in a higher MIC value.

Sometimes susceptibility breakpoints change over time. These changes often reflect new understanding of clinical pharmacology or the identification or

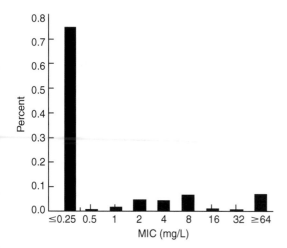

FIGURE 1 MIC distribution for clarithromycin against 1094 strains of *Streptococcus pneumoniae*; consecutive, nonduplicate clinical isolates collected in North America over 2002 by the SENTRY Surveillance Program. *Abbreviation*: MIC, Minimum inhibitory concentration. *Source*: Adapted from Ref. 34.

emergence of new resistance mechanisms. For example, given the continued emergence of cephem-resistant Enterobacteriaceae, including extended spectrum beta-lactamase (ESBL)-producing strains, the appropriateness of current Clinical and Laboratory Standards Institute (CLSI) susceptibility breakpoints has been the focus of recent attention. It is interesting to note that the original Enterobacteriaceae susceptibility breakpoint (susceptible ≤ 8 mg/L, resistant >32) for intravenous cefo-taxime, set in the early 1980s, was based on pooled analyses of data from patients infected with *Pseudomonas aeruginosa*, Enterobacteriaceae, or staphylococci (35). As there were relatively few Enterobacteriaceae with MIC values of 8 mg/L, and since most *P. aeruginosa* in the database had MIC values ≥ 16 mg/L, the current break-points for Enterobacteriaceae were actually driven by the staphylococci. Over the last two decades, we have learned that the exposures, as measured by the duration of time drug concentrations exceed the MIC (T > MIC), needed to eradicate staphy-lococci are smaller than that required to eradiate Gram-negative bacilli, indicating the need for lower breakpoints for the latter pathogen group. Indeed, pre-clinical and PK-PD target attainment (36) and clinical data (37) have emerged supporting this reduction and, in Europe, cephalosporin breakpoints have already been reduced 2- to 16-fold (38). Data such as these demonstrate that appropriately established susceptibility breakpoints are not only vital for patient care decisions but also important from an epidemiologic standpoint to accurately quantify and compare rates of antibacterial resistance. In any event, the impact of susceptibility breakpoints changing over time can best be negated by comparing shapes of MIC distributions rather than point estimates (i.e., susceptibility breakpoints) of susceptibility.

Despite the importance of using clinical response data to guide the selection of susceptibility breakpoints, one needs to be cognizant of the limitations of using traditional definitions for response in community-based infections. In a recent commentary, Powers (32) proposed that antibacterial resistance may not be as common as would be predicted by our current laboratory-based methods, thereby necessitating, perhaps, a re-definition of "resistance." As he suggested, if "true" antibacterial resistance were so prevalent, more patients would fail therapy than is currently documented, thereby resulting in more hospitalizations and possibly more deaths. However, it is important to note that for many of the community-based infections for which patients may be less immunosuppressed, it is not hospitalization or death that is likely the marker of resistance-driven failure, but rather the inability to return to normal activities soon enough or to be productive when back at work. These latter outcomes may appear much less objective but are likely more meaningful to the patient. Given the differences in severity between hospital and community-based infections, it is expected that some patients will improve clinically in the face of resistance while others may not, despite the use of potent antibacterial therapy.

MONITORING ANTIBACTERIAL USE AND RESISTANCE

The relationship between antibacterial use and the emergence of resistance is well documented (39–41), and benchmarking antimicrobial use in conjunction with antimicrobial resistance can be extraordinarily valuable for demonstrating both the need for, and the impact of, antimicrobial stewardship programs. By obtaining data from other institutions, benchmarking techniques can be used to demonstrate the impact of services not currently offered at an institution. Such data may even provide a sufficiently compelling argument to justify to administrators the need for enhanced support of such clinical programs.

In addition to curtailing antibacterial resistance, there are other compelling reasons to monitor the use of antibacterial agents. Institutional antimicrobial use has been shown to represent 16–20% of annual drug expenditures (13). Given this level of spending, even a modest improvement in prescribing has the potential to make a significant economic impact. The effectiveness of various activities aimed at reducing inappropriate antimicrobial use can also be benchmarked. Such activities might include the following: staffing levels (measured as full-time equivalents) of pharmacists, technicians, clinical pharmacists, and infection control staff; pharmacy department computing resources; programs for switching or IV-to-PO streamlining of antimicrobials; various infection control practices; computer access to microbiology results; and the impact of formulary guidelines. Many of these activities promote appropriate antimicrobial use, which will likely have a positive impact on controlling antibacterial resistance and reducing anti-bacterial-associated adverse events.

Although relationships between antimicrobial use and resistance have been described for certain agents and microorganisms, not all studies evaluating use and resistance have been able to demonstrate a statistically significant association. The results of studies in which no association is observed may be due in part to small sample size, limited duration of observation, poor quality of data and/or limitations of study design, or existence of interactions with other variables not captured by the investigator.

Perhaps the most important limitation of using surveillance data for demonstrating a relationship between antibacterial use and resistance is the qualitative nature of microbiologic data available. Microbiologic data is usually obtained from hospital antibiograms which show the proportion of isolates that were sensitive, intermediate, or resistant to a drug of interest over a given study period. Given the nature of susceptibility testing, the more quantitative form of antibacterial susceptibility data (i.e., MIC) is not often available. The problem with relying on qualitative susceptibility data is one of resolution. Only when a relatively large proportion of the bacterial population crosses the susceptibility breakpoint for resistance can one detect changes. As shown in Figure 2, large increases in MIC_{50} values may not immediately manifest with a large proportion of resistant isolates. In this example, a 59% increase in the MIC_{50} value resulted in a relatively modest (3.8%) increase in isolates falling within the resistant category. However, as the MIC_{50} value continues to increase, an unexpectedly large proportion of isolates may fall into the resistant category rather suddenly. Evaluation of actual MIC values rather than the proportion of resistant isolates allows for detection of shifts in the MIC distribution much earlier, often allowing for an intervention prior to a clinical or epidemiological crisis.

While the data collected from individual hospitals are often qualitative, sources of quantitative susceptibility data from institutions are available. A number of large and longstanding surveillance systems, such as the SENTRY Antimicrobial Surveillance Program and the Trust (TRUST) and MYSTIC Surveillance Programs, have performed extensive MIC testing for isolates collected globally. Moreover, these surveillance systems frequently collect more information about the patient and institution from which isolates were collected than is usually reported. Such data allow for multiple linear regression analyses evaluating the impact of various patient- and institution-specific variables on MIC data and, thus, represent a step forward in the effort to better understand the predictors of resistance (42–44).

One challenge in the clinical study of resistant bacteria has been the difficulty in identifying patients likely to be infected with such pathogens. In an effort to identify factors predictive of resistance, linear regression and correlation analyses have frequently been applied to epidemiologic data collected across multiple institutions (13,45–47). In these analyses, the outcome variable is typically the percentage of isolates that are nonsusceptible or resistant to a given

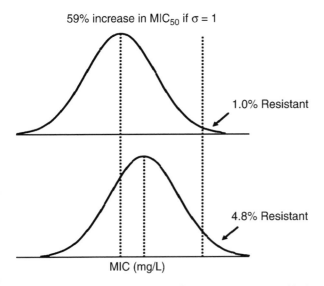

FIGURE 2   Impact of change in MIC_{50} on the proportion of isolates that are resistant. *Abbreviation*: MIC, minimum inhibitory concentration.

antibacterial agent. However, the use of qualitative susceptibility data places undue restrictions upon the sensitivity of an analysis: significant increases in MIC values within any of the qualitative susceptibility categories (susceptible, intermediate, or resistant) cannot be detected (48). Epidemiologic analyses involving quantitative MIC data overcome the latter limitation. Studies evaluating factors associated with a quantitative dependent variable such as percent of isolates that are resistant are evaluating whether or not there is significant shift in the tail of a probability distribution with and without the effect of a factor of interest (e.g., drug usage). Such a shift is often a difficult effect to detect, especially when there are few intermediate or resistant isolates within the population of interest. It is often easier to detect the effect of factors impacting the MIC_{50} value rather than those factors that shift a tail probability, since the former analysis of MIC values has greater statistical power than the latter type of analysis (49). In addition, analyses that make use of tools such as censored regression can account for the truncated nature of MIC data, allowing for better characterization of factors that affect changes in susceptibility (43).

LOCAL SURVEILLANCE AND FUTURE DIRECTIONS

National and international surveillance data are of great value for understanding global trends in antibacterial resistance and provide a repository of data for analyses to determine factors predictive of decreased susceptibility. It is, however, even more crucial to understand the pattern of antibacterial resistance trends locally and within the institution of interest in order to detect early signals of potentially serious problems. To this end, the appropriate compilation of susceptibility data is critical.

Until recently, hospitals followed their own set of guidelines for abstracting and presenting data in the form of an antibiogram. However, standardized guidelines to gather, analyze, and present cumulative antimicrobial susceptibility test data in the form of an antibiogram have been published in CLSI document M39-2A (50). Through this guideline, hospitals have a standardized methodology for data extraction for all drugs tested and for reporting results. For example, guidance is given as to which isolates should be included in the analysis (e.g., the first isolate from a patient within an analysis period), the analysis period (at least annual), population tested (e.g., inpatient, intensive care unit, or nursing home), specimen source, and a reasonable minimum of number of isolates for each organism ($n = 30$). A standardized approach to constructing antibiograms will facilitate internal and external benchmarking of antibacterial resistance patterns. The commitment to collecting antibacterial use and clinical outcome data will further enhance the value of data derived from benchmarking. Such activities will ultimately benefit and support antimicrobial stewardship activities and formulary decisions.

As described in this chapter, current susceptibility breakpoints are not optimal for all classes of agents or all patient populations and are in the process of being re-evaluated by groups such as CLSI and the European Committee on Antimicrobial Susceptibility Testing (EUCAST). As such, benchmarking of susceptibility data characterized as susceptible, intermediate, and resistant is less informative, and evaluations based on such comparisons may lead to suboptimal decisions with regard to formulary decisions and empiric prescribing. To optimize the value of data from microbiologic tests, institutions will need to implement an automated susceptibility testing methodology that can deliver MIC values, or at least a limited range of such values. Actual MIC data will allow for benchmarking of MIC distributions (including MIC_{50} and MIC_{90} values) in addition to the proportion of isolates that are resistant. The former will allow for detection of changes in susceptibility patterns prior to the occurrence of any large shift in MIC values into the resistant category. From a prescribing perspective, actual MIC data will also allow for interpretation of PK-PD target attainment analyses and, ultimately, better dose selection for an individual patient. For example, if testing for a particular microorganism demonstrates a MIC value in a higher range, dosing regimens may be optimized for the patient.

In conclusion, benchmarking can be a valuable and powerful tool in the fight against antibiotic resistance, but it is only as effective as the data used. Data from large multinational surveillance programs are of great value to understanding patterns of antibacterial resistance, and to date, these data have been under-utilized. The evaluation of MIC distributions using statistical tools that can accommodate quantitative MICs (including the pattern of MIC censoring) will allow for a better understanding of the impact of institution-, patient-, and microorganism-specific factors on changes in MIC, before high-level resistance develops in multiple regions. Future endeavors will require broad-based quality data from surveillance programs that are not dependent solely on funding from the pharmaceutical industry.

REFERENCES

1. Zetola N, Francis JS, Nuermberger EL, Bishai WR. Community-acquired methicillin-resistant *Staphylococcus aureus*: an emerging threat. Lancet Infect Dis 2005; 5:275–86.
2. Deming WE. Out of the Crisis. Cambridge: Massachusetts Institute of Technology Center for Advanced Engineering Study, 1986.
3. Woomer N, Long CO, Anderson C, Greenberg EA. Benchmarking in home health care: a collaborative approach. Caring 1999; 18:22–8.
4. Narong MN, Thongpiyapoom S, Thaikul N, Jamulitrat S, Kasatpibal N. Surgical site infections in patients undergoing major operations in a university hospital: using standardized infection ratio as a benchmarking tool. Am J Infect Control 2003; 31:274–9.
5. Bissell MG. The effect of benchmarking clinical practice with the clinical laboratory. Clin Lab Med 1999; 19:867–76.
6. Fridkin SK, Lawton R, Edwards JR, Tenover FC, McGowan JE, Gaynes RP. The Intensive Care Antimicrobial Resistance Epidemiology Project. The National Nosocomial Infections Surveillance (NNIS) Systems Hospitals. Monitoring antimicrobial use and resistance: comparison with a national benchmark on reducing vancomycin use and vancomycin-resistant enterococci. Emerg Infect Dis 2002; 8:702–7.
7. The Joint Commission. ORYX for Health Care Organizations. Using the Framework Criteria. www.jointcommission.org/AccreditationPrograms/Hospitals/ORYX/using_framework_criteria.htm. (last accessed on May 29, 2007).
8. Bhavnani SM. Benchmarking in health-system pharmacy: current research and practical applications. Am J Health-Syst Pharm 2000; 57(Suppl. 2): S13–20.
9. Rifenburg RP, Paladino JA, Hanson SC, Tuttle JA, Schentag JJ. Benchmark analysis of strategies hospitals use to control antimicrobial expenditures. Am J Health-Syst Pharm 1996; 53:2054–62.
10. Schentag JJ, Paladino JA, Birmingham MC, Zimmer G, Carr JR, Hanson SC. Use of benchmarking techniques to justify the evolution of antibiotic management programs in healthcare systems. J Pharm Technol 1995; 11:203–10.
11. Bhavnani SM, Ambrose PG. Optimizing antimicrobial use and combating bacterial resistance: benchmarking and beyond. In: Owens RC Jr, Ambrose PG, eds. Antibiotic Optimization: Concepts and Strategies in Clinical Practice. Marcel Dekker: New York 2005.

12. Benchmarking program. CPL Associates, LLC. Amherst, New York. www.cplassociates.com (last accessed on May 31, 2007).
13. Bhavnani SM, Callen WA, Forrest A, Gilliland KK, Collins DA, Paladino JA, Schentag JJ. Effect of flouroquinolone expenditures on susceptibility of *Pseudomonas aeruginosa* to ciprofloxacin in U.S. hospitals. Am J Health-Syst Pharm 2003; 60:1962–70.
14. World Health Organization. WHO global strategy for containment of antimicrobial resistance. Geneva, 2001. whqlibdoc.who.int/hq/2001/WHO_CDS_CSR_DRS_001.2a. pdf (last accessed May 31, 2007)
15. Felmingham D, White AR, Jacobs MR, et al. The Alexander Project: the benefits from a decade of surveillance. J Antimicrob Chemother 2005; 56(Suppl S2):ii3–21.
16. Turner PJ, Greenhalgh JM, Edwards JR, McKellar J. The MYSTIC (Meropenem Yearly Susceptiblity Test Information Collection) Programmer. Int J Antimicrob Agents 1999; 13:117–25.
17. Global aspects of antimicrobial resistance among key bacterial pathogens: results from the 1997–1999 SENTRY Antimicrobial Surveillance Program Clin Infect Dis 2001; 32(Suppl. 2):S81–167.
18. Karlowsky JA, Jones ME, Mayfield DC, Thornsberry C, Sahm DF. Ceftriaxone activity against Gram-positive and Gram-negative pathogens isolated in US clinical microbiology laboratories from 1996 to 2000: results from The Surveillance Network® (TSN®) Database-USA. Int J Antimicrob Agents 2002; 19:413–26.
19. Harding I, Felmingham D. PROTEKT years 1–3 (1999–2002): study design and methodology. J Chemother 2004; 16(Suppl. 6):9–18.
20. Jones ME, Karlowsky JA, Blosser-Middleton R, Critchley IA, Thornsberry C, Sahm DF. Apparent plateau in β-lactamase production among clinical isolates of *Haemophilus influenza* and *Moraxella catarrhalis* in the United States: results from the LIBRA Surveillance initiative. Int J Antimicrob Agents 2002; 19:119–23.
21. Whitney CG, Farley MM, Hadler J, et al. Increasing prevalence of multidrug-resistant *Streptococcus pneumoniae* in the United States. N Engl J Med 2000; 343:1917–24.
22. Fridkin SK, Edwards JR, Tenover FC, et al. Antimicrobial resistance prevalence rates in hospital antibiograms reflect prevalence rates among pathogens associated with hospital-acquired infections. Clin Infect Dis 2001; 33:324–30.
23. Koeth LM, Miller LA. Evolving concepts of pharmaceutical company-sponsored surveillance studies. Clin Infect Dis 2005; 41:S279–82.
24. Cornaglia G, Hryniewicz W, Jarlier V, et al. European recommendations for antimicrobial resistance surveillance. Clin Microbiol Infect 2004; 10:349–83.
25. Stelling J, Travers KU, Jones RN, et al. Advantages of a coordinated system of independent global surveillance databases: a report from the Global Advisory on Antibiotic Resistance Data (GAARD) [abstract]. International Conference on Emerging Infectious Diseases Program, (Atlanta, GA, March 24–27, 2002. www.cdc.gov.iceid/program.htm (last accessed May 31, 2007)
26. Stelling JM, Travers K, Jones RN, Turner PJ, O'Brien TF, Levy SB. Integrating *Escherichia coli* antimicrobial susceptibility data from multiple surveillance programs. Emerg Infect Dis 2005; 11:873–5.
27. Finch R. Bacterial resistance—the clinical challenge. Clin Microbiol Infect 2002; 8(Suppl. 3):21–32.
28. London Department of Health. The path of least resistance. Standing Medical Advisory Committee, Sub-group on Antimicrobial Resistance. Sep 1, 1998. www.dh.gov.uk.en/publicationsandstatistics/Publications/PublicationsPolicyandGuidance/DH_4009357 (last accessed May 31, 2007).
29. The European Antimicrobial Resistance Surveillance System (EARSS). Annual Report 2005. www.rivm.nl/earss/Images/EARSS%202005_tcm61-34899.pdf. (last accessed May 31, 2007).
30. Bronzwaer S, Cars O, Buchholz U, et al. and participants in the European Antimicrobial Resistance Surveillance System. A European study on the relationship between antimicrobial use and antimicrobial resistance. Emerg Infect Dis 2002; 8:278–82.
31. Burley CJ, Tillotson GS. Antimicrobial resistance: can we see the wood for the trees? Lancet Infect Dis 2003; 3:125–6.

32. Powers JH. Anti-infective research and development-problems, challenges, and solutions. Lancet Infect Dis 2007; 7:74–6.

33. Intensive Care Antimicrobial Resistance Evaluation (ICARE). www.sph.emory.edu/ICARE/index.php (last accessed June 1, 2007).

34. Ambrose PG. Antimicrobial susceptibility breakpoints: PK-PD and susceptibility breakpoints. Treat Respir Med. 2005; 4(Suppl. 1):5–11.

35. Fuchs PC, Barry AL, Thornsberry C, et al. Cefotaxime: in vitro activity and tentative interpretive standards for disk susceptibility testing. Antimicrob Agents Chemother 1980; 18:88–93.

36. Ambrose PG, Bhavnani SM, Jones RN, Craig WA, Dudley MN. Use of pharmacokinetics-pharmacodynamics and Monte Carlo simulation as decision support for the re-evaluation of NCCLS cephem susceptibility breakpoints for Enterobacteriaceae. 44th Interscience Conference on Antimicrobial Agents and Chemotherapy, Washington, D.C., October 30–November 2, 2004 (Abstract No. A-138).

37. Craig WA, Bhavnani SM, Ambrose PG, Dudley MN, Jones RN. Evaluation of clinical outcome among patients with ESBL-Producing Enterobacteriaceae treated with cephalosporin monotherapy. 45th Interscience Conference on Antimicrobial Agents and Chemotherapy, Washington D.C., December 16–19, 2005 (Abstract No. K-1291).

38. The European Committee on Antimicrobial Susceptibility Testing (EUCAST). www.escmid.org/sites/science/eucast/index.aspx (last accessed June 1, 2007).

39. Chen DK, McGeer A, de Azavedo JC, Low DE. Decreased susceptibility of *Streptococcus pneumoniae* to fluoroquinolones in Canada. N Engl J Med 1999; 341:233–9.

40. McGowan JE Jr. Antimicrobial resistance in hospital organisms and its relation to antibiotic use. Rev Infect Dis 1983; 5:1033–48.

41. Seppala H, Klaukka T, Lehtonen R, Nenonen E, Huovinen P. Outpatient use of erythromycin: link to increased erythromycin resistance in group A streptococci. Clin Infect Dis 1995; 21:1378–85.

42. Bhavnani SM, Hammel JP, Forrest A, Jones RN, Ambrose PG. Relationships between patient- and institution-specific variables and decreased antimicrobial susceptibility of Gram-negative pathogens. Clin Infect Dis 2003; 37:344–50.

43. Hammel JP, Bhavnani SM, Jones RN, Forrest A, Ambrose PG. Comparison of censored regression and standard regression analyses for modeling relationships between antimicrobial susceptibility and patient- and institution-specific variables. Antimicrob Agents Chemother 2006; 50:62–7.

44. Bhavnani SM, Hammel JP, Jones RN, Ambrose PG. Relationship between increased levofloxacin use and decreased susceptibility of *Streptococcus pneumoniae* in the United States. Diagn Microbiol Infect Dis 2005: 51:31–7.

45. Ballow CH, Schentag JJ. Trends in antibiotic utilization and bacterial resistance. Report of the National Nosocomial Resistance Surveillance Group. Diagn Microbiol Infect Dis 1992; 15(2 Suppl):37S–42S.

46. Lesch CA, Itokazu GS, Danziger LH, Weinstein RA. Multi-hospital analysis of antimicrobial usage and resistance trends. Diagn Microbiol Infect Dis 2001; 41:149–54.

47. Johnson CK, Polk R. Antimicrobial use in U.S. hospitals and methicillin-resistant *Staphylococcus aureus* (MRSA). 43rd Interscience Conference on Antimicrobial Agents and Chemotherapy, Chicago, IL September 14–17, 2003, (Abstract K-1399).

48. Bhavnani SM. Antimicrobial Surveillance Programs: Can these databases be helpful in identifying relationships predictive of resistance and be applied to patient care? 41st Meeting of the Infectious Diseases Society of America, San Diego, CA, October 9–12, 2003, (Abstract #1005).

49. Bhavnani SM, Hammel JP, Jones RN, Ambrose PG. Evaluating relationships between antimicrobial use and bacterial resistance: Comparison of the statistical power achieved for different regression methods. 44th Interscience Conference on Antimicrobial Agents and Chemotherapy, Washington, DC, October 30–November 2, 2004 (Abstract No. K-1550).

50. Clinical and Laboratory Standards Institute. M39-2A, Analysis and presentation of cumulative antimicrobial susceptibility test data. Wayne, PA: CLSI, 2005.

3

Antibiotic Resistance: Opportunity or Obstacle for the Pharmaceutical Industry?

Glenn S. Tillotson
Replidyne, Inc., Milford, Connecticut, U.S.A.,

INTRODUCTION

Antibiotics have been said to be the only drug class with built-in obsolescence. As with the latest Microsoft® software or Dell® personal computer, there will always be a need for something new very soon. In the case of antibiotic resistance, this is due to bacterial "ingenuity"/make-up or human predisposition to assisting the Darwinian selection process by either under-dosing and overexposure or by mere negligence and poor compliance. So, against this backdrop of opportunity, why hasn't the pharmaceutical industry consistently beaten the bacterial foe and the burgeoning resistance? In the interests of provocation, I address this question from two viewpoints, and I ask the reader to reach their own conclusions.

OPPORTUNITY

Antibiotic resistance, as opposed to antiviral or antifungal resistance, is widespread among both hospital and community pathogens. There is a thriving "cottage-industry" of susceptibility surveillance programs, some supported by government or quasi-official bodies and others funded by the pharmaceutical industry. These programs encompass respiratory, urinary, bloodstream, skin and soft tissue, and occasional other sources of pathogens. The dominant source is the respiratory tract, which accounts for 47% of antibiotic prescriptions, and thus the largest opportunity for a new antibiotic to make an impact (Fig. 1). Table 1 shows a selection of ongoing surveillance programs.

Recent data from large programs has illustrated the growing issue of anti-biotic resistance, especially among bacteria from respiratory infections. In the United States (the largest consumer of antibiotics) multi-drug resistant *Streptococcus pneumoniae* (MDRSP) now account for one in four strains from community respiratory tract infections. Thus, as an empiric prescribing physician, the odds of "picking a resistant case" are fairly high. Indeed in some areas these odds shorten from one in four to almost one in two (Fig. 2). Moreover, several metropolitan areas have rates of MDRSP, which exceed the threshold advocated by the Infectious Diseases Society of America (IDSA), > 20%, beyond which empiric reliability is poor and it is recommended that an alternative antibiotic class be used empirically (1). This same criterion has yet to be applied in other infections.

S. pneumoniae is still the most frequent bacterial pathogen in community-acquired respiratory tract infections and, as stated above, has become resistant to many antibiotics, with the newer fluoroquinolones being the possible exception. The mortality associated with this resistant organism is significant. Aspa et al.

These are the sole thoughts and comments of the author and do not represent any company or other group.

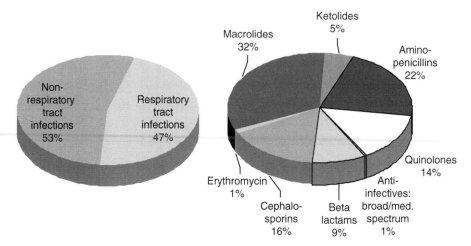

FIGURE 1 Antibiotic prescriptions, United States 2005. Respiratory tract infections account for nearly half (47%) of the uses for the selected antibiotic classes [IMS National Disease and Therapeutic Index™ (IMS Health, Norwalk, Connecticut, U.S.A.), 12 months ending September, 2005].

showed an increase of some 6% in patients with community-acquired infection (CAP) due to penicillin resistant strains (2). Additionally, Klepser et al. showed that pneumonia due to MDRSP added a growing financial burden of >$1500 per case to their treatment (3). So, in the light of this impact of resistance, one would expect the pharmaceutical industry to invest many more resources into the burgeoning resistance issue in community Respiratory Tract Infections (RTIs). However, those on major formulary committees, such as managed care or pharmacy benefit programs, do not "see these changes," so are still mandated to ensure that drug-acquisition costs do not rise, and so they "see" no need for these new agents to fight a problem that does not directly impact their consumer.

In the hospital setting, nosocomial infections account for a huge and growing burden of morbidity, mortality, and expenditure. The shifting patterns of pathogens and their resistance patterns are encouraging the use of either more broad spectrum agents or increasingly complex combinations that may carry a toxicity burden (to either the patient or the formulary) (Fig. 3) (4).

The argument for fighting resistance in the nosocomial pathogens tends to be much more high profile, despite the lower incidence, and as such has been seen as a bigger opportunity by the pharmaceutical industry. In late 2005, there were several compounds in development targeting the Gram-positive resistant problem species: oritavancin, dalbavancin, telavancin, ramoplanin, ceftibprole, and doripenem for Gram-negative infections, while in the community arena there are faropenem, cethromycin, and some early phase ketolides from Enanta and Johnson & Johnson (Table 2). So clearly there are still many opportunities available for a brave company to move into a sparse field.

OBSTACLES
Clinical Reluctance
Some 60 years ago Sir Alexander Fleming pointed out the imminent folly of antibiotic usage and the pathway we were about to embark upon:

TABLE 1 Current Multinational Antimicrobial Resistance Surveillance Program

Study	Acronym	Funding sponsor	Start date	Notes	References
Industry-supported programs					
The Alexander project		GlaxoSmithKline	1992	Initiated by SmithKline Beecham	1
The meropenem yearly susceptibility test information collection	MYSTIC	AstraZeneca	1997		2
The SENTRY antimicrobial resistance program	SENTRY	Bristol-Myers Squibb	1997	Active in 5 continents	3
The Surveillance Network	TSN	Focus Technologies	1998		4
Prospective Resistant Organism Tracking and Epidemiology for the Ketolide Telithromycin	PROTEKT	Aventis	1990	PROTEKT US program started in 2000	http://www.proteckt.org
LIBRA surveillance program	LIBRA	Bayer	2000	Compilation of studies from 1998–present	http://www.librainitiative.com
Academic/government-driven programs					
European antimicrobial resistance surveillance system	EARSS	European Commission	1998		http://www.rivm.nl/earss/
European surveillance of antibiotic resistance	ESAR	European Commission	1998		http://www.rivm.nl/earss/
Active bacterial core surveillance program	ABCs	U.S. Centers for Disease Control and Prevention	1995		5 and http://www.cdc.gov/drugresistance
Antimicrobial resistance information bank	ARInfoBank	World Health Organization	1999		http://oms2.b3e.jussieu.fr/arinfobank/
Intensive care antimicrobial resistance evaluation	ICARE	4 companies under auspices of CDC	1998	A periodic surveillance of ICUs across United States	6 and http://www.cdc.gov/drugresistance

Source: Adapted from Ref. 7.

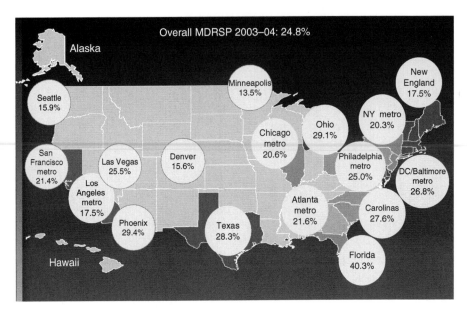

FIGURE 2 Antibiotic susceptibility among multi-drug resistant *Streptococcus pneumoniae* (MDRSP) in the United States, 2003–2004. Resistance to two or more of the following: penicillins, cephalosporins, macrolides, trimethoprim and sulfamethoxazole, or tetracycline or fluoroquinolones. *Source*: From Ref. 22.

it is not difficult to make microbes resistant to penicillin in the laboratory by exposing them to concentrations not sufficient to kill them, and the same thing has occasionally happened in the body … Moral: if you use penicillin use enough (5).

This approach was a reiteration of Ehrlich's prescient lecture in 1913 (6), and yet we still strive to ignore these prophecies. Guillemot et al. proved that low doses given often for long periods will clearly select for the "weakest link in a population" and lead to resistance emergence (7). In human medicine, 80% to 90% of antimicrobials are prescribed in the community setting; some sources estimate that almost half are dubious in their appropriateness. Indeed, the World Health Organization (WHO) estimated that respiratory tract infections, which account for many of these prescriptions, account for over 94 disability-adjusted life years lost globally, and were the fourth major cause of mortality. Thus many authorities espouse that the best way to stop or slow antimicrobial resistance is by using them less often. Most experts agree that it is the widespread, poorly controlled use of these vital agents that has led us to where we are presently in the battle against microbes, and unfortunately the microbes are winning.

From our brief seminars at Medical School we are constantly told, "when you use an antibiotic, use just enough not to make the patient sick, give it for 10 to 14 days just to be sure, and always save the new more potent drugs until the last resort."

This incantation has been ingrained into millions of prescribers for over 50 years and we are only recently realizing that this mantra is probably incorrect. However, kicking this habit will take extensive education and other incentives. Moreover, patients need to be aware that new antibiotics do not require extended courses of therapy and that shorter courses of therapy are as effective as the old

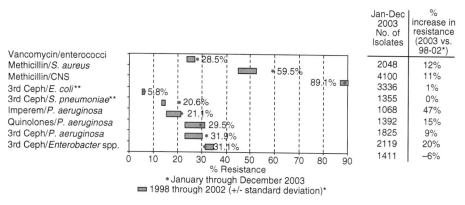

	Jan-Dec 2003 No. of Isolates	% increase in resistance (2003 vs. 98-02*)
Vancomycin/enterococci	2048	12%
Methicillin/S. aureus	4100	11%
Methicillin/CNS	3336	1%
3rd Ceph/E. coli**	1355	0%
3rd Ceph/S. pneumoniae**	1068	47%
Imperem/P. aeruginosa	1392	15%
Quinolones/P. aeruginosa	1825	9%
3rd Ceph/P. aeruginosa	2119	20%
3rd Ceph/Enterobacter spp.	1411	-6%

FIGURE 3 Changes in nosocomial pathogen incidence and antimicrobial susceptibility. Selected antimicrobial-resistant pathogens associated with noscomical infections in ICU patients, comparison of resistance rates from January through December 2003 with 1998 through 2002 using the NNIS System. *Notes*: *Percent (%) increase in resistance rate of current year (January–December 2003) compared with mean rate of resistance over previous 5 years (1998–2002): [(2003 rate–previous 5-year mean rate)/previous 5-year mean rate] X 100. **"Resistance" for *E. coli* or *K. pneumoniae* is the rate of nonsusceptibility of these organisms to either 3rd Ceph group or aztreonam. *Abbreviations*: CNS, coagulase-negative staphylococci; 3rd Ceph, resistance to 3rd generation cephalosporins (either ceftriaxone, cefotaxime, or ceftazidime); Quinolone, resistance to either ciprofloxacin or ofloxacin.

10 to 14 day standard durations of therapy. Thus, a major educational campaign to various parties is required to alter the old habits; such a change could be a major influence on antibiotic resistance.

Recent evidence has shown that, despite the best efforts of industry and U.S. Food and Drug Administration (FDA) approvals, many prescribers still follow the old adage of writing an antibiotic prescription for 10 to 14 days. A survey of prescriptions for three common RTIs shows that almost all were written for 2 to 3 days longer than approved for specific infections (Table 3). Thus, exposing the patients' normal flora to unnecessary drug levels with possible resistance selection a consequence, in addition to exacerbation of some adverse events. The industry's innovations are being wasted by prescribers who fail to follow the latest developments, despite significant educational efforts by the industry in various venues and vehicles, such as continuing medical education (CME) programs, etc.

Perhaps while waiting for this approach to be adopted we should follow Ehrlich's advice from almost a century ago to use either combinations of agents or use the highest (safe) dose quickly and briefly. This "frapper fort et frapper vite" concept has been used in the management of cancer and many viral diseases such as HIV, and yet we consider the lowly pneumococcus and other mere bacteria to simply shrivel up and die at the mere whiff of any antibiotic. Experience has shown us that these prolific organisms can very rapidly adapt to new agents and lead to their obsolescence.

What will it take to move medical attitudes and practices to new antibiotics, away from the "saving the best till last" to the new approach of "dead bugs don't mutate" and hence slow this inexorable rise in resistance, is a question I am not sure we have an answer to.

TABLE 2   Antibiotics Currently in Development or in Development October 2007

Drug name or designation (company)	Class	Status
ABT492 (Wakunaga)	Quinolone	Phase I[a,c]
WCK771A(Wockhardt)	Quinolone	Phase I[a]
PNU288034 [Pfizer (Pharmacia)]	Oxazolidinone	Phase I[a,c]
Garenoxacin [BMS284756 (Schering-Plough and Toyoma)]	Quinolone	Phase III[b,c]
Doripenem (Shionogi and Peninsula Pharma/J&J)	Carbapenem	Phase III[b,d]
CS-023 (Sankyo and Roche)	Carbapenem	Phase II[a,b]
Faropenem (Replidyne)	Penem	Phase III
Tigecycline [GAR936 (Wyeth)]	Tetracycline	Approved[d]
MC02479 [RWJ54428, RWJ442831[a] (Trine and J&J)]	Cephalosporin	Phase I[b]
MC04546 [RWJ333441, RWJ333442[a] (Trine and J&J)]	Cephalosporin	Phase I[b]
VRC4887 [LBM415 (Vicuron/Pfizer and Novartis)]	Hydroxamate	Phase I[b]
Ramoplanin [Oscient and Vicuron/Pfizer]	Glycolipodepsipeptide	Phase II–III[b]
Oritavancin [LY333328 (Intermune and Lilly)]	Glycopeptide	Phase III[b]
Rifalazil (Activbiotics)	Benzoxazinorifamycin	Phase II[b,c]
Ceftbiprole/BAL5788 (Basilea/J&J)	Cephalosporin	Phase II[b,e]
MC04,124 (Mpex Pharm, Trine and Daiichi)	Peptide	Preclinical[c]
MP60I,205 (Mpex Pharm and Daiichi)	Peptide	Preclinical[c]
Dalbavancin (Vicuron/Pfizer)	Glycopeptide	Phase III[b,d]
TD6424 Telavancin (Theravance/Astellis)	Lipoglycopeptide	Phase II[b,d]
Cethromycin (Advanced Life Sciences)	Macro/ketolide	Phase III

[a]Prodrug of active component.
[b]Discontinued development.
[c]Information acquired from Investigational Drugs database, company website, press release, or analyst meeting.
[d]Approved or "approvable."
[e]Submitted.
Abbreviations: J&J, Johnson & Johnson; Topo, topoisomerase.

Regulatory Impediments

In addition to commercial and technical issues, it is clear that ever-changing regulatory hurdles pose significant challenges to new antibiotic development. Because antibiotics can be used to treat more than one infection caused by a specific bacterial species, it is mandated that each infective indication due to *S. pneumoniae* or any other common pathogen to be treated must be studied in at least two clinical trials with a minimum number of isolates of intended species in each indication (often 10–25 strains per indication, with resistant phenotypes being considered a separate group). Yet despite the apparent prevalence of resistance, it can prove difficult to enroll enough valid patients in each indication to satisfy the needs of the regulatory authorities. This contradictory situation is due to the strict inclusion/exclusion criteria, which can markedly reduce the number of evaluable patients. Additionally, in many other diseases that are preferred by the pharmaceutical industry, e.g., diabetes, hypertension, or cancer, patients have a clinical diagnosis prior to entry to the study, whereas in antibiotic trials usually only half of enrolled patients actually have a proven bacterial species, thus leading to large studies with low "return on investment" in terms of bacterial yield for regulatory review. If we had rapid diagnostic tests, which could eliminate nonbacterial infections, this would improve the yield, but sadly this has not proven a fruitful area of research for other reasons. From both the nosocomial and community infection perspectives, the infamous Lasagna's Law frequently applies: once you begin to search for a disease or infection, it typically disappears, leading to much longer enrolment times or, in some cases, early termination of a study. Thus, in

TABLE 3 Comparison of Actual Antibiotic Use Compared with FDA Approved Durations for Specific Indications

Indication	Gemi approved	Gemi actual	Moxi approved	Moxi actual	Gati approved	Gati actual	Levo approved	Levo actual	Azithro approved	Azithro actual	Clari approved	Clari actual
ABS	NA	6.6	10	10	7 to 10	9.5	5 to 10	10.1	5	5	10	9.5
Other URTI	NA	6.3	NA	8.3	NA	7.6	NA	8.1	NA	5	NA	8.2
AECB	5	5.8	5	7.4	5	7	7	8.1	NA	5	7	8.4
CAP	7	6.8	10	9.1	7	7.3	5 or 10	9.3	5	5	10	9
All others	NA	7.7	NA	8.5	NA	4.8	NA	8.4	5		NA	
All indications		6.3		8.5		7		8.6			NA	

Abbreviations: ABS, acute bacterial sinusitis; AECB, acute exacerbations of chronic bronchitis; Azithro, azithromycin; CAP, community acquired pneumonia; Clari, clarithromycin; FDA, U.S. Food and Drug Administration; Gati, gatifloxacin; Gemi, gemifloxacin; Levo, levofloxacin; Moxi, moxifloxacin; NA, not available; URTI, upper respiratory tract infections.

2005, of the >500 drugs in clinical development with investigational new drugs, only 6 were antibiotics, this is a continuation of the trend described by Spellberg, Powers, and others (Fig. 4) (8).

To add to these fundamental dilemmas of antibiotic clinical research, the different regulatory bodies in the United States, Canada, Europe, and Japan lead to another layer of complexity in terms of what each wants in levels of detail of efficacy and safety investigations. Certainly, International Harmonization has helped reduce these issues, but nevertheless there are constantly altering "goal-posts" in Europe that do not help sponsors choose the best route for their particular new compound. Vast differences in antibiotic resistance and the perceptions towards how best to handle them underpin the different nations' attitudes to new antibiotics and further complicate the drug review process in Europe.

Finally, a recent complicating factor has been the opinion of the FDA towards certain respiratory infections in terms of their causality and bacterial infection. Three "infective" indications, acute otitis media, acute bacterial sinusitis, and acute exacerbations of chronic bronchitis, have all been questioned with regard to the value of antibiotics. Indeed we know that many such infections are probably viral in origin and thus it is proposed that exposing these patients to antibiotics merely drives the resistance crisis. The issue of wrong dose for the wrong duration does not feature in these arguments. Instead we are being recommended to simply not use antibiotics on the assumption that most patients will get better anyway on their own, the so-called "polyanna effect." However, for those that do not recover spontaneously, more protracted infection, time off work or usual activities, hospitalization or potentially death may be outcomes that could be prevented with an antibiotic. Currently (as of October 2007) the FDA is requiring that companies wishing to obtain the above indications conduct placebo-controlled studies of their investigational agents before considering such a submission. This stance is, in the case of acute exacerbations of chronic bronchitis (AECB), not based on much clinical data, and thus may be depriving patients of potentially useful new agents, as companies may decide such huge investment is not worth the possible return revenue, despite there being over 15 million patients with AECB annually in the United States alone. There is evidence from Anthonisen, Allegra, Saint, and others that, in the right types of AECB patients, antibiotics clearly exert a benefit (9,10).

Hopefully, reason and clinical data will help prevent a stand-off, and new appropriate agents will be approved for these indications, as millions of U.S. patients suffer each year from both susceptible and resistant bacterial infections.

Economic Requirements of the Industry

This section is increasingly complex from an antibiotic aspect, and I hope to give some insight into the many considerations that have to be applied when developing and subsequently marketing a new antibiotic.

Most MBA students would be surprised by neither the simple equation applied to drug development nor the common conclusions regarding antibiotics. A litany of TLAs (three letter abbreviations) are collated, correlated, confounded, and eventually concluded to reveal the death knell of most antibiotics, a negative Net Present Value (NPV)!!

How this magical number is calculated is not within the scope of this review, but rest assured it involves a mix of science, economics, and arcane witchcraft.

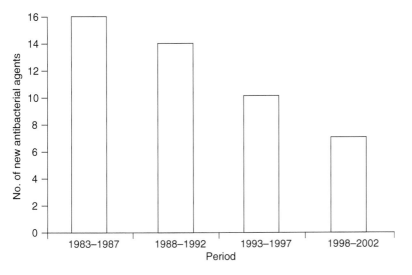

New antibacterial agents approved since 1998.

Drug	Year approved	Novel mechanism
Rifapentine	1998	No
Quinupristin/dalfopristin	1999	No
Moxifloxacin	1999	No
Gatifloxacin	1999	No
Linezolid	2000	Yes
Cefditoren pivoxil	2001	No
Ertapenem	2001	No
Gemifloxacin	2003	No
Daptomycin	2003	Yes
Tigecycline	2005	No

FIGURE 4   New antibacterial agents approved in the United States, 1983–2005.

One freakish fact, which could shift many such calculations, is the eventual price of the new antibiotic. It is staggering that patients are more prepared to pay $40 for a bottle of wine or carton of cigarettes than the co-pay for a new drug that has been shown to more rapidly get them back to normal or work. The simple fact is that many of today's new antibiotics are being priced "competitively" so as to have fair fight with older, possibly generic agents, which are probably less active in a variety of outcome measures. The price of good health seems not to have kept up with inflation and thus affects the possible asking price in the NPV estimations.

Basic Costs

Research and development (R and D) of a new drug is fraught with risks and is time-consuming. Even with an aggressive R and D program it can cost up to $800 million and at least 5 years to bring an antibiotic from lab to bedside. For single or few indications these costs can be a little lower but the timeline is still a major hurdle. This has an impact on the patent protection period of the eventual compound of 20 years, thus the longer it takes to get approval the less time there is to obtain a return on the massive investment.

Taking a New Drug to Market in the United States

As our understanding of antibiotic pharmacokinetics has improved both the dosing and duration of therapy, it has brought a dilemma: basically, we are prescribing fewer tablets per patient today than 5 years ago.

Thus, from a new business development perspective, it is less attractive to invest research dollars into a five tablet per patient/scrip drug compared with a one tablet a day for 365 days a year for the rest of a patient's life. These mathematics are fairly simple. So from this equation it is clear that there is little encouragement for the industry to develop a new antibiotic.

Once a drug is approved, another set of issues appears. These relate to pricing and availability on various formularies, which are mandated to save as much money on drugs as they can, regardless of possible savings for other areas of the healthcare system.

A silo mentality exists in many systems that maybe counterproductive to not only saving a system money but also to preventing patients from benefiting from a new therapy that may get them back to work sooner or have a longer period before their next inevitable infective attack. Perhaps as the real payors play a bigger role in determining how much is paid for which services, the real benefits, such as less absenteeism and presenteeism or improved productivity, will drive choices of certain drugs that do have data to support such novel outcomes.

Finally in this complex equation of economic considerations is the impact of marketing and prescriber exposure to drive prescriptions. One of the reasons "big pharma" walked away from developing and marketing a new antibiotic is the low return in dollar terms per field representative promoting that drug. For a company with a large field force (>1000 individuals) a drug has to be capable of generating sales of >$1 billion annually. Any drug that cannot generate such sales, based on 5 tablets per patient, is much less financially attractive than one that leads to 365 tabs/year/20 years. Thus, there is a possible opportunity for "small pharma" to get into a niche its larger cousin is not interested in. Or is it?

It all comes down to "share of voice," i.e., the number of times a company informs the prescriber about a drug each week or month compared with the competition. Repetition leads to more frequent prescribing; whether that is right or wrong is not for me to say but it does explain how some drugs are being used far more than others despite a possibly inferior profile.

Formulary Status
One major hurdle for small pharma is the ability to get your new drug onto various formularies, such as managed care or pharmacy benefit organizations, state Medicaid bodies, Veterans Administration groups, or other similar tiered systems. Often small pharma has only one or two drugs in their portfolio, thus they are less able to make deals or discounts or be able to provide rebates of one sort or another. Equally, if they are added to the formulary on Tier 3, the co-pays are so high patients often ask if there is a less expensive but effective alternative (or in some cases the pharmacist suggests such a drug). So the possible opportunities for small pharma to introduce a new antibiotic are not as easy or attractive as first appears.

Meanwhile, European and Canadian reimbursement procedures are another hurdle altogether—both are complex and time-consuming, in addition to the lengthy regulatory approval processes.

Aversion to Change by Physicians and Patients, or the Fight Against Human Nature
The final, and huge, obstacle is the lack of inertia among prescribers to want to change because they do not see resistance in their practice. Despite the data from Centers for Disease Control and Prevention (CDC), WHO, and many other experts, most primary care physicians claim not to see patients return for another antibiotic because of resistance. This may be because they do not look for it in the first place, as we know that >98% of RTI prescriptions are written empirically (so they would not know if the patient had a resistant pathogen initially or not). Indeed, if the patient does return a few days later a sputum is unlikely to be taken. Patients calling back for another antibiotic are rarely perceived to have failed because of resistance.

Add to this the medical school training of stepwise antibiotic escalation then new drugs are much less likely to be adopted early, thus resistance will continue to be encouraged by this Darwinian process of selecting out the resistant mutants in a given population. Drlica and colleagues espoused the "mutant prevention concentration" approach almost a decade ago (11), but still we dose to treat the most susceptible bug in a population, not the most resistant one. It is not surprising to understand where we are in terms of resistance today.

So, I began discussing susceptibility programs and our clear awareness of growing resistance. Human nature, being what it is, has failed to see a glaring amber signal regarding fluoroquinolone resistance in the United States regarding *S. pneumoniae*. In the early 1990s we witnessed a slow but eventually rampant resistance to penicillins, macrolides, tetracyclines, and co-trimoxazole. From 1990 to 1994 intermediate resistance slowly emerged, followed by high-level resistance, leading to levels of nonsusceptibility of 30% to 40% across the United States for the major drugs commonly used in community practice. We have seen a similar process emerge with fluoroquinolones over the period 1999–2003, but we condone the use of less potent class members because they save money (in acquisition terms only) (Fig. 5) (12–15). As this is the only class with predictable activity against

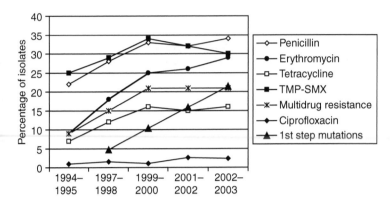

FIGURE 5 Pneumococcal Resistance to Antimicrobials Surveillance Program, 1988–2004. *Abbreviation*: TMP-SMX, trimethoprim and sulfamethoxazole.

pneumococci, *Haemophilus influenzae*, atypical species, and relevant Gram-negative species, then the class needs treating with some respect before it goes the same way as the other classes. However, industry, both big and small, needs to be reassured that this approach is being embraced before it invests another $800 million.

"Big Pharma Has Walked Away and Is Slow to Return"
Big pharmaceutical companies have undergone some remarkable changes in the last decade with respect to antibiotic R and D. First, there are simply fewer companies due to acquisitions and mergers leading to the reduction of the pharmaceutical "space" over the last decade. Second, of these organizations, several, such as Bristol-Myers Squibb, Bayer, Glaxo-Smith-Kline (GSK), and Astra Zeneca, among others, have simply elected not to pursue antibiotic R and D. Dr. Robert Ruffulo the head of research at Wyeth, was reported in the *Wall Street Journal* (WSJ) on November 8th, 2005, as saying, "making a new antibiotic that doesn't return its investment isn't good for us or for making other drugs. Other diseases need us too."

Dr. Steve Projan, former head of Wyeth's anti-infective research, calculated that the financial value of a new injectable antibiotic, best estimated at $100 million annually at peak, is minimal compared with a drug for a chronic condition such as osteoporosis, which can earn >$1.5 billion annually.

Of the major companies who have been in the field, Johnson & Johnson is still investing in antibiotic development, while Novartis and GSK are still putting money into vaccine studies. It appears that it will take some significant changes at the regulatory, federal, and medical practice levels to encourage Big Pharma to get its feet wet again.

Biotech/Small Pharma Has Picked at the Bones, but Commercialization Is Very Difficult—Share of Voice Matters (Size Does Matter!)
In contrast to the Big Pharma approach, a myriad of small companies have begun to move into the antibiotic field. However, it is very important to note that many of these drugs were generally well developed by Big Pharma prior to being shelved. It is this opportunistic approach that has tempted venture capital companies to invest in these "second phase" development programs, which have less of a risk compared

with starting from white powder to Phase 3 New Drug Application (NDA) programs costing >$800 million. Figure 6 shows the recent drug development undertaken by small biotech or pharmaceutical companies in the antibiotic field. The success stories include Cubist, who have introduced daptomycin, gemifloxacin (Oscient), and, most recently, oral vancomycin (Viropharma). Other successes include Basilea and the out-licensing of ceftibiprole to Johnson & Johnson, Peninsula with doripenem, again to Johnson & Johnson, and Vicuron, with its two agents dalbavancin and anidulafungin being acquired by Pfizer.

However, none of these small pharma companies have the sales and marketing power to ensure a major commercial success unless they enlist the promotional power of a large community-based sales force.

In the current antibiotic marketplace, several drugs dominate, mainly due to large sales forces with several "faces" to ensure constant exposure of the prescriber

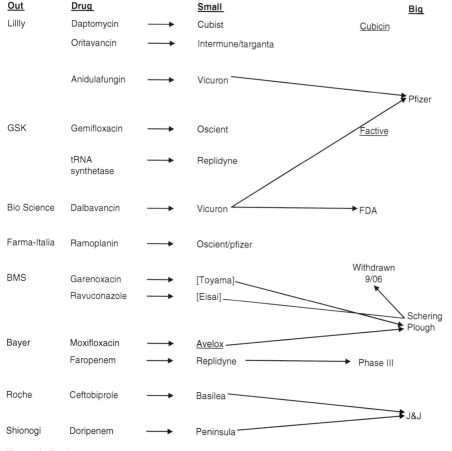

Key: underlined = approved
    FDA= New Drug Application submitted in 2005.

FIGURE 6 Compound movement among pharmaceutical companies. *Abbreviations*: BMS, Bristol-Myers Squibb; FDA, U.S. Food and Drug Administration; GSK, GlaxoSmithKline; J&J, Johnson & Johnson.

to promotional messages. It is clear that repetition of a scientific message leads to more prescriptions. Small pharma companies with sales forces of < 300 struggle to provide adequate repetition to those physicians who are regular writers of antibiotics. "Share of voice" is essential to the commercial success of an antibiotic in the larger community setting, but less so in the hospital environment, which tends to be less promotionally sensitive but more price/contract affected.

Small pharma will continue to attract venture capital hopes of a billion-dollar block-buster, but increasingly big pharma will invest in more predictable chronic condition drugs that need to be taken every day for the rest of a patient's life. Perhaps venture capital should be renamed "vulture capital" as they circle the bones of carcasses shelved/rejected by big pharma?

BIOSHIELD AND OTHER GOVERNMENT INITIATIVES

Following 9/11 and the subsequent anthrax situation, U.S. government officials began to appreciate the possibility of bacterial attacks against the nation. Thus, in February of 2003, in his State of the Union Address (16), President Bush announced Project BioShield—a comprehensive effort to develop and make available modern, effective drugs and vaccines to protect against attack by biological and chemical weapons or other dangerous pathogens. Project BioShield was intended to pay for "next-generation" medical countermeasures, and to allow the government to buy improved vaccines or drugs for smallpox, anthrax, and botulinum toxin. This would be enabled by the provision of $6 billion over ten years. Funds would also be available to buy countermeasures to protect against other dangerous pathogens, such as Ebola and plague, as soon as scientists verify the safety and effectiveness of these products.

This program was intended to provide spending authority for the delivery of next-generation medical countermeasures in addition to new relevant National Institutes of Health programs. However, this initial flurry of activity did not lead to the anticipated outcomes and was met with some criticism. Dr. John Bartlett raised the following issues in an address to a Senate hearing (17):

> I am testifying today on behalf of IDSA to communicate our strong support for the creation of new legislation that will remove financial disincentives to anti-infective R and D so that U.S. physicians will have the tools necessary to take care of very sick patients suffering from infectious diseases. New medicines and diagnostics are critically needed across all areas of infectious diseases medicine.

> As Senate leaders move forward to develop new legislation, commonly referred to as BioShield II, IDSA and its members urge you to extend the new legislation's scope beyond pathogens designated as relevant to "bioterror" and apply any new incentives broadly to cover drugs, vaccines, and diagnostics needed to treat all areas of infectious diseases, particularly antibiotics to treat antibiotic-resistant organisms. There is an inextricably linked, synergistic relationship between R and D efforts needed to protect against both natural occurring infections and bioterrorism agents. As such, we believe this approach makes perfect sense.

Background

In July 21, 2004, the same day that President Bush signed The Project BioShield Act (BioShield I), IDSA issued its landmark report entitled, "Bad Bugs, No Drugs: As

Antibiotic Discovery Stagnates, A Public Health Crisis Brews." Our report calls attention to a serious public health problem—at the same time that emerging infections and antibiotic resistance are increasing, drug companies are withdrawing from anti-infective R and D. IDSA is particularly concerned about antibiotic R and D, an area in which many pharmaceutical and biotechnology companies have shown the least commitment in recent years, either withdrawing totally or seriously downsizing their dedicated resources and staff. Infectious disease (ID) and HIV physicians on the frontline of patient care see patients every day who face lengthy hospitalizations, painful courses of treatment, and even death because of drug-resistant and other infections. We desperately need new weapons to protect our patients.

Members of Congress are beginning to see the connection between naturally occurring infections and bioterrorism and understand our vulnerability. In their reports on BioShield I in 2003, both the House Government Reform Committee and the Energy and Commerce Committee linked "natural conditions," including antimicrobial resistance and dangerous viruses, to national security concerns. The Energy and Commerce Report stated "advancing the discovery of new antimicrobial drugs to treat resistant organisms ... may well pay dividends for both national security and public health."

Policymakers have recognized the urgent need to spur R and D related to biodefense, which led to the enactment of BioShield I earlier this year. While the concern about bioterrorism is highly appropriate, it is important to keep things in perspective. Not one American has died from bioterrorism since President Bush first announced BioShield I in February of 2003, but drug-resistant bacteria and other infections have killed tens of thousands of Americans in hospitals and communities across the United States, and millions of people across the world, during that same short period of time.

Antibiotic-Resistant Bacterial Pathogens: Why IDSA Is Concerned

New treatments, preventions, and diagnostics are clearly needed in all areas of ID medicine. However, IDSA is particularly concerned that the pharmaceutical pipeline for new antibiotics is drying up. ID clinicians are alarmed by the prospect that effective antibiotics may not be available to treat seriously ill patients in the near future. There simply are not enough new drugs in the pharmaceutical pipeline to keep pace with drug-resistant bacterial infections, so-called "superbugs." Antibiotics, like other antimicrobial drugs, have saved millions of lives and eased patients' suffering. The withdrawal of companies from antibiotic R and D is a frightening twist to the antibiotic resistance problem and, we believe, one that has not received adequate attention from federal policymakers.

Until recently, pharmaceutical company R and D efforts have provided new drugs in time to treat bacteria that became resistant to older antibiotics. That is no longer the case.

Why Naturally Occurring Infections Should Be Included within BioShield I and BioShield II

IDSA strongly supports including all infectious diseases, and particularly antibiotics used to treat antibiotic-resistant organisms, within the scope of BioShield II—extending the scope of BioShield II to include infectious diseases that are naturally occurring will enhance the research needed to develop bioterrorism countermeasures and vice versa. We also urge that the "guaranteed market" provisions of BioShield I be expanded to apply to the development of all antibiotics, not just those intended to fight bioterror agents of present concern. Antibiotic-resistant organisms that currently threaten Americans in hospitals and communities can have future national and global security implications as well.

While BioShield I loosely could be applied to the development of antibiotics used to treat naturally occurring resistant organisms, it is not likely that such antibiotics will be listed as a priority of the Administration under BioShield I. BioShield I-related funding mostly or entirely will be utilized for procurement of bioterrorism countermeasures where the government is the sole market. There is a substantial civilian market for antibiotics, with the government only a marginal player. In those cases, it would not be the government that is the principal purchaser. However, the government could contribute to and administer a pool of funds from federal and charitable sources that will make up the guarantee pool. Then it can add the tax, intellectual property, and other incentives from BioShield II to make it all work. This approach would be consistent with our needs for bioterrorism preparedness and provide a much-needed benefit to our public health infrastructure.

Policymakers and the public should have no illusions that future pharmaceutical charity will be insufficient to address the existing and emerging infectious pathogens that threaten U.S. and global health. Instead, IDSA believes the onus is on the federal government to lure industry to anti-infective R and D as a means to protect U.S. public health and strengthen national security.

Potential Solutions

A list of potential legislative solutions that may help to spur R and D of drugs, vaccines, and diagnostics to treat, prevent, and detect bacteria, viruses, parasites, fungi, and other infectious organisms is shown in Table 4.

ISDA Conclusions

The time for talk has passed—it is now time to act. The federal government must take decisive action now to address the burgeoning problem of infectious diseases, particularly the lack of antibiotics to treat resistant organisms.

Strong words indeed from the IDSA. However, the limitations of BioShield have been highlighted elsewhere (18). Drug companies, however, have been markedly cool to the new law, unimpressed with the amount of money involved or assurances that their work will pay off.

The goal of BioShield I and II, explained a congressional staffer familiar with the intricacies of both, is to get the pharmaceutical industry to invest directly in the research needed to support biodefense. "The theory here is that you can shift the risk of the research to the industry," said the staffer, who asked not to be named. "If the research is not successful, then the loss is that of the companies, not the government (19)."

So far the reaction from the pharmaceutical industry has been chilly. Only a few small firms have accepted grants, said the staffer, and it is not clear if anyone will bid on a recently announced Department of Health and Human Services contract to develop and manufacture treatments for inhalation anthrax.

TABLE 4 IDSA Possible Initiatives to Develop New Antibiotics and Fight Resistance

Commission to prioritize antimicrobial discovery (Critical Priority)
    Establish and empower an independent Commission to Prioritize Antimicrobial Discovery to decide which infectious pathogens to target using the legislative research and development incentives listed below.

Supplemental intellectual property protections
    "Wild-card" patent extension (Critical Priority)
    Restoration of all patent time lost during FDA's review of and clinical trials undertaken related to priority antibiotics and anti-infectives
    Extended market and data exclusivity similar to what has been successfully implemented for pediatric and orphan drugs

Other potential statutory incentives
    Tax incentives for research and development of priority anti-infectives (Critical Priority)
    Measured liability protections (Critical Priority)
    Additional statutory flexibility at FDA regarding approval of antibiotics and other anti-infectives
    Antitrust exemptions for certain company communications
    A guaranteed market similar to that provided in BioShield I for priority antibiotics that target resistant bacterial and other anti-infectives

Establish similar statutory incentives to spur research and development for rapid diagnostic tests for targeted pathogens, which will help to reduce the cost of clinical trials

Potential statutory incentives of interest to small biopharmaceutical companies
    Waive FDA supplemental application user fees for priority antibiotics and other anti-infectives
    Tax credits specifically targeting this segment of the industry
    Small business grants

Abbreviations: IDSA, Infectious Diseases Society of America; FDA, U.S. Food and Drug Administration.

The Pharmaceutical Research and Manufacturers of America (PhRMA), which represents leading pharmaceutical research and biotechnology companies, issued a three-sentence statement after the Senate passed BioShield I, calling the bill "an important step forward." A PhRMA representative declined further comment; the statement said, however:

> We have urged, and still hope for, the enactment of additional measures, such as meaningful product liability protection for products specifically designed to be used (or used in new ways) to combat bioterrorism threats, as well as procurement provisions that more closely resemble the competitive private market in which the biotechnology and pharmaceutical industries ordinarily operate (18).

Limits on liability, as mentioned in the statement, have been broadly discussed and are being considered for BioShield II. The idea, said the staffer, would be to apply provisions of the Support Anti-terrorism by Fostering Effective Technologies Act of 2002—the SAFETY Act, now only applicable after an attack—to vaccines and other countermeasures. Such a change could shift much of the liability risk to the government, even during the clinical trial phase of a drug's development. The shift is necessary, explained the aide, because bioterror drugs cannot be fully tested on humans for ethical reasons, and side effects that would normally be detected may slip through. Companies have made it clear they will not take this risk.

"The liability issue is a big one," confirmed Dr. Fred Cohen, president of Crownstone in Bensalem, Pennsylvania. "I think having liability protection is a necessary step to get companies to seriously consider expending the resources necessary to develop these medicines," Cohen said.

New antibiotics are not being developed because, even though drug resistant diseases are emerging, there still are enough treatments in hand that any new antibiotic has a very small market. This is especially true since doctors only use new drugs as a last resort for fear of creating even more drug-resistant bacteria. There currently is just not enough financial incentive for the major firms to go after new antibiotics, Cohen said, but a patent extension could change that.

To summarize this extensive opinion on BioShield I and II, there is not much actual exchange of money to companies trying to get involved in a fairly small, and possibly redundant, market, with no liability protection if something is not detected during accelerated studies. So, although $6 billion sounds like significant government input, it has to be remembered that it is spread over 10 years and only to successful tenders/proposals. There have been very few of the latter so far, hence the IDSA's reaction. Good intentions will not slow the inexorable rise of resistance; only properly thought out and implemented ideas might be successful.

Patients Are Media-Scared and Ill-Informed

The increasing incidence or prevalence of antibiotic resistance is now an issue of major public concern. Newspaper headlines frequently carry feature stories of the impact on individuals as the doomsday scenario of widespread and untreatable drug-resistant infections in our hospitals. The extent and significance of antibiotic-resistant bacteria is clearly becoming increasingly apparent. Reports of antibiotic resistance and concerns highlighted by ID specialists over the last half century were generally unheeded until partway through the last decade (mid-1990s) when the importance of the issue finally achieved political recognition. In 1995, the American Society for Microbiology and three years later the U.K. Select Committee of the House of Lords published reports that were influential in developing national strategies. Soon after these initiatives the European Union and the WHO presented their approaches to this global problem. The latter currently has a six-part strategy for controlling antibiotic resistance (Table 5). Interestingly, the "encouragement of new drug and vaccine development" is the last part of this strategy, while other somewhat more nebulous efforts have a higher profile. Each of these five alternative approaches will involve significant changes in human habits and prescribing along with major investment to cover improved surveillance and monitoring of drug usage. Please note this was a powerful sentiment described by Dr. Gro-Harlen Brundtland of the WHO in the 2001 strategy (Fig. 7).

The fourth strand to the WHO strategy involves education of professionals and the general public; unfortunately, the latter often lacks the basic understanding of the principles required to fully appreciate the impact of inappropriate prescribing or poor compliance. On the other hand, the training the medical profession receives

TABLE 5 World Health Organization
Strategies for Reducing Resistance

Improve microbiological surveillance
Monitor drug utilization
Promote prudent prescribing
Educate professionals and general public
Promote infection control and hygiene
Encourage new drug and vaccine development

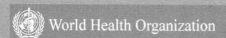

World Health Organization

- According to the report, **the most effective strategy against antimicrobial resistance is to get the job done right the first time – to unequivocally destroy microbes** – thereby defeating resistance before it starts. The challenge is to get the right treatment to the patient, each and every time.

- "Used wisely and widely, the drugs we have today can be used to prevent the infections of today and the antimicrobial-resistant catastrophes of tomorrow," said Dr. Brundtland.

- "However, if the world fails to mount a more serious effort to fight infectious diseases, antimicrobial resistance will increasingly threaten to send the world back to a pre-antibiotic age. **Our grandparents lived during an era without effective antibiotics. We don't want the same situation for our grandchildren.**"

Dr. Gro Harlem Brundtland, Director-General of WHO, 2001.

FIGURE 7 WHO's position toward antibiotic resistance. *Source*: From Ref. 21.

on antibiotics and their use is patently inadequate. However, to effect this change, medical curricula will need almost immediate "sea-changes" in terms of adopting "new" antibiotic concepts, such as those espoused by Ehrlich in 1913 to use antibiotics in an aggressive but appropriate manner by hitting the bacteria "hard and fast."

If changing medical attitudes are going to be difficult, imagine what shifting the general public ideas will take? For years, patients have been used to receiving an antibiotic for their cough, sniffle, etc., because they have an important meeting, trip, wedding, etc. We are all familiar with the poor compliance with antibiotics and the use of remnant drugs for a later time or even another family member. More educational campaigns are required.

Perhaps the recent excellent article in the WSJ on November 8th, 2005 (page A1), by Hensley and Wysocki, in which they describe the crisis unfolding in the United States and, by consequence elsewhere, with respect to influenza and resistant bacterial infections, may stimulate public awareness. The conundrum remains: how it is that the United States can produce highly rewarding chronic care drugs, such as Lipitor (which earns >$12 billion annually, an amount larger than the total vaccine market), or lifestyle compounds like Viagra, whereas several large pharmaceutical companies have stopped research into new antibiotics or vaccines because the market for a new antibiotic is small in comparison.

The public has little or no appreciation for the investment involved in developing a new antibiotic, nor the increasing constraints being applied to the possible consumption or market for antibiotics. Currently, we are seeing several campaigns to use less antibiotics. In addition, a better understanding of the pharmacodynamics of these drugs has allowed us to optimally dose them and shorten durations of therapy, thus reducing the total number of pills given to each patient, while achieving the same or better outcomes than the old three–times-a-day for 10 to 14 days regimen. This combination is obviously decreasing the potential value to a company in terms of its investment and potential profitability. The public is also unaware of the significant financial pressures being applied to pharmaceutical companies to not charge a realistic market price. This federal penny-pinching is not unique to the United States. In Canada, antibiotic prices have not increased for 7 years, while, in Europe, once a drug is approved, there follows a lengthy and convoluted process to establish reimbursement in each of the >25 nations in the centralized process. This mandatory price control may be conveyed as being in the overall interests of the country, but in reality all it has done is deter the industry from investing further in a vital area of medical care.

Unfortunately, the information in this WSJ article is unlikely to hit the masses, and thus it is probably only the financial analysts who will note the problem, not see any answers, and recommend investors to look elsewhere for their retirement plans.

However, for the public to fully grasp the significance of the impending crisis of dwindling antibiotic options, it will require a major public figure to be infected with a multi-drug resistant infection, like *S. pneumoniae*, but hopefully not die. With the subsequent media frenzy, explaining the consequences of the lack of new agents for our children and their offspring, then, and only then, will more people realize that we are looking down an empty research pipeline with the only light being the oncoming juggernaut of antibiotic resistance.

Can the Pharmaceutical Industry Play a Role in Developing New Antibiotics or Reducing Resistance?

Yes, is the simple answer, but, more importantly, where are the incentives? It is clear there is an unmet medical need; however, this need is often poorly appreciated by governments, regulators, healthcare providers and payors, physicians, and, finally, the public.

The WHO identified various strategic components in this battle, several of which the pharmaceutical industry can undertake. These include:

- Resistance surveillance
- Prescriber education toward prudent prescribing (whatever that is) via continuing medical processes
- Monitoring drug usage/utilization
- New drug development

Other approaches, in which the industry can be of less help, include better infection control and improved hygiene. However, this support would require approval by the various companies' stock holders. Perhaps the better question is, will they endorse such activities if they adversely affect the profitability and share price of the company?

The answers do not only lie with the pharmaceutical executives but their bosses, the shareholders!

Come back, Ehrlich! All is forgiven! (Fig. 8).

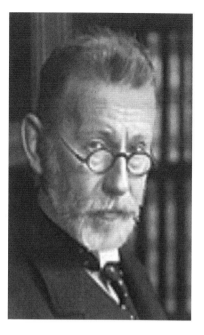

FIGURE 8   Paul Ehrlich—a prescient visionary?

REFERENCES

1. Warren JW, Abrutyn E, Hebel JR, Johnson JR, Schaeffer AJ, Stamm WE. Guidelines for antimicrobial treatment of uncomplicated acute bacterial cystitis and acute pyelonephritis in women. Infectious Diseases Society of America (IDSA). Clin Infect Dis 1999; 29(4):745–58.
2. Aspa J, Rajas O, Rodriguez de Castro F, et al. Pneumococcal Pneumonia in Spain Study Group. Drug-resistant pneumococcal pneumonia: clinical relevance and related factors. Clin Infect Dis 2004; 38(6):787–98.
3. Klepser ME, Klepser DG, Ernst EJ, et al. Health care resource utilization associated with treatment of penicillin-susceptible and—nonsusceptible isolates of *Streptococcus pneumoniae*. Pharmacotherapy 2003; 23(3):349–59.
4. National Nosocomial Infections Surveillance System. National Nosocomial Infections Surveillance (NNIS) System Report, data summary from January 1992 through June 2004, issued October 2004. Am J Infect Control 2004; 32(8):470–85.
5. Fleming A. Penicillin. Nobel Lecture, December 11, 1945. http://nobelprize.org/medicine/laureates/1945/fleming-lecture.pdf
6. Ehrlich P. Address to the International Society of Medicine. Lancet 1913; 445–52.
7. Guillemot D, Carbon C, Balkau B, et al. Low dosage and long treatment duration of beta-lactam: risk factors for carriage of penicillin-resistant *Streptococcus pneumoniae*. JAMA 1998; 279(5):365–70.
8. Spellberg B, Powers JH, Brass EP, Miller LG, Edwards JE Jr. Trends in antimicrobial drug development: implications for the future. Clin Infect Dis 2004; 38(9):1279–86.
9. Wilson R, Tillotson G, Ball P. Clinical studies in chronic bronchitis: a need for better definition and classification of severity. J Antimicrob Chemother 1996; 37(2):205–8.
10. Niederman MS. Who should receive antibiotics for exacerbations of chronic bronchitis? A plea for more outcome-based studies. Clin Infect Dis 2004; 39(7):987–9.
11. Drlica K. Refining the fluoroquinolones. ASM News 1999; 65:410–15.
12. Doern GV, Brueggemann A, Holley HP Jr, Rauch AM. Antimicrobial resistance of *Streptococcus pneumoniae* recovered from outpatients in the United States during the

winter months of 1994 to 1995: results of a 30-center national surveillance study. Antimicrob Agents Chemother 1996; 40:1208–13.

13. Doern GV, Brueggemann AB, Huynh H, Wingert E. Antimicrobial resistance with *Streptococcus pneumoniae* in the United States, 1997–98. Emerg Infect Dis 1999; 5(6):757–65.

14. Doern GV, Heilmann KP, Huynh HK, Rhomberg PR, Coffman SL, Brueggemann AB. Antimicrobial resistance among clinical isolates of *Streptococcus pneumoniae* in the United States during 1999–2000, including a comparison of resistance rates since 1994–1995. Antimicrob Agents Chemother 2001; 45(6):1721–9.

15. Doern GV, Richter SS, Miller A, et al. Antimicrobial resistance among *Streptococcus pneumoniae* in the United States: have we begun to turn the corner on resistance to certain antimicrobial classes? Clin Infect Dis 2005; 41(2):139–48.

16. http://www.whitehouse.gov/news/releases/2003/02/20030203.html

17. http://www.idsociety.org/Template.cfm?Section=Home&CONTENTID= 10303& TEMPLATE=/ContentManagement/ContentDisplay.cfm

18. http://www.washingtonpost.com/wp-dyn/articles/A13873-2004Jul25.html

19. Anonymous. Personal interview. May 2004.

20. Anonymous. Personal interview. February 2003.

21. http://www.who.int/infectious-disease-report/2000/intro.htm

22. Blosser R, Tillotson G, Flamm RK, Styers DA, Sahm DF, Jones ME. The prevalence of multidrug resistance among *Streptococcus pneumoniae* in the United States. Presentation at the 15th ECCMID. Abs P1087.

4

Understanding Studies of Resistant Organisms: Focus on Epidemiologic Methods

Ebbing Lautenbach
*Center for Clinical Epidemiology and Biostatistics, University of Pennsylvania,
Philadelphia, Pennsylvania, U.S.A.*

INTRODUCTION

An understanding of the principles of epidemiology is critical to the study of antimicrobial resistance. The value of epidemiological methods in the study of healthcare infections and antimicrobial resistance has been recognized for some time (1–4). The ability to accurately quantify new patterns of healthcare infections and resistance, design and carry out rigorous studies to identify factors associated with disease, and devise and evaluate interventions to address emerging issues are vital to the study of antimicrobial resistance. In recent years, there has been renewed interest in efforts to explore previously unstudied aspects of epidemiological methods in the study of healthcare infections and antimicrobial resistance (5–8).

This chapter reviews the advantages and disadvantages of various study designs. In addition, current epidemiologic issues in the study of antimicrobial resistance are discussed. These include: (*i*) quasi-experimental study design, (*ii*) control group selection in studies of antimicrobial resistance, (*iii*) definitions of antibiotic exposure, and (*iv*) assessment of mortality as an outcome of infection.

STUDY DESIGN

Various study designs may be chosen when seeking to address a clinical question. These study designs, in order of increasing methodological rigor, include: case report, case series, ecologic study, cross-sectional study, case-control study, cohort study, and randomized controlled trial. Randomized controlled trials, case-control studies, and cohort studies are considered analytic studies while the other designs are considered descriptive studies.

Case Report/Case Series

A case report is the clinical description of a single patient [e.g., a single patient with a bloodstream infection due to fluoroquinolone (FQ)-resistant *Escherichia coli* (FQREC)]. A case series is a report of several patients with the disease of interest. A case report/series can function to generate hypotheses that may then be tested in future analytic studies. The primary limitation of a case report/series is that it describes at most a few patients and may not be generalizable. In addition, since a case report/series does not include a comparison group, one cannot determine which characteristics in the description of the cases are unique to the illness.

Ecologic Study

In an ecologic study, one compares geographic and/or time trends of an illness to trends in risk factors (e.g., a comparison of annual hospital-wide use of FQs with annual prevalence of FQREC). Ecologic studies often use aggregate data collected for other purposes (e.g., antimicrobial susceptibility patterns from a hospital's clinical microbiology laboratory). Thus, one advantage of an ecologic study is that it is often quick and easy to carry out. Such a study may provide early support for or against a hypothesis. However, one cannot distinguish between various hypotheses that might be consistent with the data. Perhaps most importantly, ecologic studies do not incorporate patient level data. With such a study, one only knows that there is a correlation between annual hospital-wide use of FQs and yearly prevalence of FQREC, but not that the actual patients infected with FQREC received FQs.

Cross-Sectional Study

A cross-sectional study assesses the status of subjects with regard to the risk factor and disease at the same point in time. A cross-sectional study to investigate FQREC might assess all patients currently hospitalized with regard to whether they have a FQREC infection as well as whether they are receiving FQs. A cross-sectional study is relatively easy to carry out since all subjects are assessed at only one point in time. As such, this type of study may provide early evidence for or against a hypothesis. A major disadvantage of a cross-sectional study is that it does not capture the concept of elapsed time (i.e., it is not possible to determine whether the risk factor or the outcome came first). Furthermore, a cross-sectional study does not provide information about the transition between health states.

Case-Control Study

In comparing the various types of analytic studies (e.g., case-control, cohort, experimental-randomized controlled trial) one should consider the traditional two by two table (Fig. 1). While all three study designs seek to investigate the association between a risk factor (or exposure) and an outcome of interest, they differ fundamentally in how patients are enrolled into the study. In a case-control

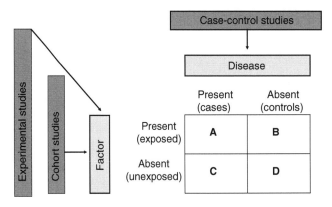

FIGURE 1   Study designs. *Source*: Adapted from Ref. 46.

study, patients are entered into the study based on the presence or absence of the outcome (or disease) of interest. These two groups (i.e., those with the disease and those without the disease) are then compared to determine if they differ with regard to the presence of risk factors of interest.

A case-control study design is particularly useful when the outcome being studied is rare, since one may enroll all patients with the outcome of interest. This study design is much more efficient than the comparable cohort study, in which a group of patients with and without an exposure of interest would need to be followed for a period of time to determine who develops the outcome of interest. One limitation of a case-control study is that only one outcome may be studied. Another disadvantage of this approach is that one cannot directly calculate the incidence or relative risk because the investigator fixes the number of cases and controls to be studied.

Of great importance in a case-control study is the process by which cases and controls are selected. Cases may be restricted to any group of diseased individuals. However, they must arise from a theoretical source population such that a diseased person not selected is presumed to have arisen from a different source population. For example, in studying risk factors for nosocomial FQREC infection, the theoretical source population could be considered to be the population of patients hospitalized at the institution. Thus, a patient at that institution with a clinical isolate demonstrating FQREC would be included as a case. However, a patient with FQREC infection at a different hospital would not be included. Cases must also be chosen in a manner independent of their status with regard to an exposure of interest.

Controls should also be representative of the theoretical source population that gave rise to the cases. Thus, if a control were to have developed the disease of interest, they would have been selected as a case. In the example above, controls may be randomly selected from among all non-FQREC infected patients in the hospital. In investigating the association between FQ use and FQREC infection, these two groups (i.e., patients with FQREC infection and a random sample of all other hospitalized patients) could be compared to determine what proportion of patients in each group had experienced recent FQ exposure. Finally, like cases, controls must be chosen in a manner independent of their status with regard to an exposure of interest and should not be selected because they have characteristics similar to cases. The selection of controls in case-control studies of antimicrobial resistance are discussed in greater detail in a later section of this chapter.

Cohort Study

In a cohort design, patients are entered into the study based on the presence or absence of an exposure (or risk factor) of interest (Fig. 1). These two groups (i.e., those with the exposure and those without the exposure) are then compared to determine if they differ with regard to development of the outcome of interest. Whether a cohort study is prospective or retrospective depends on when it is conducted with regard to when the outcome of interest occurs. If patients are identified as exposed or unexposed and then followed forward in time to determine whether they develop the outcome, it is a prospective cohort study. If the study is conducted after all outcomes have already occurred, it is a retrospective cohort study. As an example, one might identify all patients who receive a FQ in the hospital (i.e., the exposed) and compare them to patients who do not receive a FQ (i.e., the unexposed). These groups could then be followed forward to determine what proportion of patients in each group develops the outcome of interest (i.e., FQREC infection).

An advantage of a cohort study is that one may study multiple outcomes from a single exposure. Also, this study design allows the investigator to calculate an incidence as well as a relative risk in comparing the two groups. Potential limitations of a cohort study include substantial time and cost requirements due to often prolonged follow up of subjects. In addition, if the outcome is rare, a large number of subjects would need to be followed to ensure adequate sample size. Finally, the longer the study duration, the more likely subjects will be lost to follow up, potentially biasing the study results. Some of these limitations are lessened in a retrospective cohort study, since outcomes have already occurred and patients do not need to be followed prospectively.

Randomized Controlled Trial
The randomized controlled trial is very similar to the cohort study (Fig. 1). However, in a cohort study patients are enrolled already with or without the exposure of interest. In a randomized controlled trial, the investigator assigns the exposure randomly. This study design provides the most convincing demonstration of causality because patients in both groups should (provided randomization has worked appropriately) be equal with regard to all important variables except the one variable (exposure) manipulated by the investigator. While randomized controlled trials may provide the strongest support for or against an association of interest, they are costly studies, and there may be ethical issues that preclude their conduct.

BIAS

Bias is the systematic error in the collection or interpretation of data. Types of bias include information bias (i.e., distortion in the estimate of effect due to measurement error or misclassification of subjects on one or more variables) and selection bias (i.e., distortion in the estimate of effect resulting from the manner in which subjects are selected for the study). For example, a common type of information bias in case-control studies is recall bias. One may compare patients with a FQREC infection to a random sample of noninfected controls in an effort to identify risk factors for FQREC infection. If patients with a FQREC infection are aware of their diagnosis, they may be more likely to try to identify possible reasons for why they experienced a resistant infection. If this group is more likely to remember recent antibiotic use than are controls, the association between recent antibiotic use and FQREC infection will be spuriously strengthened.

Potential bias must be addressed at the time the study is designed since it cannot be corrected during the analysis of the study. In addition to evaluating whether bias may exist, one must also consider the likely impact of the bias on the study results. Bias may be nondifferential (i.e., biasing toward the null hypothesis and making the two groups being compared look artificially similar) or differential (i.e., biasing away from the null hypothesis and making the two groups being compared look artificially dissimilar).

CONFOUNDING

Confounding occurs when the association observed between an exposure and outcome is due, in part, to the effect of some other variable. To be a confounder, a variable must be associated with both the exposure and outcome of interest, but cannot be a result of the exposure. Confounding can result in an over- or under-estimate of the effect of the exposure of interest. For example, in assessing the association between a FQREC infection and mortality, one must consider under-lying severity of illness as a potential confounder. Patients with greater severity of illness are more likely to develop FQREC infection. In addition, greater severity of illness is also more likely to result in mortality. Thus, severity of illness, because it is associated with both the exposure and outcome of interest, is a potential confounding variable. Unlike bias, a confounding variable may be controlled for in the study analysis. However, in order to do this, data regarding the presence or absence of the confounder must be collected during the study.

MEASURES OF THE STRENGTH OF ASSOCIATION

p Value

The chi-square test for comparison of two binomial proportions is the most common method of measuring strength of association in a two by two table. A *p* value of <.05 indicates that an effect at least as extreme as that observed in the study is unlikely to have occurred by chance alone, given that there is truly no relationship between the exposure and the disease. Although this is the conventional interpreta-tion, there is nothing magical about the 0.05 cutoff for statistical significance. One limitation of the *p* value is that this value reflects both the magnitude of the difference between the groups as well as the sample size. Consequently, even a small difference between groups (if the sample size is large) may be statistically significant, even if it is not clinically important. Conversely, a larger effect that would be clinically important may not be statistically significant if the sample size is small.

95% Confidence Interval

Recognizing the limitations of the *p* value noted above, it is preferable to report the 95% confidence interval (CI) for a given relative risk or odds ratio. The 95% CI provides a range within which the true magnitude of the effect lies with a certain degree of assurance. Observing whether the 95% CI crosses 1.0 (i.e., the value of null effect) provides the same information as the *p* value. If the 95% CI crosses 1.0, the *p* value will almost never be <0.05. The impact of the sample size can be ascertained from the width of the confidence interval. The narrower the confidence interval, the less variability was present in the estimate of the effect, reflecting a larger sample size. The wider the CI, the smaller the sample size. When interpreting results that are not statistically significant, the width of the CI may be helpful. A narrow CI implies there is most likely no real effect, whereas a wide interval suggests the data are also compatible with a true effect and that the sample size was simply inadequate.

SPECIAL ISSUES IN HEALTHCARE EPIDEMIOLOGY METHODS

Quasi-Experimental Study Design

In addition to the study designs reviewed previously, the quasi-experimental study design is often utilized in studies of antimicrobial resistance (9). This design is also referred to as a "before-after" or "pre-post intervention" study (10,11). The goal of a quasi-experimental study is typically to evaluate an intervention without using randomization. The most basic type of quasi-experimental study involves the collection of baseline data, the implementation of an intervention, and the collection of the same data following the intervention. For example, the baseline prevalence of FQREC in a hospital would be calculated, an intervention to improve FQ use would then be instituted, and the prevalence of FQREC would again be measured after a prespecified time period. Many different variations of quasi-experimental studies exist and include: (*i*) institution of multiple pre-tests (i.e., collection of baseline data on more than one occasion); (*ii*) repeated interventions (i.e., instituting and removing the intervention sequentially); and (*iii*) inclusion of a control group (i.e., a group on which baseline and subsequent data are collected but on which no intervention is implemented) (Table 1) (9,12).

While often employed in evaluations of interventions addressing emerging resistance, critical evaluation of the advantages and disadvantages of quasi-experimental studies has only recently been conducted (9,12). Indeed, a recent systematic review of four infectious diseases journals found that during a two-year period, 73 articles focusing on infection control and/or antimicrobial resistance used a quasi-experimental study design (9). Of these articles, only twelve (16%) used a control group, three (4%) provided justification for the use of the quasi-experimental study design, and 17 (23%) mentioned at least one of the potential limitations of such a design (9).

There are several advantages to the quasi-experimental study design. In general, a well-designed and adequately powered randomized controlled trial provides the strongest evidence for or against the efficacy of an intervention. However, there are several reasons why a randomized controlled trial may not be

TABLE 1 Hierarchy of Quasi-Experimental Study Designs

A. Quasi-experimental designs without control groups

1. One-group pre-test–post-test design	O1 X O2
2. One-group pre-test–post-test design using a double pre-test	O1 O2 X O3
3. One-group pre-test–post-test design using a nonequivalent dependent variable	(O1a, O1b) X (O2a, O2b)
4. Removed-treatment design	O1 X O2 O3 remove X O4
5. Repeated-treatment design	O1 X O2 remove X O3 X O4

B. Quasi-experimental designs with control groups

1. Post-test-only design with nonequivalent groups	X O1 ——— O2
2. Untreated control group design with dependent pre-test and post-test samples	O1a X O2a O1b X O2b
3. Untreated control group design with dependent pre-test and post-test samples and a double pre-test	O1a O2a X O3a O1b O2b O3b
4. Untreated control group design with dependent pre-test and post-test samples and switching replications	O1a X O2a O3a O1b O2b X O3b

Note: In general, studies in category B are of higher design quality than those in category A. Also, as one moves down within each category, the studies become of higher quality; e.g., study 5 in category A is of higher study design quality than study 4, etc. Time moves from left to right.
Abbreviations: O, observational measurement; X, intervention under study.
Source: Adapted from Ref. 9.

feasible in the study of interventions designed to curb antimicrobial resistance. Randomizing individual patients to an intervention is often not a reasonable approach, given the person to person transmission of resistant pathogens. One might consider randomizing specific units or floors within one institution to receive the intervention. However, these units are not self-contained and patients and healthcare workers frequently move from unit to unit. Thus, any effect on reduced transmission/acquisition of new resistant infections noted in the intervention units are likely to also result in some reduction in resistant infections in nonintervention areas (i.e., contamination). This would bias the results toward the null hypothesis (i.e., no effect of the intervention). In such a situation, a well designed quasi-experimental study offers a compelling alternative approach. In addition, this study design is frequently used when it is not ethical to conduct a randomized controlled trial. Further, when an intervention must be instituted rapidly in response to an emerging issue (e.g., an outbreak), the first priority is to address and resolve the issue. In this case, it would be unethical to randomize an intervention across patient groups.

Limitations of quasi-experimental studies include regression to the mean, uncontrolled confounding, and maturation effects. Implementation of an intervention is often triggered in response to a rise in the rate above the norm (13). Regression to the mean predicts that these elevated rates will tend to decline, even without intervention. This may serve to bias the results of a quasi-experimental study, as it may be falsely concluded that an effect is due to the intervention (10,11). Several approaches may be employed to address this potential limitation. First, incorporating a prolonged baseline period prior to the intervention permits an evaluation of the natural fluctuation in rates of the outcome over time. Second, changes in the outcome of interest may be measured at a control site (e.g., another institution) during the same time period. Finally, the use of segmented regression analysis may assist in addressing possible regression to the mean in that not only will the immediate change in prevalence coincident with the intervention be assessed, but also the change in slope over time (14–16).

Another potential limitation in quasi-experimental studies is uncontrolled confounding. This is most likely to occur when variables other than the intervention change over time (10,11). This limitation can be addressed by measuring known confounders (e.g., hospital census) and controlling for them in analyses. However, not all confounders are known or easily measured (e.g., quality of medical and nursing care). To address this, one may assess a nonequivalent dependent variable to evaluate the possibility that factors other than the intervention influenced the outcome (9,12). A nonequivalent dependent variable should have similar potential causal and confounding variables as the primary dependent variable except for the effect of the intervention. For example, in assessing the impact of an intervention to limit FQ use on FQREC prevalence, one might consider incidence of catheter-associated bloodstream infections as a nonequivalent dependent variable. While FQREC prevalence and catheter-associated bloodstream infection might both be affected by such factors as patient census, it is unlikely that FQ use specifically would affect the incidence of catheter-associated bloodstream infections.

Finally, maturation effects are related to natural changes that patients experience with the passage of time (10,11). In addition, there are cyclical trends (e.g., seasonal variation) that may be a threat to the validity of attributing an observed outcome to an intervention. This potential limitation may be addressed through approaches noted above including assessment of a prolonged baseline period, use of control sites, implementing interventions at different time periods at different sites, and assessing a nonequivalent dependent variable.

Control Group Selection in Studies of Antimicrobial Resistance

Numerous studies have focused on identifying risk factors for antimicrobial resistance. The majority of these studies have been case-control designed studies and how controls are selected in such studies is critical in ensuring the validity of study results. Recent work has highlighted this issue of control group selection specifically for studies of antibiotic resistance (5,17–20).

Traditionally, two types of control groups have been used in studies of antimicrobial resistant organisms (5). The first type of control group is selected from patients who do not harbor the resistant pathogen. The second type of control group is selected from among subjects with a susceptible form of the infection. For example, in a study of risk factors for infection with FQREC in hospitalized patients, the first type of control group would be selected from among the general hospitalized patient population while the second control group would be selected from among those patients with a FQ-susceptible *E. coli* (FQSEC) infection. The choice of control group should be based primarily on the clinical question being asked. While use of this second type of control group has historically been more common, it has recently been demonstrated that use of this type of control group (e.g., patients infected with the susceptible form of the organism) may result in an overestimate of the association between antimicrobial exposure and resistant infection (19,20). Using the example above, the explanation for this finding has been stated as follows: if the controls are represented by patients with FQSEC infections, it is very unlikely that these patients would have recently received FQs (i.e., the risk factor of interest) since exposure to FQs may have eradicated FQSEC colonization. Thus, the association between FQ use and FQREC would be overestimated (21). A limitation of using the first type of approach (i.e., using patients without infection as controls) is that, in addition to identifying risk factors for resistance, this approach also identifies risk factors for infection with that organism in general (regardless of whether the infection is resistant or susceptible). Thus, there is no way to distinguish the degree to which a risk factor is associated with the resistance phenotype versus associated with the infecting organism in general (18).

A concern with using the second type of control group (i.e., selecting from all hospitalized patients) is potential misclassification bias. Subjects selected as controls who have never had a clinical culture obtained may in fact harbor unrecognized colonization with the resistant organism under study (17). Since it is probable that patients colonized with the resistant organism would likely have had greater prior antimicrobial exposure than subjects not colonized, this misclassification would likely result in a bias toward the null (i.e., the cases and controls would appear falsely similar with regard to prior antimicrobial use). Another concern with using the second type of control group and identifying as controls those patients who have never had a clinical culture is that differences between cases and controls may reflect the fact that clinical cultures were performed for case patients but not for controls. Since procurement of cultures is not a random process but based on clinical characteristics, it is possible that the severity of illness or antibiotic exposure may be greater among cases, regardless of the presence of antibiotic-resistant infection (5). One potential approach would be to limit eligible controls to those patients for whom at least one clinical culture has been performed and does not reveal the resistant organism of interest. Such a negative culture would suggest that the patient is likely not colonized with the resistant organism. However, recent work has demonstrated that using clinical cultures to identify eligible controls leads to the selection of a control group with a higher comorbidity score and greater exposure to antibiotics compared with a control group for which clinical cultures were not performed (17).

One approach for addressing the issues in control group selection in studies of antimicrobial resistance is the case-case-control study design (18,22–24). In this design, effectively two case-control studies are performed. In the first, cases are defined as those patients harboring the resistant organism while controls are those patients without the pathogen of interest. In the second, cases are instead defined as those patients harboring the susceptible bacteria while controls, similar to the first approach, are those patients without the pathogen of interest (18). These two separate studies are then carried out with risk factors from the two studies compared qualitatively. This approach allows for the comparison of risk factors identified from the two studies to indicate the relative contribution of the resistant infection over and above simply having the susceptible infection. A potential limitation in this approach is the difficulty in matching for potential confounders because of the use of only one control group (18). Since there are two different case groups, case variables (e.g., duration of hospitalization, patient location) cannot be used for matching. In addition, the qualitative comparison of results from the two studies in this design leaves open the question as to how much of a difference in results is meaningful.

Definitions of Antibiotic Exposure in Study of Resistance

Numerous studies have sought to identify risk factors for infection or colonization with resistant organisms (8,25). Elucidating such risk factors is essential to inform interventions designed to curb further emergence of resistance. Past studies have particularly focused on antimicrobial use as a risk factor because it can be modified in the clinical setting (26,27). However, the approaches used to define prior antibiotic exposure vary considerably across studies (5). More importantly only recently have attempts been made to identify the impact of differences in these approaches on study conclusions.

One recent study investigated methods used in past studies to describe the extent of prior antibiotic use (e.g., exposure yes/no vs. duration of exposure) as well as the impact of using different methods on study conclusions (28). A systematic review of all studies investigating risk factors for extended-spectrum beta-lactamase-producing *Escherichia coli* and *Klebsiella* species (ESBL-EK) was conducted. Among the 25 included studies, prior antibiotic use was defined as a categorical variable in 18 studies, four studies defined prior antibiotic exposure as a continuous variable, and three studies included both a categorical and a continuous variable to describe prior antibiotic exposure. Only one paper provided an explicit justification for its choice of variable to describe prior antibiotic exposure. The authors then re-analyzed a dataset from a prior ESBL-EK risk factor study (29), developing two separate multivariable models, one in which prior antibiotic use was described as a categorical variable (e.g., exposure yes/no) and one in which antibiotic use was described as a continuous variable (e.g., antibiotic days). Results of the two multivariable models using different methodological approaches differed substantially. Specifically, third-generation cephalosporin use was a risk factor for ESBL-EK when antibiotic use was described as a continuous variable but not when antibiotic use was described as a categorical variable (28).

These results suggest that describing prior antibiotic use as a categorical variable may mask significant associations between prior antibiotic use and resistance. For example, when the categorical variable is used, a subject who received only one day of an antibiotic would be considered identical to a subject who received 30 days of the same antibiotic. However, the risk of resistance is almost certainly not the same in these two individuals. Describing prior antibiotic use as a continuous variable allows for a more detailed characterization of the association between length of exposure and resistance. Recent work in the medical statistics literature emphasizes that the use of cut points can result in misinterpretation of data and that dichotomizing continuous variables reduces analytic power and makes it impossible to detect nonlinear relationships (30). Indeed, the relationship between prior antimicrobial use and resistance may not be linear (i.e., the risk of resistance may not increase at a constant rate with increasing antimicrobial exposure). It is possible that the risk of resistance does not increase substantially until a certain amount of antimicrobial exposure has been attained (e.g., a "lower threshold").

Another issue regarding defining prior antimicrobial use centers on how specific agents are grouped. For example, antibiotic use could be classified by agent (e.g., cefazolin), class (e.g., cephalosporins), or spectrum of activity (e.g., Gram-negative). Antibiotics are frequently grouped together in classes even though individual agents within the class may differ significantly (31), and such categorizations may mask important associations. It is unknown if using different categorization schemes results in different conclusions regarding the association between antibiotic use and resistance. A recent study explored these issues, focusing on ESBL-EK as a model (32). In a systematic review, 20 studies of risk factors for ESBL-EK that met inclusion criteria revealed tremendous variability in how prior antibiotic use was categorized. Categorization of prior antibiotic use was defined in terms of the specific agents, drug class, and often a combination of both. No study justified its choice of categorization method. There was also marked variability across studies with regard to which specific antibiotics or antibiotic classes were assessed. As expected, a majority of the studies ($n = 16$) specifically investigated the use of beta-lactam antibiotics as risk factors for ESBL-EK. A variable number of studies also examined the association between use of other antibiotics and ESBL-EK infection: aminoglycosides (9 studies), FQs (10 studies), and trimethoprim-sulfamethoxazole (7 studies). In a reanalysis of data from a prior study of risk factors for ESBL-EK (29), two separate multivariable models of risk factors for ESBL-EK were constructed: one with prior antibiotic use categorized by class and the other with prior antibiotic use categorized by spectrum of activity (32). The results of these multivariable models differed substantially.

A final issue is how remote antibiotic use is assessed. A systematic review of studies investigating risk factors for ESBL-EK (28), found that the time window during which antibiotic use was reviewed ranged from 48 hr to one year prior to the resistant infection. Furthermore, studies often did not explicitly state how far back in time prior antibiotic use was assessed (28).

The Association Between Resistance and Mortality

Increasingly, studies have focused on more clearly identifying the impact of antimicrobial resistance (33). Increasing attention has recently been paid to potential methodological issues in assessing the relationship between an antimicrobial-resistant infection and mortality (5,33). One important issue is the need to control for severity of illness. An oft-noted risk factor for resistant infection is greater underlying severity of illness. However, severity of illness is also a predictor of mortality. These characteristics suggest that severity of illness is likely to be an important confounder in the association between resistant infection and mortality. There are several measures that assess severity of illness, including the Acute Physiology and Chronic Health Evaluation (APACHE) II score (34) and the McCabe-Jackson Score (35). However, no severity of illness score has been developed or validated specifically to predict outcome in patients with infection. Regardless of the measure used, it is critical to control for severity of illness in studies assessing the impact of resistant infection on mortality.

It is important to carefully consider when severity of illness is assessed (36). The vast majority of studies have assessed severity of illness at the time the infection is diagnosed (i.e., when the culture is initially drawn). However, the culture is generally obtained because of clinical suspicion of infection suggesting that infection has already progressed at some time point prior to the culture being obtained. Since infection will typically also lead to worse severity of illness it is likely that severity of illness measured on the day the culture is obtained is more accurately an intermediate variable (e.g., infection leads to a greater severity of illness, which then ultimately leads to death). Controlling for an intermediate variable in this way usually causes an underestimate of the effect of the exposure of interest on the outcome (37). It has been suggested that results of studies that control for severity of illness on the day the culture is obtained should be interpreted with caution since they may represent an underestimate of the true association between resistant infection and mortality (36). However, recent work focusing on FQREC has noted that APACHE II scores calculated on the day of culture, one day prior to culture, and two days prior to culture do not differ substantively (38). Furthermore, when assessing the adjusted association between FQ resistance and mortality, there were no substantive differences across multivariable models incorporating APACHE II calculated at different time points (38).

The choice of control group is also relevant in studies of outcomes (36). Since studies addressing outcomes related to infection are primarily cohort studies, "controls" in these studies are more appropriately referred to as the "unexposed" or "reference" group. As in case-control studies of antibiotic resistance, there are effectively two choices for a reference group. In the first, patients with a resistant infection (e.g., FQREC) are compared with patients with the susceptible counterpart (e.g., FQSEC). In the second type of control group, patients with a resistant infection (e.g., FQREC) are compared with patients with no infection. Although either approach is valid, they address slightly different clinical questions. In the first, the result provides an assessment of the added impact of harboring a resistant infection versus a susceptible infection. In the second, the impact of having a resistant infection versus no infection is ascertained. It has been demonstrated that the latter type of comparison typically results in a higher estimate of the impact of resistance on mortality (39,40).

Finally, an important issue concerns how mortality is defined. Crude in-hospital mortality has been the most common measure of mortality likely because it is the least subjective in its assessment. However, this definition of mortality fails to distinguish those cases in which resistant infection clearly resulted in death as opposed to those cases in which infection occurred but was likely unrelated to mortality. Some studies have proposed approaches to categorizing the outcome of mortality relative to how likely it is to have resulted from an infection. One approach would be to assign an arbitrary time period after the infection (e.g., one week) beyond which the occurrence of mortality would be assumed to be independent of the infection. Another approach has proposed categories designed to assess attributable mortality as an outcome (29,41–43). In this definition, the possible outcomes are classified as follows: (*i*) mortality directly attributable to infection: death during hospitalization in the setting of clinical evidence of active infection and a positive culture result; (*ii*) mortality indirectly attributable to infection: failure or further compromise of an organ system due to infection and death occurring during hospitalization as a result of organ failure; (*iii*) mortality unrelated to infection: death occurring during hospitalization after an episode of infection but due to causes independent of the infectious process; and (*iv*) survival: patient discharged alive from the hospital. The proportion of deaths directly and indirectly attributable to infection defines the attributable mortality. While this approach may more appropriately designate mortality as attributable to infection, many of the criteria remain quite subjective. Of note, recent studies, using both this approach as well as crude in-hospital mortality as outcomes, found no substantive differences in final study results when using both approaches (44,45).

SUMMARY

The study of antimicrobial resistance has become increasingly complex. To better understand the existing literature, and to optimally design future studies to elucidate the nature of these infections, a strong understanding of epidemiologic principles and approaches is essential. Although recent years have witnessed a resurgence in the study of epidemiological methodology in antimicrobial resistance, this field of inquiry must continue to expand in the future. Only through the most rigorously derived evidence can we hope to devise and implement successful strategies to limit future antimicrobial resistance.

REFERENCES

1. Haley RW, Quade D, Freeman HE and Bennett JV. The SENIC Project. Study on the efficacy of nosocomial infection control (SENIC Project). Summary of study design. Am J Epidemiol 1980; 111:472–85.
2. Haley RW, Schaberg DR, McClish DK, et al. The accuracy of retrospective chart review in measuring nosocomial infection rates. Results of validation studies in pilot hospitals. Am J Epidemiol 1980; 111:516–33.
3. Freeman J, McGowan JE Jr. Methodologic issues in hospital epidemiology. I. Rates, case-finding, and interpretation. Rev Infect Dis 1981; 3:658–67.
4. Freeman J, McGowan JE Jr. Methodologic issues in hospital epidemiology. II. Time and accuracy in estimation. Rev Infect Dis 1981; 3:668–77.
5. D'Agata EM. Methodologic issues of case-control studies: a review of established and newly recognized limitations. Infect Control Hosp Epidemiol 2005; 26:338–41.
6. Paterson DL. Looking for risk factors for the acquisition of antibiotic resistance: A 21st century approach. Clin Infect Dis 2002; 34:1564–7.

7. Schwaber MJ, De-Medina T, Carmeli Y. Epidemiological interpretation of antibiotic resistance studies—what are we missing? Nat Rev Microbiol 2004; 2:979–83.

8. Harbarth S, Samore M. Antimicrobial resistance determinants and future control. Emerg Inf Dis 2005; 11:794–801.

9. Harris AD, Lautenbach E, Perencevich E. A systematic review of quasi-experimental study designs in the fields of infection control and antibiotic resistance. Clin Infect Dis 2005; 41:77–82.

10. Shadish WR, Cook TD, Campbell DT. Experimental and Quasi-experimental Designs for Generalized Causal Inference. Boston: Houghton Mifflin Company, 2002.

11. Cook TD, Campbell DT. Quasi-experimentation: Design and Analysis Issues for Field Settings. Chicago: Rand McNally Publishing, 1979.

12. Harris AD, Bradham DD, Baumgarten M, Zuckerman IH, Fink JC, Perencevich EN. The use and interpretation of quasi-experimental studies in infectious diseases. Clin Infect Dis 2004; 38:1586–91.

13. Morton V, Torgerson DJ. Effect of regression to the mean on decision making in health care. BMJ 2003; 326:1083–4.

14. Ramsay CR, Matowe L, Grilli R, Grimshaw JM, Thomas RE. Interrupted time series designs in health technology assessment: lessons from two systematic reviews of behavior change strategies. Int J Technol Assess Health Care 2003; 19:613–23.

15. Wagner AK, Soumerai SB, Zhang F, Ross-Degnan D. Segmented regression analysis of interrupted time series studies in medication use research. J Clin Pharm Ther 2002; 27:299–309.

16. Matowe LK LC, Crivera C, Korth-Bradley JM. Interrupted time series analysis in clinical research. Ann Pharmacother 2003; 37:1110–6.

17. Harris AD, Carmeli Y, Samore MH, Kaye KS, Perencevich E. Impact of severity of illness bias and control group misclassification bias in case-control studies of antimicrobial-resistant organisms. Infect Control Hosp Epidemiol 2005; 26:342–5.

18. Kaye KS, Harris AD, Samore M, Carmeli Y. The case-case-control study design: addressing the limitations of risk factor studies for antimicrobial resistance. Infect Control Hosp Epidemiol 2005; 26:346–51.

19. Harris AD, Karchmer TB, Carmeli Y, Samore MH. Methodological principles of case-control studies that analyzed risk factors for antibiotic resistance: a systematic review. Clin Infect Dis 2001; 32:1055–61.

20. Harris AD, Samore MH, Lipsitch M, Kaye KS, Perencevich E, Carmeli Y. Control-group selection importance in studies of antimicrobial resistance: examples applied to *Pseudomonas aeruginosa*, *Enterococci*, and *Escherichia coli*. Clin Infect Dis 2002; 34: 1558–63.

21. Carmeli Y, Samore MH, Huskins C. The association between antecedent vancomycin treatment and hospital-acquired vancomycin-resistant enterococci. Arch Intern Med 1999; 159:2461–8.

22. Kaye KS, Harris AD, Gold H, Carmeli Y. Risk factors for recovery of ampicillin-sulbactam-resistant Escherichia coli in hospitalized patients. Antimicrob Agents Chemother 2000; 44:1004–9.

23. Harris AD, Smith D, Johnson JA, Bradham DD, Roghmann MC. Risk factors for imipenem-resistant *Pseudomonas aeruginosa* among hospitalized patients. Clin Infect Dis 2002; 34:340–5.

24. Harris AD, Perencevich E, Roghmann MC, Morris G, Kaye KS, Johnson JA. Risk factors for piperacillin-tazobactam-resistant *Pseudomonas aeruginosa* among hospitalized patients. Antimicrob Agents Chemother 2002; 46:854–8.

25. Livermore DM. Can better prescribing turn the tide of resistance? Nat Rev Microbiol 2004; 2:73–8.

26. Patterson JE. Antibiotic utilization: is there an effect on antimicrobial resistance? Chest 2001; 119(Suppl. 2):426S–30S.

27. Safdar N, Maki DG. The commonality of risk factors for nosocomial colonization and infection with antimicrobial-resistant *Staphylococcus aureus*, *enterococcus*, Gram-negative bacilli, *Clostridium difficile*, and *Candida*. Ann Intern Med 2002; 136:834–44.

28. Hyle EP, Bilker WB, Gasink LB, Lautenbach E. Impact of different methods for describing the extent of prior antibiotic exposure on the association between antibiotic use and antibiotic-resistant infection. Infection Control and Hospital Epidemiology 2007; 28:647–54.

29. Lautenbach E, Patel JB, Bilker WB, Edelstein PH, Fishman NO. Extended-spectrum B-lactamase-producing *Escherichia coli* and *Klebsiella pneumoniae*: risk factors for infection and impact of resistance on outcomes. Clin Infect Dis 2001; 32:1162–71.

30. Royston P, Altman D, Sauerbrei W. Dichotomizing continuous predictors in multiple regression: a bad idea. Stat Med 2006; 25:127–41.

31. Donskey CJ. The role of the intestinal tract as a reservoir and source for transmission of nosocomial pathogens. Clin Infect Dis 2004; 39:219–26.

32. MacAdam H, Zaoutis TE, Gasink LB, Bilker WB, Lautenbach E. Investigating the association between antibiotic use and antimicrobial resistance: impact of different methods of categorizing prior antibiotic use. Int J Antimicrob Agents 2006; 28:325–32.

33. Cosgrove SE. The relationship between antimicrobial resistance and patient outcomes: mortality, length of hospital stay, and health care costs. Clin Infect Dis 2006; 42(Suppl. 2):S82–9.

34. Knaus WA, Drapier EA, Wagner DP, Zimmerman JE. APACHE II: A severity of disease classification system. Crit Care Med 1985; 13:818–29.

35. McCabe WR, Jackson GG. Gram-negative bacteremia Etiology and ecology. Arch Intern Med 1962; 110:847–55.

36. Cosgrove SE, Carmeli Y. The impact of antimicrobial resistance on health and economic outcomes. Clin Infect Dis 2003; 36:1433–7.

37. Robins JM. The control of confounding by intermediate variables. Stat Med 1989; 8:679–701.

38. Hamilton KW, Bilker WB, Lautenbach E. Controlling for severity of illness in assessment of the association between antimicrobial-resistant infection and mortality: Impact of calculating Acute Physiology and Chronic Health Evaluation (APACHE) II scores at different time points. Infection Control and Hospital Epidemiology 2007; 28:832–6.

39. Engemann JJ, Carmeli Y, Cosgrove SE, et al. Adverse clinical and economic outcomes attributable to methicillin resistance among patients with *Staphylococcus aureus* surgical site infection. Clin Infect Dis 2003; 36:592–8.

40. Kaye KS, Engemann JJ, Mozaffari E, Carmeli Y. Reference group choice and antibiotic resistance outcomes. Emerg Inf Dis 2004; 10:1125–8.

41. Noskin GA, Peterson LR, Warren JR. *Enterococcus faecium* and *Enterococcus faecalis* bacteremia: acquisition and outcome. Clin Infect Dis 1995; 20:296–301.

42. Lautenbach E, Schuster MG, Bilker WB, Brennan PJ. The role of chloramphenicol in the treatment of bloodstream infection due to vancomycin-resistant *Enterococcus*. Clin Infect Dis 1998; 27:1259–65.

43. Weinstein MP, Murphy JR, Reller LB, Lichtenstein KA. The clinical significance of positive blood cultures: a comprehensive analysis of 500 episodes of bacteremia and fungemia in adults. II. Clinical observations, with special reference to factors influencing prognosis. Rev Infect Dis 1983; 5:54–70.

44. Lautenbach E, Metlay JP, Bilker WB, Edelstein PH, Fishman NO. Association between fluoroquinolone resistance and mortality in *Escherichia coli* and *Klebsiella pneumoniae* infections: role of inadequate empiric antimicrobial therapy. Clin Infect Dis 2005; 41:923–9.

45. Hyle EP, Lipworth AD, Zaoutis TE, Nachamkin I, Bilker WB, Lautenbach E. Impact of inadequate initial antimicrobial therapy on mortality in infections due to extended-spectrum beta-lactamase-producing enterobacteriaceae: variability by site of infection. Arch Intern Med 2005; 165:1375–80.

46. Lautenbach E. Epidemiological methods in infection control. In: Lautenbach E, Woeltje K, eds. Practical Handbook for Healthcare Epidemiologists. Thorofare, New Jersey: Slack Inc, 2004.

Part II: Contemporary Antimicrobial Resistance Issues:
Gram-Positive, Gram-Negative, and Miscellaneous Pathogens

5 *Staphylococcus aureus*: Resistance Update and Treatment Options

Pamela A. Moise
Department of Pharmacy Practice, Thomas J. Long School of Pharmacy and Health Sciences, University of the Pacific, Stockton, California, U.S.A.

George Sakoulas
Department of Medicine, Division of Infectious Diseases, New York Medical College, Valhalla, New York, U.S.A.

INTRODUCTION

The complex relationship between *Homo sapiens* and *Staphylococcus aureus* has undoubtedly existed for millennia. While controversial, a theory was proposed in 1985 implicating staphylococcal toxic shock syndrome, possibly following influenza infection, as the etiology of the Thucydides syndrome, a series of plagues that, under conditions of population crowding, inflicted a greater than 25% mortality on the Athenians during the early years of war with Sparta in the Peloponnesian Wars (431–404 B.C.) (1,2). It was not coincidental that the emergence of this hypothesis fell on the heels of the widely publicized surge in menstrual toxic shock cases in the 1980s associated with hyperabsorbent tampons. For, in both illnesses, "people in good health were all of a sudden attacked by violent heats in the head, and redness and inflammation in the eyes, the inward parts, such as the throat or tongue and... severe diarrhea, this brought on a weakness which was generally fatal."

Whether the illness described by Thucydides truly represented staphylococcal toxic shock syndrome versus some other infectious agent will never be known for sure. However, its emergence and partial acceptance as a plausible theory for a catastrophic event on a human society shows that we accept the notion that *S. aureus* has been with us as long as civilization itself. This relationship can be best pictured as a pyramid, whereby 20% to 40% of the general population serves as the pyramid base, through permanent or transient colonization of the mucocutaneous barrier, with "hotspots" of colonization in the anterior nares, axillae, perineum, and hands (3). Although an effective barrier, violation of the mucocutaneous membrane via macroscopic or microscopic trauma sets the stage for one to move up the pyramid. Higher on the pyramid denotes less common but more severe infection, from superficial skin infections, more severe soft tissue infections, lower respiratory tract infections, deep-seeded abscesses, bone and joint infections, and finally culminating in bloodstream infections and endocarditis. Hosts as well as bacterial factors are important in colonization and progression to invasive disease.

As we discuss current concepts in the treatment of *S. aureus* infections, it is important for the reader to understand that, throughout history, the pathogen and the host in this relationship have evolved in parallel in the context of pathogenesis and antimicrobial therapeutics via virulence factors and antimicrobial resistance. For example, after the global availability of penicillin around 1950, virulent *S. aureus* strains such as phage-type strain 80/81 emerged penicillin resistant in the 1950s, causing serious infections worldwide. This strain was successfully suppressed in the 1960s with the development of antistaphylococcal beta-lactams, like methicillin, and remained insignificant until the new century, where it has re-emerged as one of the community-acquired (CA) methicillin-resistant *S. aureus* (MRSA) clones.

S. *aureus* has also found a niche well-suited to it in nosocomial environments worldwide. Advances and application of surgical techniques, increased physiologic immunosuppression via the aging population and obesity-driven diabetes mellitus, iatrogenic immunosuppression via chemotherapy or organ transplantation, large-scale implementation of intravascular catheters, aggressive medical care offered in intensive care units, and long-term care in subacute nursing facilities (SNFs) that help prolong the lives of even the most moribund of hosts for months, frequently under considerable antimicrobial selection pressure, have worked together to generate today's formidable nosocomial MRSA. It is clear that as we have evolved in our therapeutics, *S. aureus* continues to match up to us along the way.

S. AUREUS HETEROGENEITY

The name of the organism, *S. aureus*, serves to describe well the microscopic and macroscopic characteristics of the organism. The term "*Staphylococcus*" is derived from the Greek "staphyle," which means "grape." One who has seen a Gram stain of a specimen teeming with Gram-positively stained staphylococci would understand why this name was given to the organisms in this genus, with organisms clumped together like clumps of purple grapes on a vine. The term "aureus" is derived from the Latin term meaning "gold coin" and "aurum," or "gold." Simply looking at the colonies of bacterial growth of a *S. aureus* skin abscess culture on a blood agar plate under aerobic conditions in the clinical microbiology laboratory will give the reader an obvious explanation on the organism's name. This pigment is generated by production of caretinoids by the organism and may be enhanced by longer incubation.

The appearance of *S. aureus* on blood agar plates is an interesting place to begin the discussion of the organism. Most classical descriptions of the organism will state that the organism forms convex, sharp, and smooth colonies 1 to 2 mm in diameter after 24 hr of growth at 35°C under aerobic conditions, with creamy yellow or gold colonies producing beta-hemolysis on sheep blood agar. However, discussions with several experienced microbiologists will reveal that this classical description may not apply for many clinical isolates, particularly those acquired from hospital infections and those of nosocomial MRSA. Many of these colonies may be smaller, heterogeneous in size, and produce minimal hemolysis of sheep blood, if at all. Similar descriptions have been given to so-called "small colony variants" of *S. aureus* that have been associated with persistent, recurrent infections caused by organisms with multiple antibiotic resistance. These mutants were found to result from defects in electron transport (4).

TREATMENT

Treatment of *S. aureus* infections can be quite challenging. MRSA has emerged in the community. And, although resistance rates vary, *S. aureus* have developed resistance to virtually every antimicrobial agent available for clinical use. The threat posed by vancomycin resistance in clinically significant *S. aureus* infections, and the emergence of MRSA in the community, led to the development of new antimicrobial agents and a renewed interest in older active against these pathogens. The pharmacologic parameters, U.S. Food and Drug Administration (FDA)-approved indications, and advantages and disadvantages of vancomycin and the newly available *S. aureus* active antimicrobial agents are displayed in Tables 1 and 2.

S. aureus is a major pathogen in bloodstream and endovascular, skin and soft tissue, respiratory, and bone and joint infections (5). The discussion below focuses on the management of these infections.

Bloodstream Infections Including Endocarditis

While the spectrum of causative pathogens in bloodstream infections continues to change, *S. aureus* remains one of the most common organisms isolated (6–12). Mortality associated with *S. aureus* bacteremia is significant, and is more common with MRSA bacteremia (12–14). Management of *S. aureus* bacteremia depends on the severity of the infection and if it is considered complicated or not. *S. aureus* bacteremia may be considered "uncomplicated" in the case of catheter-related bacteremia or other identified focus of infection. Successful treatment of uncomplicated *S. aureus* bacteremia requires removal of the identified focus of infection (the catheter) and 2 weeks of parenteral antimicrobial therapy. Patients with complicated *S. aureus* bacteremia are at high risk for developing endocarditis and/or other complications.

Complicated *S. aureus* bacteremia requires 4 to 6 weeks of antimicrobial therapy, and should be considered in patients with positive blood cultures after 48 hr of treatment (despite removal of catheter, if suspected source), persistent fever after 72 hr, skin examination suggestive of acute systemic infection, community-acquired infection, and the presence of an orthopedic or other prosthetic device (15). Those with an unknown focus of bacteremia or endocarditis also require 4 to 6 weeks of treatment (Tables 3 and 4). In addition, patients who are quantitatively (i.e., primary hematology) or qualitative (i.e., diabetes and renal failure) immunodeficient require special attention, and 4 to 6 weeks of treatment should be considered.

Given elevated rates of vancomycin treatment failures in MRSA bacteremia caused by organisms with vancomycin MIC of >1 mg/L, it is suggested that clinicians should obtain a quantitative vancomycin MIC for patients with these infections and consideration be given for alternative therapy for such organisms. Furthermore, patients who have a higher risk of such organisms (i.e., patients recently treated with vancomycin) should also be considered for alternative empiric anti-MRSA therapy.

Skin and Skin Structure Infections

S. aureus represents a common etiologic agent of skin and skin structure infection (SSSI), ranging in severity from mild to life-threatening disease and in community as well as nosocomial settings. The first step in management is to strotify by the presence or absence of systemic toxicity (e.g., hemodynamic instability,

(text continues on p.82)

TABLE 1 Features and Properties of Three Newer Gram-Positive Antibiotics

Antibiotic details	Quinupristin/dalfopristin (Synercid)	Linezolid (Zyvox)	Daptomycin (Cubicin) (29)	Tigecycline (Tigecyl)
FDA-approved indications	VRE faecium bacteremia Complicated SSSIs (MSSA or *Streptococcus pyogenes*)	VRE faecium infections, including bacteremia Nosocomial pneumonia (MSSA, MRSA, or PCN-S *S. pneumoniae*) Complicated SSSIs (MSSA, *S. pyogenes*, or *S. agalactiae*), including diabetic foot infections, without osteomyelitis Uncomplicated SSSIs (MSSA or *S. pyogenes*) CAP (PCN-S *S. pneumoniae* or MSSA), including bacteremia	Complicated SSSIs Bacteremia, including right-sided endocarditis	Complicated SSSIs (MSSA and MRSA, *E. faecalis, E. coli, S. agalactiae, S. pyogenes, B. fragilis*, etc.) Complicated intra-abdominal infections (MSSA, *E. coli, B. fragilis*, etc.)
Mechanism of action	Inhibits protein synthesis by binding to the peptidyltransferase domain of the bacterial ribosome (30)	Inhibits bacterial protein translation at the initiation phase of protein synthesis (31)	Disruption of bacterial cell membrane potential	Inhibits protein synthesis by binding to the bacterial ribosome
Dosage regimen	7.5 mg/kg IV q8 h	Adults and adolescents (>12 yr): 600 mg IV or PO q12 h Birth to 11 yr: 10 mg/kg IV or PO q8 h	4 mg/kg IV q24 h (SSSI) 6 mg/kg IV q24 h (bacteremia and right-sided endocarditis) Interval should be increased to q48 h in patients with creatinine clearance <30 mL/min	100 mg IV ×1, followed by 50 mg IV q12 h Dose should be decreased to 25 mg IV q12 h in patients with severe hepatic insufficiency (Child Pugh C)

PK parameters	Quinupristin—Vd 0.45 L/kg Dalfopristin—Vd 0.24 L/kg	600 mg IV q12 h: C_{max} 15.1 µg/mL $AUC_{0-\tau}$ 89.7 µg h/mL $T_{1/2}$ 4.8 hr 600 mg PO q12 h: C_{max} 21.2 µg/mL $AUC_{0-\tau}$ 138 µg h/mL $T_{1/2}$ 5.4 hr	4 mg/kg IV QD at steady state: C_{max} 57.8 µg/mL AUC_{0-24} 494 µg h/mL Vd 0.1 L/kg $T_{1/2}$ 8.1 h	Multiple 50 mg q12 h dose: C_{max} 0.87 µg/mL (after 30 min infusion); 0.63 (after 60 min infusion) AUC_{0-24} 4.70 µg h/mL V_{ss} 639 L $T_{1/2}$ 42.4 hr
Plasma protein binding	Quinupristin—55% to 78% Dalfopristin—11% to 26%	31%	92%	71% to 89%
Most common adverse events	Venous irritation Arthralgia Myalgia Nausea Diarrhea Vomiting Rash	Nausea Vomiting Thrombocytopenia (~2.4%) Myelosuppression	Constipation Injection-site reactions Nausea Headache Diarrhea Vomiting CPK elevation (2–3%)	Nausea Vomiting Diarrhea SGPT increase (5.6%) SGOT increase (4.3%)

Abbreviations: CAP, community-acquired pneumonia; CPK, creatinine phosphokinase; FDA, U.S. Food and Drug Administration; IV, intravenous; MRSA, methicillin-resistant *Staphylococcus aureus*; MSSA, methicillin-sensitive *Staphylococcus aureus*; PCN-S, penicillin-sensitive; PK, pharmacokinetic; PO, oral therapy; SGOT, serum glumatic oxaloacetic transaminase; SGPT, serum glumatic pyruvic transaminase; SSSI, skin and skin structure infection; VRE, vancomycin-resistant enterococci.

TABLE 2 Advantages and Disadvantages of Five *Staphylococcus aureus* Active Parenteral Antimicrobial Agents: The Bottom Line

	Vancomycin (Vancocin)	Quinupristin/dalfopristin (Synercid)	Linezolid (Zyvox)	Daptomycin (Cubicin)	Tigecycline (Tygacil)
The "Good"	With the exception of the small incidences of VRSA and VISA, virtually all strains of *S. aureus* are susceptible to vancomycin The vast majority of CoNS are susceptible Inexpensive	The total treatment duration required may be 1 to 2 days shorter compared to vancomycin (for MRSA), oxacillin, or cefazolin (32)	PO formulation 100% bioavailable Hospital length of stay is 1 to 2.5 days shorter compared with vancomycin (13,33,34)	Administered once daily over 30 minutes Exhibits rapid bactericidal action Penetrates well into pus (~68%) More rapid clinical response and a 1-day shorter duration of therapy for complicated SSSIs (35) FDA approved for endocarditis (right sided only)	Expanded spectrum of activity against Gram-positive, Gram-negative, and anaerobic bacteria Not affected by extended-spectrum beta-lactamases Enhanced penetration into many tissues
The "Bad"	Outpatients must receive IV therapy; PO form not absorbed Requires therapeutic drug monitoring (vancomycin	Bacteriostatic against *E. faecium* Inhibits the cytochrome P450 3A4 pathway, and caution is warranted with concomitant use of other	The cost of IV or PO is approximately $140 or $106 per day (36) Requires weekly CBCs in patients on prolonged therapy (>2 weeks)	Requires weekly CPK determinations in patients receiving >1 week of therapy	Bacteriostatic against most pathogens Structurally similar to tetracycline antibiotics, and therefore may have similar adverse effects

serum concentrations) in many patients Poor lung tissue penetration Bacteriostatic against *Enterococcus* and many clinical MRSA	medications eliminated via this pathway (may increase concentrations of cyclosporine, nifedipine, and midazolam) IV therapy is approximately $320 per day (36)	Reversible, nonselective MAO inhibitor; therefore has potential to interact with adrenergic and serotonergic agents	Not an option for pneumonia (35); inactivated by lung surfactant Slower bactericidal activity against MRSA than against MSSA	(photosensitivity, pseudotumor cerebri, pancreatitis, and anti-anabolic action).
The "Ugly" Enhances the toxicities of aminoglycosides (37) Significant mortality rate in patients treated with vancomycin for MRSA pneumonia VISA and VRSA In 2002, 37.5% of enterococcal isolates causing infection in U.S. ICUs were VRE (38)	*Enterococcus faecalis* is resistant in vitro to quinupristin/dalfopristin Arthralgias and myalgias can be severe Drug is rarely used because of adverse effects	Can suppress the bone marrow in a time-dependent manner (39) Can cause optic neuritis/optic neuropathy (40–42)	Associated with an occasional elevation in CPK levels in patients and volunteers, resulting in transient muscle weakness and myalgia (29)	Limited clinical data

Abbreviations: CBC, complete blood count; CoNS, coagulase-negative staphylococci; CPK, creatine phosphokinase; FDA, U.S. Food and Drug Administration; IV, intravenous; MAO, monoamine oxidase; PO, oral therapy; VRE, vancomycin-resistant enterococci; VISA, vancomycin-intermediate *Staphylococcus aureus*; VRSA, vancomycin-resistant *Staphylococcus aureus*.

TABLE 3 Antibiotic Regimens for *Staphylococcus aureus* Native Valve Endocarditis

	Dose	Duration (wks)	Weekly labs
Methicillin-susceptible			
Nafcillin or oxacillin[a]	2 g IV q 4 h	4–6	CBC, creat, LFT
Cefazolin[a]	2 g IV q 8 h	4–6	CBC, creat, LFT
Vancomycin[a]	15–20 mg/kg IV 12 h	4–6	CBC, creat, trough (15–20 µg/mL)
Methicillin-resistant			
Vancomycin[a]	15–20 mg/kg IV 12 h	4–6	CBC, creat, trough (15–20 µg/mL)
Daptomycin[a]	6 mg/kg/day	4–6	CBC, creat, LFT, CPK
Glycopeptide-resistant (vancomycin MIC >2 µg/ml[b])			
Daptomycin	6–8 mg/kg/day	6	CBC, creat, LFT, CPK
Linezolid	600 mg IV q 12 h	6	CBC, creat, LFT

Note: For methicillin-susceptible strains where beta-lactamase production is ruled out by nitrocefin disk, use Penicillin G 3 to 4 million units IV q 4 hr. Vancomycin should be infused over 60–90 minutes to avoid histamine reactions causing "redman syndrome." For patients with this reaction despite slow infusion, the author has administered vancomycin as a continuous infusion successfully.
[a]Optional but highly recommended: gentamicin 1 mg/kg IV q 8–2 hr to maintain serum peak concentrations 3–4 µg/mL and trough concentrations 0.2–0.6 µg/mL. Duration of 4–7 days or until bacteremia quenched.
[b]No formal studies available. Recommendations are based on case reports and animal model experiments.
Abbreviations: CBC, complete blood count; CPK, creatinine phosphokinase; creat, creatinine; IV, intravenous; LFT, liver function test; MIC, minimum inhibitory concentration.

tachycardia, fever, or hypothermia). Patients demonstrating systemic toxicity should be admitted to an intensive care setting and evaluated by blood culture, hematology, and chemistry labs including a creatinine phosphokinase (CPK) level, and radiographic imaging of the involved site where indicated. Note, however, that even in cases of toxic shock syndrome caused by *S. aureus* soft tissue infection, the yield from blood cultures is very low (< 1%).

TABLE 4 Antibiotic Regimens for *Staphylococcus aureus* Prosthetic Valve Endocarditis

	Dose	Duration (wks)	Weekly labs
Methicillin-susceptible			
Nafcillin or oxacillin	2 g IV q 4 h	6–6	CBC, creat, LFT
PLUS			
Gentamicin	1 mg/kg IV q 8–12 h	2	Creat, peak (3–4 µg/mL), trough (0.3–0.6 µg/mL)
PLUS			
Rifampin[a]	300 mg PO/IV q 8 h	6–8	CBC, LFT
Methicillin-resistant			
Vancomycin	15–20 mg/kg IV 12 h	4–6	CBC, creat, trough (15–20 µg/mL)
PLUS			
Gentamicin	1 mg/kg IV q 8–12 h	2	Creat, peak (3–4 µg/mL), trough (0.3–0.6 µg/mL)
PLUS			
Rifampin[a]	300 mg PO/IV q 8 h	6–8	CBC, LFT

[a]Generally added 5 days after initiation of antimicrobial therapy or preferably after bacteremia clears.
Abbreviations: CBC, complete blood count; creat, creatinine; IV, intravenous; LFT, liver function test; PO, oral therapy.

For patients without systemic symptoms, additional queries and exam findings should be entertained looking for more severe infection. This is particularly important in the ever-increasing medically (e.g., elderly and rheumatologic disease) and pharmacologically (e.g., organ transplant patients and those on glucocorticoid therapy) immunosuppressed patient population where systemic signs of inflammation may not be present despite severe infection. These include:

- Careful history to determine the rate of progression or spread,
- Pain out of proportion to cutaneous findings, suggestive of severe deep infection such as fasciitis or pyomyositis,
- Formation of bullae or cutaneous hemorrhage, and
- Anesthesia of the skin overlying disease.

Note that patients with underlying neuropathy may tend to underestimate severity of infection as gauged by pain and those with severe peripheral vascular disease may not develop marked warmth and erythema.

Basic management principles surrounding all soft tissue infection, regardless of the microbiology, is prompt surgical debridement of devitalized tissues, drainage of abscess fluid, and removal of associated prosthetic devices in cases of severe infection. Failure to adhere to this principle will severely hamper the efficacy of therapy. Controversies may arise, as these decisions are frequently made at the discretion of individual physician clinical judgment. It is important to understand that infection may initially continue to evolve even in the presence of appropriate antimicrobial therapy and daily assessment for development of complications requiring surgical debridement.

A list of available systemic agents for the treatment of *S. aureus* soft tissue infection is given in Table 5. Note that the choices of therapy will be individualized based on severity of infection, patient allergies, and the presence other co-pathogens such as Gram-negatives and/or anaerobes. Rigorous clinical data are lacking to guide many practitioners facing soft tissue infections caused by community-associated MRSA organisms harboring Panton-Valentine leukocidin. After drainage of abscesses where appropriate, patients with residual cellulitis should be considered for parenteral or oral antimicrobial therapy based on severity of infection. The majority of these infections can be treated with oral antibiotics. The authors have successfully employed minocycline with the option od additional rifampin with chlohexidine-based skin baths. For centers where a D-test has confirmed the absence of inducible resistance to clindamcyin in most CA-MRSA, clindamycin offers a therapeutic option.

Bone and Joint Infections

S. aureus is the most common pathogen in osteomyelitis, septic arthritis, and prosthetic joint infections. Mortality for bone and joint infections is typically not very high; however, morbidity and long-term functional impairment is. Management consists of a combination of surgery to remove devitalized bone and prolonged intravenous (IV) antibiotic therapy, typically for 6 weeks. Limited high-quality data exists with antimicrobial therapy used for bone and joint infections, and therefore it is nearly impossible to make evidence-based recommendations. Our antibiotic recommendations are shown in Table 6.

TABLE 5 Antimicrobial Therapy for Skin and Skin Structure Infections Due to
Staphylococcus aureus

	Dose	Comment
Methicillin-susceptible		
Nafcillin/oxacillin	1–2 g IV q 4 h	Preferred agent
Cefazolin	2 g IV q 8 h[a]	
Clindamycin	600 mg IV q 8 h	Must request "D-test"
	450 mg PO q 8 h	if macrolide-R
Dicloxacillin	500 mg PO q 6 h	
Cephalexin	500 mg PO q 6 h[a]	
Minocycline	100 mg PO q 12 h	
TMP-SMZ	2 doses PO q 12 h or	
	1 dose PO q 12 h[a]	
Methicillin-resistant		
Vancomycin	30 mg/kg/day in 2 or 3 divided	Trough 10–20 µg/mL
	doses[a]	
Linezolid	600 mg IV or PO q 12 h	
Daptomycin	4–6 mg/kg IV qd[a]	Author prefers 6 mg/kg
Tigecycline	100 mg IV x1, followed by 50 mg IV	Dose should be 25 mg
	q 12 h	IV q 12 h in severe hepatic
		impairment
Minocycline	100 mg PO q 12 h	
Clindamycin	600 mg IV q 8 h	Must request "D-test" if
	450 mg PO q 8 h	macrolide-R
TMP-SMZ	2 doses PO q 12 h or	
	1 dose PO q 12 h[a]	

Note: Duration of therapy is usually 7 to 14 days.
[a]Regimens require dose adjustment for renal insufficiency.
Abbreviations: IV, intravenous; PO, oral therapy; TMP-SMZ, trimethoprim-sulfamethoxazole.

Patients with infections of the spine require special mention, particularly those with underlying comorbidities like diabetes and end-stage renal disease who have infections caused by MRSA. It has been the experience of many clinicians, including the authors, that 6–8 weeks of parenteral antimicrobial therapy may not suffice to eradicate infection, and relapses of infections are seen. We have had success by employing an extended (3–6 months) of oral minocycline and rifampin combination therapy for susceptible organisms if significant radiographic disease persists by MRI or if the sedimentation rate remains markedly elevated at the end of parenteral therapy. Patients who do not respond to this approach would be re-evaluated for surgical therapy.

Respiratory Tract Infections

S. aureus, including MRSA, is among the most common cause of nosocomial pneumonia (16). In addition, recent reports have shown that *S. aureus* and MRSA have been associated with severe community-acquired pneumonia in previously healthy children and adults (17,18).

A list of agents available for the treatment of *S. aureus* soft pneumonia is given in Table 7. Currently, vancomycin is the first choice at many institutions for the treatment of nosocomial pneumonia due to MRSA. However, poor response to

TABLE 6 Antimicrobial Therapy for Osteomyelitis Due to *Staphylococcus aureus*

	Dose	Comment
Methicillin-susceptible		
Nafcillin or oxacillin	2 g IV q 4 h	Preferred agent
Cefazolin	2 g IV q 8 h[a]	
Clindamycin	600 mg IV q 8 h	Must request "D-test" if macrolide-R
	450 mg PO q 8 h	
Dicloxacillin	500 mg PO q 6 h	
Cephalexin	500 mg PO q 6 h[a]	
Minocycline	100 mg PO q 12 h	
TMP-SMZ	2 doses PO q 12 h[a]	
Rifampin	300 mg PO/IV q 8 h	Optional adjuvant therapy
Methicillin-resistant		
Vancomycin	15–20 mg/kg q 12 h[a]	Trough 15–20 μg/mL
Linezolid	600 mg IV or PO q 12 h	
Clindamycin	600 mg IV q 8 h	Must request "D-test" if macrolide-R
	450 mg PO q 8 h	
Minocycline	100 mg PO q 12 h	
TMP-SMZ	2 doses PO q 12 h[a]	
Rifampin	300 mg PO/IV q 8 h	Optional adjuvant therapy

Note: There is minimal high-quality evidence on the optimal antimicrobial therapy for osteomyelitis. Duration of therapy is usually 6 weeks. Osteomyelitis with implanted hardware may require up to 6 months of therapy. Removal of hardware is essential.
[a]Regimens require dose adjustment for renal insufficiency.
Abbreviations: IV, intravenous; PO, oral therapy; TMP-SMZ, trimethoprim-sulfamethoxazole.

vancomycin may occur in a significant number of patients with MRSA pneumonia (19,20). This viewpoint has prompted a variety of strategies to improve the results of vancomycin therapy. We recently recommended dosing vancomycin to achieve a total 24-hr AUC/MIC (area under the concentration time curve divided by the minimum inhibitory concentration) of approximately 400 for management of *S. aureus* pneumonia (21). The most recent American Thoracic Society and Infectious Disease Society of America guidelines now recommend higher vancomycin trough levels of 15 to 20 μg/mL (22), which would require doses of approximately 20 mg/kg every 12 hr in patients with normal renal function. Vancomycin dosing to achieve peaks and troughs of 15 to 20 μg/mL when the

TABLE 7 Antimicrobial Therapy for *Staphylococcus aureus* Pneumonia

	Dose	Comment
Methicillin-susceptible		
Nafcillin/oxacillin	2 g IV q 4 h	Preferred agent
Clindamycin	600 mg IV q 8 h	Must request "D-test" if macrolide-R
	450 mg PO q 8 h	
Dicloxacillin	500 mg PO q 6 h	
Methicillin-resistant		
Vancomycin	15–20 mg/kg IV q12 h[a]	Trough 15–20 μg/mL
Linezolid	600 mg IV or PO q 12 h	

Note: Duration of therapy is usually 7 to 14 days.
[a]Regimen requires dose adjustment for renal insufficiency.
Abbreviations: IV, intravenous; PO, oral therapy.

vancomycin MIC is 0.5 or $1.0\,\mu g/mL$ would typically achieve a threshold 24-hr AUC/MIC ratio of 400. However, when the MIC is $2.0\,\mu g/mL$, a 24-hr AUC of 800, or an average steady state concentration of $33\,\mu g/mL$, would be required; which is typically not achieved clinically. Not surprisingly, a recent investigation found that vancomycin efficacy was significantly lower for MRSA pneumonia when vancomycin MIC values were $2.0\,\mu g/mL$, despite achieving target trough concentrations of $>15\,\mu g/mL$ (23).

THE FUTURE IN *S. AUREUS* TREATMENT

Dalbavancin, telavancin, and ceftobiprole are currently under clinical investigation for the management of *S. aureus* infections. Dalbavancin (once-weekly) and telavancin (once-daily) are semisynthetic lipoglycopeptides that are under investigation for the management of skin and soft tissue infections, bacteremia (dalbavancin only), and pneumonia (24–26). Ceftobiprole is an anti-MRSA beta-lactam in Phase III clinical trials (27) that also has an extended spectrum of Gram-negative activity (28). It will be interesting to observe the evolution of the antimicrobial repertoire against *S. aureus,* as this pathogen continues to adapt to our therapeutic strategies.

REFERENCES

1. Langmuir AD, Worthen TD, Solomon J, Ray CG, Petersen E. The Thucydides syndrome. A new hypothesis for the cause of the plague of Athens. N Engl J Med 1985; 313(16):1027–30.
2. Olson PE, Hames CS, Benenson AS, Genovese EN. The Thucydides syndrome: Ebola deja vu? (or Ebola reemergent?). Emerg Infect Dis 1996; 2(2):155–6.
3. Peacock SJ, de Silva I, Lowy FD. What determines nasal carriage of *Staphylococcus aureus*? Trends Microbiol 2001; 9(12):605–10.
4. Proctor RA. Respiration and small-colony variants of *Staphylococcus aureus*. In: Fischetti VA, Novick RP, Ferretti JJ, Portnoy DA, Rood JI, eds. Gram-Positive Pathogens. Washington D.C.: ASM Press, 2000.
5. Moreillon P, Que YA, Glauser MP. *Staphylococcus aureus* (including Staphylococcal toxic shock). In: Mandell GL, Bennett JE, Dolin R, eds. Principles and Practices of Infectious Diseases. 6th ed. Philadelphia, PA: Elsevier Inc, 2005; 2321–50.
6. Lyytikainen O, Ruotsalainen E, Jarvinen A, Valtonen V, Ruutu P. Trends and outcome of nosocomial and community-acquired bloodstream infections due to *Staphylococcus aureus* in Finland, 1995-2001. Eur J Clin Microbiol Infect Dis 2005; 24(6):399–404.
7. Albrecht SJ, Fishman NO, Kitchen J, et al. Reemergence of Gram-negative health care-associated bloodstream infections. Arch Intern Med 2006; 166(12):1289–94.
8. Falagas ME, Bakossi A, Pappas VD, Holevas PV, Bouras A, Stamata E. Secular trends of blood isolates in patients from a rural area population hospitalized in a tertiary center in a small city in Greece. BMC Microbiol 2006; 6:41.
9. Safdar A, Rodriguez GH, Balakrishnan M, Tarrand JJ, Rolston KV. Changing trends in etiology of bacteremia in patients with cancer. Eur J Clin Microbiol Infect Dis 2006; 25(8):522–6.
10. Wu CJ, Lee HC, Lee NY, et al. Predominance of Gram-negative bacilli and increasing antimicrobial resistance in nosocomial bloodstream infections at a university hospital in southern Taiwan, 1996-2003. J Microbiol Immunol Infect 2006; 39(2):135–43.
11. Steinberg JP, Clark CC, Hackman BO. Nosocomial and community-acquired *Staphylococcus aureus* bacteremias from 1980 to 1993: impact of intravascular devices and methicillin resistance. Clin Infect Dis 1996; 23(2):255–9.

12. Wisplinghoff H, Bischoff T, Tallent SM, Seifert H, Wenzel RP, Edmond MB. Nosocomial bloodstream infections in US hospitals: analysis of 24,179 cases from a prospective nationwide surveillance study. Clin Infect Dis 2004; 39(3):309–17.
13. Cosgrove SE, Sakoulas G, Perencevich EN, Schwaber MJ, Karchmer AW, Carmeli Y. Comparison of mortality associated with methicillin-resistant and methicillin-susceptible *Staphylococcus aureus* bacteremia: a meta-analysis. Clin Infect Dis 2003; 36(1):53–9.
14. Whitby M, McLaws ML, Berry G. Risk of death from methicillin-resistant *Staphylococcus aureus* bacteraemia: a meta-analysis. Med J Aust 2001; 175(5):264–7.
15. Fowler VG Jr, Olsen MK, Corey GR, et al. Clinical identifiers of complicated *Staphylococcus aureus* bacteremia. Arch Intern Med 2003; 163(17):2066–72.
16. National Nosocomial Infections Surveillance (NNIS) System Report, data summary from January 1992 through June 2004, issued October 2004. Am J Infect Control 2004; 32(8):470–85.
17. Johnston BL. Methicillin-resistant *Staphylococcus aureus* as a cause of community-acquired pneumonia–a critical review. Semin Respir Infect 1994; 9(3):199–206.
18. Hageman JC, Uyeki TM, Francis JS, et al. Severe community-acquired pneumonia due to *Staphylococcus aureus*, 2003-04 influenza season. Emerg Infect Dis 2006; 12(6):894–9.
19. Moise PA, Schentag JJ. Vancomycin treatment failures in *Staphylococcus aureus* lower respiratory tract infections. Int J Antimicrob Agents 2000; 16(Suppl. 1):S31–4.
20. Moise PA, Forrest A, Birmingham MC, Schentag JJ. The efficacy and safety of linezolid as treatment for *Staphylococcus aureus* infections in compassionate use patients who are intolerant of, or who have failed to respond to, vancomycin. J Antimicrob Chemother 2002; 50(6):1017–26.
21. Moise-Broder PA, Forrest A, Birmingham MC, Schentag JJ. Pharmacodynamics of vancomycin and other antimicrobials in patients with *Staphylococcus aureus* lower respiratory tract infections. Clin Pharmacokinet 2004; 43(13):925–42.
22. Guidelines for the management of adults with hospital-acquired, ventilator-associated, and healthcare-associated pneumonia. Am J Respir Crit Care Med 2005; 171(4):388–416.
23. Hidayat LK, Hsu DI, Quist R, Shriner KA, Wong-Beringer A. High-dose vancomycin therapy for methicillin-resistant *Staphylococcus aureus* infections: efficacy and toxicity. Arch Intern Med 2006; 166(19):2138–44.
24. Scheinfeld N. Dalbavancin: a review for dermatologists. Dermatol Online J 2006; 12(4):6.
25. Van Bambeke F. Glycopeptides and glycodepsipeptides in clinical development: a comparative review of their antibacterial spectrum, pharmacokinetics and clinical efficacy. Curr Opin Investig Drugs 2006; 7(8):740–9.
26. Kanafani ZA. Telavancin: a new lipoglycopeptide with multiple mechanisms of action. Expert Rev Anti Infect Ther 2006; 4(5):743–9.
27. Page MG. Anti-MRSA beta-lactams in development. Curr Opin Pharmacol 2006; 6(5):480–5.
28. Chambers HF. Ceftobiprole: in-vivo profile of a bactericidal cephalosporin. Clin Microbiol Infect 2006; 12(Suppl. 2):17–22.
29. Fenton C, Keating GM, Curran MP. Daptomycin. Drugs 2004; 64(4):445–55.
30. Barriere JC, Berthaud N, Beyer D, Dutka-Malen S, Paris JM, Desnottes JF. Recent developments in streptogramin research. Curr Pharm Des 1998; 4(2):155–80.
31. Shinabarger DL, Marotti KR, Murray RW, et al. Mechanism of action of oxazolidinones: effects of linezolid and eperezolid on translation reactions. Antimicrob Agents Chemother 1997; 41(10):2132–6.
32. Carbon C. Costs of treating infections caused by methicillin-resistant staphylococci and vancomycin-resistant enterococci. J Antimicrob Chemother 1999; 44(Suppl. A):31–6.
33. Li Z, Willke RJ, Pinto LA, et al. Comparison of length of hospital stay for patients with known or suspected methicillin-resistant *Staphylococcus* species infections treated with linezolid or vancomycin: a randomized, multicenter trial. Pharmacotherapy 2001; 21(3):263–74.

34. Willke RJ, Glick HA, Li JZ, Rittenhouse BE. Effects of linezolid on hospital length of stay compared with vancomycin in treatment of methicillin-resistant *Staphylococcus* infections. An application of multivariate survival analysis. Int J Technol Assess Health Care 2002; 18(3):540–54.
35. Pegues DA. Daptomycin: a viewpoint by david a. Pegues. Drugs 2004; 64(4):457–8.
36. Fowler VG Jr, Boucher HW, Corey GR, et al. Daptomycin versus standard therapy for bacteremia and endocarditis caused by *Staphylococcus aureus*. N Engl J Med 2006; 355(7):653–65.
37. Rybak MJ, Abate BJ, Kang SL, Ruffing MJ, Lerner SA, Drusano GL. Prospective evaluation of the effect of an aminoglycoside dosing regimen on rates of observed nephrotoxicity and ototoxicity. Antimicrob Agents Chemother 1999; 43(7):1549–55.
38. National Nosocomial Infections Surveillance (NNIS) System Report, data summary from January 1992 through June 2003, issued August 2003. Am J Infect Control 2003; 31(8):481–98.
39. Gerson SL, Kaplan SL, Bruss JB, et al. Hematologic effects of linezolid: summary of clinical experience. Antimicrob Agents Chemother 2002; 46(8):2723–6.
40. Frippiat F, Bergiers C, Michel C, Dujardin JP, Derue G. Severe bilateral optic neuritis associated with prolonged linezolid therapy. J Antimicrob Chemother 2004; 53(6):1114–5.
41. McKinley SH, Foroozan R. Optic neuropathy associated with linezolid treatment. J Neuroophthalmol 2005; 25(1):18–21.
42. Saijo T, Hayashi K, Yamada H, Wakakura M. Linezolid-induced optic neuropathy. Am J Ophthalmol 2005; 139(6):1114–6.

6 Enterococci: Resistance Update and Treatment Options

Peter K. Linden
*Department of Critical Care Medicine, University of Pittsburgh Medical Center,
Pittsburgh, Pennsylvania, U.S.A.*

INTRODUCTION

Enterococci are Gram-positive, facultative bacteria that comprise part of the normal colonizing microflora of the human intestines with variable secondary reservoirs in the oropharynx, female genital tract, and skin surface (1). The genus *Enterococcus* was recognized as a distinct taxonomy only as recently as 1984 and consists of at least 17 species (2). It has long been reported that the vast majority of human infections are caused by *E. faecalis* (80–90%) and *E. faecium* (5–10%) strains followed by infrequent infection due to *E. raffinosus*, *E. avium*, *E. durans*, *E. gallinarum,* and other species. More recently, however, some centers have noted an increase in *E. faecium* isolates to as high as 22% of all enterococcal isolates (3). Although enterococci may possess virulence properties including hemolysins, aggregation substance, gelatinase, proadherence factors, and others, they are generally considered to be of relatively low virulence and invasiveness but still capable of producing a wide range of opportunistic infections when anatomic breaches occur. Enterococci are also quite capable of promulgating systemic inflammatory response, severe sepsis, and septic shock and have been a frequent inciting blood pathogen in recent sepsis trials (4). Such infections can be monomicrobial (i.e., endocarditis) but are often polymicrobial due to the presence of other enteric pathogens, particularly in the hepatobiliary tree and other intra-abdominal sites.

Based on serial surveillance data since the 1980s, the epidemiologic impact from enterococcal infection has dramatically increased particularly in the nosocomial setting and become a significant public health concern due principally to newly acquired resistance; in a nationwide surveillance study [Surveillance and Control of Pathogens of Epidemiological (SCOPE) Importance] between 1995 and 2002 enterococci were the third most frequent cause of nosocomial bloodstream infection and high-level vancomycin resistance was present in 60% of *E. faecium* strains but only 2% of *E. faecalis* (5). A Centers for Disease Control and Prevention surveillance program during the same time period showed that vancomycin-resistant enterococci (VRE) accounted for 27.5% of ICU nosocomial bacteremic and nonbacteremic infections (6). The principal forces behind this important trend include the increased prevalence and greater longevity of immunocompromised hosts due to native or iatrogenic immunosuppression, the increased use of antimicrobials that are devoid of enterococcal activity (cephalosporins, quinolones) or selective for more resistant phenotypes, and, most importantly, the appearance of new resistance mechanisms (i.e., high-level vancomycin resistance) that confer resistance to previously effective antimicrobial classes. This chapter focuses on the important trends in enterococcal antimicrobial resistance, particularly glycopeptide resistance, their clinical impact, and strategies for effective treatment, prevention, and control.

ENTEROCOCCAL RESISTANCE
Intrinsic Resistance Mechanisms
Enterococci possess a broad array of constitutive, nontransferable resistance mechanisms against a variety of antimicrobials, which both reduces baseline therapeutic options and magnifies the effect of superimposed acquired resistance traits (Table 1). Relative or absolute resistance to the beta-lactams (penicillin, ampicillin, antipseudomonal penicillins, cephalosporins) is expressed in all enterococci including those strains without prior beta-lactam exposure due to structural changes of the inner-cell wall low molecular weight penicillin-binding proteins (PBPs), which confer low affinity for these compounds (7). Exposure of such enterococcal strains to an effective beta-lactam results in inhibitory but not bactericidal activity as measured by time-killing kinetic curves (8). This "tolerance" property has clinical import only in those clinical scenarios where eradication of the infection requires bactericidal effect (endovascular infection, meningitis) but which is not required for the majority of enterococcal infections.

Low-level resistance to aminoglycosides derive from their low penetrability through the outer perimeter envelope of the organism, a property that can be overcome with the synergistic activity of an effective cell wall active agent such as a penicillin or vancomycin (9). Although the majority of enterococci exhibit in vitro susceptibility to trimethoprim/sulfamethoxazole their ability to utilize exogenous folate in vivo precludes the clinical utility of trimethoprim-sulfamethoxazole and other agents which impair folate synthesis (10). A significant percentage of enterococci may also possess constitutive resistance to macrolides (erythromycin, azithromycin) and lincosamides (clindamycin) primarily mediated by ribosomal modifications (11).

Acquired Resistance Mechanisms
There are few other species of bacteria that have the proclivity and efficiency of the *Enterococcus* to acquire new and multiple antimicrobial resistance mechanisms (Table 1).

TABLE 1 Intrinsic and Acquired Resistance Mechanisms Among Enterococci

Antimicrobial	Mechanism(s)	Comments
Ampicillin, penicillin	Altered binding protein	
Aminoglycosides (LL)	Decreased permeability	High level gentamicin strains may be
	Altered ribosomal binding	susceptible to high level streptomycin
Clindamycin	Altered ribosomal binding	
Tetracyclines	Efflux pump	
Trimethoprim	Can utilize folate	
Acquired		
Ampicillin, penicillin (HL)	Mutation of PPB 5	95% of *E. faecium*
		<5% *E. faecalis*
Aminoglycoside (HL)	Enzyme modification	
Quinolones	DNA gyrase mutation	
Chloramphenicol	Efflux pump	
Glycopeptide	Altered cell wall binding	Transposon *1546*
Quinupristin/dalfopristin	Ribosomal modification	*ermB* gene
	Efflux pump	*vatD, vatE* gene
Linezolid	Point mutation	G2476U mutation
Daptomycin	Unknown	

Abbreviations: HL, high level; LL, low level; PPB, pencillin-binding protein.

The genomic elements, which encode for resistance are carried on plasmids or larger transposon elements, are stable, and often carry multiple resistance determinants that culminate in multidrug-resistant strains. Enterococci acquire resistance to chloramphenicol (mediated by chloramphenicol acetyltransferase), quinolones (by gyrase mutations), rifampin (by mutation of the gene that encodes for RNA polymerase), and to tetracyclines by a variety of mechanisms (12). However, the most clinically important antimicrobials to which enterococci have acquired resistance are discussed in more detail below.

High-Level Beta-Lactam Resistance

Overproduction and/or mutation of the PBP 5 receptor leading to diminished affinity for beta-lactams has increased dramatically in *E. faecium* but remains uncommon (<5%) among *E. faecalis* strains (13,14). This property is expressed constitutively and carried by resistance genes located on chromosomal elements. *E. faecium* strains with acquired high-level ampicillin resistance have ampicillin minimum inhibitory concentrations (MICs) >128 µg/mL and are neither inhibited nor killed by ampicillin, penicillin or other beta-lactams. The ubiquity of high-level ampicillin resistance has been a major step toward the eventual evolution of multidrug resistance among *E. faecium* as the superimposition of other resistance traits have appeared in such strains.

High-Level Aminoglycoside Resistance

The first reports of high-level gentamicin resistant (HLGR) strains in the United States were in 1979, appearing in both *E. faecalis* and *E. faecium* (15). More recent surveillance data from the SCOPE program between the years 1997 and 1999 showed 69–71% of all U.S. enterococcal strains were HLGR and 40% of all tested were VRE strains (16). Enterococci acquire resistance to aminoglycosides via (*i*) changes in the ribosomal attachment sites; (*ii*) diminished aminoglycoside transport into the cell; (*iii*) aminoglycoside-modifying enzymes (adenyltransferase, phosphotransferase, and bifunctional acetyl-phosphotransferase). The first two mechanisms are encoded by chromosomal mutations while the modifying enzymes are mediated by plasmids. Although the majority of HLGR strains also exhibit high-level streptomycin resistance, a minority retain sensitivity to streptomycin and thus susceptibility testing to high-level streptomycin is worthwhile in HLGR strains (18,19). No reliable bactericidal activity can be achieved with any antimicrobial combination against strains with high-level aminoglycoside resistance. Thus an optimal antimicrobial regimen for such enterococcal infections that require bactericidal activity, i.e., endocarditis, does not exist. Valve replacement may be required if a trial of high dose ampicillin is unsuccessful (20).

Beta-Lactamase Production

Penicillinase-producing strains of *E. faecalis* were first described in 1979, however this phenomenon has remained quite localized and rare to the present time and confined to *E. faecalis* species only (21). Specific penicillinase detection using routine laboratory testing methods may fail to detect such strains since the quantity of penicillinase production is small (22). Penicillinase-inhibitors (clavulanate, sulbactam, tazobactam) do restore susceptibility to the parent beta-lactams (amoxicillin, ampicillin, piperacillin) and are clinically effective in combination therapy. Vancomycin is also a feasible therapeutic alternative in beta-lactam allergic or -intolerant individuals.

Vancomycin and Other Glycopeptide Resistance
Epidemiology
Without question, the appearance of E. faecium strains with high-level vancomycin resistance in France and England in 1986 was a major watershed mark in the evolution of enterococcal antimicrobial resistance and the final step toward the subsequent establishment of endemic multidrug-resistant enterococci (22,23). VRE strains did not first appear in the United States until 1989, but thereafter their incidence rapidly increased from 0.3% of all enterococci in 1989 to 7.9% in 1993 (24). During this early period the majority of reported VRE isolates were almost exclusively E. faecium, were mono- or pauciclonal in origin, and predominantly originated from ICU patients in tertiary care centers particularly in the northeastern United States. Both vanA and vanB genotype outbreaks were observed; however, there was no discernible epidemiologic or clinical differentiation between the two types. Local enhancement of contact precautions usually aborted or significantly modified such outbreaks.

A more contemporaneous surveillance study of bloodstream isolates have shown a steady decrease in vancomycin susceptibility among E. faecium strains from 60% in 1997 to only 39.1% in 2002, while the vast majority (96.1–99.4%) of E. faecalis strains continue to remain vancomycin susceptible over this 5-year period (25). Although the incidence of VRE remains highest in the ICU unit setting, it has increased to a greater relative extent on hospital floors and parahospital centers such as long-term acute care facilities (LTAC) and skilled care nursing facilities which often receive patients from hospitals with endemic VRE epidemiology (26).

Genetic Basis of Vancomycin Resistance
Six distinct glycopeptide resistance phenotypes have been discovered; VanA, VanB, VanC, VanD, VanE, and VanG, distinguished based on gene content, glycopeptide MICs, inducibility, and transferability properties (Table 2) (27). The VanA and VanB phenotypes uniformly confer high-level vancomycin resistance

TABLE 2   Level and Type of Vancomycin Resistance in Enterococci

Strain characteristic	Acquired resistance level, type				Intrinsic resistance, low level, type VanC1/C2/C3	
	High, VanA	Variable, VanB	Moderate, VanD	Low	VanG	VanE
MIC, mg/L						
Vancomycin	64–100	4–1000	64–128	16	8–32	2–32
Teicoplanin	16–512	0.5–1	4–64	0.5	0.5	0.5–1
Conjugation	Positive	Positive	Negative	Positive	Negative	Negative
Mobile element	Tn *1548*	Tn *1547* or Tn *1549*	—	—	—	—
Expression	Inducible	Inducible	Constitutive	Inducible	inducible	Constitutive inducible
Location	Plasmid chromosome	Plasmid chromosome	Chromosome	Chromosome	Chromosome	Chromosome
Modified target	D-Ala-D-Lac	D-Ala-D-Lac	D-Ala-D-Lac	D-Ala-D-Ser	D-Ala-D-Ser	D-Ala-D-Ser

Abbreviations: D-Ala-D-Lac, D-alanine-D-lactate; D-Ala-D-Ser, D-alanine-D-serine; MIC, minimum inhibitory concentration.
Source: From Ref. 27.

(MIC > 64 μg/mL) and have the highest prevalence and clinical importance. Although VanB strains retain susceptibility to teicoplanin, this agent was never commercially available in the United States and rapid resistance has been described when VanB strains undergo teicoplanin exposure (28). Transposon 1546 (Tn1546) contains the *vanA* gene complex, which encodes for an 8-peptide sequence culminating in ligase-mediated modification of the cell wall target for vancomycin from a high affinity D-alanine–D-alanine linkage to a low affinity D-alanine–D-lactate linkage on the cell wall peptidoglycan terminus (29). The *vanB* gene cluster has partial DNA homology with the *vanA* gene cluster and similarly encodes for ligase modification of the vancomycin target. The *vanA* gene has been shown to be transferable in vitro to *Staphylococcus aureus* and naturally occurring *vanA* gene-mediated vancomycin resistance probably due to horizontal transposon transmission has been reported in four methicillin-resistant *S. aureus* (MRSA) strains in three patients with protracted vancomycin exposure for MRSA infection and a fourth patient without prior vancomycin exposure (30–35).

Dynamics and Risk Factors for VRE Colonization and Infection

Colonization with VRE is a necessary prerequisite for VRE superinfection, which arises only when anatomic or other predisposing factors become manifest. Similar to the more susceptible enterococcal strains, the natural colonizing reservoir for VRE is the intestinal tract, with secondary contiguous reservoirs on the skin, genitourinary tract, and oropharynx (36,37). There are three sequential processes leading to detectable VRE colonization and potential subsequent infection with multiple modifiers (Fig. 1): (*i*) Exposure to enterococci containing the vancomycin-resistant genome via contact with an animate or inanimate source. It should be emphasized that the *vanA* gene does not arise from a spontaneous or antibiotic-induced mutation. (*ii*) Amplification of the VRE inoculum within the gastrointestinal reservoir usually due to antimicrobial selective pressures. Prior or ongoing antimicrobials may also enhance the risk of VRE colonization by reducing naturally competing gut flora. (*iii*) Natural or iatrogenic anatomic or immune defects that lead to bloodstream or nonbloodstream (tissue) invasion. Perirectal, rectal, or preferentially stool cultures have been the traditional sites to detect VRE colonization (38,39). Broth pre-enrichment and a selective VRE culture media containing vancomycin maximize both sensitivity and specificity, respectively, although enrichment may lengthen the testing period by 1 to 2 days compared to direct plating of the specimen. Microbroth dilution methods appear superior to agar dilution and automated systems. Media with a higher vancomycin concentration (15 μg/mL) may reduce the isolation of VanC enterococcal strains, which are of lower clinical importance (40). The lower limits of fecal VRE inoculum detection are generally in the range of 10^2 to 10^3 log cfu/g with such methods. Novel and more rapid techniques such as real-time *vanA* or *vanB* gene polymerase chain reaction methods are now commercialized and continue to gain wider acceptance (41).

The duration of VRE intestinal colonization is variable and can last for months to years and may be indefinite, in part due to the inoculum-detection threshold of the testing method employed (42–44). Spontaneous clearance of intestinal colonization only occurs in the minority of patients in several studies analyzing serial cultures both in antimicrobial and nonantimicrobial exposed patients.

Multiple case control and cohort studies have analyzed risk factors for either VRE colonization, VRE superinfection, or both (45–48). Two fundamental

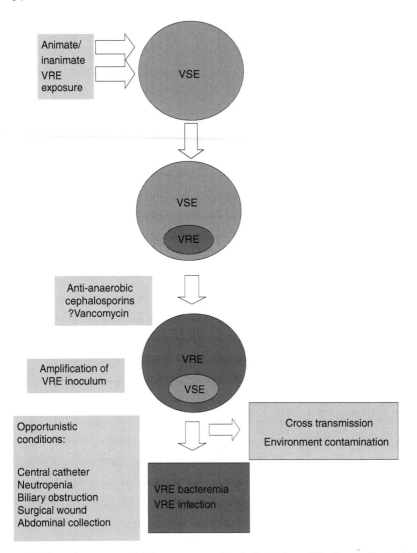

FIGURE 1 Sequence of VRE exposure and antimicrobial amplification leading to VRE super-infection and increased VRE transmission. *Abbreviations*: VRE, vancomycin-resistant enterococci; VSE, vancomycin-susceptible enterococci.

risk factor categories are demographic/illness severity variables and the type, intensity, and duration of recent antimicrobial exposure. Demographic risks include duration of hospitalization and ICU length of stay, physical proximity to VRE colonized patients in the same unit, hospitalization in units with a high prevalence of VRE, and "colonization pressure." Prior administration of multiple antibiotics, third-generation cephalosporins, antimicrobials with anaerobic spectrums (metronidazole, clindamycin), and parenteral vancomycin have been implicated in case-control analyses of colonization or superinfection. Such antimicrobials probably exert a selective effect and amplify otherwise undetectable or smaller VRE inocula in the intestines and other secondary

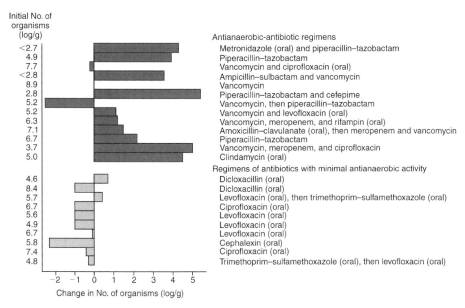

Initial No. of organisms (log/g)

<2.7
4.9
7.7
<2.8
8.9
2.8
5.2
5.2
6.3
7.1
6.7
3.7
5.0

4.6
8.4
5.7
6.7
5.6
4.9
6.7
5.8
7.4
4.8

Antianaerobic-antibiotic regimens
Metronidazole (oral) and piperacillin–tazobactam
Piperacillin–tazobactam
Vancomycin and ciprofloxacin (oral)
Ampicillin–sulbactam and vancomycin
Vancomycin
Piperacillin–tazobactam and cefepime
Vancomycin, then piperacillin–tazobactam
Vancomycin and levofloxacin (oral)
Vancomycin, meropenem, and rifampin (oral)
Amoxicillin–clavulanate (oral), then meropenem and vancomycin
Piperacillin–tazobactam
Vancomycin, meropenem, and ciprofloxacin
Clindamycin (oral)

Regimens of antibiotics with minimal antianaerobic activity
Dicloxacillin (oral)
Dicloxacillin (oral)
Levofloxacin (oral), then trimethoprim–sulfamethoxazole (oral)
Ciprofloxacin (oral)
Levofloxacin (oral)
Levofloxacin (oral)
Levofloxacin (oral)
Cephalexin (oral)
Ciprofloxacin (oral)
Trimethoprim–sulfamethoxazole (oral), then levofloxacin (oral)

Change in No. of organisms (log/g)

FIGURE 2 Effect of exposure to various antimicrobial(s) on the fecal VRE inoculum. *Abbreviation*: VRE, vancomycin-resistant enterococci. *Source*: From Ref. 49.

reservoirs. Donskey and colleagues have demonstrated that the density of VRE as measured by serial quantitative stool cultures increased significantly when patients received ≥ 1 antianaerobic antimicrobial (Fig. 2), while this effect was not seen in patients receiving antimicrobials with minimal antianaerobic activity (50). Interestingly, parenteral vancomycin administration resulted in no increase in the stool VRE density. Moreover, patients with high VRE density coupled with fecal incontinence were also more likely to have positive environmental cultures for VRE. The "VRE-selective" effects of antimicrobials and other risk factors become relatively diminished when the proportion of patients already colonized with VRE is 50% or greater, which may explain some studies where newly introduced antibiotic control measures may only yield modest reductions in VRE colonization and infection rates in hyperendemic settings (51). Patients with comorbidities including oncologic conditions, especially neutropenia, and prior solid organ transplantation, especially liver transplantation, appear to have the highest rates of VRE bacteremia and poorest outcomes.

GENERAL ISSUES IN THE TREATMENT OF ENTEROCOCCAL INFECTION

The treatment of serious enterococcal infection is challenging from several aspects. Since enterococci may colonize skin, wound, and mucosal surfaces, and their isolation is often accompanied by more virulent pathogens, a careful clinical assessment of whether the reported isolate is a likely cause of the patient's clinical syndrome and merits specific treatment is always warranted. Realistically, however, it may be difficult to make this distinction, particularly in patients who have major comorbid conditions or critical illness, which is naturally coupled with colonization or infection due to multidrug-resistant enterococcal infection. Secondly, the clinician must decide whether the patient's condition requires bactericidal (combination) antimicrobial activity, the length of such treatment, and whether nonantimicrobial interventions are needed, such as catheter removal, surgical or radiologic drainage or debridement, or valve replacement.

Does the Isolate Require Antimicrobial Treatment?

Microbiologic culture data that report the presence of enterococci always require some level of clinical discrimination to determine whether they merit treatment. Enterococcal isolates from a respiratory specimen (sputum, endotracheal aspirate, bronchoalveolar lavage), and skin, wound, or musocal surfaces almost always represent colonization. Urine cultures obtained via indwelling bladder (Foley) catheters often represent asymptomatic bacteriuria. Wound and intra-abdominal drains often become colonized with skin flora including enterococci. However, such isolates may be significant when the character of the drainage fluid reveals evidence of inflammatory response, i.e., leukocytes, purulence. Although enterococci may be blood culture contaminants, particularly when specimens are obtained from indwelling intravascular catheters, the appropriate clinical bias should be that such cultures represent true pathogens in most instances. Finally, simple nonantimicrobial interventions may obviate the need for antienterococcal therapy such as removal of intravascular or bladder catheters or superficial wound debridement (52,53).

Is Bactericidal Therapy Required?

The majority of enterococcal infections are not proven to require bactericidal treatment and can be managed successfully with a single effective agent (54,55). Either native- or prosthetic-valve endocarditis is the prototype enterococcal infection for which bactericidal antimicrobial therapy is required, usually achieved with the combination of a cell wall active agent such as ampicillin, penicillin, or vancomycin combined with an aminoglycoside such as gentamicin or streptomycin (1). Other sites of infection for which bactericidal treatment is probably merited include enterococcal meningitis and enterococcemia in a neutropenic host (54). However, a bactericidal combination is not possible to achieve with enterococci exhibiting both high-level aminoglycoside resistance and almost all strains of *E. faecium* strains with high-level vancomycin resistance. An uncommon exception is vancomycin-resistant *E. faecalis* strains that retain ampicillin and high-level gentamicin susceptibility. Successful treatment of such cases has been reported with ampicillin and gentamicin, ampicillin + ofloxacin, penicillin + streptomycin, and linezolid + gentamicin (56). Limited clinical experience is available for the treatment of vancomycin-resistant enterococcal endocarditis with the newer agents, which is detailed below.

TREATMENT OF VRE

Despite the established high prevalence of multidrug-resistant enterococcal strains with high-level vancomycin resistance, there is a remarkable paucity of controlled, comparative trial data on its antimicrobial treatment. Major obstacles have been the slow development of novel agents with VRE activity; high levels of comorbidity, which confounds outcome interpretation; complex surgical infection for which

TABLE 3 Therapeutic Antimicrobial Options for VRE Infection

Antimicrobial(s)	Reported evidence	Comments
High dose ampicillin or ampicilin-sulbactam	Case reports	May be effective with VRE strains with ampicillin MIC 32–64 µg/mL
Chloramphenicol	Case series	Resistance reported
Tetracycline, doxycyline	Case reports	± Rifampin or ciprofloxacin
Novobiocin	Anecdotal	No longer manufactured
Nitrofurantoin	Small case series	Only for UTI
Teicoplanin	Case reports	Not active against VanA Resistance in VanB reported
Quinupristin/dalfopristin	Large case series but noncomparative	Bacteriostatic Not active against *E. faecalis* Resistance reported
Linezolid	1. Dose comparative trial 2. Large compassionate use series	Bacteriostatic Resistance reported
Daptomycin	Case report + series	Bactericidal Resistance reported
Tigecycline	In vitro data only	Bacteriostatic
Dalbavancin	In vitro data only	VanA strains resistant
Telavancin	In vitro data only	
Oritavancin	In vitro data only	

Abbreviations: UTI, urinary tract infection; VRE, vancomycin-resistant enterococci.

antimicrobial therapy alone is not curative; and the polymicrobial nature of many VRE infections, particularly, those occurring in the abdomen.

Both approved and nonapproved treatment options for VRE are summarized in Table 3. At present there are only two FDA-approved treatments for VRE (*E. faecium*) infection, quinupristin/dalfopristin (Q/D, Synercid®) and linezolid (Zyvox®), and two other approved agents that have in vitro activity against VRE but are not approved for VRE infection, daptomycin (Cidecin®), which is approved for complicated skin–skin structure infection (CSSSI) and *S. aureus* bacteremia, and tigecycline (Tygacil®), which is approved for CSSSI and intra-abdominal infection.

Prior to the availability of Q/D and linezolid approval, several centers published their experience with a variety of available agents or combinations that demonstrated in vitro activity. Clinical success was described with high parenteral dosages of ampicillin or ampicillin/sulbactam (18–24 g/day), even including endocarditis. Such a strategy appears limited to those uncommon VRE strains with ampicillin MICs of 32 to 64 µg/mL, a target range for which plasma ampicillin levels can exceed with high-dose therapy (57–59). Since no beta-lactamase elaboration occurs with VRE, the mechanism of sulbactam activity is not known; a plausible explanation is its intrinsic PBP properties.

Chloramphenicol has bacteriostatic activity against enterococci and VRE strains; however, its in vivo efficacy was never established. In a retrospective study of 80 cases of VRE bacteremia, 51 patients were treated with chloramphenicol, from which 22/36 (61%) evaluable patients demonstrated a clinical response (60). A microbiologic response was also observed in 33/43 (79%) of the microbiologically evaluable patients. No survival benefit was observed compared with VRE bacteremic patients in the study cohort who did not receive chloramphenicol. Subsequently at the same center, the prevalence of chloramphenicol resistance among

VRE strains over a 10-year period (1991–2000) were observed to increase from 0% to 11%, a trend that correlated significantly with prior chloramphenicol or quinolone exposure (61). Isolated reports of favorable outcome for VRE infection have also been reported with the use of tetracycline, doxycycline, and oral novobiocin combined with either ciprofloxacin or doxycycline; however, such experience has never been reproduced in larger clinical series of prospective trials (62–65).

Teicoplanin, a glycopeptide not commercially available in the United States, does have in vitro activity versus VanB phenotypic enterococci. In a European study of 63 patients with vancomycin-susceptible enterococcal (VSE) infection, clinical and microbiologic responses were observed in 84% and 87% of cases, respectively (66). This agent remains unstudied for VanB enterococcal infection, perhaps in part to the development of teicoplanin resistance among VanB E. faecalis during teicoplanin therapy (67,68).

Nitrofurantoin has in vitro activity against both VanA and VanB enterococci (69). Due to its ability to achieve high urinary concentrations, nitrofurantoin has been shown to be effective in VRE urinary tract infection (53,70). Nitrofurantoin cannot be employed for VRE outside the urinary tract and in patients with a creatinine clearance < 30 mL/min, since elevated blood concentrations are associated with hepatic, pulmonary, hematologic, and other toxicities.

Quinupristin/Dalfopristin

Quinupristin/Dalfopristin (Q/D) is a semisynthetic parenteral streptogramin combination compound, which is derived from its parent natural compound pristinamycin, a product of Streptomyces pristinaspiralis, an oral and topical anti-staphylococcal agent that has been in clinical use since the 1980s in Europe. The major properties of this compound are summarized in Table 4. This antimicrobial is a 30:70 mixture of quinupristin and dalfopristin, which are semisynthetic derivatives of streptogramin types B and A, respectively. It is a unique antimicrobial since it acts through sequential ribosomal binding and is internally synergistic to produce a bactericidal action. Dalfopristin initially binds to the 50S bacterial ribosome, which induces a permanent conformational change that accelerates quinupristin ribosomal binding (71). Protein synthesis is impaired via both the interruption of peptide chain elongation, and the inhibition of formed peptide extrusion. Such synergism results in bactericidal activity against some important Gram-positive species including S. pneumoniae, S. agalacticae, and some strains of S. aureus. However, only bacteriostatic activity is present for the majority of E. faecium strains by time-killing curve studies. 23S ribosomal modification MLSb phenotype resistant, primarily encoded for by the ermB gene (erythromycin methylase), modifies the ribosomal attachment site for quinupristin, which limits protein-inhibitory activity to only the dalfopristin moiety (72). Erythromycin resistance serves as an excellent surrogate marker for the presence of the MLSb phenotype among enterococci. Q/D is also unique as an antienterococcal agent based on its marked disparity in in vitro susceptibility between E. faecium (MIC90 = 1–2 µg/mL) and E. faecalis (MIC90 = 8–16 µg/mL). This disparity is most likely due to altered ribosomal binding or presence of an active efflux pump. Clinical interest in the utility of Q/D for serious VRE infection began in the mid-1990s with a large-scale, noncomparative, open-label, emergency use program for multiresistant Gram-positive infection, principally vancomycin-resistant E. faecium and MRSA infection refractory or intolerant to vancomycin (73,74). The patient populations in both series had a high prevalence

TABLE 4 Major Features of Quinupristin/Dalfopristin and Linezolid

Feature	Quinupristin/dalfopristin	Linezolid
Antimicrobial class	Streptogramin	Oxazolidinone
Peak serum concentrations (mg/L)	10–12	15.1
Elimination half-life (hr)	0.8 (Q), 0.6 (D)	5.5
Major metabolic routes	Hepatobiliary	Peripheral non-oxidative
Major elimination routes	Fecal (70–75%)	Nonrenal (65%)
	Urinary (19%)	Urinary (30%)
Protein binding (%)	30 (Q) 70 (D)	31
Mechanism of action	Protein synthesis inhibition	Protein synthesis inhibition
Site of action	50S ribosome	70S initiation complex
Post-antibiotic effect (h)	6–8	1
Bactericidal (vs. VRE)	No	No
Cytochrome P-450 inhibition	Yes	No
Formulations	Parenteral	Parenteral + oral
Dose and administration	5–7.5 mg/kg q 8–12h	600 mg q 12h
Dosage adjustment	None	None
Approved indications	VRE	VRE
	Complicated SSSI	Complicated SSSI
	Nosocomial pneumonia	Nosocomial pneumonia
Major adverse effects	Phlebitis (peripheral)	Myelosuppression
	Myalgia/arthralgia	
Cost ($US per day; 2000 values)	$300–350	$115 (parenteral)
		$80 (oral)

Abbreviations: D, dalfopristin; Q, quinupristin; qXh, every X hours; SSSI, skin and skin structure infection; VRE, vancomycin-resistant enterocooci.
Source: From Ref. 17.

of acute and chronic comorbidities including diabetes, oncologic conditions, chronic liver disease, dialysis, mechanical ventilation, and prior organ transplantation. Q/D was administered at 7.5 mg/kg intravenously every 8 hr to patients with documented VRE bacteremia or nonbacteremic VRE infection, with the duration of treatment determined by the primary treating physicians. The overall success rate, defined as both clinical success and bacteriologic eradication, was 65.8% in the initial study and 65.6% in the follow-up study. There have been several reports of clinical cure combining Q/D with doxycycline or high dose-ampicillin in endocarditis; however, no larger scale experience has been performed (75–77).

As Q/D usage increased both before and after its regulatory approval in 1999, several important clinical limitations became apparent. Peripheral intravenous administration was associated with a high rate of phlebitis, necessitating central venous administration. Myalgia and arthralgia unassociated with objective inflammatory signs was observed in 7% to 10% of patients in the emergency use program, with much higher rates in oncologic patients and liver transplant recipients (78,79). Although the precise reason for this toxicity is unknown, a neuropathic cause is suspected. Its higher incidence in populations with diminished metabolism and excretion suggest it is due to either native drug or metabolite accumulation.

Phenotypic resistance to Q/D among *E. faecium* (MIC $\geq 4\,\mu g/mL$) was observed in 6 (1.8%) and 5 (1.3%) of VRE cases either during or after treatment from both published emergency use series (73,74). Clonal dissemination of

Q/D-resistant strains, despite the absence of Q/D or other streptogramin exposure, has been described among pediatric patients (80). Three fundamental resistance mechanisms have been discovered: enzymatic modification (acetylation) of dalfopristin encoded by the *vatD* or *vatE* genes, active efflux by an ATP-binding protein encoded by the *msrC* or *lsa* genes, and alteration of the ribosomal target site encoded for by the *erm* genes (72). Since phenotypic resistance requires the presence of resistance mechanisms to both the quinupristin and dalfopristin components, at least 2 or more resistance genes are present. Several surveillance studies have uncovered large Q/D resistance reservoirs among *E. faecium* isolated from both domestic poultry and livestock in the United States (81). Multiple resistance mechanisms including the *ermB*, *vatA*, *vatB*, and as yet unknown mechanisms appear to be responsible for this phenomenon. Virginiamycin, a streptogramin food additive in use since 1974, may be in part responsible for this observation. In vivo transfer of the *vanA* gene from an *E. faecium* isolate of animal origin to a human *E. faecium* strain has been shown in normal volunteers who ingested both strains (82). Vertical food chain transmission to humans is theoretically possible but does not appear to be common to the present time based on the continued low prevalence of Q/D resistance in human surveillance studies and the distinct pulse-field patterns seen in animal VRE isolates (81).

Linezolid

Linezolid is an oxazolidinedinone compound, a novel synthetic class that inhibits bacterial protein synthesis in a unique fashion via inhibiting the formation of the 70S initiation complex (50S and 30S ribosomes, mRNA, initiation factors 2 and 3, and fMet-tRNA) (83). The major properties of linezolid are summarized in Table 4. Linezolid exhibits a broad Gram-positive spectrum but has only bacteriostatic activity against VRE or VSE with an MIC90 of 2 µg/mL, which is right at the susceptibility breakpoint. FDA approval was granted in 2000 for vancomycin-resistant *E. faecium* infection, as well as for other site indications including community and nosocomial pneumonia, and CSSSI. Due to the lack of an approved comparator agent, linezolid was evaluated for patients with clinical and microbiologic evidence of serious VRE infection in a blinded parenteral dose-comparative trial comparing 66 patients randomized to 200 mg q 12 hr to 79 patients treated with 600 mg q 12 hr (84). Among evaluable patients at end-of-treatment, a modest dose response was observed with 67% and 52% response rates seen in the high-dose and low-dose groups, respectively. In addition, efficacy and safety was also demonstrated in a large study ($n = 796$ patients) emergency use program for resistant, treatment refractory, or intolerant patients with serious Gram-positive infection (85). Among 549 cases of VRE infection, there was an 81.4% clinical cure rate at end-of-therapy. Since linezolid is a bacteriostatic agent that displays no synergistic activity with other agents, its efficacy in VRE native- or prosthetic-valve endocarditis remains questionable. Both clinical success and failure have been reported when linezolid has been used as a first-line therapy or salvage treatment. However, no large-scale randomized trial experience is yet available (86–88).

In recent years linezolid has become the dominant agent for the treatment of serious VRE infection. Multiple reports of linezolid resistance (MIC ≥ 8 µg/mL) occurring in VRE (*E. faecium*) and VSE (*E. faecalis*) strains that were susceptible (MIC 1–2 µg/mL) at baseline but developed a four-fold or greater rise in MIC to 8 to 32 µg/mL (89–92). Common to most cases where linezolid resistance appeared has been a protracted length of therapy (>28 days) associated with retained foci of VRE infection, such as abscesses, devitalized tissue, or foreign materials. The majority of linezolid-resistant isolates contain a single base-pair mutation in the genome encoding for domain V of the 23S ribosomal-binding site (G2476U mutation). The phenotypic level of resistance as determined by elevation in MIC level has been shown to correlate with the "gene dose" or number of copies 23S rDNA containing the G2466U mutation (93). Notably, this mutation was predicted by earlier in vitro spiral plate serial passage experiments with linezolid (94). Horizontal cross-transmission of an identical clone of linezolid-resistant *E. faecium* among linezolid-naïve patients within the same ICU or hospital center have also been described (95,96). A case-control study revealed that a longer course of linezolid (38 vs. 11 days) and linezolid exposure prior to hospitalization were risk factors for the emergence of linezolid-resistant VRE (97). Thus, repeat linezolid susceptibility testing is advisable in patients who have had prior linezolid exposure, persistent isolation of a VRE strain on therapy, or in patients treated in a nosocomial setting with prior linezolid resistance.

Although gastrointestinal symptoms are the most common reported toxicity, reversible myelosuppression (thrombocytopenia, leukopenia, and/or anemia) has been the most important treatment-limiting side effect, with higher rates observed than the original registration studies. Bone marrow examination has shown changes similar to those observed with reversible chloramphenicol toxicity (98,99). Such toxicity is usually observed only with linezolid treatment that exceeds 2 weeks. Other reported toxicities of note include gastrointestinal upset, rare cases of serotonin syndrome, optic and peripheral neuropathy, and lactic acidosis (100–103).

Daptomycin

Daptomycin is a novel cyclic lipopeptide compound with a broad Gram-positive spectrum and rapid bactericidal activity currently approved for CSSSI and *S. aureus* bacteremia, including right-sided endocarditis (104). Its apparent mechanism of action includes attachment to the exterior of the bacterial cytoplasmic membrane with membrane penetration of a lipophilic tail with disruption of the transmembrane potential due to ion efflux, an effect that is both concentration- and calcium ion-dependent and leads to nonlytic bacterial cell death. In vitro studies have shown near-uniform activity against vancomycin-resistant *E. faecium* and *E. faecalis* strains, with an MIC 90 of 4–8 μg/mL (105,106). In one recent study examining only VRE strains which were either linezolid- or Q/D-resistant, daptomycin demonstrated susceptibility using a 4 μg/mL provisional breakpoint (107). The MIC breakpoint is 4 μg/mL for vancomycin-susceptible *E. faecalis*; however, there is no established breakpoint for vancomycin-susceptible or -resistant *E. faecium*. Regardless of the testing method (E-test, disk diffusion, or broth dilution) the zone size or MIC result can be significantly elevated by a two- to eightfold magnitude with inadequate calcium supplementation. At the present time, clinical experience with daptomycin for serious VRE infection remains quite limited. The optimal dosing for enterococcal infection is not yet established; however, daily dosing at 6 mg/kg in the absence of renal insufficiency has been the most common dosing scheme. A randomized phase III trial versus linezolid in VRE infection was aborted due to enrollment difficulties. In a study of nine neutropenic patients with VRE bacteremia treated with daptomycin at 4 or 6 mg/kg/day, a clinical and/or microbiologic response was observed in only 4/9 (44%) (108). In a second report a similar response rate of 5/11 (45%) was observed in patients with VRE bacteremia and endocarditis treated with 6 mg/kg/day of daptomycin (109). Unfortunately, daptomycin resistance has been reported during treatment for vancomycin-resistant *E. faecalis*, *E. faecium*, and *E. durans* infection with a rise in the MIC to $\geq 8\,\mu g/mL$ (110–112).

Tigecycline
Tigecycline is the first approved agent of the glycylcycline class, a group closely related to the tetracyclines but synthetically modified to achieve an enhanced spectrum of activity against MRSA, other multi-resistant Gram-positive species, and many Gram-negative bacilli (113). Tigecycline is currently approved for CSSSI and intra-abdominal infection based on phase III studies showing comparability to standard comparator regimens. VRE were not included in these registration trials. However, tigecycline exhibits very low MICs for both vancomycin-susceptible and vancomycin-resistant clinical strains of *E. faecium* and *E. faecalis* (MIC90 = 0.012 $\mu g/mL$), although National Committee for Clinical Laboratory Standards breakpoints for vancomycin-resistant *E. faecium* strains are not yet established (114,115). Although clinical experience with tigecycline for VRE infection is not yet available, it appears to be a promising option particularly for intra-abdominal sites where it has shown comparable efficacy to meropenem in non-VRE monomicrobial and polymicrobial infection.

Novel Glycopeptides (Oritavancin, Dalbavancin, and Telavancin)
Several new glycopeptide derivatives have in vitro bactericidal activity against VRE. Dalbavancin is a long-acting derivative (half-life 7–10 days) of teicoplanin that has received approval for the treatment of CSSSI; however, similarly to teicoplanin this agent lacks in vitro activity against the more prevalent VanA enterococcal strains (116).

Oritavancin is a semisynthetic glycopeptide that blocks peptidoglycan synthesis and exerts bactericidal activity across a broad Gram-positive spectrum (117). It has superior activity against VanA and VanB enterococci compared with dalbavancin and telavancin with both concentration-dependent bactericidal activity against both *E. faecium* and *E. faecalis* strains (MIC90 = 1–2 $\mu g/mL$) and is synergistic with ampicillin against the majority of isolates (118). This agent has completed phase III trials in CSSSI; however, concerns pertaining to its long half-life, high protein binding, and reports of spontaneous resistance may limit its development.

Telavancin, a long-acting lipoglycopeptide with multiple sites of action at the cell membrane and cell wall, has shown noninferiority versus standard therapy in Gram-positive CSSSI including MRSA; however, clinical data for VRE is not yet available (119,120).

INTESTINAL ERADICATION OF VRE
Eradicating or suppressing VRE carriage in the intestinal tract is a theoretically attractive approach if targeted to patients at high risk for VRE superinfection with discrete at-risk periods, i.e., oncologic patients with neutropenia and mucositis or liver and other abdominal solid organ recipients during the early post-transplant period. Decolonization has been studied in both animal models and humans with a variety of agents and combinations. The combination of oral bacitracin (25,000 U 3× day), gentamicin (80 mg 3× day), and doxycycline failed to show a difference

in either VRE eradication or VRE bacteremia during a 3-month follow-up period versus untreated controls (121). A similar study employing bacitracin (75,000 U 4× day) and doxycyline 100 mg/day for 14 days did show a 3.1 log decrease in the quantitative stool VRE inoculum; however, there was no difference at end of follow-up in the rates of VRE persistence versus a control group (122). Ramoplanin, a nonabsorbed glycolipodepsipeptide compound with potent VRE activity, was studied in a blinded placebo-controlled study at two dosages 100 or 400 mg every 12 hr for 7 days (123). VRE suppression was observed at 7 days after treatment; however, this effect waned rapidly such that all groups had equivalent rates of VRE colonization by 21 days after treatment.

Ramoplanin is currently undergoing a phase III blinded, placebo-controlled trial in neutropenic oncology patients with intestinal VRE colonization. At present there is no evidence that therapy directed at systemic VRE infection with Q/D, linezolid, or other nonapproved agents serendipitously terminates or shortens the duration of intestinal VRE colonization.

CONTROL AND PREVENTION OF VRE

In the United States, VRE acquisition occurs almost exclusively in healthcare centers and has been shown by epidemiologic typing methods to transfer both within and between healthcare facilities (124–126). Large-scale investigations to control VRE have produced widely disparate results and have been recently summarized in an evidence-based guideline from the Society for Healthcare Epidemiology of America (SHEA) directed at the control of both multidrug-resistant *S. aureus* and *Enterococcus* (127). It is important to discriminate whether control efforts are directed at aborting or modifying a short-term epidemic outbreak usually related to a single VRE clone or an established endemic setting with a multiclonal VRE since the latter poses a much greater challenge and probably requires a broader spectrum of collaborative effort (128).

The fundamental control approaches have included interventions to control physical exposure of patients to the VRE genome from contaminated healthcare workers or contaminated inanimate surfaces that may be stationary or mobile objects such as healthcare equipment. The major categories of recommendations include: (*i*) requirement for an active surveillance program to identify colonized patients; (*ii*) hand hygiene with an alcohol-based preparation and routine monitoring of hand hygiene compliance; (*iii*) barrier precautions including gloves and gowns for patients known or suspected to be colonized with VRE or universal gown and gloving in high risk units; (*iv*) disinfecting hospital surfaces with effective agents and methods; and (*v*) use of dedicated equipment or adequately cleaning them before use on another patient. In addition, "antibiotic stewardship" is needed, particularly directed at reducing the use of antibiotics with antianaerobic activity and late-generation cephalosporins that amplify the VRE intestinal inoculum and enhance the risk of environmental contamination and superinfection. Antibiotic controls can be exerted by either manipulation of the central antibiotic formulary or controlling individual antibiotic prescription.

FUTURE PERSPECTIVE

The antimicrobial therapeutic options for enterococcal infection have expanded remarkably in the past 10 years and promise to expand even further. Nevertheless it is sobering that new resistance mechanisms have appeared during the early part of the learning curve with these novel compounds. Moreover, the appearance of the *vanA* gene in MRSA due to horizontal transmission from co-colonizing VRE strains exemplifies that the *Enterococcus* is both an efficient donor and receptacle for the gene pool encoding for antimicrobial resistance. VRE has become a "way of life" in our hospitals and will no doubt continue to exert a significant effect on antimicrobial practices, infection control efforts, and the clinical outcomes of our most compromised patients for the foreseeable future.

REFERENCES

1. Murray BE. The life and times of the *Enterococcus*. Clin Microbiol Rev 1990; 3:46–65.
2. Facklam RR, Sahm DA. *Enterococcus*. In: Murray PR, Baron EJ, Pfaller MA, Tenover FC, Yolken RH, eds. Manual of Clinical Microbiology. Washington, D.C.: American Society of Microbiology, 1995:308–14.
3. Treitmen AN, Yarnold PR, Warren J, Noskin GA. Emerging incidence of *Enterococcus faecium* among hospital isolates (1993–2002). J Clin Microbiol 2005; 43:462–3.
4. Linden PK. Can enterococcal infections initiate sepsis syndrome? Curr Inf Dis Reports 2003; 5:372–78.
5. Centers for Disease Control and Prevention. National Nosocomial Surveillance (NNIS) system Report, Data summary from January 1992 through June 2003, issued August 2003. Am J Infect Control 2003; 31:481–98.
6. Wisplinghoff H, Bischoff T, Tallent SM, Seiferd H, Wenzel RP, Edmond MB. Nosocomial bloodstream infections in US hospitals: analysis of 24, 179 cases from a prospective nationwide surveillance study. Clin Infect Dis 2004; 39:309–17.
7. Hoffman SA, Moellering RC Jr. The *Enterococcus*: "putting the bug in our ears". Ann Intern Med 1987; 106:757–61.
8. Moellering RC. The Garrod Lecture. The *Enterococcus*: a classic example of the impact of antimicrobial resistance on therapeutic options. J Antimicrob Chemother 1991; 21:1–12.
9. Hodges TL, Zighelboim-Daum S, Eliopoulos GM, Wennersten C, Moellering RC Jr. Antimicrobial susceptibility changes in *Enterococcus faecalis* following various penicillin exposure regimens. Antimicrob Agents Chemother 1992; 36:121–5.
10. Hamilton-Miller JM, Purves D. Enterococci and antifolate antibotics. Eur J Clin Microbiol 1986; 5:391–94.
11. LeClercq R, Couvalin P. Bacterial resistance to macrolide, lincosamide and streptogramin antibiotics by target modification. Antimicrob Agents Chemother 1991; 35:1267–72.
12. Lefort A, Mainardi JL, Tod M, Lotholary O. Antienterococcal antibiotics. Med Clin N Am 2000; 84(6):1471–95.
13. Rubkine T, Mainardi JL, Sougakoff W, Collatz E, Gutmann L. Penicillin-binding protein 5 sequence alterations in clinical isolates of *Enterococcus faecium* with different levels of B-lactam resistance. J Infect Dis 1998; 178:159–63.
14. Grayson ML, Eliopoulos GM, Wennersten CB, et al. Increasing resistance to B-lactam antibiotics amongst clinical isolates of *Enterococcus faecium*: a 22-year review at one institution. Antimicrob Agents Chemother 1991; 35:2180–4.
15. Horodniceanu T, Bougueleret L, El-Solh N, Bieth G, Delbos F. High level resistance to gentamicin in *Streptococcus faecalis* subsp. *zymogenes*. Antimicrob Agents Chemother 1979; 16:686–9.
16. Mederski-Samoraj BD, Murray BE. High level resistance to gentamicin in clinical isolates of enterococci. J Infect Dis 1983; 147:751–7.
17. Linden A. Rationale for targeting interleukin-17 in the lungs. Curr Opin Invest Drugs 2003; 4(11):1304–12.
18. Leclercq R, Dutka-Malen S, Brisson-Noel A, et al. Resistance of enterococci to aminoglycosides and glycopeptides. Clin Infect Dis 1992; 15:495–501.

19. Spiegel CA, Hucyke M. Endocarditis due to streptomycin-susceptible *Enterococcus faecalis* with high-level gentamicin resistance. Arch Intern Med 1989; 149:1873–5.
20. Eliopoulos GM. Aminoglycoside resistant enterococcal endocarditis. Infect Dis Clin North Am 1993; 7:117–33.
21. Murray BE. B-lactamase producing enterococci. Antimicrob Agents Chemother 1992; 36:2355–9.
22. Methods for dilution of antimicrobial susceptibility tests for bacteria that grow aerobically, 4th ed. Vol 17. Villanova, PA: National Committee for Clinical Laboratory Standards, 1997:1–29 (Publications no. M7-A4).
23. Leclercq R, Derlot E, Duval J, Courvalin P. Plasmid mediated resistance to vancomycin and teicoplanin in *Enterococcus faecium*. N Engl J Med 1988; 319:157–61.
24. Centers for Disease Control and Prevention. Nosocomial enterococci resistant to vancomycin—United States 1989–1993. MMWR Mort Mortal Wkly Rep. 1993; 42:597–9.
25. Biedenbach DJ, Moet GJ, Jones RN. Occurrence and antimicrobial resistance pattern comparisons among bloodstream infection isolates from the SENTRY Antimicrobial Surveillance Program (1997–2002). Diag Microbiol Infect Dis 2004; 50:59–69.
26. Lai KK, Fontecchio SA, Kelly AL, Baker S, Melvin ZS. The changing epidemiology of vancomycin-resistant enterococci. Infect Control Hosp Epidemiol 2003; 24:264–8.
27. Courvalin P. Vancomycin resistance in Gram-positive cocci. Clin Infect Dis 2006; 42: S25–34.
28. Handwerger S, Skoble J. Identification of chromosomal mobile element conferring high-level vancomycin resistance in *Enterococcus faecium*. Antimicrob Agents Chemother 1995; 39:2446–53.
29. Gold HS. Vancomycin resistant enterococci: mechanisms and clinical observations. Clin Infect Dis 2001; 33:210–19.
30. Noble WC, Virani Z, Cree RG. Co-transfer of vancomycin and other resistance genes from *Enterococcus faecalis* NYTC 12201 to *Staphylococcus aureus*. FEMS Microbiol Lett 1992; 72:195–8.
31. Chang S, Sievert DM, Hageman JC, et al. Infection with vancomycin-resistant *Staphylococcus aureus* containing the *vanA* resistance gene. N Engl J Med 2003; 348:1342–7.
32. Kacica M, McDonald LC. Vancomycin-resistant *Staphylococcus aureus*—New York, 2005. MMWR Morb Mortal Wkly Rep 2005; 53:322–3.
33. Miller D, Urdaneta V, Weltman A. Vancomycin-resistant *Staphylococcus aureus*-Pennsylvania 2002. MMWR Morb Mortal Wkly Rep 2002; 51:902.
34. Sievert DM, Boulton ML, Stolzman G, et al. *Staphylococcus aureus* resistant to vancomycin—United States 2002. MMWR Morb Mortal Wkly Rep 2002; 51:565–7.
35. Whitener CJ, Park SY, Browne FA, et al. Vancomycin-resistant Staphylococcus aureus in the absence of vancomycin exposure. Clin Infect Dis 2004; 38:1049–55.
36. Donskey CJ. The role of the intestinal tract as a reservoir and source for transmission of nosocomial pathogens. Clin Infect Dis 2004; 39:219–26.
37. Beezhold DW, Slaughter S, Hayden MK, et al. Skin colonization with vancomycin-resistant enterococci among hospitalized patients with bacteremia. Clin Infect Dis 1997; 24:704–6.
38. D'Agasta EM, Gautam S, Green WK, Tang YW. High rate of false-negative results of the rectal swab culture method in detection of gastrointestinal colonization with vancomycin-resistant enterococci. Clin Infect Dis 2002; 34:167–72.
39. Weinstein JW, Tallapragada S, Farrel P, Dembry LM. Comparison of rectal and perirectal swabs for detection of colonization with vancomycin-resistant enterococci. J Clin Microbiol 1996; 34:210–2.
40. Novicki TJ, Schapiro JM, Ulness BK, et al. Convenient selective differential broth for isolation of vancomycin-resistant *Enterococcus* from fecal material. J Clin Microbiol 2004; 42:1637–40.
41. Paule SM, Trick WE, Tenover FC, et al. Comparison of PCR assay to culture for surveillance detection of vancomycin-resistant enterococci. J Clin Microbiol 2003; 41:4805–7.

42. Montecalvo MA, Lencastre H, Carraher M, et al. Natural history of colonization with vancomycin-resistant *Enterococcus faecium*. Infect Control Hosp Epidemiol 1995; 16:680–5.

43. Baden LR, Thiemke W, Skolnik A, et al. Prolonged colonization with vancomycin-resistant *Enterococcus faecium* in long-term care patients and the significance of "clearance". Clin Infect Dis 2001; 33:1654–60.

44. Roghmann MC, Aquiyumi S, Schwalbe R, Morris JG Jr. Natural history of colonization with vancomycin-resistant *Enterococcus faecium*. Infect Control Hosp Epidemiol 1997; 18:679–80.

45. Tornieporth NG, Roberts RB, Hafner JJ, Riley LW. Risk factors associated with vancomycin-resistant *Enterococcus faecium* infection or colonization in 145 matched case and control patients. Clin Infect Dis 1996; 23:767–72.

46. Bonten MJ, Hayden MK, Nathan C, et al. Epidemiology of colonization of patients and environment with vancomycin-resistant enterococci. Lancet 1996; 348:1615–9.

47. Morris JG, Shay DK, Hebden JN, et al. Enterococci resistant to multiple antimicrobial agents including vancomycin, establishment of endemicity in a university medical center. Ann Intern Med 1995; 123:250–9.

48. Warren DK, Kollef MH, Seiler SM, Fridkin SK, Fraser VJ. The epidemiology of vancomycin-resistant *Enterococcus* in a medical intensive care unit. Infect Control Hosp Epidemiol 2003; 24:238–41.

49. Donskey CJ, Chowdhry T, Hecker M, et al. Effect of antibiotic therapy on the density of vancomycin-resistant enterococci in the stool of colonized patients. N Engl J Med 2000; 343:1925–32.

50. Bonten MJ, Slaughter S, Ambergen AW, et al. The role of "colonization pressure" in the spread of vancomycin-resistant enterococci: an important infection control variable. Arch Intern Med 1998; 158:1127–32.

51. Lautenach E, LaRosa LA, Marr AM, et al. Changes in the prevalence of vancomycin-resistant enterococci in response to antimicrobial formulary interventions: impact of progressive restrictions on use of vancomycin and third-generation cephalosporins. Clin Infect Dis 2003; 36:440–6.

52. Quale J, Landman D, Atwood E, et al. Experience with a hospital-wide outbreak of vancomycin-resistant enterococci. Am J Infect Control 1996; 24:372–9.

53. Lai KK. Treatment of vancomycin resistant *Enterococcus faecium* infections. Arch Intern Med 1996; 156:2579–84.

54. Pankey GA, Sabath LD. Clinical relevance of bacteriostatic versus bactericidal mechanisms of action in the treatment of Gram-positive bacterial infections. Clin Infect Dis 2004; 38:864–70.

55. Finberg RW, Moellering RC, Tally FP, et al. The importance of bactericidal drugs, future directions in infectious diseases. Clin Infect Dis 2004; 39:1314–20.

56. Tsigrelis C, Singh KV, Coutinho TD, Murray BE, Baddour LM. Vancomycin-resistant *Enterococcus faecalis* endocarditis: linezolid failure and strain characterization of virulence factors. J Clin Microbiol 2007; 45:631–5.

57. Mekonen ET, Noskin GA, Hacek DM, Peterson LR. Successful treatment of persistent bacteremia due to vancomycin resistant ampicillin resistant *Enterococcus faecium*. Microb Drug Resist 1995; 1:249–53.

58. Dodge RA, Daly JS, Davaro R, Glew RH. High dose ampicillin plus streptomycin for treatment of a patient with severe infection due to multi-drug resistant enterococci. Clin Infect Dis 1997; 25:1269–70.

59. Murray BE. Vancomycin-resistant enterococcal infections. N Engl J Med 2000; 342: 710–21.

60. Lautenbach E, Schuster MG, Biler WB, et al. The role of chloramphenicol in the treatment of bloodstream infection due to vancomycin-resistant *Enterococcus*. Clin Infect Dis 1998; 27:1259–65.

61. Gould CV, Fishman NO, Nakamkin NI, Lautenbach E. Chloramphenicol resistance in vancomycin resistant enterococcal bacteremia: impact of prior fluoroquinolone use. Infect Cont Hosp Epidemiol 2004; 25:138–45.

62. Howe RA, Robson M, Oakhill A, et al. Successful use of tetracycline as therapy of an immunocompromised patient with septicemia caused by a vancomycin-resistant Enterococcus. J Antimicrob Chemother 1997; 40:144–5.
63. Linden PK, Pasculle AW, Manez R, et al. Utilization of novobiocin and ciprofloxacin for the treatment of serious infection due to vancomycin-resistant *Enterococcus faecium*. In: Program and Abstracts of the Thirty-Third Interscience Conference on Antimicrobial Agents and Chemotherapy, New Orleans, LA. Washington, D.C.: American Society for Microbiology, 1993; 1027(Abstract):307.
64. Montecalvo MA, Horowitz H, Wormser GP, et al. Effect of novobiocin-containing antimicrobial regimens on infection and colonization with vancomycin resistant *Enterococcus faecium*. Antimicrob Agents Chemother 1995; 39:794.
65. Taylor SE, Paterson DL, Yu VL. Treatment options for chronic prostatitis due to vancomycin-resistant *Enterococcus faecium*. Eur J Clin Microbiol Infect Dis 1998; 17:798–800.
66. Schmidt JL. Efficacy of teicoplanin for enterococcal infections: 63 cases and review. Clin Infect Dis 1992; 15:302–6.
67. Aslangul E, Baptista M, Fantin B, et al. Selection of glycopeptide-resistant mutants of VanB type *Enterococcus faecalis* BM4281 in vitro and in experimental endocarditis. J Infect Dis 1997; 175:598–605.
68. Hayden MK, Trenholme GM, Schultz JE, et al. In vivo development of teicoplanin resistance in a VanB *Enterococcus faecalis*. J Infect Dis 1993; 167:1224–7.
69. Zhanel GG, Hoban DJ, Karlowsky JA. Nitrofurantoin is active against vancomycin-resistant enterococci. Antimicrob Agents Chemother 2001; 45:324–6.
70. Linden P, Coley K, Kusne S. Bacteriologic efficacy of nitrofurantoin for the treatment of urinary tract infection due to vancomycin-resistant *Enterococcus faecium*. Clin Infect Dis 1999; 29:999.
71. Cocito C, DiGiambattista M, Nyssen E, Vannuffel P. Inhibition of protein synthesis by streptogramins and related antibiotics. J Antimicrob Chemother 1997; 39(Suppl. A): 7–13.
72. Hershberger E, Donabedian S, Konstantinou K, Zervos MJ. Quinupristin-dalfopristin resistance in Gram-positive bacteria: mechanism of resistance and epidemiology. Clin Infect Dis 2004; 38:92–8.
73. Moellering RC, Linden PK, Reinhardt J, et al. The efficacy and safety of quinupristin/dalfopristin for the treatment of vancomycin-resistant *Enterococcus faecium*. J Antimicrob Chemother 1999; 44:251–71.
74. Linden PK, Moellering RC, Wood CA, et al. Treatment of vancomycin-resistant *Enterococcus faecium* infections with quinupristin/dalfopristin. Clin Infect Dis 2001; 33:1816–23.
75. Brown J, Freeman BB. Combining quinupristin/dalfopristin with other agents for resistant infections. Ann Pharmacother 2004; 38:677–85.
76. Bethea JA, Walko CM, Targos PA. Treatment of vancomycin-resistant enterococcus with quinupristin/dalfopristin and high dose-ampicillin. Ann Pharmacother 2004; 38:998–91.
77. Thompson RL, Lavin B, Talbot GH. Endocarditis due to vancomycin-resistant *Enterococcus faecium* in an immunocompromised patient: cure by administering combination therapy with quinupristin/dalfopristin and high-dose ampicillin. South Med J 2003; 96:818–20.
78. Raad I, Hachem R, Hanna H, et al. Treatment of vancomycin-resistant enterococcal infections in the immunocompromise host: quinupristin-dalfopristin in combination with minocycline. Antimicrob Agents Chemother 2001; 45:3202–4.
79. Olsen KM, Rebuck JA, Rupp ME. Arthralgias and myalgias related to quinupristin-dalfopristin administration. Clin Infect Dis 2001; 32:e83–6.
80. Klare WG, Spnecker FB, Witte W. Intra-hospital dissemination of quinupristin-dalfopristin- and vancomycin-resistant *Enterococcus faecium* in a paediatric ward of a German hospital. J Antimicrob Chemother 2003; 52:113–5.
81. Donabedian SM, Perri MB, Vager D, et al. Quinupristin-dalfopristin resistance in *Enterococcus faecium* isolates from humans, farm animals, and grocery store meat in the United States. J Clin Microbiol 2006; 44:3361–5.

82. Lester CH, Frimodt-Moller N, Sorensen TL, Monnet DL, Hammerum AM. In vivo transfer of the *vanA* resistance gene from an *Enterococcus faecium* isolate of animal origin to an *E. faecium* isolate of human origin in the intestines of human volunteers. Antimicrob Agents Chemother 2006; 50:596–9.

83. Moellering RC. Linezolid: the first oxazolidinone antimicrobial. Ann Intern Med 2003; 138:135–42.

84. Pharmacia and Upjohn. Linezolid for the treatment of vancomycin resistant enterococcal infections: a double-blind trial comparing 600 mg linezolid every 12 hr with 200 mg linezolid every 12 hr (study report M/1260/0054A). Peapack, NJ: Pharmacia Upjohn, 1999.

85. Birmingham MC, Raynes CR, Meagher AK, Flavin SM, Batts DH, Schentag JJ. Linezolid for the treatment of multidrug-resistant Gram-positive infections: experience from a compassionate use program. Clin Infect Dis 2003; 36:159–68.

86. Stevens MP, Edmond MB. Endocarditis due to vancomycin-resistant enterococci: case report and review of the literature. Clin Infect Dis 2005; 41:1134–42.

87. Archuleta S, Murphy B, Keller MJ. Successful treatment of vancomycin-resistant *Enterococcus faecium* endocarditis with linezolid in a renal transplant recipient with human immunodeficiency virus infection. Transpl Infect Dis 2004; 6:117–9.

88. Babcock HM, Ritchie DJ, Christiansen E, Starlin R, Little R, Stanley S. Successful treatment of vancomycin-resistant *Enterococcus* endocarditis with oral linezolid. Clin Infect Dis 2001; 32:1373–5.

89. Zimmer SM, Caliendo AM, Thigpen MC, Somani J. Failure of linezolid treatment for enterococcal endocarditis. Clin Infect Dis 2003; 37:e29–30.

90. Gonzales RD, Schreckenberger PK, Graham MB, et al. Infections due to vancomycin-resistant *Enterococcus faecium* resistant to linezolid [letter]. Lancet 2001; 357:1179.

91. Seedat J, Zick G, Klare I, et al. Rapid emergence of resistance to linezolid during linzolid therapy of an *Enterococcus faecium* infection. Antimicrob Agents Chemother 2006; 50:4217–9.

92. Marra AR, Major Y, Edmond MD. Central venous catheter colonization by linezolid-resistant, vancomycin-susceptible *Enterococcus faecalis*. J Clin Microbiol 2006; 44:1915–16.

93. Rahim S, Pillai SK, Gold HS, Venkataraman L, Inglima K, Press RA. Linezolid-resistant, vancomycin-resistant *Enterococcus faecium* infection in patients without prior exposure to linezolid. Clin Infest Dis 2003; 36(11):E146–8. Epub 2003 May 20.

94. Swaney SM, Shinabarger DL, Schaadt RD, Bock JH, Slightom JL, Zurenko GE. Oxazolidinone resistance is associated with a mutation in the peptidyl transferase region of 23S rRNA (abstract C-104). In: Program and Abstracts of the 38th Interscience Conference on Antimicrobial Agents and Chemotherapy (San Diego), Washington, D.C.: American Society for Microbiology, 1998:98–9.

95. Herrero IA, Issa NC, Patel R. Nosocomial spread of linezolid-resistant vancomycin-resistant *Enterococcus faecium*. N Engl J Med 2002; 346:867–9.

96. Marshall SH, Donskey CJ, Hutton-Thomas R, Salata RA, Rice LB. Gene dosage and linezolid resistance in *Enterococcus faecium* and *Enterococcus faecalis*. Antimicrob Agents Chemother 2002; 46:3334–6.

97. Pai MP, Rodvold KA, Schreckenbefger PC, Gonzales RD, Petrolatti JM, Quinn JP. Risk factors associated with the development of infection with linezolid- and vancomycin-resistant *Enterococcus faecium*. Clin Infect Dis 2002; 35:1269–72.

98. Green SL, Maddox JC, Huttenbach ED. Linezolid and reversible myelosuppression. JAMA 2001; 286:1974.

99. Halpern M. Linezolid-induced pancytopenia. Clin Infect Dis 2002; 35:347–8.

100. Wigen CL, Goetz MB. Serotonin syndrome and linezolid. Clin Infect Dis 2002; 34:1651–2.

101. Saijo T, Hayashi K, Yamada H, Wakakura M. Linezolid-induced optic neuropathy. Am J Opthamol 2005; 139:1114–16.

102. Bressler AM, Zimmer SM, Gilmore JL, Somani J. Peripheral neuropathy associated with prolonged use of linezolid. Lancet Infect Dis 2004; 4:528–31.

103. Apodaca AA, Rakita RM. Linezolid-induced lactic acidosis. N Engl J Med 2003; 348:86–7.
104. Carpenter CF, Chambers HF. Daptomycin: another novel agent for treating infections due to drug-resistant Gram-positive pathogens. Clin Infect Dis 2004; 38:994–1000.
105. Pfaller MA, Sader HS, Jones RN. Evaluation of the in vitro activity of daptomycin against 19615 clinical isolates of Gram-positive cocci collected in North American hospitals (2002–2005). Diagn Microbiol Infect Dis 2007; Jan 18 (epub).
106. Jorgensen JH, Crawford SA, Kelly CC, Patterson JE. In vitro activity of daptomycin against vancomycin-resistant enterococci of various Van types and comparison of susceptibility testing methods. Antimicrob Agents Chemother 2003; 47:3760–3.
107. Anastasiou DM, Thorne GM, Luperchio SA, Alder JD. In vitro activity of daptomycin against clinical isolates with reduced susceptibility to linezolid and quinupristin/dalfopristin. Int J Antimicrob Agents 2006; 28:385–8.
108. Poutsiaka DD, Skiffingeron S, Miller KB, Hadley S, Snydman DR. Daptomycin in the treatment of vancomycin-resistant *Enterococcus faecium* bacteremia in neutropenic patients. J Infect 2007; 54(6):567–71. Epub 2006 Dec 26.
109. Segreti JA, Crank CW, Finney MS. Daptomycin for the treatment of Gram-positive bacteremia and infective endocarditis: a retrospective case series of 31 patients. Pharmacotherapy 2006; 26:47–52.
110. Long JK, Choueiri TK, Hall GS, Avery RK, Sekeres MA. Daptomycin-resistant *Enterococcus faecium* in a patient with acute myeloid leukemia. Mayop Clin Proc 2005; 80:1215–16.
111. Munoz-Price LS, Lolans K, Quinn JP. Emergence of resistance to daptomycin during treatment of vancomycin-resistant *Enterococcus faecalis* infection. Clin Infect Dis 2005; 41:565–6.
112. Lewis JS II, Owens A, Cadena J, et al. Emergence of daptomycin resistance in *Enterococcus faecium* during daptomycin therapy. Antimicrob Agents Chemother 2005; 49:1664–5.
113. Stein GE, Craig WA. Tigecycline: a critical analysis. Clin Infect Dis 2006; 43:518–24.
114. Sader HS, Jones RN, Stilwell MG, Dowzicky MJ, Fritsche TR. Tigecycline activity tested against 26,474 bloodstream infection isolates: a collection from 6 continents. Diagn Microbiol Infect Dis 2006; 52:181–6.
115. Waites KB, Duffy LB, Dowzicky MJ. Antimicrobial susceptibility amongst pathogens collected from hospitalized patients in the United States and in vitro activity of tigecycline, a new glycylcycline antimicrobial. Antimicrob Agents Chemother 2006; 50:3479–84.
116. Streit JM, Sader HS, Fritsche TR, Jones RN. Dalbabancin activity against selected populations of antimicrobial resistant Gram-positive pathogens. Diagn Microbiol Infect Dis 2005; 53:307–10.
117. Barrett JF. Recent developments in glycopeptide antibacterials. Curr Opin Invest Drugs 2005; 6:781–90.
118. Baltch AL, Smith RP, Ritz WJ, Bopp LH. Comparison of inhibitory and bactericidal activities and postantibiotic effects of LY-333328 and ampicillin used singly and in combination against *Enterococcus faecium*. Antimicrob Agents Chemother 1998; 42:2564–8.
119. Styjewski ME, Chu VH, O'Riordan WD, et al. Telavancin versus standard therapy for treatment of complicated skin and skin structure infections caused by Gram-positive bacteria: FAST 2 Study. Antimicrob Agents Chemother 2006; 50:862–7.
120. Poulakou G, Giamarellou H. Investigational treatments for postoperative surgical site infections. Expert Opin Investig Drugs 2007; 16:137–55.
121. Weinstein MR, Dedier H, Brunton J, Campbell I, Conly JM. Lack of efficacy of oral bacitracin plus doxycycline for the eradications of stool colonization with vancomycin-resistant *Enteroocus faecium* clin Infect Dis 1999; 29:361–6.
122. Hachem R, Radd I. Failure of oral antimicrobial agents in eradicating gastrointestinal colonization with vancomycin-resistant enterococci. Infect Cont Hosp Epidemiol 2002; 23:43–4.

123. Wong MT, Kauffman CA, Standiford HC, et al. Effective suppression of vancomycin-resistant *Enterococcus* in asymptomatic gastrointestinal carriers by a novel glycolipo-depsipeptide, ramoplanin. Clin Infect Dis 2001; 33:1476–82.

124. Martone WJ. Spread of vancomycin-resistant enterococci: why did it happen in the United States? Infect Cont Hosp Epidemiol 1998; 19:539–45.

125. Clark NC, Cooksey RC, Hill BC, Swenson JM, Tenover FC. Characterization of glycopeptide-resistant enterococci from U.S. hospitals. Antimicrob Agents Chemother 1993; 37:2311–7.

126. Livonrnese LL, Dias S, Romanowski B, et al. Hospital-acquired infection with vancomycin-resistant *Enterococcus faecium* transmitted by electronic thermometers. Ann Intern Med 1992; 117:112–16.

127. Muto CA, Jernigan JA, Ostrowsky BE, et al. SHEA Guidelines for the preventing, nosocomial transmission of multidrug-resistant strains of *Staphylococcus aureus* and *Enterococcus*. Infect Control Hosp Epidemiol 2003; 24:362–86.

128. Armeanu E, Bonten MJ. Control of vancomycin-resistant enterococci: one size fits all? Clin Infect Dis 2005; 41:210–6.

7   *Streptococcus pneumoniae*: Resistance Update and Treatment Options

Nicole Akar and William R. Bishai
Center for Tuberculosis Research, Johns Hopkins University School of Medicine, Baltimore, Maryland, U.S.A.

Sanjay K. Jain
Department of Pediatrics and Center for Tuberculosis Research, Johns Hopkins University School of Medicine, Baltimore, Maryland, U.S.A.

INTRODUCTION

Streptococcus pneumoniae is a major worldwide bacterial pathogen responsible for a variety of infections including pneumonia, bacteremia, otitis media, meningitis, sinusitis, and other infections. It is the most common pathogen causing bacterial community-acquired pneumonia (CAP) (1). Pneumococcal pneumonia has always been responsible for significant morbidity and mortality. In the pre-antibiotic era, it carried a 25% to 35% case fatality rate, which increased to 80% if bacteremia was present (2). Following the introduction of penicillin, mortality rates were reduced to below 10% (3). Sixty years later, mortality rates still remain around 12% for all hospitalized patients (1) and up to 25% for those with bacteremia (1,4). The continued significant mortality of pneumococcal disease despite the advances in antimicrobial therapy and intensive care management over the past half-century underscores the innate pathogenicity of this organism.

S. pneumoniae has evolved and shows extensive resistance to penicillin and other antimicrobials (5,6). The situation is made worse by the concurrent rise of resistance to other antimicrobials, particularly in isolates that are already penicillin-resistant. Multi-drug resistant *S. pneumoniae* (MDRSP), defined as resistance to penicillin and at least 2 other antibiotic classes, was first reported from South Africa in 1978 (7), but has now spread to every continent. MDRSP now comprise nearly 31% of pneumococcal isolates in the United States (6).

In a study done in 1998, the annual cost of treating CAP in the United States was estimated to be $8.4 billion (8). In this study, the social costs, including lost work time and lost wages for patients as well as their caretakers (in the case of affected children), were not taken into account. Therefore, actual healthcare costs may be substantially higher. Since *S. pneumoniae* is the most common pathogen causing bacterial CAP, it is a significant contributor to the cost of treating CAP. Furthermore, as the antimicrobial resistance of the pathogens responsible for CAP increase, the costs associated with these infections are likely to continue to rise.

PREVALENCE OF RESISTANCE
Penicillin Resistance

Published surveillance data suggest that approximately 35% to 38% of *S. pneumoniae* isolates in the United States are penicillin non-susceptible. Of these, approximately

22% have high-level resistance (Table 1) (6). Certain areas of the world, such as Spain, Hungary, and South Africa, have reported rates of reduced susceptibility to penicillin as high as 40% to 70% (9–11).

The mechanism of penicillin resistance in *S. pneumoniae* consists of stepwise mutations in one or more of the five major penicillin binding-proteins (PBPs) in the bacterial cell wall that serve as targets for beta-lactam action. In general, alterations of more than one PBP are needed to reduce susceptibility to penicillin, whereas high-level resistance requires mutations in at least four PBPs. All beta-lactams utilize similar targets; as a result, resistance to cephalosporins and carbapenems has emerged together with penicillin resistance.

TABLE 1 Summary of Major Antimicrobial Classes for Treatment of CAP

Antimicrobial class	Rates of *Streptococcus pneumoniae* resistance in United States	Mechanism of resistance	Advantages to use	Disadvantages to use
Penicillins[a]	35–38%	Stepwise mutations in one or more of the 5 penicillin binding proteins	High-dose amoxicillin is active against most *S. pneumoniae* strains	Lacks activity against atypical agents; high doses lead to more gastrointestinal intolerance
Macrolides[b]	28–30%	Modification of the ribosomal target site, conferred by the *ermB* gene; Active drug efflux, mediated by the *mefA* gene	Achieve high tissue and ELF concentrations; clarithromycin and azithromycin can be given once daily	Macrolide resistance is high and breakthrough pneumococcal bacteremia with macrolide-resistant strains is more common than other classes
Fluoroquinolones[c]	2–3%	Stepwise chromosomal mutations *gyrA* or *parC*; Active drug efflux mediated by the multi-drug transporter, *pmrA*	Active against most *S. pneumoniae* strains in United States, including penicillin-resistant strains; can be given once daily	Very broad-spectrum agents that are extensively used for several indications other than CAP; Possibility of abuse with risk of increasing resistance by *S. pneumoniae*; Are not used in children

[a]Data From Ref. 6.
[b]Data From Refs. 6,12.
[c]Data From Refs. 24,25.
Abbreviations: CAP, community acquired pneumonia; ELF, epithelial lining fluid.

Macrolide Resistance

The prevalence of macrolide resistance has increased markedly in *S. pneumoniae* in the last decade. Approximately 28% to 30% of *S. pneumoniae* currently exhibit resistance to erythromycin, clarithromycin, dirithromycin, or azithromycin (6,12). Breakthrough pneumococcal bacteremia may now be more common with macrolide-resistant strains than with beta-lactam- or fluoroquinolone-resistant strains (13). Exceedingly high rates are reported from countries in Europe, Asia, and South America (14).

Macrolides exert their activity by binding to specific domains of the 50S ribosomal subunit and block the extension of the nascent polypeptide chain through the exit tunnel in the ribosome. Resistance to macrolides occurs by one of two mechanisms. The first mechanism is modification of the ribosomal target site, conferred by the *ermB* gene, which may be constitutively or inducibly expressed in *S. pneumoniae*. The *ermB* gene codes for a ribosomal methylase that methylates a single adenine residue, markedly reducing the affinity of macrolides for the target site. This mechanism results in high-level macrolide resistance that is erythromycin minimum inhibitory concentration (MIC) $\geq 64\,\mu g/mL$, and cross-resistance with lincosamides such as clindamycin and streptogramins (so-called "MLS" resistance) due to overlapping binding sites. Rarely, mutations in the 23S rRNA or the ribosomal proteins L4 or L22 may also alter the target site and result in MLS resistance. The second common mechanism of macrolide resistance in pneumococci is active drug efflux, mediated by an efflux pump encoded by the *mefA* gene. This pump confers resistance to 14- and 15-member macrolides, but not to 16-member macrolides (e.g., spiramycin and josamycin), clindamycin, or streptogramins. This mechanism results in low- to mid-level resistance, with MICs for erythromycin between 1 and $32\,\mu g/mL$, although the MICs appear to be increasing over time (15). The prevalence of the respective macrolide resistance mechanisms varies by geography. The efflux mechanism accounts for more than two-thirds of resistant isolates in North America, but <20% in Europe and South Africa (14). Most of the dramatic rise in macrolide resistance in the United States during the last decade is attributable to the efflux mechanism (15,16).

Ketolides are a new class of macrolides and are semi-synthetic derivates of erythromycin A. Their defining characteristic is the removal of the neutral sugar, L-cladinose, from the three position of the ring and subsequent oxidation of the 3-hydroxyl to a 3-keto functional group. Telithromycin is the first of this new class of drugs to be approved for clinical use. Ketolides have excellent microbiologic activity against drug-resistant *S. pneumoniae*. Efflux-mediated resistance is less effective against ketolides because they are poor substrates for the efflux pumps. Within their binding site on the bacterial ribosome, ketolides interact with two regions of the 23S rRNA. Telithromycin binds to A752 in addition to A2058 bound by erythromycin and other macrolides and azalides (17,18). In addition, ketolides lack the capacity to induce *erm* expression, and therefore are active against inducibly resistant macrolide strains (19). For these reasons, ketolides retain their activity against most *S. pneumoniae* regardless of their erythromycin susceptibility and are active against isolates constitutively expressing *ermB* (20,21). Ketolide-resistant strains of *S. pneumoniae* have, however, been described and these strains often have *ermB* and may also harbor 23S rRNA mutations and/or have altered L4 and L22 ribosomal proteins (22,23).

Fluoroquinolone Resistance

Rates of resistance to fluoroquinolones are 2% to 3% in U.S.-based surveillance studies (24,25). These rates are higher in parts of Asia (Hong Kong, 14.3%; South Korea, 2.9%) (26).

The development of resistance to fluoroquinolones arises by one of two mechanisms: (*i*) stepwise accumulation of chromosomal mutations in the quinolone resistance determining regions (QRDRs) of *gyrA* or *parC* encoding the respective enzymes; or (*ii*) active drug efflux mediated by the multi-drug transporter, *pmrA*. Spontaneous mutations occur in the QRDRs of *gyrA* and *parC* of S. *pneumoniae* with frequencies varying from 1 in 10^6 to 1 in 10^9 (27). The first mutation to confer a survival advantage over the "wild-type" during fluoroquinolone exposure occurs predictably in the preferred enzymatic target (i.e., *gyrA* or *parC*) for the particular fluoroquinolone providing the selection pressure. These first-step mutations are generally associated with a 4- to 8-fold elevation in the MIC for all fluoroquinolones that preferentially target the mutated enzyme, but have little impact on the activity of fluoroquinolones that prefer the other enzyme as a target. When a population of such first-step mutants again reaches a density of 10^6 to 10^9 organisms, it becomes probable that a second mutation in the other enzyme will occur. The double mutant will now display more complete resistance to any one fluoroquinolone and cross-resistance to all fluoroquinolones. If, as suggested by some investigators, more than 10^9 organisms may be present in the lungs of patients with acute exacerbations of chronic bronchitis or pneumonia, then there is ample opportunity to select for mutants that occur with a frequency of one in 10^6 to 10^9 (28). Continued or repetitive fluoroquinolone exposure may then select increasingly resistant isolates. A fluoroquinolone with comparable potent activity for both enzymes should be less likely to select drug-resistant mutants, since spontaneous mutations in both enzymes are necessary to become resistant, an event that occurs with a frequency less than one in 10^{12}. However, no clinically available agent has been clearly demonstrated to have such dual activity (29). Alternatively, a fluoroquinolone that is able to achieve concentrations at the site of infection sufficient to inhibit the growth of all first-step mutants should severely restrict the stepwise selection of double mutants. Assuming that first-step mutants are usually 4 to 8 times less susceptible than wild-type bacteria, the fluoroquinolone of choice should achieve a concentration at the site of infection that is at least 8-fold higher than the wild-type MIC in order to restrict mutant selection (30). On the other hand, over-reliance on less potent fluoroquinolones may well facilitate the stepwise selection of fluoroqui-nolone-resistant pneumococci. Further clinical data indicate that use of older fluor-oquinolones (ciprofloxacin, levofloxacin) against resistant strains of S. *pneumoniae* results in clinical failure (28,31,32).

RISK FACTORS FOR RESISTANCE

Risk factors for the presence of penicillin-resistant isolates in children include daycare attendance, recent antimicrobial treatment (<90 days), and age younger than 2 years (33). Similarly, in adults, the risk factors for infection with DRSP center on the two factors most important to the spread of DRSP: antibiotic selection pressure and exposure to carriers. Not surprisingly, recent beta-lactam therapy (within 3 months) has been identified as a major risk factor for both carriage of and infection with beta-lactam resistant S. *pneumoniae* in multiple studies (34–36). Recent hospitalization, alcoholism, institutional residence, immunosuppressive illness such as HIV infection, extremes of age, and exposure to children in day care are markers for exposure to carriers and also risk factors for DRSP (35,37–39). The introduction of the pneumococcal conjugate vaccine has led to a decrease in DRSP (40,41), though one recent study shows that it may have increased the antimicrobial resistance among non-vaccine serotypes (41).

Previous antibiotic use is the major risk factor for macrolide resistance (42). As a result, the prevalence of resistance is higher in children (particularly those with recurrent otitis media or in day care), recently hospitalized patients, and patients with penicillin-resistant isolates (14). In a study of adults with bacteremic pneumococcal pneumonia, prior exposure to a macrolide antimicrobial agent, failure to complete the course of prescribed drugs, prior flu vaccination, and Hispanic ethnicity were associated with an increased probability of macrolide resistance (43). However, in the same study, 55% of patients with macrolide-resistant infections reported no antimicrobial drug exposure in the preceding 6 months. Increasing use of new longer-acting macrolides has been strongly correlated with increasing resistance rates (16,44,45). It has been suggested that long-acting macrolides are more likely to lead to resistance due to lower peak serum concentrations and longer periods with sub-MIC levels (14,44). Azithromycin use has repeatedly been associated with pharyngeal carriage of resistant pneumococci (46–48).

Fluoroquinolones are not commonly used for pediatric infections, due to concerns of cartilage toxicity. Risk factors for resistance include old age, prior fluoroquinolone exposure, chronic obstructive pulmonary disease, nursing home residence, and nosocomial acquisition of infection (31,49,50). Ironically, many of these risk factors are also risk factors for respiratory tract infections caused by Gram-negative rods and are frequently cited as indications for empiric fluoroquinolone therapy (51). In fact, there seems to be a direct relationship between the amounts of fluoroquinolone use and development of resistance (52). Further, a recent study indicates that many patients receiving outpatient fluoroquinolones may not have required antimicrobial therapy and that the dose and duration were often incorrect (53). This has therefore led to a growing concern that overuse of fluoroquinolones may lead to the demise of this class (54).

CLINICAL IMPLICATIONS OF RESISTANCE

S. pneumoniae is a virulent human pathogen and the benefits of antimicrobial therapy on mortality from bacteremic disease are well known (55). Meehan et al. showed that a delay in the initiation of antibiotic therapy for CAP was also associated with an increase in mortality (56). Despite the obvious concerns regarding the emergence of DRSP and the risk that initial empiric regimens may include drugs to which the infecting organism is resistant, the real clinical impact of pneumococcal resistance has been difficult to measure.

A number of studies have been conducted to determine the effect of penicillin-susceptible versus penicillin non-susceptible strains of *S. pneumoniae* on clinical outcomes. However, there is no clear consensus on this ongoing debate. Several studies and reviews suggest that clinical outcomes do not differ significantly between patients with pneumonias due to penicillin-susceptible versus penicillin non-susceptible strains (57–61). However, a recent meta-analysis of prospective cohort studies to examine the association between penicillin resistance and short-term all-cause mortality for pneumococcal pneumonia suggested that penicillin resistance is associated with a higher mortality rate than is penicillin susceptibility in hospitalized patients with pneumococcal pneumonia (62). These data are conflicting even for patients with bacteremic pneumococcal pneumonia (63,64). Further, there seems to be a paradox in which the interpretation of in vitro resistance profiles may not appear to predict the in vivo outcome of pneumococcal pneumonia (61). Several possible reasons for such a paradox exist, including the fact that accepted susceptibility breakpoints may not be appropriate for pneumococcal pneumonia. The stepwise accumulation of PBP mutations means that susceptibility to beta-lactams is not an all-or-none phenomenon but, rather, concentration-dependent. Up until recently, the National Committee for Clinical Laboratory Standards (NCCLS), now the Clinical Laboratory Standards Institute (CLSI), recommended that isolates with penicillin MICs <0.06 µg/mL be considered susceptible, isolates with MICs of 0.12 to 1 µg/mL intermediate, and isolates with MICs ≥2 µg/ml resistant to penicillin. These guidelines were based on achievable concentrations of penicillin in the cerebrospinal fluid (CSF), and intended to prevent clinical failures in the treatment of meningitis caused by penicillin-intermediate isolates (65). Since the levels of penicillin obtained in the lung parenchyma are higher than those in CSF and similar to those in serum, the designations of susceptibility based on these guidelines are not appropriate for pneumococcal pneumonia and may have overstated the problem as it relates to pneumonia caused by penicillin non-susceptible *S. pneumoniae* (54). In fact, Turett et al. have shown that in their study, higher mortality was noted only for patients harboring *S. pneumoniae* with penicillin MIC ≥4 µg/mL (66). An additional caveat in determining the effect of DRSP concerns the sensitivity of the outcome variables used to detect clinical failures. Previous work has suggested that mortality from bacteremic pneumococcal pneumonia within the first 5 days of presentation is independent of the administration of antibiotics (55). Therefore, a true association between drug resistance and mortality may only become apparent 5 or more days from presentation. In an analysis of nearly 6000 patients with pneumococcal pneumonia, Feikin et al. failed to link penicillin resistance to mortality (67). However, if deaths in the first 4 days were excluded as likely refractory to any effective antimicrobial therapy, mortality was significantly associated with penicillin MIC ≥4 µg/mL or cefotaxime MIC ≥2 µg/mL. This study is limited, however, by the fact that information about the severity of illness on presentation and whether the specific antimicrobial agents received were active in vitro was not included in the analysis. A final limitation of the studies assessing the impact of resistance on outcomes is that the in vitro activity of the actual antibiotic regimen the patients received has not been correlated with outcomes. One would expect that clinical failures could only be ascribed to drug resistance for patients receiving discordant therapy (i.e., the infecting organism is resistant to all drugs used) rather than concordant therapy. However, studies have not found an association between discordant therapy and an increased risk of clinical failure (37,60,68).

The MICs associated with *ermB*-mediated resistance are often ≥128 µg/mL. These levels are far greater than the drug levels routinely achieved in serum or epithelial lining fluid (ELF). As a result, the resistance conferred by this mechanism would be expected to be clinically relevant. For a majority of isolates with *mefA*-mediated macrolide-resistance, the MICs are within a range of drug concentrations achievable in the ELF by routine dosing of clarithromycin or, possibly, azithromycin. However, in a prospective study of pneumococcal bacteremia, macrolide resistance was found to contribute to an increased risk of macrolide failure, irrespective of the underlying resistance mechanism or of the degree of elevation in erythromycin MIC (69). Current data suggest that, unlike penicillin resistance, macrolide resistance is more likely to be clinically relevant and may lead to clinical failures (48,69–71).

Microbiologic failures and the selection of resistant organisms during therapy for CAP and acute exacerbations of chronic bronchitis (AECB) with ciprofloxacin and ofloxacin have been well described (72). Clinical failures have been reported for patients receiving levofloxacin for AECB or pneumonia in the setting of fluoroquinolone resistance (72–74). Most failures have occurred in older adults with underlying lung disease and recent exposure to fluoroquinolones. Failure has occurred despite intravenous administration and most patients reported have responded to agents of another antibiotic class, suggesting that failure was related to resistance.

NEW THERAPIES OR THERAPEUTIC STRATEGIES

Optimal use of antimicrobials begins by selecting the most potent agent as the first choice for therapy. Pharmacodynamic data from experimental models and clinical studies allow comparisons among members of each antibiotic class to predict the agents that are most likely to effect the greatest bacterial eradication and result in the least selection of resistant mutants (75,76). Sub-optimal exposure to any antimicrobial may occur through inadequate dosing, duration of administration, and failure to consider the antimicrobial concentrations at the site of infection. Inadequate antibiotic therapy contributes to carriage of DRSP that in turn promotes spread of resistant clones (77–79).

Beta-lactams work in a time-dependent manner, which means that the duration of time during which their concentration stays above the MIC at the site of infection is critical to their success. Currently, all parenteral beta-lactams recommended for the treatment of pneumococcal pneumonia can achieve a time above MIC of 40% to 50% against organisms with a MIC of $\leq 2\,\mu g/mL$ using standard dosing, although some, such as cefuroxime, barely reach this critical value (54). Largely on the basis of the clinical and pharmacodynamic data presented thus far, the CLSI has instituted new interpretive breakpoints against non-meningeal isolates. Using these new breakpoints, a much greater proportion of pneumococci are now considered susceptible (80). Since, penicillin-resistance in *S. pneumoniae* is due to step-wise alteration in PBPs, and not due to beta-lactamases, administration of higher doses of beta-lactams would therefore overcome resistance. Highly active beta-lactams effective against *S. pneumoniae* include high-dose amoxicillin (90–100 mg/kg/day), cefdinir, cefpodoxime, cefprozil, and cefuroxime. Effective parenteral agents include ceftriaxone and cefotaxime, while ceftazidime and ticarcillin should be avoided.

It is important to evaluate the in vitro activity of an antimicrobial against the pathogen in conjunction with achievable concentrations at the site of infection. Through exceptional tissue penetration and long tissue elimination half-lives, macrolides may achieve concentrations at the site of infection that are substantially greater than serum levels. In the case of pneumonia caused by *S. pneumoniae*, antimicrobial levels in the alveolar ELF (and, to a lesser extent, within leukocytes and alveolar macrophages) are thought to be more important in determining therapeutic efficacy than serum levels (81–83). Macrolides such as clarithromycin and azithromycin are concentrated in leukocytes and have higher concentrations in alveolar ELF tissues compared with plasma (84). Therefore, these agents are very active for pneumonias. The treatment of uncomplicated pneumonia caused by isolates with MICs as high as 4 μg/mL or even 8 to 16 μg/mL may be possible due to the exceptional tissue penetration of the macrolides. For now, macrolide monotherapy remains a reasonable alternative for outpatients without comorbidities. Continued monitoring of the clinical efficacy of the macrolides will be important as the prevalence and the magnitude of macrolide resistance continues to increase. Ketolides are generally active against MLS-resistant pneumococci due to a greater affinity for the ribosomal binding site and weaker induction of inducible *erm* expression. Telithromycin is also a weak inducer and poor substrate for the *mefA* efflux pump (85). In April 2004, telithromycin was approved in the United States for the treatment of CAP, AECB, and acute bacterial sinusitis. Despite the advanced targeting of telithromycin, safety signals have been detected with respect to blurry vision, unmasking and worsening of myasthenia gravis, and acute hepatotoxicity. This has led to loss of its indication for AECB and acute bacterial sinusitis. Though it still has an indication for CAP, it is not to be used in patients with myasthenia gravis. In the latest CAP guidelines, final recommendations for telithromycin are pending safety evaluation by the U.S. Food and Drug Administration (FDA) (86).

The newer fluoroquinolones, gemifloxacin and moxifloxacin, possess improved activity against *S. pneumoniae*. They have proven effective against penicillin-resistant, macrolide-resistant, and multidrug-resistant *S. pneumoniae*. High clinical cure and bacterial eradication rates have been observed in clinical trials using fluoroquinolones for the treatment of community-acquired respiratory infections (87). For patients in which fluoroquinolones have been used to treat CAP or acute exacerbation of chronic bronchitis, the clinical cure rates are typically 90% (88). Moreover, the new fluoroquinolones may be dosed once-daily, increasing patient compliance (87). However, fewer genetic barriers are likely to result in more rapid development of resistance in *S. pneumoniae* under conditions of expanded use. The newer fluoroquinolones moxifloxacin and gemifloxacin combine the highest in vitro potency and the best pharmacokinetic profiles. These drugs require two spontaneous mutations (typically, 1 in *gyrA*, 1 in *parC*) before a "wild-type" organism develops clinically significant resistance. Thus these agents should not only be more effective, but also less likely to select for resistance. Peak levels for these drugs in serum exceed the MIC for first-step *gyrA* mutants (89,90). This rationale for preferential use of moxifloxacin and gemifloxacin is undermined if the infecting isolate already harbors a mutation in *parC*, as might occur after ciprofloxacin exposure. This isolate, while still susceptible to gemifloxacin and moxifloxacin, then requires only a single mutation in *gyrA* to acquire resistance to these agents. For reasons already discussed, such an event is probable during the treatment of CAP and may set the stage for selective amplification of the double mutant under continued fluoroquinolone pressure. Unfortunately, current routine methods for susceptibility testing are not sufficiently sensitive to detect such isolates harboring *parC* mutations (91). This logic therefore suggests that we should not be saving the most potent agents under the premise that patients who fail a less potent fluoroquinolone should still respond to most potent agents. It will be difficult to preserve the efficacy of the latter agents if resistance mutations enriched by less potent fluoroquinolones continues to increase in prevalence.

TABLE 2   List of Various Options for Empiric Antimicrobial Treatment of
Community-Acquired Pneumonia

Outpatient
Healthy and no antimicrobial use within 3 months
    Macrolide
    Doxycyline
Presence of comorbidities (chronic heart, lung, liver, renal disease; diabetes mellitus; alcoholism;
  malignancies; asplenia; immunosuppressing conditions or use of immunosuppressing drugs)
  or antimicrobial use within past 3 months
    Respiratory fluoroquinolone (moxifloxacin, gemifloxacin, or levofloxacin)
    Beta-lactam and macrolide
Inpatient
Non-ICU treatment
    Respiratory fluoroquinolone
    Beta-lactam and macrolide
ICU treatment
    Beta-lactam (cefotaxime, ceftriaxone, or ampicillin-sulbactam) and azithromycin
    Above beta-lactam and respiratory fluoroquinolone
If *Pseudomonas* is a concern
    Antipneumococcal, antipseudomonal beta-lactam (piperacillin/tazobactam, cefepime,
      imipenem, or meropenem), and fluoroquinolone (ciprofloxacin
      or levofloxacin—750mg)
    Above beta-lactam and aminoglycoside and azithromycin
    Above beta-lactam and aminoglycoside and antipneumococcal fluoroquinolone

Abbreviation: ICU, intensive care unit.
Source: Adapted from Ref. 86.

    In March 2007, new guidelines for the treatment of CAP were released by the American Thoracic Society (ATS), the Infectious Diseases Society of America (IDSA), and the Centers for Disease Control and Prevention (CDC) (86). The guidelines for treatment of empiric outpatient and inpatient CAP were not changed significantly from previous guidelines. Ertapenem was added as an acceptable beta-lactam alternative for hospitalized patients with risk factors for Gram-negative infections other than *Pseudomonas*. Table 2 summarizes the 2007 CAP recommendations for outpatient and inpatient treatment.

    Current immunization against pneumococcal pneumonia and influenza should reduce the incidence of CAP and other respiratory tract infections. Immunization against *S. pneumoniae*, with Pneumovax^{TM} (pneumococcal vaccine polyvalent; Merck and Co., Inc., Whitehouse Station, New Jersey, U.S.A.) for adults or Prevnar^{TM} (pneumococcal 7-valent conjugate vaccine; Wyeth pharmaceuticals, Inc., Philadel-phia, Pennsylvania, U.S.A.) for children, can reduce the incidence of invasive infections as well as reduce nasopharyngeal carriage (92,93). Since more than 80% of resistant pneumococci and all six of the predominant MDRSP clones in the United States are covered by the vaccines (94), more appropriate use of both vaccines could play a very valuable role in reducing the spread of drug-resistant *S. pneumoniae* (40).

CONCLUSION

Streptococcus pneumoniae is the bacterial pathogen responsible for a number of infections, particularly CAP. These bacterial infections are a significant cause of morbidity and contribute significantly to health costs in the United States; rates of antimicrobial-resistant *S. pneumoniae* are on the rise. Despite rising rates of resistant

S. pneumoniae, beta-lactams, macrolides, and fluoroquinolones are likely to be effective for empiric treatment of CAP. However, pharmacokinetic and pharmaco-dynamic parameters need to be considered during the selection of the appropriate antimicrobial. Use of a narrow/spectrum but highly potent agent is likely to be most successful in treatment and for the prevention of development of resistance. Fluoroquinolone use must be monitored, as overuse of these antimicrobials may eventually contribute to their premature demise. Preventive strategies include vaccination against influenza and *S. pneumoniae*, which may be very valuable in the management of *S. pneumoniae* and resistance.

REFERENCES

1. Fine MJ, Smith MA, Carson CA, et al. Prognosis and outcomes of patients with community-acquired pneumonia. A meta-analysis. JAMA 1996; 275:134–41.
2. File TM Jr. *Streptococcus pneumoniae* and community-acquired pneumonia: a cause for concern. Am J Med 2004; 117(Suppl. 3A):39S–50S.
3. Austrian R. Confronting drug-resistant pneumococci. Ann Intern Med 1994; 121:807–9.
4. Plouffe JF, Breiman RF, Facklam RR. Bacteremia with *Streptococcus pneumoniae*. Impli-cations for therapy and prevention. Franklin County Pneumonia Study Group. JAMA 1996; 275:194–8.
5. Jacobs MR. *Streptococcus pneumoniae*: epidemiology and patterns of resistance. Am J Med 2004; 117(Suppl. 3A):3S–15S.
6. Jenkins SG, Farrell DJ, Patel M, Lavin BS. Trends in anti-bacterial resistance among *Streptococcus pneumoniae* isolated in the USA, 2000–2003: PROTEKT US years 1–3. J Infect 2005; 51:355–63.
7. Jacobs MR, Koornhof HJ, Robins-Browne RM, et al. Emergence of multiply resistant pneumococci. N Engl J Med 1978; 299:735–40.
8. Niederman MS, McCombs JS, Unger AN, Kumar A, Popovian R. The cost of treating community-acquired pneumonia. Clin Ther 1998; 20:820–37.
9. Fenoll A, Martin Bourgon C, Munoz R, Vicioso D, Casal J. Serotype distribution and antimicrobial resistance of *Streptococcus pneumoniae* isolates causing systemic infections in Spain, 1979–1989. Rev Infect Dis 1991; 13:56–60.
10. Marton A, Gulyas M, Munoz R, Tomasz A. Extremely high incidence of antibiotic resistance in clinical isolates of *Streptococcus pneumoniae* in Hungary. J Infect Dis 1991; 163:542–8.
11. Friedland IR, Klugman KP. Antibiotic-resistant pneumococcal disease in South African children. Am J Dis Child 1992; 146:920–3.
12. Farrell DJ, Jenkins SG. Distribution across the USA of macrolide resistance and macrolide resistance mechanisms among *Streptococcus pneumoniae* isolates collected from patients with respiratory tract infections: PROTEKT US 2001–2002. J Antimicrob Chemother 2004; 54(Suppl. 1):i17–22.
13. Mandell LA, Bartlett JG, Dowell SF, File TM Jr, Musher DM, Whitney C. Update of practice guidelines for the management of community-acquired pneumonia in immu-nocompetent adults. Clin Infect Dis 2003; 37:1405–33.
14. Lynch IJ, Martinez FJ. Clinical relevance of macrolide-resistant *Streptococcus pneumoniae* for community-acquired pneumonia. Clin Infect Dis 2002; 34(Suppl. 1):S27–46.
15. Gay K, Baughman W, Miller Y, et al. The emergence of *Streptococcus pneumoniae* resistant to macrolide antimicrobial agents: a 6-year population-based assessment. J Infect Dis 2000; 182:1417–24.
16. Hyde TB, Gay K, Stephens DS, et al. Macrolide resistance among invasive *Streptococcus pneumoniae* isolates. JAMA 2001; 286:1857–62.
17. Hansen LH, Mauvais P, Douthwaite S. The macrolide-ketolide antibiotic binding site is formed by structures in domains II and V of 23S ribosomal RNA. Mol Microbiol 1999; 31:623–31.

18. Xiong L, Shah S, Mauvais P, Mankin AS. A ketolide resistance mutation in domain II of 23S rRNA reveals the proximity of hairpin 35 to the peptidyl transferase centre. Mol Microbiol 1999; 31:633–9.
19. Champney WS, Tober CL, Burdine R. A comparison of the inhibition of translation and 50S ribosomal subunit formation in Staphylococcus aureus cells by nine different macrolide antibiotics. Curr Microbiol 1998; 37:412–7.
20. Giovanetti E, Montanari MP, Marchetti F, Varaldo PE. In vitro activity of ketolides telithromycin and HMR 3004 against italian isolates of Streptococcus pyogenes and *Streptococcus pneumoniae* with different erythromycin susceptibility. J Antimicrob Chemother 2000; 46:905–8.
21. Davies TA, Dewasse BE, Jacobs MR, Appelbaum PC. In vitro development of resistance to telithromycin (HMR 3647), four macrolides, clindamycin, and pristinamycin in *Streptococcus pneumoniae*. Antimicrob Agents Chemother 2000; 44:414–7.
22. Reinert RR, van der Linden M, Al-Lahham A. Molecular characterization of the first telithromycin-resistant *Streptococcus pneumoniae* isolate in Germany. Antimicrob Agents Chemother 2005; 49:3520–2.
23. Al-Lahham A, Appelbaum PC, van der Linden M, Reinert RR. Telithromycin-nonsusceptible clinical isolates of *Streptococcus pneumoniae* from Europe. Antimicrob Agents Chemother 2006; 50:3897–900.
24. Doern GV, Richter SS, Miller A, et al. Antimicrobial resistance among *Streptococcus pneumoniae* in the United States: have we begun to turn the corner on resistance to certain antimicrobial classes? Clin Infect Dis 2005; 41:139–48.
25. Doern GV, Brown SD. Antimicrobial susceptibility among community-acquired respiratory tract pathogens in the USA: data from PROTEKT US 2000–01. J Infect 2004; 48:56–65.
26. Canton R, Morosini M, Enright MC, Morrissey I. Worldwide incidence, molecular epidemiology and mutations implicated in fluoroquinolone-resistant *Streptococcus pneumoniae*: data from the global PROTEKT surveillance programme. J Antimicrob Chemother 2003; 52:944–52.
27. Fukuda H, Hiramatsu K. Primary targets of fluoroquinolones in *Streptococcus pneumoniae*. Antimicrob Agents Chemother 1999; 43:410–2.
28. Davidson R, Cavalcanti R, Brunton JL, et al. Resistance to levofloxacin and failure of treatment of pneumococcal pneumonia. N Engl J Med 2002; 346:747–50.
29. Smith HJ, Nichol KA, Hoban DJ, Zhanel GG. Dual activity of fluoroquinolones against *Streptococcus pneumoniae*: the facts behind the claims. J Antimicrob Chemother 2002; 49:893–5.
30. Sanders CC. Mechanisms responsible for cross-resistance and dichotomous resistance among the quinolones. Clin Infect Dis 2001; 32(Suppl. 1):S1–8.
31. Chen DK, McGeer A, de Azavedo JC, Low DE. Decreased susceptibility of *Streptococcus pneumoniae* to fluoroquinolones in Canada. Canadian Bacterial Surveillance Network. N Engl J Med 1999; 341:233–9.
32. Ho PL, Yung RW, Tsang DN, et al. Increasing resistance of *Streptococcus pneumoniae* to fluoroquinolones: results of a Hong Kong multicentre study in 2000. J Antimicrob Chemother 2001; 48:659–65.
33. Block SL, Harrison CJ, Hedrick JA, et al. Penicillin-resistant *Streptococcus pneumoniae* in acute otitis media: risk factors, susceptibility patterns and antimicrobial management. Pediatr Infect Dis J 1995; 14:751–9.
34. Dowell SF, Schwartz B. Resistant pneumococci: protecting patients through judicious use of antibiotics. Am Fam Physician 1997; 55:1647–54, 1657–8.
35. Clavo-Sanchez AJ, Giron-Gonzalez JA, Lopez-Prieto D, et al. Multivariate analysis of risk factors for infection due to penicillin-resistant and multidrug-resistant *Streptococcus pneumoniae*: a multicenter study. Clin Infect Dis 1997; 24:1052–9.
36. Vanderkooi OG, Low DE, Green K, Powis JE, McGeer A. Predicting antimicrobial resistance in invasive pneumococcal infections. Clin Infect Dis 2005; 40:1288–97.
37. Ewig S, Ruiz M, Torres A, et al. Pneumonia acquired in the community through drug-resistant *Streptococcus pneumoniae*. Am J Respir Crit Care Med 1999; 159:1835–42.

38. Nava JM, Bella F, Garau J, et al. Predictive factors for invasive disease due to penicillin-resistant *Streptococcus pneumoniae*: a population-based study. Clin Infect Dis 1994; 19:884–90.

39. Campbell GD Jr, Silberman R. Drug-resistant *Streptococcus pneumoniae*. Clin Infect Dis 1998; 26:1188–95.

40. Kyaw MH, Lynfield R, Schaffner W, et al. Effect of introduction of the pneumococcal conjugate vaccine on drug-resistant *Streptococcus pneumoniae*. N Engl J Med 2006; 354:1455–63.

41. Farrell DJ, Klugman KP, Pichichero M. Increased antimicrobial resistance among nonvaccine serotypes of *Streptococcus pneumoniae* in the pediatric population after the introduction of 7-valent pneumococcal vaccine in the United States. Pediatr Infect Dis J 2007; 26:123–8.

42. Moreno S, Garcia-Leoni ME, Cercenado E, Diaz MD, Bernaldo de Quiros JC, Bouza E. Infections caused by erythromycin-resistant *Streptococcus pneumoniae*: incidence, risk factors, and response to therapy in a prospective study. Clin Infect Dis 1995; 20:1195–200.

43. Metlay JP, Fishman NO, Joffe MM, Kallan MJ, Chittams JL, Edelstein PH. Macrolide resistance in adults with bacteremic pneumococcal pneumonia. Emerg Infect Dis 2006; 12:1223–30.

44. Baquero F. Evolving resistance patterns of *Streptococcus pneumoniae*: a link with long-acting macrolide consumption? J Chemother 1999; 11(Suppl. 1):35–43.

45. Bergman M, Huikko S, Huovinen P, Paakkari P, Seppala H. Macrolide and azithromycin use are linked to increased macrolide resistance in *Streptococcus pneumoniae*. Antimicrob Agents Chemother 2006; 50:3646–50.

46. Leach AJ, Shelby-James TM, Mayo M, et al. A prospective study of the impact of community-based azithromycin treatment of trachoma on carriage and resistance of *Streptococcus pneumoniae*. Clin Infect Dis 1997; 24:356–62.

47. Morita JY, Kahn E, Thompson T, et al. Impact of azithromycin on oropharyngeal carriage of group A Streptococcus and nasopharyngeal carriage of macrolide-resistant *Streptococcus pneumoniae*. Pediatr Infect Dis J 2000; 19:41–6.

48. Malhotra-Kumar S, Lammens C, Coenen S, Van Herck K, Goossens H. Effect of azithromycin and clarithromycin therapy on pharyngeal carriage of macrolide-resistant streptococci in healthy volunteers: a randomised, double-blind, placebo-controlled study. Lancet 2007; 369:482–90.

49. Ho PL, Tse WS, Tsang KW, et al. Risk factors for acquisition of levofloxacin-resistant *Streptococcus pneumoniae*: a case-control study. Clin Infect Dis 2001; 32:701–7.

50. Linares J, de la Campa AG, Pallares R. Fluoroquinolone resistance in *Streptococcus pneumoniae*. N Engl J Med 1999; 341:1546–7; author reply 1547–8.

51. Niederman MS, Mandell LA, Anzueto A, et al. Guidelines for the management of adults with community-acquired pneumonia. Diagnosis, assessment of severity, antimicrobial therapy, and prevention. Am J Respir Crit Care Med 2001; 163:1730–54.

52. Bhavnani SM, Hammel JP, Jones RN, Ambrose PG. Relationship between increased levofloxacin use and decreased susceptibility of *Streptococcus pneumoniae* in the United States. Diagn Microbiol Infect Dis 2005; 51:31–7.

53. Lautenbach E, Larosa LA, Kasbekar N, Peng HP, Maniglia RJ, Fishman NO. Fluoroquinolone utilization in the emergency departments of academic medical centers: prevalence of, and risk factors for, inappropriate use. Arch Intern Med 2003; 163:601–5.

54. Heffelfinger JD, Dowell SF, Jorgensen JH, et al. Management of community-acquired pneumonia in the era of pneumococcal resistance: a report from the Drug-Resistant *Streptococcus pneumoniae* Therapeutic Working Group. Arch Intern Med 2000; 160:1399–408.

55. Austriam R, Gold J. Pneumococcal bacteremia with especial reference to bacteremic pneumococcal pneumonia. Ann Intern Med 1964; 60:759–76.

56. Meehan TP, Fine MJ, Krumholz HM, et al. Quality of care, process, and outcomes in elderly patients with pneumonia. Jama 1997; 278:2080–4.

57. Tan TQ, Mason EO Jr, Barson WJ, et al. Clinical characteristics and outcome of children with pneumonia attributable to penicillin-susceptible and penicillin-nonsusceptible *Streptococcus pneumoniae*. Pediatrics 1998; 102:1369–75.

58. Falco V, Almirante B, Jordano Q, et al. Influence of penicillin resistance on outcome in adult patients with invasive pneumococcal pneumonia: is penicillin useful against intermediately resistant strains? J Antimicrob Chemother 2004; 54:481–8.
59. Aspa J, Rajas O, Rodriguez de Castro F, et al. Drug-resistant pneumococcal pneumonia: clinical relevance and related factors. Clin Infect Dis 2004; 38:787–98.
60. Falagas ME, Siempos, II, Bliziotis IA, Panos GZ. Impact of initial discordant treatment with beta-lactam antibiotics on clinical outcomes in adults with pneumococcal pneumonia: a systematic review. Mayo Clin Proc 2006; 81:1567–74.
61. Bishai W. The in vivo–in vitro paradox in pneumococcal respiratory tract infections. J Antimicrob Chemother 2002; 49:433–6.
62. Tleyjeh IM, Tlaygeh HM, Hejal R, Montori VM, Baddour LM. The impact of penicillin resistance on short-term mortality in hospitalized adults with pneumococcal pneumonia: a systematic review and meta-analysis. Clin Infect Dis 2006; 42:788–97.
63. Metlay JP, Hofmann J, Cetron MS, et al. Impact of penicillin susceptibility on medical outcomes for adult patients with bacteremic pneumococcal pneumonia. Clin Infect Dis 2000; 30:520–8.
64. Ho PL, Que TL, Ng TK, Chiu SS, Yung RW, Tsang KW. Clinical outcomes of bacteremic pneumococcal infections in an area with high resistance. Eur J Clin Microbiol Infect Dis 2006; 25:323–7.
65. Musher DM, Bartlett JG, Doern GV. A fresh look at the definition of susceptibility of *Streptococcus pneumoniae* to beta-lactam antibiotics. Arch Intern Med 2001; 161:2538–44.
66. Turett GS, Blum S, Fazal BA, Justman JE, Telzak EE. Penicillin resistance and other predictors of mortality in pneumococcal bacteremia in a population with high human immunodeficiency virus seroprevalence. Clin Infect Dis 1999; 29:321–7.
67. Feikin DR, Schuchat A, Kolczak M, et al. Mortality from invasive pneumococcal pneumonia in the era of antibiotic resistance, 1995–1997. Am J Public Health 2000; 90:223–9.
68. Pallares R, Linares J, Vadillo M, et al. Resistance to penicillin and cephalosporin and mortality from severe pneumococcal pneumonia in Barcelona, Spain. N Engl J Med 1995; 333:474–80.
69. Daneman N, McGeer A, Green K, Low DE. Macrolide resistance in bacteremic pneumococcal disease: implications for patient management. Clin Infect Dis 2006; 43:432–8.
70. Musher DM, Dowell ME, Shortridge VD, et al. Emergence of macrolide resistance during treatment of pneumococcal pneumonia. N Engl J Med 2002; 346:630–1.
71. Lonks JR, Garau J, Gomez L, et al. Failure of macrolide antibiotic treatment in patients with bacteremia due to erythromycin-resistant *Streptococcus pneumoniae*. Clin Infect Dis 2002; 35:556–64.
72. Chodosh S, Schreurs A, Siami G, et al. Efficacy of oral ciprofloxacin vs. clarithromycin for treatment of acute bacterial exacerbations of chronic bronchitis. The Bronchitis Study Group. Clin Infect Dis 1998; 27:730–8.
73. Urban C, Rahman N, Zhao X, et al. Fluoroquinolone-resistant *Streptococcus pneumoniae* associated with levofloxacin therapy. J Infect Dis 2001; 184:794–8.
74. Kuehnert MJ, Nolte FS, Perlino CA. Fluoroquinolone resistance in *Streptococcus pneumoniae*. Ann Intern Med 1999; 131:312–3.
75. Schentag JJ, Gilliland KK, Paladino JA. What have we learned from pharmacokinetic and pharmacodynamic theories? Clin Infect Dis 2001; 32(Suppl. 1):S39–46.
76. Craig WA. Pharmacokinetic/pharmacodynamic parameters: rationale for antibacterial dosing of mice and men. Clin Infect Dis 1998; 26:1–10; quiz 11–2.
77. Dagan R, Klugman KP, Craig WA, Baquero F. Evidence to support the rationale that bacterial eradication in respiratory tract infection is an important aim of antimicrobial therapy. J Antimicrob Chemother 2001; 47:129–40.
78. Yagupsky P, Porat N, Fraser D, et al. Acquisition, carriage, and transmission of pneumococci with decreased antibiotic susceptibility in young children attending a day care facility in southern Israel. J Infect Dis 1998; 177:1003–12.

79. Dabernat H, Geslin P, Megraud F, et al. Effects of cefixime or co-amoxiclav treatment on nasopharyngeal carriage of *Streptococcus pneumoniae* and Haemophilus influenzae in children with acute otitis media. J Antimicrob Chemother 1998; 41:253–8.
80. Doern GV, Heilmann KP, Huynh HK, Rhomberg PR, Coffman SL, Brueggemann AB. Antimicrobial resistance among clinical isolates of *Streptococcus pneumoniae* in the United States during 1999–2000, including a comparison of resistance rates since 1994–1995. Antimicrob Agents Chemother 2001; 45:1721–9.
81. Amsden GW. Pneumococcal macrolide resistance—myth or reality? J Antimicrob Chemother 1999; 44:1–6.
82. Baldwin DR, Honeybourne D, Wise R. Pulmonary disposition of antimicrobial agents: in vivo observations and clinical relevance. Antimicrob Agents Chemother 1992; 36:1176–80.
83. Baldwin DR, Honeybourne D, Wise R. Pulmonary disposition of antimicrobial agents: methodological considerations. Antimicrob Agents Chemother 1992; 36:1171–5.
84. Rodvold KA, Gotfried MH, Danziger LH, Servi RJ. Intrapulmonary steady-state concentrations of clarithromycin and azithromycin in healthy adult volunteers. Antimicrob Agents Chemother 1997; 41:1399–402.
85. Leclercq R, Courvalin P. Resistance to macrolides and related antibiotics in *Streptococcus pneumoniae*. Antimicrob Agents Chemother 2002; 46:2727–34.
86. Mandell LA, Wunderink RG, Anzueto A, et al. Infectious Diseases Society of America/American Thoracic Society consensus guidelines on the management of community-acquired pneumonia in adults. Clin Infect Dis 2007; 44(Suppl. 2):S27–72.
87. Zhanel GG, Fontaine S, Adam H, et al. A review of new fluoroquinolones: focus on their use in respiratory tract infections. Treat Respir Med 2006; 5:437–65.
88. Shams WE, Evans ME. Guide to selection of fluoroquinolones in patients with lower respiratory tract infections. Drugs 2005; 65:949–91.
89. Blondeau JM, Zhao X, Hansen G, Drlica K. Mutant prevention concentrations of fluoroquinolones for clinical isolates of *Streptococcus pneumoniae*. Antimicrob Agents Chemother 2001; 45:433–8.
90. Smith HJ, Walters M, Hisanaga T, Zhanel GG, Hoban DJ. Mutant prevention concentrations for single-step fluoroquinolone-resistant mutants of wild-type, efflux-positive, or ParC or GyrA mutation-containing *Streptococcus pneumoniae* isolates. Antimicrob Agents Chemother 2004; 48:3954–8.
91. Richardson DC, Bast D, McGeer A, Low DE. Evaluation of susceptibility testing to detect fluoroquinolone resistance mechanisms in *Streptococcus pneumoniae*. Antimicrob Agents Chemother 2001; 45:1911–4.
92. Black S, Shinefield H, Fireman B, et al. Efficacy, safety and immunogenicity of heptavalent pneumococcal conjugate vaccine in children. Northern California Kaiser Permanente Vaccine Study Center Group. Pediatr Infect Dis J 2000; 19:187–95.
93. Dagan R, Melamed R, Muallem M, et al. Reduction of nasopharyngeal carriage of pneumococci during the second year of life by a heptavalent conjugate pneumococcal vaccine. J Infect Dis 1996; 174:1271–8.
94. Whitney CG, Farley MM, Hadler J, et al. Increasing prevalence of multidrug-resistant *Streptococcus pneumoniae* in the United States. N Engl J Med 2000; 343:1917–24.

Acinetobacter Species: Resistance Update and Treatment Options

Lisa L. Maragakis and Trish M. Perl

Department of Medicine, Division of Infectious Diseases, and Department of Hospital Epidemiology and Infection Control, Johns Hopkins Medical Institutions, Baltimore, Maryland, U.S.A.

INTRODUCTION

Multidrug-resistant (MDR) *Acinetobacter baumannii* has been reported worldwide and is now recognized to be among the most difficult antimicrobial-resistant Gram-negative bacilli (GNB) to control and treat. While definitions of antimicrobial resistance vary in the literature, increasing antimicrobial resistance among isolates of *Acinetobacter* has been clearly documented. The organism is a rapidly emerging pathogen in the healthcare setting, where it causes healthcare-associated infections including bacteremia, pneumonia, meningitis, urinary tract infections, and wound infections. Properties of *A. baumannii*, such as its ability to survive under a wide range of environmental conditions and to persist for extended periods of time on environmental surfaces, make it a frequent cause of outbreaks as well as an endemic pathogen in the healthcare setting. Risk factors for colonization or infection with *A. baumannii* include prolonged length of hospital stay, exposure to intensive care units (ICUs) and mechanical ventilation, antimicrobial use, recent surgery, invasive procedures, and underlying severity of illness. An increase in the level of antimicrobial resistance greatly limits the therapeutic options for patients infected with this organism, especially when isolates are resistant to the carbapenem class of antibiotics. Carbapenems remain the treatment of choice when isolates are susceptible and colistin has made a resurgence for use against MDR-*Acinetobacter* infections that have developed high-level resistance to all other conventional agents. Even though some data support the use of sulbactam, rifampin, and tigecycline, the available literature cannot provide clear answers about these agents as therapeutic options due to lack of controlled clinical studies. Furthermore, it is not clear if combination therapy is more effective than monotherapy. These uncertainties and the lack of therapeutic options make infection control measures and prevention strategies that are effective for controlling transmission of antimicrobial-resistant *Acinetobacter* essential.

THE ORGANISM

Acinetobacter spp. are non–lactose-fermenting, Gram-negative, aerobic coccobacilli. *A. baumannii* is the species that is most associated with clinical infections and outbreaks (1). This pathogen has a complicated taxonomic history and is sometimes referred to as the *A. calcoaceticus–A. baumannii* complex (2). *Acinetobacter* spp. are generally considered to be of low virulence, though they do possess virulence factors including a polysaccharide capsule and endotoxin (1). *Acinetobacter* spp. can be found on healthy human skin, particularly in the groin, axilla, and toe webs, but most are species other than *A. baumannii* (3). The organism is ubiquitous in environmental soil and water and can survive in the environment for long periods of time even under adverse conditions such as desiccation (2,4).

EPIDEMIOLOGY

Acinetobacter is a rapidly emerging pathogen in the healthcare setting, where it causes healthcare-associated infections including bacteremia, pneumonia, meningitis, urinary tract infections, and wound infections. Properties of *A. baumannii*, such as its ability to survive under a wide range of environmental conditions and to persist for extended periods of time on environmental surfaces, make it a frequent cause of outbreaks as well as an endemic pathogen in the healthcare setting (2). Risk factors for colonization or infection with *A. baumannii* include prolonged length of hospital stay, exposure to ICUs and mechanical ventilation, antimicrobial use, recent surgery, invasive procedures, and underlying severity of illness (Table 1) (2).

Outbreaks

Antimicrobial-resistant *A. baumannii* has been responsible for numerous outbreaks in acute care hospitals. *Acinetobacter's* ability to survive on environmental surfaces for months makes nosocomial transmission extremely difficult to control. The costs associated with control of an outbreak can be staggering, and some institutions have been forced to close entire units in order to interrupt transmission of *Acinetobacter*. Most reported outbreaks occur in ICUs, burn units, and settings with high-risk patients. Outbreaks have been traced to respiratory care equipment, curtains, wound care procedures, humidifiers, as well as other patient care items and widespread environmental contamination is often reported (5–9). Generally, outbreaks are caused by one or more epidemic clones of *Acinetobacter*, though outbreak strains can co-exist with endemic strains, making it more difficult to detect and control transmission.

Endemic *Acinetobacter*

In many cases, MDR-*Acinetobacter* has become endemic in healthcare institutions demonstrating complex epidemiology, co-existence of multiple strain types, and a combination of "imported" organisms and transmission among patients. Once MDR organisms are introduced into the healthcare environment, several factors

TABLE 1 Risk Factors for Colonization or Infection with *Acinetobacter baumannii*

Prolonged length of hospital stay
Exposure to intensive care units
Exposure to mechanical ventilation
Antimicrobial use
Recent surgery
Invasive procedures
Severity of illness

work together to maintain their presence, including the presence of susceptible patients, selective pressure from antimicrobial use, the presence of patients already colonized or infected (colonization pressure), and incomplete compliance with infection control procedures (10). New York has had some of the most extensive experience in the United States to date dealing with antimicrobial resistant GNB, including *Acinetobacter* spp. and *Pseudomonas* spp. In a report of citywide clonal spread, 53% of *A. baumannii* and 24% of *P. aeruginosa* isolates were resistant to carbapenems, while 12% and 29%, respectively, were resistant to all standard antimicrobial agents (11). Abbo et al. studied 118 patients with MDR *Acinetobacter* in Israel and found ten different pulsed field gel electrophoresis (PFGE) clones, two predominant clones, and many small clusters of patients with no common source identified despite molecular testing and extensive investigation (12). This type of scenario illustrates how the complex epidemiology of the endemic organism makes it even more difficult to control.

Inter-institutional Spread

The *Acinetobacter* literature demonstrates inter-institutional transmission highlighting the need for effective control strategies and a coordinated public health response to this growing threat. Molecular-based typing of strains such as PFGE or other methods can be used to identify outbreaks and to monitor inter-institutional, regional, and international transmission (13). Using ribotyping, amplified fragment length polymorphism (AFLP) fingerprinting, and cluster analysis, Nemec and Dijkshoorn et al. demonstrated the broad genetic relatedness of carbapenem-susceptible *Acinetobacter* isolates that have caused outbreaks in Western Europe (14). Investigators have used PFGE to demonstrate inter-institutional spread of carbapenem-resistant *Acinetobacter* among multiple acute care hospitals in many locales including New York, Argentina, the United Kingdom, and the Iberian Peninsula, among others (15–18). Gales et al. used PFGE to demonstrate the spread of epidemic *Acinetobacter* clones between Brazil and Argentina (19).

MDR *Acinetobacter* has been reported in patients residing in rehabilitation and long-term-care facilities (LTCFs) as well as in acute care hospitals (20,21). LTCFs face special infection control challenges due to a multitude of factors including lack of on-site laboratory facilities and limited resources (22). Urban et al. has called for further study to determine if colonization of patients in LTCFs is a source of transmission to patients in acute care hospitals and vice versa (23). Patient movement between healthcare facilities and among different levels of care, including acute care hospitals, community hospitals, and LTCFs, likely represents an important source of healthcare-associated transmission of MDR organisms (Fig. 1). Furthermore, rehabilitation and some LTCFs are accepting patients with increasing illness severity who require advanced medical support such as mechanical ventilation, adding a new risk population to these facilities.

U.S. Military Experience

An increased number of *A. baumannii* infections have been noted in U.S. military personnel wounded during the conflicts in Iraq and Afghanistan (24,25). These infections are generally extremely resistant to a variety of antimicrobial agents, are commonly associated with traumatic injuries, and include deep wound infections, osteomyelitis, respiratory infections, and bacteremia (24–27). There are three main

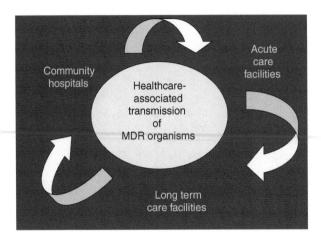

FIGURE 1   Inter-institutional spread of MDR organisms. *Abbreviation*: MDR, multidrug resistant.

hypotheses for how wounded soldiers acquire *Acinetobacter* (28). The first is that soldiers are previously colonized with the organism, perhaps on their skin or in their nares, and are auto-inoculated during a penetrating traumatic injury. However, cultures taken prior to deployment from healthy soldiers' skin and nares found no *Acinetobacter* in the nares, and though skin colonization was common, strain types did not match the strains that infect returning wounded soldiers (29,30). Therefore, it is less likely that prior colonization explains *Acinetobacter* infected war wounds. The second hypothesis is that *Acinetobacter* from the local environment (soil or water) is introduced during traumatic injury. Two studies showed that cultures of war wounds taken in Iraq soon after injuries grew primarily low virulence Gram-positive organisms. The few Gram-negative organisms recovered were susceptible to many antimicrobial agents (28,31), which does not support the hypothesis of environmental contamination at the time of injury. The third hypothesis is that *Acinetobacter* is healthcare-associated, acquired by soldiers in medical facilities during the process of stabilization, emergency treatment, and evacuation through the military medical system. Though investigation is ongoing and the true source of *Acinetobacter* infections in soldiers remains uncertain, current literature favors this third hypothesis of healthcare-associated transmission (25,26,29,31). A retrospective study of cultures in a deployed, military, tertiary care hospital in Iraq found that while newly injured U.S. soldiers' cultures grew mostly coagulase-negative staphylococcus, cultures from non-U.S. patients (mostly Iraqi civilians) grew significantly more antimicrobial-resistant Gram-negative organisms including *Acinetobacter* (31). The hospital received soldiers soon after their injuries and most soldiers were transferred out of the facility within 72 hours (31). Deployed military healthcare facilities increasingly provide humanitarian care to local populations as well as military personnel (31). This allows increased opportunities for transmission of endemic pathogens. In addition, these military medical facilities often operate in existing local hospitals that may have endemic sources of antimicrobial resistant organisms, and infection control efforts are limited by the facilities, conflict, and other local conditions (31). The U.S. military has implemented additional infection control procedures and active surveillance cultures for *Acinetobacter* (25). The potential for introduction of new, virulent strains of MDR *Acinetobacter* into U.S. and U.K. hospitals by returning soldiers is a major concern that warrants ongoing surveillance and careful attention to infection control measures (26,32,33).

IMPACT ON PATIENT OUTCOMES AND COSTS

As described earlier, *Acinetobacter* infections usually occur in severely ill patients who undergo invasive procedures, including mechanical ventilation in the ICU. Consistent with this vulnerable patient population, the crude mortality rate in patients with *Acinetobacter* infections is high, with estimates ranging from 26% to 68% (34–36). However, since the severity of underlying illness is a significant risk factor for *Acinetobacter* infection, it has proved difficult to determine the attributable mortality of these infections independent of patients' severe underlying illnesses. A recent systematic review of matched case-control and cohort studies concluded that the available evidence suggests that infection or colonization with *Acinetobacter* is associated with increased mortality (37). Many studies attempting to answer the question of attributable mortality were, however, limited by small sample sizes, methodological differences, and failure to adequately control for patients' severity of illness (37). Other experts have concluded that *Acinetobacter* infection is not independently associated with increased mortality (2), and several studies that rigorously controlled for severity of illness did not find *Acinetobacter* infection to be associated with significantly increased mortality (34,38,39). An alternative explanation is that *Acinetobacter* infection is a marker of increased mortality in patients with severe underlying illness, injury, or burns but is not an independent predictor of mortality (38). The risk of mortality may be different for various types of *Acinetobacter* infection. Studies have found that *Acinetobacter* bacteremia secondary to pneumonia has a higher mortality rate than catheter-associated bacteremia (40,41). It is also important to consider how antimicrobial resistance is defined in these studies, since mortality may be related to the extent of antimicrobial resistance, the effectiveness of empiric therapy before susceptibility testing is complete, and the availability of definitive therapeutic options. One might imagine that *Acinetobacter* infection due to an MDR strain would lead to higher mortality due to the choice of ineffective empiric antimicrobial agents (agents to which the infection is not susceptible). Interestingly, several studies have found poor correlation between the empiric choice of antimicrobial agents to which the infection was resistant and patient mortality (34,38,40–42). However, a recent matched cohort study in Korea found that ineffective empiric antimicrobial therapy was significantly higher in patients with carbapenem-resistant *Acinetobacter* bacteremia than in patients with carbapenem-susceptible *Acinetobacter* bacteremia, and ineffective empiric therapy was an independent predictor of 30-day mortality (along with age, immunosuppression, and severity of illness) (36). In summary, the crude mortality of *Acinetobacter* infection is extremely high, it is difficult to distinguish the attributable mortality of *Acinetobacter* infection from that of the severity of underlying illnesses, and mortality may vary significantly depending on the type of infection and the extent of antimicrobial resistance.

In contrast to its debatable independent association with mortality, *Acinetobacter* infection is more convincingly associated with increased morbidity, prolonged stays in the hospital and ICU, and increased costs. A retrospective, matched cohort study found that patients with *Acinetobacter* bacteremia had a

5 days excess length of mechanical ventilator dependence and ICU stay compared to critically ill patients without *Acinetobacter* infection (39). Infection with a MDR strain of *Acinetobacter* may have an even greater impact and was found to significantly prolong ICU length of stay by 6 days and median hospital length of stay by 18 days (34,43). One study found no evidence of prolonged ICU length of stay in patients with ventilator-associated pneumonia (VAP) due to *Acinetobacter* (44). Again, the impact on length of stay may depend on the type of infection and the extent of antimicrobial resistance of the organism. Increased time on mechanical ventilation and lengths of stay for patients with healthcare-associated *Acinetobacter* infections imply that patients suffer increased morbidity from these infections. In addition, increased lengths of stay clearly indicate that these healthcare associated infections compromise the quality of care provided, which leads to increased healthcare costs and diverts resources away from other critical areas of healthcare (45). Though more difficult to quantify, these infections and their associated morbidity undoubtedly increase costs to patients, their families, and communities as well.

ANTIMICROBIAL RESISTANCE

Both *Acinetobacter* and *Pseudomonas* have high levels of intrinsic antimicrobial resistance, and increasing resistance has been documented for isolates worldwide. This extensive antimicrobial resistance may be due in part to the organisms' relatively impermeable outer membrane and its existence in soil and water where it is exposed to many environmental challenges and a large reservoir of resistance genes (46). Definitions of MDR *Acinetobacter* vary in the medical literature, referring to a wide array of genotypes and phenotypes that can be confusing to both researchers and clinicians (47). Two of the most common criteria for MDR are carbapenem resistance or resistance to three or more antimicrobial classes (47). Carbapenem-resistant *Acinetobacter* has been reported by tertiary-care hospitals, usually in the setting of nosocomial outbreaks. Some strains of MDR *Acinetobacter* are susceptible only to colistin or polymyxin B, peptide antibiotics not routinely used due to earlier reports of toxicities (sometimes these isolates are referred to as polymyxin-only-susceptible or POS *Acinetobacter*). Strains that demonstrate resistance to all antimicrobial agents including polymyxin (sometimes referred to as pan-drug-resistant, or PDR, *Acinetobacter*) have also been reported making treatment of these infections extremely difficult and in some cases impossible to treat.

Mechanisms of Resistance

Resistance mechanisms in *Acinetobacter* are similar to those of *Pseudomonas* though less is known about *Acinetobacter* because it has not been studied as extensively (Table 2) (48,49). The mechanisms of resistance generally fall into three categories: (*i*) antimicrobial inactivating enzymes, (*ii*) reduced access to bacterial targets, or (*iii*) mutations that change targets or cellular functions (Table 2) (49). In the first category of antimicrobial inactivating enzymes, *Acinetobacter* possesses a wide array of beta-lactamases that serve to hydrolyze and confer resistance to penicillins, cephalosporins, and carbapenems. There are four classes of beta-lactamases (A–D). *Acinetobacter* possesses class C enzymes (Amp C cephalosporinases) that are chromosomally encoded and confer resistance to broad-spectrum

TABLE 2 Mechanisms of Antimicrobial Resistance in *Acinetobacter* spp.

Antimicrobial inactivating enzymes	Beta-lactamases that hydrolyze and confer resistance to penicillins, cephalosporins, and carbapenems
	Class C enzymes, such as AmpC cephalosporinases (46,48)
	Class D OXA-type enzymes (50,51)
	Class B metallo-beta-lactamases, such as VIM and IMP (46,48)
	Aminoglycoside-modifying-enzymes (46)
Reduced access to bacterial targets	Loss or modification of porin channels which are important for transport of antimicrobial agents into the cell (46,48,54,55)
	Efflux pumps capable of actively removing a broad range of antimicrobial agents from the bacterial cell (46)
Mutations that change cellular targets or functions	Altered bacterial targets that decrease affinity for antimicrobial agents
	Changes in the bacterial cell membrane that interfere with colistin binding (56)
	Mutations in the bacterial targets *gyrA* and *parC* topoisomerase confer resistance to quinolone agents (46)

cephalosporins (46,48). Recently, in the setting of emerging carbapenem resistance among *Acinetobacter* species, a large number of class D OXA-type enzymes with activity against carbapenem agents have been characterized from diverse locations, including Scotland, Spain, France, Japan, Singapore, China, Brazil, Cuba, and Kuwait, among others (50,51). Some strains of *Acinetobacter*, like *Pseudomonas*, also express class B metallo-beta-lactamases (MBLs) that have a much greater power to hydrolyze a broad array of antimicrobial agents including carbapenems (48). The activity of MBLs, such as those belonging to the VIM and IMP families, depends on zinc ions. MBLs are much more efficient and potent than other beta-lactamases and pose a significant threat because they are often located on mobile genetic elements (class 1 integrons) that can be easily transferred among bacteria on plasmids (46,48). Many variants exist and both IMP and VIM beta-lactamases have been found in a wide array of bacterial species, including *Acinetobacter*, in many countries around the globe (48,52,53). Surveillance is needed to monitor the spread of MBLs, as this represents an emerging public health threat with implications for antimicrobial use and infection control (13). Aminoglycoside resistance can also be mediated by the mechanism of inactivating enzymes called aminoglycoside-modifying-enzymes (AMEs) (46) and genes conferring aminoglycoside resistance often co-exist with MBLs (13).

The second category of resistance mechanisms reduces the ability of antimicrobial agents to reach their intended bacterial target(s). Porin channels and other outer membrane proteins in the bacterial cell membrane are important for transport of antimicrobial agents into the cell to gain access to bacterial targets. Carbapenem resistance in *Acinetobacter* has been linked to the loss of proteins from the outer membrane of the bacterium and these proteins are thought to be porin channels (48,54,55). It is likely that beta-lactamases and outer membrane alterations such as modified porin channels work together to confer resistance to beta-lactam agents (46). Efflux pumps also work to reduce the ability of antimicrobial agents to reach their intended bacterial target by removing or expelling the agents. Similar to *Pseudomonas, Acinetobacter* possesses efflux pumps that are capable of actively removing a broad range of antimicrobial agents from the bacterial cell (46).

The third category of mechanisms of resistance involves point mutations that alter bacterial targets or functions, sometimes decreasing the affinity for antimicrobial agents or upregulating other cellular functions such as the production of efflux pumps or other proteins. Resistance to colistin is thought to be mediated by changes in the bacterial cell membrane that interfere with the agent's ability to bind bacterial targets (56). This type of mechanism is also seen in *Acinetobacter*'s resistance to quinolone agents from mutations in the bacterial targets *gyrA* and *parC* topoisomerase enzymes (46).

The origin of various mechanisms of resistance remains unclear but is generally one of three types. *Acinetobacter* species can acquire resistance genes from other organisms, mutations leading to resistance can develop over time within *Acinetobacter* strains, or small subpopulations with pre-existing resistance mechanisms may emerge and become dominant under the selective pressure of antimicrobial use (50). These three processes are not mutually exclusive and likely function together to explain the emerging resistance among *Acinetobacter* species. A recent study using a comparative genomic approach to study an epidemic MDR-*Acinetobacter* strain in France found a large genomic "resistance island" containing 45 resistance genes, many of which appeared to have been acquired from *Pseudomonas*, *Salmonella*, or *Escherichia* genera (57). In the healthcare setting, the emergence of antimicrobial resistant *Acinetobacter* is due to both selective pressure exerted by the use of broad-spectrum antibiotics and the transmission of antimicrobial-resistant strains among patients, though the amount that each contributes is not yet known (58).

TREATMENT
Carbapenems

Overall, increasing antimicrobial resistance of *Acinetobacter* species leaves few therapeutic options for infected patients. There are no well-designed clinical trials to compare regimens for treating MDR-*Acinetobacter* infections. Available data on various therapeutic regimens comes from in vitro studies, animal studies, and uncontrolled trials. Due to extensive antimicrobial resistance to other antimicrobial classes, clinicians rely heavily on carbapenems for these infections. Meropenem and imipenem remain the treatment of choice for MDR-*Acinetobacter* infections caused by isolates that retain susceptibility to this antimicrobial class. Colistin, amikacin, sulbactam (available as ampicillin/sulbactam), rifampin, and tetracycline are other agents that often have activity against MDR-*Acinetobacter* isolates. The Meropenem Yearly Susceptibility Test Information Collection (MYSTIC) surveillance program has documented discordance between *Acinetobacter* species' susceptibility to carbapenems in favor of imipenem as more potent than meropenem against these organisms [lower minimum inhibitory concentration (MIC) and higher percentage of susceptible isolates] (59,60). However, the converse result was reported for 320 *A. baumannii* isolates in Greece where meropenem was found to have superior activity compared with imipenem (61). It is thought that specific mechanisms of resistance such as efflux pumps may affect meropenem to a greater degree than imipenem while specific beta-lactamases hydrolyze imipenem more efficiently than meropenem (61). Distribution of these resistance mechanisms vary in different geographic locations. Susceptibility testing of imipenem does not predict susceptibility to meropenem or vice versa (59). Unfortunately, carbapenem-resistant *Acinetobacter* isolates are increasingly reported worldwide.

Beta-Lactamase Inhibitors

Beta-lactamase inhibitors alone, particularly sulbactam, have intrinsic activity against many *Acinetobacter* strains. The presence of a beta-lactam agent (i.e., ampicillin) in combination with the beta-lactamase inhibitor does not appear to contribute any activity or synergy (62,63). Sulbactam is not generally clinically available alone (without ampicillin) and monotherapy with sulbactam is not recommended for severe *Acinetobacter* infections. However, Wood et al. did report successful use of sulbactam to treat 14 patients with VAP due to MDR *Acinetobacter*, finding no difference in clinical outcomes compared to 63 patients who received imipenem therapy (64). Antimicrobial susceptibility testing of beta-lactam–beta-lactamase combinations at fixed concentrations (such as agar dilution or the E test) must be interpreted with caution as they may be misleading by indicating susceptibility when an isolate is actually resistant (63). Levin et al. reported a cure rate of 67.5% using ampicillin/sulbactam clinically for treatment of severe, carbapenem-resistant *Acinetobacter* infections (65). However, good patient outcomes in this case series were significantly associated with a lower severity of illness [measured by Acute Physiology and Chronic Health Evaluation II (APACHE II) score], and colistin was not studied as it was not clinically available in Brazil at the time of the study. Sulbactam may have a role in combination therapy for severe MDR-*Acinetobacter* infections, though more study is needed (see below).

Tigecycline

Tigecycline, a relatively new glycylcycline agent, has activity against MDR *Acinetobacter* (66) and has been used clinically despite the lack of established breakpoints to determine susceptibility of *Acinetobacter* isolates (67). However, like other agents in this class, tigecycline is bacteriostatic, not bactericidal, against *Acinetobacter* isolates (67). High-level resistance to tigecycline has been detected among some *Acinetobacter* isolates, raising concern that the organism will evade this antimicrobial agent by up-regulating chromosomally mediated efflux pumps (49,68–70). Peleg et al. recently reported two cases of MDR-*Acinetobacter* bloodstream infection that occurred while patients were receiving tigecycline for other indications (70). The isolates demonstrated high levels of tigecycline resistance apparently due to an efflux pump mechanism. Given this finding and concern over whether adequate peak serum concentrations can be achieved, tigecycline is best reserved for salvage therapy in consultation with an infectious diseases specialist until more data are available (70).

Aminoglycosides

Aminoglycoside agents such as tobramycin or amikacin may be a treatment option for MDR-*Acinetobacter* isolates that retain susceptibility. These agents are usually used in conjunction with another active antimicrobial agent. Many isolates of MDR *Acinetobacter* retain at least intermediate susceptibility to amikacin or tobramycin, but resistance to this class of agents is also increasing largely due to aminoglycoside-modifying enzymes or efflux pump mechanisms.

Polymyxin Therapy

Given the limited therapeutic options for the most resistant *Acinetobacter* infections, clinicians have returned to the use of polymyxin B or polymyxin E (colistin) as the best therapeutic option for severe *Acinetobacter* infections that demonstrate broad antimicrobial resistance to other available classes of agents including carbapenems (71,72). Polymyxins are polypeptide antibiotics originally discovered in 1947 but largely abandoned for clinical use more than 20 years ago due to reports of serious nephrotoxicity and neurotoxicity (71). Colostin is the most common form used clinically. Colistin acts by disturbing the bacterial cell membrane, thus increasing permeability and leading to cell death (71). Colistin's positive electrostatic charge is attracted to the negatively charged lipopolysaccharide (LPS) molecule in the outer membrane of GNB. This attraction facilitates disruption of the cell envelope and also enables the agent to bind and neutralize endotoxin, which is a component of LPS (71). Bacterial resistance to colistin and polymyxins is relatively rare but has been reported (73,74). The disk diffusion method (based on colistin sulfate) can be used to determine isolates' susceptibility to colistin and the suggested breakpoint for susceptibility is ≤2 mg/L. Bacterial resistance to polymyxin is generally due to alterations in the outer cell membrane or to an efflux pump mechanism that removes the agent from the bacterial cell (71,72). Colistin is bactericidal against *Acinetobacter* and its effect is concentration-dependent (72). Clinically, intravenous colistin is an option for treatment of *Acinetobacter* infections when isolates are not susceptible to other available antimicrobial agents or when treatment with conventional agents is not effective. Observational clinical studies have reported favorable responses (cure or improvement) from 57% to 77% among severely ill patients in the ICU with MDR-*Acinetobacter* infections including pneumonia, bacteremia, sepsis, intra-abdominal infections, and central nervous system (CNS) infections (75–78). Though high-quality pharmacokinetic data are lacking, colistin is reported to have relatively poor distribution into the lungs and cerebrospinal fluid (CSF). Clinical outcomes therefore likely vary for different types of infections. Despite an overall "good outcome" rate of 67%, Levin et al. found a much lower response rate of 25% for patients with MDR-GNB pneumonia treated with parenteral colistin (75). Several other studies have reported more favorable clinical response rates, between 56% and 61%, for parenteral colistin treatment of VAP due to MDR *Acinetobacter* (79–82). Garnacho-Montero et al. concluded that intravenous colistin was a safe and effective alternative to imipenem for the treatment of VAP due to carbapenem-resistant *Acinetobacter* (79). The crude VAP-related mortality in this study remained quite high (38%) whether treated with intravenous imipenem or colistin. It must be noted that the majority of studies on the clinical efficacy of colistin are observational and no data are currently available from controlled clinical trials.

With regard to CNS infections, there are case reports of successful treatment of MDR-*Acinetobacter* meningitis with parenteral colistin but it has poor CNS penetration and its efficacy in this setting remains unclear (83,84). Several case reports and case series report the use of intraventricular or intrathecal therapy with polymyxins (with or without parenteral therapy) for the treatment of GNB meningitis (83,85–87). Falagas et al. recently reviewed clinical evidence from 64 reports involving 31 episodes of GNB meningitis to determine the safety and effectiveness of intraventricular or intrathecal therapy with polymyxins (88). Overall, cure was achieved in 51/64 (80%) of patients with GNB meningitis, including 10/11 (91%) of patients with *Acinetobacter* meningitis. The majority of patients received systemic polymyxins or other antimicrobial therapy in addition to the local administration of polymyxins. Twenty-eight percent had neurological toxicity (mostly meningeal irritation) that was apparently reversible. The authors conclude that intraventricular or intrathecal polymyxin therapy is effective against GNB meningitis and though toxicity is common, it appeared to be dose-dependent and reversible (88). Because the majority of patients also received systemic antimicrobial therapy, it is not clear how much additional effect was achieved by the local administration of polymyxin in the CSF. At least one case report indicated that polymyxin was a useful adjunct to systemic therapy for treatment of MDR-*Acinetobacter* meningitis in a patient with an indwelling ventricular-peritoneal shunt and other foreign material that could not be removed (85). Overall, there is insufficient evidence to draw conclusions regarding the efficacy, safety, or pharmacokinetic properties of colistin for treatment of CNS infections, though it remains an important option for salvage therapy when *Acinetobacter* strains are resistant to conventional regimens (83).

In addition to the parenteral, intrathecal, and intraventricular routes, colistin may also be administered by aerosolization. Most clinical experience with nebulized colistin has been in cystic fibrosis (CF) patients with MDR *Pseudomonas* or other MDR-GNB (71,72). There is far less experience with inhaled colistin therapy in patients without CF. Kwa et al. reported a case series of 21 non-CF patients with nosocomial pneumonia due to MDR *Acinetobacter* or *Pseudomonas* and found a clinical response rate of 57% with aerosolized colistin alone (89). Many of the patients received parenteral antibiotics to which the infection was resistant but none received parenteral colistin (89). Michalopolous et al. found that seven of eight patients treated with nebulized colistin had a good clinical response (90). Most patients in this study received concurrent parenteral therapy with colistin or another agent with activity against the infection. Bronchospasm is a potential complication of treatment with aerosolized colistin but only one patient experienced it in the Kwa series and it was not seen in the second study (89,90). From these limited data and prior experience in CF patients, it appears that nebulized colistin may provide benefit in the treatment of MDR-GNB nosocomial pneumonia, especially if used as an adjunct to parenteral therapy (72).

The parenteral form of colistin is colistimethate sodium. Unfortunately, useful data on the pharmacokinetics, pharmacodynamics, and toxicodynamics of colistin are lacking. This is primarily because colistin was originally introduced over 50 years ago, before the implementation of current drug approval requirements. In addition, earlier methods of measuring serum concentrations of the drug were inaccurate and unable to adequately distinguish concentrations of colistimethate (the nonactive pro-drug) from colistin (72). The recommended dosing of colistin depends on the specific product being used. There are inconsistencies among various manufacturers and the labeling of different formulations varies using international units, milligrams (mg) of colistin base activity, or other units. This variation makes it difficult to interpret and compare studies' results, especially when research occurs in different parts of the world and specific formulations are not fully described (72). When the units of measurement are converted to milligrams of colistimethate sodium, different manufacturers' recommended doses and maximum daily doses vary substantially (72). Data suggest that current recommended dosing regimens may often lead to serum levels of colistin that are below the MIC of the infecting organism (72). These problems highlight the urgent need for careful pharmacologic studies using the best available techniques and the importance of attention to formulation and dosing in clinical care and research studies. Polymyxin nephrotoxicity usually manifests as acute tubular necrosis, and a variety of neurologic toxicities has been reported, including dizziness, parathesias, confusion, and neuromuscular blockade. Nephrotoxicity of colistin may be potentiated by concurrent therapy with aminoglycoside agents (72). Both nephrotoxicity and neurotoxicity are usually reversible and appear to be dose-dependent (71,72). Generally, recent reports have found less polymyxin toxicity than was originally reported and authors conclude that colistin is both safe and effective (72,78,79). Polymyxin dosing must be adjusted in renal insufficiency. Unfortunately, the lack of accurate pharmacokinetic data means that appropriate dosing in renal failure remains unclear, especially for patients receiving dialysis therapy (72).

Synergy and Combination Therapy

As noted previously, controlled clinical trials have not been performed to evaluate various therapies for MDR *Acinetobacter* so it is difficult to evaluate the role of synergy or combination therapy to treat MDR-*Acinetobacter* infections. For *Acinetobacter* isolates that are susceptible to only polymyxins, it is not clear if colistin should be used alone or in combination with other agents. For isolates resistant to all available agents including colistin, combination therapy is the last remaining option. Most available data regarding synergy or combination therapy are from case series, animal models, or in vitro studies. One such study demonstrated in vitro synergy between colistin and rifampin against MDR-*Acinetobacter* (91). Other studies have also explored the effectiveness of combination regimens that include rifampin. A clinical case series reported microbiological cure in 64% of 14 patients with VAP due to MDR-*Acinetobacter* or *Pseudomonas* treated with parenteral colistin plus rifampin; however, interpretation of these findings is limited by the lack of a comparison group (92). Recently, an animal study found that colistin prolonged survival in neutropenic rats with experimental MDR-*Acinetobacter* thigh infections and colistin's efficacy was enhanced by the addition of rifampin (93). One case report attributes successful treatment of *Acinetobacter* meningitis to the addition of rifampin to meropenem when treatment with meropenem alone had been ineffective (94). Montero et al. studied a mouse model of MDR-*Acinetobacter* pneumonia and found that the combinations of rifampin with imipenem, tobramycin, or colistin were the most effective regimens against an isolate with high-level carbapenem-resistance (95). A follow-up clinical pilot study, however, cautions against the use of imipenem plus rifampin for treatment of carbapenem-resistant *Acinetobacter* infections because the authors observed a high failure rate and documented emergence of rifampin resistance in 70% of the patients treated with this regimen (96).

Aminoglycoside agents have also been studied in various combination therapeutic regimens. In the Montero mouse model, the combination of imipenem plus tobramycin was the best regimen against an isolate with moderate carbapenem resistance (95). Another study, however, found that the addition of amikacin did not improve the outcome over imipenem monotherapy in a mouse pneumonia model (97). The combination of imipenem and amikacin was worse than imipenem alone for treatment of imipenem-resistant pneumonia in a guinea pig model despite a demonstration of in vitro synergy between the agents (98). In vitro data from 10 isolates of imipenem-resistant *Acinetobacter* showed synergy between imipenem and either colistin or amikacin (99), though the clinical utility of this synergy also remains unclear. It is thought that colistin may enhance imipenem's activity by increasing permeability of the bacterial cell wall (100).

Sulbactam has also been studied in various combination regimens against *Acinetobacter*. In vitro testing with time-kill curves of an endemic strain of

MDR *Acinetobacter* from Taiwan [susceptible to only meropenem and sulbactam (colistin was not tested)] showed that only the combination of meropenem and sulbactam was bactericidal (101). The survival of mice infected with the isolate was significantly higher if treated with both meropenem and sulbactam than with either agent alone (101). Kiffer et al. also found synergy or partial synergy in vitro between meropenem and sulbactam in 37 of 48 MDR-*Acinetobacter* isolates (102). Sulbactam appears to enhance therapy with other agents by attaching to penicillin-binding proteins (100). The combination of cefepime and ampicillin/sulbactam has also been reported to have in vitro synergy (103). A case series in Athens reported that in 67% of 50 patients who received parenteral colistin in combination with other antimicrobial agents (meropenem, imipenem, aminoglycosides, ampicillin-sulbactam, pipericillin-clavulanate, or ciprofloxacin) for severe MDR-*Acineto-bacter* and -*Pseudomonas* infections were "cured or improved" (81). Another case series of 25 patients with MDR *Pseudomonas* or *Acinetobacter* pneumonia found similar results, with 79% surviving until the end of therapy when treated with parenteral colistin plus 1 or more other agents (104). These results are comparable to cure rates reported for parenteral colistin alone, and the wide variety of other agents employed limits the ability to draw conclusions regarding combination therapy. Clinical studies are needed to determine whether any of these combinations translates into a useful therapeutic strategy.

In other settings, combination therapy is used to prevent the development of resistance to an active antimicrobial agent (or agents). Colistin is often used alone to treat MDR-*Acinetobacter* infections. Li et al. recently published disturbing information about the discovery of heteroresistance (subpopulations of *Acinetobacter* with varying levels of resistance) to colisitin in 15 of 16 *Acinetobacter* colistin-susceptible isolates studied in vitro (105). Serial passage of the isolates in the presence of colistin increased the proportion of subpopulations that were colistin resistant. Owen et al. also found in vitro evidence of heteroresistance and this suggests that combination therapy may be advisable to prevent the emergence of colistin resistance during monotherapy (105,106).

Summary of Therapy

In summary, the choice of therapy for severe infections due to the most resistant strains of MDR *Acinetobacter* is difficult, options are limited, and the available literature cannot provide clear answers due to the lack of controlled clinical studies. When isolates are susceptible to carbapenems, these remain the treatment of choice. Colistin has made a resurgence as the treatment of choice for MDR-*Acinetobacter* infections with high-level resistance to all other conventional agents. It is not clear if combination therapy is more effective than monotherapy. There is some suggestion, however, that combinations that include sulbactam, aminoglycoside agents, or rifampin may add efficacy to colistin and carbapenems against these infections. More data are needed on the pharmacokinetics, pharmacodynamics, and appropriate dosing of colistin especially in light of the discovery of heteroresistance. There is variation in the recommended dosing regimens of different formulations of colistin, and studies suggest that at recommended doses colistin serum levels may often be sub-therapeutic and low enough to foster resistance. Given the lack of good therapeutic options, the development or discovery of new therapies and greater emphasis on the prevention of healthcare-associated transmission of MDR *Acinetobacter* are essential.

INFECTION CONTROL AND PREVENTION

The many reported outbreaks of *Acinetobacter* demonstrate this organism's ability for epidemic spread and illustrate a variety of ways that lapses in proper infection control procedures can lead to transmission. When a specific point source is identified, source-specific infection control measures can be implemented to correct the problem and end transmission. However, the majority of outbreak investigations does not reveal a particular source but suggests that transmission occurs via healthcare workers' hands from the environment and fomites. Investigators often describe success with re-enforcement of existing infection control and prevention standards such as hand hygiene compliance, barrier precautions, and thorough environmental cleaning and disinfection. Other outbreaks are much more difficult to halt and require cohorting of patients, dedicated staff assignments, active surveillance cultures, and in some cases closure of entire ICUs (23,107). The presence of endemic MDR *Acinetobacter* poses even more challenges to healthcare facilities that must control multifactorial transmission of the organism over long periods of time. The Centers for Disease Control and Prevention (CDC) Healthcare Infection Control Practices Advisory Committee recently released guidelines on the control of multidrug-resistant organisms (MDROs) in healthcare settings (10). The document offers a thorough review of various infection control measures and the available supporting evidence (10). Some of these measures are briefly discussed below.

Standard Precautions and Hand Hygiene

Standard precautions are essential to the prevention of MDRO transmission in the healthcare setting. These precautions are the mainstay of prevention before MDROs are present in a healthcare environment, in the endemic MDRO setting, and in the outbreak setting (10). Routine hand hygiene and consistent and correct glove use are essential components of standard precautions. Despite being among the most important infection control measures, hand hygiene adherence among healthcare workers has been shown to be extremely low, usually less than 50% (108,109). Pittet et al. reports that hand hygiene adherence is associated with awareness of being observed, belief in being a role model for colleagues, and easy access to alcohol-based hand rubs (108). Appropriate use of gowns to prevent contamination of healthcare workers' clothes or uniform and appropriate use of masks, eye protection, and face shields are also essential. Re-enforcement and re-education of the basic tenets of standard precautions and hand hygiene are almost always components of multi-faceted interventions to control the spread of MDROs (10).

Isolation Precautions

As many as twenty years ago, the CDC recommended using transmission-based precautions such as contact isolation precautions and dedicating equipment and individual items to care for patients with epidemiologically important antibiotic-resistant organisms. These measures are intended to prevent transmission of the organisms to other patients (110). Nonetheless, antimicrobial-resistant organisms continue to pose a significant threat of healthcare-associated infections to patients. Contact isolation precautions are designed to prevent direct or indirect transmission of organisms from patients or their environment by the assignment of patients to private rooms and the use of gowns and gloves by healthcare workers upon entry to the patient isolation room (10). The Emerging Infections Network recently surveyed its members to ask if they endorsed contact isolation precautions for control of MDROs (111). Most (79%) infectious disease consultants supported contact precautions for MDR-GNB and 66% work in hospitals that use contact precautions for MDR-GNB on at least one unit (111).

Cohorting of Patients and/or Staff

In addition to contact isolation precautions, cohorting of patients on designated units has been used to prevent additional transmission in outbreaks of MDR-*Acinetobacter* (112). Such strategies are helpful logistically when large numbers of patients are involved. Some groups have also reported cohorting of staff to care for only patients colonized or infected with MDR *Acinetobacter* and even closure of entire ICUs to interrupt transmission in outbreaks (17,113–116).

Environmental Cleaning and Disinfection

Many outbreak reports have documented extensive environmental contamination with *Acinetobacter* and support the role of environment in transmission (6,7,9,112,113,117,118). Wilks et al. reported a recent outbreak of MDR *Acinetobacter* in London with environmental contamination found on curtains, laryngoscope blades, patient lifting equipment, door handles, mops, buckets, and keyboards (9). The authors report that reinforcement of proper cleaning and disinfection and clarification of responsibility for cleaning equipment and the environment interrupted transmission without the need for contact isolation precautions (9). Equipment has been implemented in a variety of outbreaks, emphasizing the need for special attention to disinfection of shared items and extra caution with respiratory care and wound care procedures (5,6,8). Environmental cleaning and disinfection are often part of interventions designed to interrupt outbreaks, but the role of the environment is likely also important in the endemic setting.

Antimicrobial Management/Stewardship

In addition to transmission among patients, healthcare workers, and the environment, MDR *Acinetobacter* can also be the result of emergence of resistance in the setting of selective pressure from antimicrobial therapy. Judicious use of antimicrobial agents, especially broad-spectrum ones, is therefore an integral part of the strategy to limit the emergence of MDR pathogens (10). Evidence-based guidelines and implementation tools can be found in the CDC's Campaign to Prevent Antimicrobial Resistance at www.cdc.gov/drugresistance/healthcare and include strategies to limit the antimicrobial treatment of culture contaminants, narrow the spectrum of therapy, limit the duration of therapy, and restrict broad-spectrum agents for appropriate indications (119). The Infectious Diseases Society of America (IDSA) recently issued guidelines for developing an institutional program of antimicrobial stewardship with the primary goal of maximizing clinical outcomes while preventing unintended consequences of antimicrobial use such as emergence of resistance (120). Antimicrobial management strategies have been used to successfully control MDR-GNB, often as one component among other interventions (114,121). The relative contributions of antimicrobial selective pressure and transmission between patients on the emergence of MDR *Acinetobacter* are not known.

Surveillance

Routine surveillance for MDROs involves monitoring microbiology clinical culture results for organisms such as MDR *Acinetobacter* passively to detect outbreaks or emerging trends so that interventions can be implemented promptly.
Active surveillance is a systematic process of performing surveillance cultures in
a defined patient population (such as all patients upon admission to a given
unit) or a targeted group of high-risk patients in order to detect asymptomatic
colonization with antimicrobial resistant organisms. In order to be effective
against transmission of MDROs, active surveillance cultures (ASC) must be
combined with isolation precautions (or another intervention) for colonized or
infected patients and there are at least two strategies. The first strategy is to
perform ASC, wait for the result (usually 24–48 hr), and then place patients
whose cultures grow MDR-GNB on isolation precautions. The second strategy is
to place all patients in the group targeted for ASC on isolation precautions at the
time of the culture (usually upon admission) and then remove patients from
isolation precautions if their surveillance culture does not grow MDR-GNB. In a
recent article, Perencevich et al. used mathematical modeling to evaluate various
interventions to control nosocomial transmission of vancomycin-resistant *Enterococcus* (VRE) in an ICU (122). The authors determined that passive surveillance,
using isolation precautions for those patients who are discovered to be colonized
through clinical cultures, offered no advantage. However, they found that active
surveillance with contact precautions for colonized patients predicted a 39%
reduction in the annual incidence of VRE in an ICU as compared to no active
surveillance (122). Furthermore, they determined that presumptive isolation of
patients pending the results of active surveillance cultures added significantly to
the control, with a predicted 65% reduction in VRE colonization (122). ASC are
often used successfully in the outbreak setting to interrupt transmission of
resistant organisms and have also been used with success to control healthcare-
associated transmission of endemic organisms (10). However, data are lacking
regarding the efficacy and cost-effectiveness of ASC for patients colonized
with antimicrobial-resistant GNB, and active surveillance remains an area of
controversy and investigation. In contrast to their strong support of contact
precautions for controlling MDR-GNB, only 37% of infectious disease specialists
surveyed by the Emerging Infections Network support ASC to prevent transmission of MDR-GNB and only 12% work in hospitals that use ASC for MDR-
GNB (111).

Which Interventions to Choose?

Harris recently published a useful paradigm for determining which infection
control interventions should be used for MDR-GNB (58). He asserts that we need
organism-specific data on the proportion of antibiotic resistance that is attributable
to antibiotic-selective pressure versus patient-to-patient transmission. These data
would help to decide whether to focus effort and resources primarily on antimicrobial management strategies or on interventions designed to interrupt transmission (58). Knowledge about the "undetected ratio" (undetected by clinical cultures
alone) could be used to predict the efficacy of ASC, and data on the duration of
colonization would help to predict the efficacy of isolation precautions. Currently
there are insufficient data to make these decisions or to evaluate the cost-effectiveness of various strategies. Almost all reports of successful control of MDROs use

a combination of multiple interventions, making it difficult to evaluate and compare the efficacy of each individually (10).

FUTURE DIRECTIONS

Further investigation of alternative infection control strategies and analysis of the cost-effectiveness of various methods to prevent transmission of antimicrobial-resistant GNB are needed. Inter-institutional spread and the prospect of transmissible resistance indicates the need for continued surveillance for plasmid-mediated metalloenzymes and a coordinated approach of healthcare providers, epidemiologists, hospital administrators, and public health officials at the institutional, city, state, and federal levels to the prevention and control of healthcare-associated MDR *Acinetobacter*. There is a need for regional strategies that extend beyond the confines of individual healthcare institutions. To facilitate treatment, existing antimicrobial agents alone and in combination need to be studied in randomized controlled clinical trials. More data are needed on the pharmacokinetics, pharmacodynamics, and appropriate dosing regimens of colistin. New antimicrobial agents are needed to treat pan-resistant *Acinetobacter* that is resistant to all existing classes of antimicrobials including colistin. Dr. Louis B. Rice recently succinctly described why development of new antibiotics against MDR *Acinetobacter* (and other MDR-GNB) is such a daunting challenge. He said, "Not only must the antibiotic be active against its intended target, but it must be able to enter the cells, remain long enough to interact with the target, and avoid expulsion by one of the multidrug efflux systems" (49). There is a glimmer of hope in antimicrobial peptides with mechanisms of action that are somewhat different from the polymyxins (74). Four members of the cecropin A-melittin peptide group were recently tested against colistin-resistant *Acinetobacter* and all showed bactericidal activity in time-kill curves (123). Though much investigation remains to be completed, these or other antimicrobial peptides may be promising alternatives to overcome polymyxin resistance in *Acinetobacter*. Otherwise, the lack of drugs in the development "pipeline" with activity against MDR-GNB is extremely disturbing.

CONCLUSIONS

Despite its reputation for relatively low virulence, MDR *Acinetobacter* poses a formidable threat to patients. Occurring most frequently in the most severely ill patients, the crude mortality of these infections is extremely high. Though the attributable mortality of MDR-*Acinetobacter* infections is debatable, these infections are clearly associated with increased morbidity and increased time on mechanical ventilation, in the ICU, and in the hospital. The cause of many outbreaks, this organism is increasingly becoming endemic in the healthcare setting. Antimicrobial resistance is increasing, likely due to both the emergence of resistance in the setting of antimicrobial pressure and to transmission of resistant organisms from patient to patient. Treatment options are severely limited and there are no controlled trials to guide therapeutic choices. Carbapenems and colistin are the agents of choice for the most resistant infections. The role of other agents and combination therapy remains unclear. The emergence of this organism challenges us to discover new antimicrobial agents, conduct well-controlled clinical trials on existing regimens and combinations, optimize dosing of agents such as colistin, and control transmission through effective infection control measures.

REFERENCES

1. Bergogne-Berezin E, Towner KJ. *Acinetobacter* spp. as nosocomial pathogens: microbiological, clinical, and epidemiological features. Clin Microbiol Rev 1996; 9(2):148–65.
2. Fournier PE, Richet H. The epidemiology and control of *Acinetobacter baumannii* in health care facilities. Clin Infect Dis 2006; 42(5):692–9.
3. Seifert H, Dijkshoorn L, Gerner-Smidt P, Pelzer N, Tjernberg I, Vaneechoutte M. Distribution of *Acinetobacter* species on human skin: comparison of phenotypic and genotypic identification methods. J Clin Microbiol 1997; 35(11):2819–25.
4. Jawad A, Heritage J, Snelling AM, Gascoyne-Binzi DM, Hawkey PM. Influence of relative humidity and suspending menstrua on survival of *Acinetobacter* spp. on dry surfaces. J Clin Microbiol 1996; 34(12):2881–7.
5. Bernards AT, Harinck HI, Dijkshoorn L, van der Reijden TJ, van den Broek PJ. Persistent *Acinetobacter baumannii*? Look inside your medical equipment. Infect Control Hosp Epidemiol 2004; 25(11):1002–4.
6. Maragakis LL, Cosgrove SE, Song X, Kim D, Rosenbaum P, Ciesla N, et al. An outbreak of multidrug-resistant *Acinetobacter baumannii* associated with pulsatile lavage wound treatment. JAMA 2004; 292(24):3006–11.
7. Das I, Lambert P, Hill D, Noy M, Bion J, Elliott T. Carbapenem-resistant *Acinetobacter* and role of curtains in an outbreak in intensive care units. J Hosp Infect 2002; 50(2):110–4.
8. Villegas MV, Hartstein AI. *Acinetobacter* outbreaks, 1977–2000. Infect Control Hosp Epidemiol 2003; 24(4):284–95.
9. Wilks M, Wilson A, Warwick S, et al. Control of an outbreak of multidrug-resistant *Acinetobacter baumannii-calcoaceticus* colonization and infection in an intensive care unit (ICU) without closing the ICU or placing patients in isolation. Infect Control Hosp Epidemiol 2006; 27(7):654–8.
10. Siegel JD, Rhinehart E, Jackson M, Chiarello L. The Healthcare Infection Control Practices Advisory Committee. Management of Multidrug-Resistant Organisms in Healthcare Settings, 2006. The Centers for Disease Control and Prevention website December 6 (cited Mar 9) (Accessed at http://www.cdc.gov/ncidod/dhqp/pdf/ar/mdroGuideline2006.pdf).
11. Landman D, Quale JM, Mayorga D, et al. Citywide clonal outbreak of multiresistant *Acinetobacter baumannii* and *Pseudomonas aeruginosa* in Brooklyn, NY: the preantibiotic era has returned. Arch Intern Med 2002; 162(13):1515–20.
12. Abbo A, Navon-Venezia S, Hammer-Muntz O, Krichali T, Siegman-Igra Y, Carmeli Y. Multidrug-resistant *Acinetobacter baumannii*. Emerg Infect Dis 2005; 11(1):22–9.
13. Cornaglia G, Akova M, Amicosante G, et al. Metallo-beta-lactamases as emerging resistance determinants in Gram-negative pathogens: open issues. Int J Antimicrob Agents 2007.
14. Nemec A, Dijkshoorn L, van der Reijden TJ. Long-term predominance of two pan-European clones among multi-resistant *Acinetobacter baumannii* strains in the Czech Republic. J Med Microbiol 2004; 53(P. 2):147–53.
15. Manikal VM, Landman D, Saurina G, Oydna E, Lal H, Quale J. Endemic carbapenem-resistant *Acinetobacter* species in Brooklyn, New York: citywide prevalence, interinstitutional spread, and relation to antibiotic usage. Clin Infect Dis 2000; 31(1):101–6.
16. Barbolla RE, Centron D, Di MA, et al. Identification of an epidemic carbapenem-resistant *Acinetobacter baumannii* strain at hospitals in Buenos Aires City. Diagn Microbiol Infect Dis 2003; 45(4):261–4.
17. Coelho JM, Turton JF, Kaufmann ME, et al. Occurrence of carbapenem-resistant *Acinetobacter baumannii* clones at multiple hospitals in London and Southeast England. J Clin Microbiol 2006; 44(10):3623–7.
18. Da Silva GJ, Quinteira S, Bertolo E, et al. Long-term dissemination of an OXA-40 carbapenemase-producing *Acinetobacter baumannii* clone in the Iberian Peninsula. J Antimicrob Chemother 2004; 54(1):255–8.
19. Gales AC, Pfaller MA, Sader HS, Hollis RJ, Jones RN. Genotypic characterization of carbapenem-nonsusceptible *Acinetobacter* spp. isolated in Latin America. Microb Drug Resist 2004; 10:286–91.

20. Bonomo RA. Multiple antibiotic-resistant bacteria in long-term-care facilities: an emerging problem in the practice of infectious diseases. Clin Infect Dis 2000; 31(6):1414–22.
21. Mody L, Bradley SF, Strausbaugh LJ, Muder RR. Prevalence of ceftriaxone- and ceftazidime-resistant gram-negative bacteria in long-term-care facilities. Infect Control Hosp Epidemiol 2001; 22(4):193–4.
22. Bradley SF. Issues in the management of resistant bacteria in long-term-care facilities. Infect Control Hosp Epidemiol 1999; 20(5):362–6.
23. Urban C, Segal-Maurer S, Rahal JJ. Considerations in control and treatment of nosocomial infections due to multidrug-resistant *Acinetobacter baumannii*. Clin Infect Dis 2003; 36(10):1268–74.
24. Centers for Disease Control and Prevention. *Acinetobacter baumannii* infections among patients at military medical facilities treating injured U.S. service members, 2002–2004. Morbidity and Mortality Weekly Report 2004; 53:1063–6.
25. Davis KA, Moran KA, McAllister CK, Gray PJ. Multidrug-resistant *Acinetobacter* extremity infections in soldiers. Emerg Infect Dis 2005; 11(8):1218–24.
26. Hujer KM, Hujer AM, Hulten EA, et al. Analysis of antibiotic resistance genes in multidrug-resistant *Acinetobacter* sp. isolates from military and civilian patients treated at the Walter Reed Army Medical Center. Antimicrob Agents Chemother 2006; 50(12):4114–23.
27. Hawley JS, Murray CK, Griffith ME, et al. Susceptibility of acinetobacter strains isolated from deployed U.S. military personnel. Antimicrob Agents Chemother 2007; 51(1):376–8.
28. Murray CK, Roop SA, Hospenthal DR, et al. Bacteriology of war wounds at the time of injury. Mil Med 2006 Sep; 171(9):826–9.
29. Griffith ME, Ceremuga JM, Ellis MW, Guymon CH, Hospenthal DR, Murray CK. *Acinetobacter* skin colonization of US Army Soldiers. Infect Control Hosp Epidemiol 2006; 27(7):659–61.
30. Griffith ME, Ellis MW, Murray CK. *Acinetobacter* nares colonization of healthy US soldiers. Infect Control Hosp Epidemiol 2006; 27(7):787–8.
31. Yun HC, Murray CK, Roop SA, Hospenthal DR, Gourdine E, Dooley DP. Bacteria recovered from patients admitted to a deployed U.S. military hospital in Baghdad, Iraq. Mil Med 2006; 171(9):821–5.
32. Jones A, Morgan D, Walsh A, et al. Importation of multidrug-resistant *Acinetobacter* spp infections with casualties from Iraq. Lancet Infect Dis 2006; 6(6):317–8.
33. Turton JF, Kaufmann ME, Gill MJ, et al. Comparison of *Acinetobacter baumannii* isolates from the United Kingdom and the United States that were associated with repatriated casualties of the Iraq conflict. J Clin Microbiol 2006; 44(7):2630–4.
34. Sunenshine RH, Wright MO, Maragakis LL, et al. Multidrug-resistant *Acinetobacter* Infection Mortality Rate and Length of Hospitalization. Emerg Infect Dis 2007; 13(1):97–103.
35. Seifert H, Strate A, Pulverer G. Nosocomial bacteremia due to *Acinetobacter baumannii*. Clinical features, epidemiology, and predictors of mortality. Medicine (Baltimore) 1995; 74(6):340–9.
36. Kwon KT, Oh WS, Song JH, et al. Impact of imipenem resistance on mortality in patients with *Acinetobacter* bacteraemia. J Antimicrob Chemother 2007; 59(3):525–30.
37. Falagas ME, Kopterides P, Siempos II. Attributable mortality of *Acinetobacter baumannii* infection among critically ill patients. Clin Infect Dis 2006; 43(3):389–90.
38. Albrecht MA, Griffith ME, Murray CK, et al. Impact of *Acinetobacter* infection on the mortality of burn patients. J Am Coll Surg 2006; 203(4):546–50.
39. Blot S, Vandewoude K, Colardyn F. Nosocomial bacteremia involving *Acinetobacter baumannii* in critically ill patients: a matched cohort study. Intensive Care Med 2003; 29(3):471–5.
40. Chen HP, Chen TL, Lai CH, et al. Predictors of mortality in *Acinetobacter baumannii* bacteremia. J Microbiol Immunol Infect 2005; 38(2):127–36.
41. Choi JY, Park YS, Kim CO, et al. Mortality risk factors of *Acinetobacter baumannii* bacteraemia. Intern Med J 2005; 35(10):599–603.

42. Falagas ME, Kasiakou SK, Rafailidis PI, Zouglakis G, Morfou P. Comparison of mortality of patients with *Acinetobacter baumannii* bacteraemia receiving appropriate and inappropriate empirical therapy. J Antimicrob Chemother 2006; 57(6):1251-4.

43. The cost of antibiotic resistance: effect of resistance among Staphylococcus aureus, Klebsiella pneumoniae, *Acinetobacter baumannii*, and Pseudmonas aeruginosa on length of hospital stay. Infect Control Hosp Epidemiol 2002; 23(2):106-8.

44. Garnacho J, Sole-Violan J, Sa-Borges M, Diaz E, Rello J. Clinical impact of pneumonia caused by *Acinetobacter baumannii* in intubated patients: a matched cohort study. Crit Care Med 2003; 31(10):2478-82.

45. Ward WJ Jr, Spragens L, Smithson K. Building the business case for clinical quality. Healthc Financ Manage 2006; 60(12):92-8.

46. Bonomo RA, Szabo D. Mechanisms of multidrug resistance in *Acinetobacter* species and *Pseudomonas aeruginosa*. Clin Infect Dis 2006; 43(Suppl. 2):S49-56.

47. Falagas ME, Koletsi PK, Bliziotis IA. The diversity of definitions of multidrug-resistant (MDR) and pandrug-resistant (PDR) *Acinetobacter baumannii* and *Pseudomonas aeruginosa*. J Med Microbiol 2006; 55(Pt 12):1619-29.

48. Thomson JM, Bonomo RA. The threat of antibiotic resistance in Gram-negative pathogenic bacteria: beta-lactams in peril! Curr Opin Microbiol 2005; 8(5):518-24.

49. Rice LB. Challenges in identifying new antimicrobial agents effective for treating infections with *Acinetobacter baumannii* and *Pseudomonas aeruginosa*. Clin Infect Dis 2006; 43(Suppl. 2):S100-5.

50. fzal-Shah M, Woodford N, Livermore DM. Characterization of OXA-25, OXA-26, and OXA-27, molecular class D beta-lactamases associated with carbapenem resistance in clinical isolates of *Acinetobacter baumannii*. Antimicrob Agents Chemother 2001; 45(2):583-8.

51. Brown S, Amyes S. OXA (beta)-lactamases in *Acinetobacter*: the story so far. J Antimicrob Chemother 2006; 57(1):1-3.

52. Walsh TR, Toleman MA, Poirel L, Nordmann P. Metallo-beta-lactamases: the quiet before the storm? Clin Microbiol Rev 2005; 18(2):306-25.

53. Lee K, Lee WG, Uh Y, Ha GY, Cho J, Chong Y. VIM- and IMP-type metallo-beta-lactamase-producing *Pseudomonas* spp. and *Acinetobacter spp.* in Korean hospitals. Emerg Infect Dis 2003; 9(7):868-71.

54. Bou G, Oliver A, Martinez-Beltran J. OXA-24, a novel class D beta-lactamase with carbapenemase activity in an *Acinetobacter baumannii* clinical strain. Antimicrob Agents Chemother 2000; 44(6):1556-61.

55. Mussi MA, Limansky AS, Viale AM. Acquisition of resistance to carbapenems in multidrug-resistant clinical strains of *Acinetobacter baumannii*: natural insertional inactivation of a gene encoding a member of a novel family of beta-barrel outer membrane proteins. Antimicrob Agents Chemother 2005; 49(4):1432-40.

56. Li J, Nation RL, Milne RW, Turnidge JD, Coulthard K. Evaluation of colistin as an agent against multi-resistant Gram-negative bacteria. Int J Antimicrob Agents 2005; 25(1):11-25.

57. Fournier PE, Vallenet D, Barbe V, et al. Comparative genomics of multidrug resistance in *Acinetobacter baumannii*. PLoS Genet 2006; 2(1):e7.

58. Harris AD, McGregor JC, Furuno JP. What infection control interventions should be undertaken to control multidrug-resistant Gram-negative bacteria? Clin Infect Dis 2006; 43(Suppl. 2):S57-61.

59. Jones RN, Sader HS, Fritsche TR, Rhomberg PR. Carbapenem susceptibility discords among *Acinetobacter* isolates. Clin Infect Dis 2006; 42(1):158.

60. Jones RN, Deshpande L, Fritsche TR, Sader HS. Determination of epidemic clonality among multidrug-resistant strains of *Acinetobacter* spp. and *Pseudomonas aeruginosa* in the MYSTIC Programme (USA, 1999–2003). Diagn Microbiol Infect Dis 2004; 49(3):211-6.

61. Ikonomidis A, Pournaras S, Maniatis AN, Legakis NJ, Tsakris A. Discordance of meropenem versus imipenem activity against *Acinetobacter baumannii*. Int J Antimicrob Agents 2006; 28(4):376-7.

62. Brauers J, Frank U, Kresken M, Rodloff AC, Seifert H. Activities of various beta-lactams and beta-lactam/beta-lactamase inhibitor combinations against *Acinetobacter baumannii* and *Acinetobacter* DNA group strains. Clin Microbiol Infect 2005; 11(1):24–30.
63. Higgins PG, Wisplinghoff H, Stefanik D, Seifert H. In vitro activities of the beta-lactamase inhibitors clavulanic acid, sulbactam, and tazobactam alone or in combination with beta-lactams against epidemiologically characterized multidrug-resistant *Acinetobacter baumannii* strains. Antimicrob Agents Chemother 2004; 48(5):1586–92.
64. Wood GC, Hanes SD, Croce MA, Fabian TC, Boucher BA. Comparison of ampicillin-sulbactam and imipenem-cilastatin for the treatment of acinetobacter ventilator-associated pneumonia. Clin Infect Dis 2002; 34(11):1425–30.
65. Levin AS, Levy CE, Manrique AE, Medeiros EA, Costa SF. Severe nosocomial infections with imipenem-resistant *Acinetobacter baumannii* treated with ampicillin/sulbactam. Int J Antimicrob Agents 2003; 21(1):58–62.
66. Seifert H, Stefanik D, Wisplinghoff H. Comparative in vitro activities of tigecycline and other antimicrobial agents against epidemiologically defined multidrug-resistant *Acinetobacter baumannii* isolates. J Antimicrob Chemother 2006; 58(5):1099–100.
67. Pachon-Ibanez ME, Jimenez-Mejias ME, Pichardo C, Llanos AC, Pachon J. Activity of tigecycline (GAR-936) against *Acinetobacter baumannii* strains, including those resistant to imipenem. Antimicrob Agents Chemother 2004; 48(11):4479–81.
68. Insa R, Cercenado E, Goyanes MJ, Morente A, Bouza E. in vitro activity of tigecycline against clinical isolates of *Acinetobacter baumannii* and Stenotrophomonas maltophilia. J Antimicrob Chemother 2007; 59(3):583–5.
69. Jones RN, Ferraro MJ, Reller LB, Schreckenberger PC, Swenson JM, Sader HS. Multi-center Studies of Tigecycline Disk Diffusion Susceptibility Results for *Acinetobacter* spp. J Clin Microbiol 2007; 45(1):227–30.
70. Peleg AY, Potoski BA, Rea R, Adams J, Sethi J, Capitano B, et al. *Acinetobacter baumannii* bloodstream infection while receiving tigecycline: a cautionary report. J Antimicrob Chemother 2007; 59(1):128–31.
71. Falagas ME, Kasiakou SK. Colistin: the revival of polymyxins for the management of multidrug-resistant Gram-negative bacterial infections. Clin Infect Dis 2005; 40(9):1333–41.
72. Li J, Nation RL, Turnidge JD, et al. Colistin: the re-emerging antibiotic for multidrug-resistant Gram-negative bacterial infections. Lancet Infect Dis 2006; 6(9):589–601.
73. Gales AC, Jones RN, Sader HS. Global assessment of the antimicrobial activity of polymyxin B against 54731 clinical isolates of Gram-negative bacilli: report from the SENTRY antimicrobial surveillance programme (2001–2004). Clin Microbiol Infect 2006; 12(4):315–21.
74. Urban C, Mariano N, Rahal JJ, et al. polymyxin B-resistant *Acinetobacter baumannii* clinical isolate susceptible to recombinant BPI and cecropin P1. Antimicrob Agents Chemother 2001; 45(3):994–5.
75. Levin AS, Barone AA, Penco J, et al. Intravenous colistin as therapy for nosocomial infections caused by multidrug-resistant *Pseudomonas aeruginosa* and *Acinetobacter baumannii*. Clin Infect Dis 1999; 28(5):1008–11.
76. Garnacho-Montero J, Ortiz-Leyba C, Fernandez-Hinojosa E, et al. *Acinetobacter baumannii* ventilator-associated pneumonia: epidemiological and clinical findings. Intensive Care Med 2005; 31(5):649–55.
77. Holloway KP, Rouphael NG, Wells JB, King MD, Blumberg HM. Polymyxin B and doxycycline use in patients with multidrug-resistant *Acinetobacter baumannii* infections in the intensive care unit. Ann Pharmacother 2006; 40(11):1939–45.
78. Kallel H, Bahloul M, Hergafi L, et al. Colistin as a salvage therapy for nosocomial infections caused by multidrug-resistant bacteria in the ICU. Int J Antimicrob Agents 2006; 28(4):366–9.
79. Garnacho-Montero J, Ortiz-Leyba C, Jimenez-Jimenez FJ, et al. Treatment of multidrug-resistant *Acinetobacter baumannii* ventilator-associated pneumonia (VAP) with intravenous colistin: a comparison with imipenem-susceptible VAP. Clin Infect Dis 2003; 36(9):1111–8.

80. Linden PK, Paterson DL. Parenteral and inhaled colistin for treatment of ventilator-associated pneumonia. Clin Infect Dis 2006; 43(Suppl. 2):S89–94.

81. Kasiakou SK, Michalopoulos A, Soteriades ES, Samonis G, Sermaides GJ, Falagas ME. Combination therapy with intravenous colistin for management of infections due to multidrug-resistant Gram-negative bacteria in patients without cystic fibrosis. Antimicrob Agents Chemother 2005; 49(8):3136–46.

82. Markou N, Apostolakos H, Koumoudiou C, et al. Intravenous colistin in the treatment of sepsis from multiresistant Gram-negative bacilli in critically ill patients. Crit Care 2003; 7(5):R78–83.

83. Katragkou A, Roilides E. Successful treatment of multidrug-resistant Acinetobacter baumannii central nervous system infections with colistin. J Clin Microbiol 2005; 43(9):4916–7.

84. Fulnecky EJ, Wright D, Scheld WM, Kanawati L, Shoham S. Amikacin and colistin for treatment of Acinetobacter baumannii meningitis. J Infect 2005; 51(5):e249–51.

85. Benifla M, Zucker G, Cohen A, Alkan M. Successful treatment of Acinetobacter meningitis with intrathecal polymyxin E. J Antimicrob Chemother 2004; 54(1):290–2.

86. Al SN, Memish ZA, Cherfan A, Al SA. Post-neurosurgical meningitis due to multidrug-resistant Acinetobacter baumanii treated with intrathecal colistin: case report and review of the literature. J Chemother 2006; 18(5):554–8.

87. Ng J, Gosbell IB, Kelly JA, Boyle MJ, Ferguson JK. Cure of multiresistant Acinetobacter baumannii central nervous system infections with intraventricular or intrathecal colistin: case series and literature review. J Antimicrob Chemother 2006; 58(5):1078–81.

88. Falagas ME, Bliziotis IA, Tam VH. Intraventricular or intrathecal use of polymyxins in patients with Gram-negative meningitis: a systematic review of the available evidence. Int J Antimicrob Agents 2007; 29(1):9–25.

89. Kwa AL, Loh C, Low JG, Kurup A, Tam VH. Nebulized colistin in the treatment of pneumonia due to multidrug-resistant Acinetobacter baumannii and Pseudomonas aeruginosa. Clin Infect Dis 2005; 41(5):754–7.

90. Michalopoulos A, Kasiakou SK, Mastora Z, Rellos K, Kapaskelis AM, Falagas ME. Aerosolized colistin for the treatment of nosocomial pneumonia due to multidrug-resistant Gram-negative bacteria in patients without cystic fibrosis. Crit Care 2005; 9(1):R53–9.

91. Giamarellos-Bourboulis EJ, Xirouchaki E, Giamarellou H. Interactions of colistin and rifampin on multidrug-resistant Acinetobacter baumannii. Diagn Microbiol Infect Dis 2001; 40(3):117–20.

92. Petrosillo N, Chinello P, Proietti MF, et al. Combined colistin and rifampicin therapy for carbapenem-resistant Acinetobacter baumannii infections: clinical outcome and adverse events. Clin Microbiol Infect 2005; 11(8):682–3.

93. Pantopoulou A, Giamarellos-Bourboulis EJ, Raftogannis M, et al. Colistin offers prolonged survival in experimental infection by multidrug-resistant Acinetobacter baumannii: the significance of co-administration of rifampicin. Int J Antimicrob Agents 2007; 29(1):51–5.

94. Gleeson T, Petersen K, Mascola J. Successful treatment of Acinetobacter meningitis with meropenem and rifampicin. J Antimicrob Chemother 2005; 56(3):602–3.

95. Montero A, Ariza J, Corbella X, et al. Antibiotic combinations for serious infections caused by carbapenem-resistant Acinetobacter baumannii in a mouse pneumonia model. J Antimicrob Chemother 2004; 54(6):1085–91.

96. Saballs M, Pujol M, Tubau F, Pena C, Montero A, Dominguez MA, et al. Rifampicin/imipenem combination in the treatment of carbapenem-resistant Acinetobacter baumannii infections. J Antimicrob Chemother 2006; 58(3):697–700.

97. Rodriguez-Hernandez MJ, Pachon J, Pichardo C, et al. Imipenem, doxycycline and amikacin in monotherapy and in combination in Acinetobacter baumannii experimental pneumonia. J Antimicrob Chemother 2000; 45(4):493–501.

98. Bernabeu-Wittel M, Pichardo C, Garcia-Curiel A, et al. Pharmacokinetic/pharmacodynamic assessment of the in-vivo efficacy of imipenem alone or in combination with amikacin for the treatment of experimental multiresistant Acinetobacter baumannii pneumonia. Clin Microbiol Infect 2005; 11(4):319–25.

99. Haddad FA, Van HK, Carbonaro C, guero-Rosenfeld M, Wormser GP. Evaluation of antibiotic combinations against multidrug-resistant *Acinetobacter baumannii* using the E-test. Eur J Clin Microbiol Infect Dis 2005; 24(8):577–9.

100. Rahal JJ. Novel antibiotic combinations against infections with almost completely resistant *Pseudomonas aeruginosa* and *Acinetobacter* species. Clin Infect Dis 2006; 43(Suppl. 2):S95–9.

101. Ko WC, Lee HC, Chiang SR, et al. in vitro and in vivo activity of meropenem and sulbactam against a multidrug-resistant *Acinetobacter baumannii* strain. J Antimicrob Chemother 2004; 53(2):393–5.

102. Kiffer CR, Sampaio JL, Sinto S, et al. in vitro synergy test of meropenem and sulbactam against clinical isolates of *Acinetobacter baumannii*. Diagn Microbiol Infect Dis 2005; 52(4):317–22.

103. Sader HS, Jones RN. Comprehensive in vitro evaluation of cefepime combined with aztreonam or ampicillin/sulbactam against multi-drug resistant *Pseudomonas aeruginosa* and *Acinetobacter* spp. Int J Antimicrob Agents 2005; 25(5):380–4.

104. Sobieszczyk ME, Furuya EY, Hay CM, et al. Combination therapy with polymyxin B for the treatment of multidrug-resistant Gram-negative respiratory tract infections. J Antimicrob Chemother 2004; 54(2):566–9.

105. Li J, Rayner CR, Nation RL, et al. Heteroresistance to colistin in multidrug-resistant *Acinetobacter baumannii*. Antimicrob Agents Chemother 2006; 50(9):2946–50.

106. Owen RJ, Li J, Nation RL, Spelman D. in vitro pharmacodynamics of colistin against *Acinetobacter baumannii* clinical isolates. J Antimicrob Chemother 2007; 59(3):473–7.

107. Simor AE, Lee M, Vearncombe M, et al. An outbreak due to multiresistant *Acinetobacter baumannii* in a burn unit: risk factors for acquisition and management. Infect Control Hosp Epidemiol 2002; 23(5):261–7.

108. Pittet D, Simon A, Hugonnet S, Pessoa-Silva CL, Sauvan V, Perneger TV. Hand hygiene among physicians: performance, beliefs, and perceptions. Ann Intern Med 2004; 141(1):1–8.

109. Boyce JM, Pittet D. Guideline for Hand Hygiene in Health-Care Settings. Recommendations of the Healthcare Infection Control Practices Advisory Committee and the HICPAC/SHEA/APIC/IDSA Hand Hygiene Task Force. Society for Healthcare Epidemiology of America/Association for Professionals in Infection Control/Infectious Diseases Society of America. MMWR Recomm Rep 2002; 51(RR-16):1–45 g(quiz).

110. Garner JS, Simmons BP. Guideline for isolation precautions in hospitals. Infect Control 1983; 4(Suppl 4):245–325.

111. Sunenshine RH, Liedtke LA, Fridkin SK, Strausbaugh LJ. Management of inpatients colonized or infected with antimicrobial-resistant bacteria in hospitals in the United States. Infect Control Hosp Epidemiol 2005; 26(2):138–43.

112. Podnos YD, Cinat ME, Wilson SE, Cooke J, Gornick W, Thrupp LD. Eradication of multi-drug resistant *Acinetobacter* from an intensive care unit. Surg Infect (Larchmt) 2001; 2(4):297–301.

113. Aygun G, Demirkiran O, Utku T, et al. Environmental contamination during a carbapenem-resistant *Acinetobacter baumannii* outbreak in an intensive care unit. J Hosp Infect 2002; 52(4):259–62.

114. Corbella X, Montero A, Pujol M, et al. Emergence and rapid spread of carbapenem resistance during a large and sustained hospital outbreak of multiresistant *Acinetobacter baumannii*. J Clin Microbiol 2000; 38(11):4086–95.

115. Ling ML, Ang A, Wee M, Wang GC. A nosocomial outbreak of multiresistant *Acinetobacter baumannii* originating from an intensive care unit. Infect Control Hosp Epidemiol 2001; 22(1):48–9.

116. Wang SH, Sheng WH, Chang YY, et al. Healthcare-associated outbreak due to pan-drug resistant *Acinetobacter baumannii* in a surgical intensive care unit. J Hosp Infect 2003; 53(2):97–102.

117. Denton M, Wilcox MH, Parnell P, et al. Role of environmental cleaning in controlling an outbreak of *Acinetobacter baumannii* on a neurosurgical intensive care unit. Intensive Crit Care Nurs 2005; 21(2):94–8.

118. de JG, Duse A, Richards G, Marais E. Back to basics–optimizing the use of available resources during an outbreak of multi-drug resistant *Acinetobacter* spp. J Hosp Infect 2004; 57(2):186–7.

119. Brinsley K, Srinivasan A, Sinkowitz-Cochran R, et al. Implementation of the Campaign to Prevent Antimicrobial Resistance in Healthcare Settings: 12 Steps to Prevent Antimicrobial Resistance Among Hospitalized Adults—experiences from 3 institutions. Am J Infect Control 2005; 33(1):53–4.

120. Dellit TH, Owens RC, McGowan JE Jr, et al. Infectious Diseases Society of America and the Society for Healthcare Epidemiology of America guidelines for developing an institutional program to enhance antimicrobial stewardship. Clin Infect Dis 2007; 44(2):159–77.

121. Rahal JJ, Urban C, Segal-Maurer S. Nosocomial antibiotic resistance in multiple Gram-negative species: experience at one hospital with squeezing the resistance balloon at multiple sites. Clin Infect Dis 2002; 34(4):499–503.

122. Perencevich EN, Fisman DN, Lipsitch M, Harris AD, Morris JG Jr, Smith D. Projected benefits of active surveillance for vancomycin-resistant enterococci in intensive care units. Clin Infect Dis 2004; 38(8):1108–15.

123. Rodriguez-Hernandez MJ, Saugar J, Docobo-Perez F, et al. Studies on the antimicrobial activity of cecropin A-melittin hybrid peptides in colistin-resistant clinical isolates of *Acinetobacter baumannii*. J Antimicrob Chemother 2006; 58(1):95–100.

9   *Pseudomonas aeruginosa*: An Understanding of Resistance Issues

Karen Lolans
Chicago Infectious Disease Research Institute, Chicago, Illinois, U.S.A.

Maria Virginia Villegas
CIDEIM, International Center for Medical Research and Training, Cali, Columbia

John P. Quinn
Chicago Infectious Disease Research Institute, John H. Stroger Jr. Hospital of Cook County, and Rush University Medical Center, Chicago, Illinois, U.S.A.

EPIDEMIOLOGY

Pseudomonas aeruginosa is a nonfermenting Gram-negative bacterium that has minimal nutritional requirements and can survive on a wide variety of surfaces and in aqueous environments. The organism is ubiquitous in the natural environment and can be isolated from soil, water, and animals, including humans. Due to its minimal nutritional requirements, it can grow in diverse environments with a predilection for moist conditions that is probably a reflection of its natural habitat and plays a critical role in its epidemiology.

Pseudomonas has numerous reservoirs in the hospital, including sinks, respiratory equipment, cleaning solutions, flowers, and uncooked vegetables, and it occasionally may be recovered from the hands of medical personnel (1,2). Human colonization begins within the gastrointestinal tract, with subsequent spread to patients' skin and moist cutaneous sites such as the perineum and axilla (3). Olson et al. found that colonization was common from patients admitted to the intensive care unit (ICU). Using detection by surveillance and clinical cultures, they found that, of 270 patients tested, 100 were colonized with *P. aeruginosa*. Sixty-three were colonized at the time of admission, and 37 acquired the organism during hospitalization. As only 80% of these would have been first detected by rectal surveillance cultures, and only 43% first identified by throat cultures, most of this carriage would have gone undetected. Clinical infection in association with preceding gastrointestinal colonization developed in 20 patients (4). These data suggest that the occurrence of *P. aeruginosa* in ICUs is and will continue to be difficult to control, as many patients arrive colonized, and most carriage is not recognized.

As such, *P. aeruginosa* has become an effective opportunistic nosocomial pathogen, rarely causing disease in healthy persons. Hospitalization increases the carriage rate, particularly among severely burned patients, among patients receiving mechanical ventilation, and in those on broad-spectrum antibiotics. Some of the invasive infections, include nosocomial pneumonia, especially ventilator-associated pneumonia, urinary tract infections, burn wound infections, and septicemia (2,4–6).

PATHOGENESIS

The pathogenesis of *P. aeruginosa* may be divided into three stages: (*i*) bacterial attachment and colonization, (*ii*) local invasion and dissemination, and (*iii*) systemic disease; although disease progression can stop at any stage. The organism is well endowed with diverse virulence factors that promote colonization and/or infection. For example, pili or fimbriae (which are specialized attachment organelles) and mucoid exopolysaccharide allow for adherence of *P. aeruginosa* to epithelial cells (1,7). In addition, exoenzyme S, which is displayed on the bacterial cell surface, appears also to mediate bacterial attachment to respiratory epithelium (8). In combination with an array of others, these secreted virulence factors and endotoxins collectively contribute to the *Pseudomonas'* pathogenic versatility (9).

Finally, no discussion would be complete without the acknowledgement of *P. aeruginosa* as a classic example of an organism that forms a biofilm. These biofilms develop preferentially on inert surfaces, such as endotracheal tubes, on dead tissue, such as sequestra of bone, and on lung tissue, particularly in those suffering from cystic fibrosis. They are developed communities of individual bacterial cells embedded in an extracellular polysaccharide matrix that can provide protection from phagocytosis, restrict the diffusion of substances, and bind antimicrobials (10). Bacteria living in biofilms usually have significantly different properties from free-floating bacteria of the same species. This protected mode of growth allows for survival in a hostile environment, and bacterial growth in biofilms is a contributing factor to resistance to antimicrobial treatment. This increased resistance has been attributed to many factors, including reduced growth rate and reduced antimicrobial penetration within the biofilm, among others (10). However, the exact nature of this remains unclear and is an area of active investigation.

Chronic bacterial infections often involve biofilm formation (10,11). The *P. aeruginosa* isolated from the sputum of patients with cystic fibrosis are commonly mucoid variants that produce the exopolysaccharide alginate. The presence of these mucoid variants has correlated with the formation of bacterial biofilms (10–12). A specific regulatory protein, PvrR, studied in *P. aeruginosa* isolates from cystic fibrosis patients was recently shown to regulate the conversion between antibiotic susceptible and resistant forms as well as affect biofilm formation (13). This evidence indicates that biofilm formation and antibiotic resistance are interrelated.

CURRENT RESISTANCE RATES

Sepsis is the most common cause of death in ICU patients worldwide. In vitro surveys show that *P. aeruginosa* is the dominant Gram-negative pathogen in this setting and a common cause of morbidity and mortality in hospitalized patients in the United States (14). According to the Center for Disease Control and Prevention's National Nosocomial Infection Surveillance (NNIS) survey, which surveys pathogens from ICUs, *P. aeruginosa* was nationwide the most frequently recovered Gram-negative pathogen independent of infection type, constituting 7.5% of strains (14). Each year from 1986 to 2003, pneumonia data from the NNIS system show that *P. aeruginosa* has accounted for the greatest proportion of Gram-negative organisms recovered from pneumonia (14). As a result, an analysis of current resistance rates is clinically important.

A large-scale survey of antibiotic susceptibility of Gram-negative aerobes (35,790 organisms from 396 ICUs in the United States) was conducted from 1994 to 2000 (15). During that period, antimicrobial resistance rates in *P. aeruginosa* remained relatively stable for most beta-lactam agents, with ceftazidime resistance occurring in approximately 15% of isolates (Table 1). These resistance data were comparable to other published national data from the NNIS survey (16), showing that in contrast to the stability of beta-lactam resistance, fluoroquinolone resistance in *P. aeruginosa* was increasing rapidly.

In a number of the most recent surveys, this trend towards escalating resistance has continued, irrespective of the antimicrobial class evaluated. Antimicrobial susceptibility data analyzed from the Intensive Care Unit Surveillance Study (ISS) gathered from 1993 to 2002 (representing 13,999 non-duplicate isolates) showed that nationwide *P. aeruginosa* susceptibilities declined significantly for all drug classes (17). In that 9-year period, significant increases in antimicrobial resistance were noted for ciprofloxacin (15–32%), imipenem (15–23%), tobramycin (9–16%), and aztreonam (26–32%). Susceptibility to cefepime was not tracked through that entire period, although a significant increase in resistance was shown for the time period in which data was available (16% in 1998 to 25% in 2002) (17). Jones et al. reported similar resistance rates for ciprofloxacin and imipenem, although a lower incidence of cefepime resistance (12.4%) was described (18).

When the NNIS survey compared the rate of *P. aeruginosa* resistance to various antimicrobials in 2003 with the mean rate of resistance over the previous 5 years, they found that quinolone resistance increased by 9%, imipenem resistance by 15%, and resistance to third generation-cephalosporins had increased by 20% (16). This data potentially identifies a break in the stability of beta-lactam resistance rates that had previously been reported, while identifying additional losses in quinolone susceptibility.

TABLE 1 Overall Antimicrobial Susceptibility Rates for *Pseudomonas aeruginosa*, 1994–2000, Intensive Care Unit Surveillance

Antimicrobial by class	*P. aeruginosa* (*n* = 8244)
Amikacin	90
Tobramycin	87
Gentamicin	68
Imipenem	83
Ciprofloxacin	76
Cefepime	71
Ceftazidime	80
Ceftriaxone	17
Cefotaxime	13
Aztreonam	67
Piperacillin	74
Ticarcillin	43
Ampicillin/sulbactam	2
Piperacillin/tazobactam	78
Ticarcillin/clavulanate	42

Note: Numbers indicated for each antimicrobial are percentages.
Source: Adapted from Ref. 15.

Further challenging the treatment choices available for *P. aeruginosa* is the noted increase in multidrug resistance (MDR) (resistance to ≥ 3 antipseudomonal drugs). Data from the ISS study indicated that the prevalence of MDR in the United States rose from 4% (in 1993) to 14% (in 2002) (17). In another long-itudinal analysis, of non-repeat nosocomial isolates from a single hospital, similar increases over that same 9-year time frame were observed (19). Also, another study found a slightly lower increase from 7.2% (in 2001) to 9.9% (in 2003) in the prevalence of the MDR phenotype (20). Overall, these studies indicate potentially increasing rates of not only single drug, but MDR phenotypes as well, and are of concern as they will affect selection of empiric therapy in critically ill patients.

EMERGENCE OF ANTIBIOTIC RESISTANCE DURING TREATMENT WITH SPECIFIC DRUGS

Antibiotic resistance in *P. aeruginosa* is an increasing problem, posing many therapeutic challenges. In addition, initially susceptible strains may acquire drug resistance during treatment, often with a relatively high frequency (21–23). This emergence of resistance has been reported with virtually all classes of drugs including beta-lactams, aminoglycosides, and quinolones (24,25).

Many strains of *P. aeruginosa* exhibiting beta-lactam resistance reflect a prior exposure of the patients to broad-spectrum beta-lactams. For example, a signifi-cant correlation was noted in a single medical center between antecedent use of ceftriaxone, cefotaxime, ceftazidime, and piperacillin and resistance to these com-pounds among bacterial strains that typically produce a type I chromosomal AmpC beta-lactamase, including 155 isolates of *P. aeruginosa* (26). Similarly, Manian et al. (23) analyzed resistance rates among 594 initial and repeat Gram-negative isolates from 287 patients in ICUs. Sixty-one percent of these were *Enterobacter* and *P. aeruginosa* isolates. These investigators reported rates of resis-tance to cephalosporins and penicillins that were significantly higher among repeat isolates and that this resistance was statistically linked to prior treatment with third-generation cephalosporins.

An interesting study examined the relative risk of emergence of resistance in *P. aeruginosa* isolates exposed to four different antimicrobial agents: ceftazi-dime, ciprofloxacin, piperacillin, and imipenem (27). Overall, 10% of 271 patients with a *P. aeruginosa* infection studied experienced an emergence of resistance during treatment. Pulsed-field gel electrophoresis (PFGE) typing confirmed that these resistant organisms represented the emergence of resistance from an initially susceptible population. Imipenem had the highest overall risk for emer-gence of resistance; ceftazidime had the lowest, with ciprofloxacin and piperacil-lin intermediate in this regard. Although this was an observational study with a relatively small number of patients (for example, 37 patients received imipenem), a prior randomized trial comparing imipenem to ciprofloxacin for the treatment of nosocomial pneumonia also showed a somewhat higher risk of emergence of resistance in the carbapenem arm (22).

MECHANISMS OF RESISTANCE TO SPECIFIC DRUGS

P. aeruginosa is often resistant to a variety of broad-spectrum antimicrobial agents, making it a formidable pathogen. Its nonsusceptibility generally results from a combination of intrinsic and acquired resistance. The *Pseudomonas'* innate resistance to multiple antimicrobial drug classes is multifactorial. Most small hydrophilic molecules, including antibiotics, enter the cell via nonspecific porin channels present in the outer membrane. The outer membrane permeability of *P. aeruginosa* has been shown to be 10- to 100-fold less efficient than, e.g., in *Escherichia coli* (28). This high intrinsic antibiotic resistance that typifies *P. aeruginosa* is recognized to be the result of synergy between this highly impermeable outer membrane and the expression of broad-spectrum multidrug efflux systems (Table 2). These efflux systems serve the physiological function of preventing toxic compounds from entering the cell in significant concentrations. They actively remove biocides, dyes, detergents, organic solvents, and metabolites as well as antibiotics from the cytoplasm or periplasmic space (29). The most important and well-studied family of these is the resistance-nodulation-cell division (RND)-type family of pumps. There are, in addition, at least four other pump families encompassing both many characterized as well as predicted efflux pump systems, based on genomic data, present in this bacterium (30). *P. aeruginosa* possesses the additional capacity to acquire resistance via mutational changes that occur in the organisms' genome along with the capacity to acquire extrachromosomal genetic material, for example, plasmids or transposons carrying resistance determinants (28,31).

CHROMOSOMAL MECHANISMS OF RESISTANCE
Beta-Lactams
Beta-lactam resistance in *P. aeruginosa* is usually mediated by overproduction of the chromosomal AmpC beta-lactamase. This overexpression results from mutations in regulatory genes (e.g., *ampR, ampD,* or *ampE*), conferring clinically significant resistance to antipseudomonal penicillins and all third generation cephalosporins (28,32). The so-called fourth generation cephalosporins, cefepime, and cefpirome are less susceptible to the chromosomal AmpC and remain somewhat more active than the third-generation compounds under these circumstances. Primarily because of their higher outer membrane permeability, lower affinity for beta-lactamase, and higher avidity for penicillin-binding proteins, only modest inactivation may result (33). However, strains of *P. aeruginosa* may acquire clinically significant resistance even to these agents by a combination of upregulation of efflux and hyperproduction of AmpC beta-lactamase (25,34).

It has been noted in *P. aeruginosa* that cefepime and ceftazidime commonly display similar MIC distribution patterns (35,36). The occurence of isolates more resistant to cefepime (FEP) than to ceftazidime (CAZ) (FEP^R/CAZ^S profile) have typically been attributed to errors in the automated testing systems used in susceptibility determinations (37). However, Hocquet et al. recently demonstrated the contribution of stable overexpression of the efflux pump system, MexXY-OprM, to this discrepant phenotype (38).

Unlike the cephalosporins and piperacillin, the carbapenems are stable to hydrolysis by AmpC and unaffected by most of the acquired beta-lactamases that occur in the species (25,39). For imipenem, the major resistance mechanism is loss of the specific porin, OprD, which serves as the primary route of entry for carbapenems. OprD loss may occur in up to 50% of patients treated with imipenem for more than one week (40). Studies in which OprD is overexpressed show that it is relatively specific for carbapenems and does not mediate passage of other beta-lactams or quinolones (41). While the loss of OprD confers resistance to imipenem, it is only associated with reduced susceptibility to meropenem.

TABLE 2 Mutational Resistances in *Pseudomonas Aeruginosa*

Mechanism	Mutation site	Effect on strain according to antipseudomonal drug								
		Fq	Carb-Tic	Pip-Azl	Czid-Atm	Cpm-Cpr	Imi	Mero	Agl	Pm
Reduced affinity										
Of topoisomerase II	*gyrA*	r/R	–	–	–	–	–	–	–	–
Of topoisomerase IV	*parC*	r/R	–	–	–	–	–	–	–	–
Derepression of AmpC										
Partial	*ampD*	–	R	R	R	r	–	–	–	–
Total	*ampD*+other	–	R	R	R	R	–	–	–	–
Upregulation										
Of MexAB-OprM	*nalB* at *mexR*; *nalC* at other	R/R	R	r/R	r/R	r/R	–	r	–	–
Of MexCD-OprJ	*nfxB*	r/R	r/R	r/R	r/R	R	–	r	–	–
Of MexEF-OprN	*nfxC* at *mexT*	r/R	r/R	r/R	r/R	r/R	r	r	–	–
Of MexXY-OprM		r/R	r/R	r/R	r/R	r/R	–	–	r/R	–
Reduced aminoglycoside transport		–	–	–	–	–	–	–	r/R	–
Loss of OprD	*oprD*; *nfxC* at *mexT*	–	–	–	–	–	R	r	–	–
Membrane changes		–	–	–	–	–	–	–	–	R

Abbreviations: Agl, aminoglycosides; Azl, azlocillin; Atm, aztreonam; Carb, carbenicillin; Czid, ceftazidime; Cpm, cefepime; Cpr, cefpirome; Fq, fluoroquinolone; Imi, imipenem; Mero, meropenem; Pip, piperacillin; Pm, polymyxin; r, reduced susceptibility; R, frank resistance (which may vary in its distinction from "r", according to the breakpoints adopted); Tic, ticarcillin.
Source: From Ref. 25.

However, it has been demonstrated that the MexAB-OprM efflux system includes most beta-lactams, including meropenem, in its substrate spectrum (42). Based on this finding, Kohler et al. (43) examined the respective contributions of OprD and efflux on carbapenem resistance in *P. aeruginosa*. By constructing mutants with varying combinations of OprD and MexAB-OprM expressions, they showed that meropenem minimum inhibitory concentrations (MICs) were strongly influenced by efflux while imipenem remained unaffected. Full resistance to meropenem thus requires two separate mutations: loss of OprD plus overexpression of an efflux system active against meropenem, and as a result, emergence of resistance to meropenem may occur less commonly than to imipenem (25).

Quinolones

Quinolone-resistant strains of *P. aeruginosa* are relatively common (15–16,18). Mechanistically, resistance in *Pseudomonas* is traditionally mediated by chromosomal target-based mutations in either DNA gyrase and/or topoisomerase genes (44), or genes regulating expression of efflux pumps (45) and sometimes both. The expression level of efflux pumps normally present in *P. aeruginosa* is not usually sufficient by itself to produce resistance to antipseudomonal drugs. The acquisition or selection of mutants overexpressing efflux pumps has been implicated in resistance to most classes of antibiotic drugs, including fluoroquinolones, antipseudomonal penicillins and cephalosporins, carbapenems and aminoglycosides (28). The combined overexpression of efflux pumps along with DNA gyrase mutations has been shown to confer high-level fluoroquinolone resistance in *P. aeruginosa* (46,47). Within the RND-type pump family, there are six naturally occurring broadly-specific multidrug-efflux (Mex) pumps identified thus far in *Pseudomonas*. While each pump has a preferential set of antimicrobial agent substrates, the fluoroquinolones are universal substrates for all known Mex pumps (42). While surveillance studies have tracked the changes in fluoroquinolone susceptibilities over time, the majority have not evaluated the mechanisms responsible for resistance (15–18). One epidemiologic study investigated the contribution of efflux pump overexpression in fluoroquinolone resistance among clinical isolates of *P. aeruginosa* from 12 countries (48). Efflux contributions to resistance varied widely by country, but indicated that efflux pump overexpression was widespread. Of the 258 strains from the United States, 50% were found to overexpress

TABLE 3 Rates of Cross-Resistance Among *Pseudomonas aeruginosa* Isolates, 1994–2000, Intensive Care Unit Surveillance

	Ciprofloxacin	
Antimicrobial	Resistant ($n = 1946$)	Susceptible ($n = 6298$)
Gentamicin	66.0	21.7
Ceftazidime	39.8	14.0
Imipenem	37.6	10.9
Amikacin	26.0	5.6

Note: Numbers indicated for each antimicrobial are percentages.
Source: Adapted from Ref. 15.

the MexAB-OprM efflux pump while 32% of isolates expressed a combination of efflux pumps and/or target mutations.

Cross-resistance may be observed when drug efflux is the resistance mechanism as efflux pumps can extrude structurally-unrelated compounds (Table 3). Quinolones may select for mutants, called Mar (multiple antibiotic resistance) mutants, that are resistant to other classes of antibiotics. At least three related efflux mutations have been observed in the laboratory. These are identified as *nalB*, *nfxB*, and *nfxC*; all of which affect regulatory genes of different efflux pumps, thus leading to their overexpression (49,50). The *nfxC* (also known as *mexT*) mutation is particularly interesting because it leads to overproduction of another protein, OprN, which is the outer membrane component of an efflux system that pumps quinolones. These strains simultaneously underexpress OprD, due to coregulation of the genes. As a result, these mutants are cross-resistant to quinolones, chloramphenicol, tetracycline and carbapenems (50).

Recently, a new mechanism of quinolone resistance—*qnr*, a plasmid-mediated horizontally-transferable gene—has been identified in Gram-negative bacteria (51). Although this phenomenon has not yet been described in *P. aeruginosa*, a number of Enterobacteriaceae have been identified expressing *qnr* genes. This mechanism provides low level of resistance to fluoroquinolones, but can enhance the level of resistance that is conferred by the target mutations. The *qnr* gene has been located within integrons on plasmids (linking it to transferable multidrug resistance) and, given the ability for gene transfer between Gram-negative bacteria, it seems likely that this resistance determinant will eventually appear in *P. aeruginosa*.

Aminoglycosides

It has long been documented that reduced penetration across the outer membrane leads to low level aminoglycoside resistance, particularly in cystic fibrosis patients and in ICUs (52,53). Recent evidence has shown that the efflux pump, MexXY, also contributes to reduced aminoglycoside accumulation in *P. aeruginosa* (53). However, the most common mechanism for aminoglycoside resistance in *P. aeruginosa* is enzymatic modification by plasmid- or chromosomally-mediated acetylating, adenylating, or phosphorylating enzymes. Carriage of multiple modifying enzymes, increasingly identified in *P. aeruginosa* strains, has lead to consequential broad aminoglycoside resistance (53).

MULTIPLE MUTATIONS AND MULTIDRUG RESISTANCE

One of the most striking characteristics of *P. aeruginosa* is its extraordinary ability for acquisition of antibiotic resistance determinants (31). No mutation has the capacity to single-handedly compromise every antipseudomonal antibiotic. However, comprehensive resistance to therapeutically useful agents is possible as a result of the convergence of multiple factors. Efflux-based resistance may have an additive or even multiplicative effects with decreased permeability, beta-lactamase expression, or target-mediated resistance so as to enhance drug resistance (54).

The rate at which a single mutation occurs is very low (say 1 per 10^8 cells). Thus, the likelihood of simultaneous emergence of these various mutations seems biologically and mathematically improbable. However, a patient's bacterial flora most frequently encounters not just a single antibiotic pressure but mixed and varying antibiotic pressures. Failure of one antibiotic regimen leads to sequential antibiotic therapy resulting in the same bacterial organism challenged by these different antibiotics. These fluctuating environments select for different bacterial variants, making sequential emergence all too likely.

The accumulation of sequential mutations is more common in hypermutator strains. These strains either lack the ability to perform DNA proofreading or mismatch repair, or use DNA polymerases with a reduced copying fidelity (55). The genetic backgrounds of these strains are primed for selecting some antibiotic-resistance mutations since mutation frequencies up to 1000-fold higher than in normal strains have been reported (56). In *P. aeruginosa* strains from chronically infected patients, as well as in other natural bacterial populations (56), the most frequently involved system is the mismatch repair system, and *mutS* is the most frequently affected gene (55,57). A recent in vitro work in *P. aeruginosa* has shown that due to defects in these systems, a population of seemingly susceptible bacteria can develop resistance to every single antipseudomonal agent due to the proliferation of resistant mutants in a few hours during drug exposure (58). In one study, these hypermutators were found in sputum samples obtained from 11 of 30 cystic fibrosis patients with chronic *P. aeruginosa* infections, versus 0 of 75 samples from patients without cystic fibrosis having acute infections (57). In recent years, hypermutation has been acknowledged as a potentially concerning problem in antibiotic resistance development (56,59).

Resistance to multiple antipseudomonal drugs can occur via a single mutation. For example, the fluoroquinolones and most beta-lactams can be simultaneously compromised by a number of mutations that result in upregulated efflux. Combine up-regulated efflux with loss of OprD and impermeability to aminoglycosides, and resistance to every drug class except the polymyxins might result.

ACQUIRED GENES AND MULTIDRUG RESISTANCE

P. aeruginosa commonly harbor acquired beta-lactamases and aminoglycoside-modifying enzymes. These are particularly prevalent among isolates from Southern Europe, Turkey, and Southeast Asia; they appear to be rare in the United States and United Kingdom. The most frequently acquired beta-lactamases are PSE-1 and PSE-4. Like most other serine-based enzymes, the resistance mediated by PSE enzymes can be overcome by the use of carbapenems, oxymino-aminothiazolyl cephalosporins (e.g., ceftazidime, cefepime, or cefpirome) or monobactams (60). However, other beta-lactamases mediating resistance are emerging in *P. aeruginosa*. We will discuss the PER-1 beta-lactamase, the extended-spectrum oxacillinase (OXA) types (known as OXA-extended-spectrum beta-lactams, or OXA-ESBLs) as well as the IMP and VIM families of metallo-beta-lactamases (MβLs).

PER-1 is a class A beta-lactamase of notable clinical importance, due to its high level of activity toward oxyimino-cephalosporins; the preferred substrate being ceftazidime (61,62). The carbapenems, however, remain active. PER-1 is commonly isolated from *P. aeruginosa* from Turkey (62,63), but otherwise has a limited geographic distribution. There have been occasional reports of isolates, outside this geographical area of origin, from areas of France and Italy (64,65). The related enzyme, PER-2, has 86% amino acid homology to PER-1 and has been sporadically identified in *P. aeruginosa* isolates only in South America (66,67). The

OXA-ESBLs, like PER-1, have primarily been reported in *P. aeruginosa* from Turkey (68). As in the case of the classic ESBLs like TEM and SHV, the OXA-ESBLs have minor sequence substitutions that greatly extend their hydrolytic activity. Most arise from point mutations among the narrow spectrum beta-lactamases, OXA-2 or OXA-10. These OXA-ESBLs confer resistance to oxyimino-aminothiazolyl cephalosporins, monobactams, and penicillins but not to carbapenems; they are only weakly inhibited by clavulanic acid (68,69). Most oxacillinase genes are plasmid-, transposon- and integron-located, facilitating dispersion (69). A few *P. aeruginosa* isolates from Turkey have been identified producing both PER enzymes and ESBLs, often together with potent aminoglycoside-modifying enzymes (70).

IMP and VIM constitute the two dominant groups of MβLs; their hydrolytic spectrum includes penicillins, cephalosporins, and carbapenems but not aztreonam (71). This phenotype may be helpful in identifying these strains in the lab. Resistance to penicillins and cephalosporins usually accompanies production of these MβLs, but carbapenem susceptibilities can be quite variable (from remaining susceptible to becoming highly resistant). This suggests that acquisition alone of a MβL does not always confer carbapenem resistance and may require the concomitant loss of OprD.

The first indication of these MβLs came in 1988 with the discovery of IMP-1 in Japan. Since then, it has predominantly been found in Japan, and multifocal outbreaks have been described (72). Although, remaining rare among *P. aeruginosa* strains in Japan, IMP-1 has also been noted among *P. aeruginosa* strains from Brazil and Korea (73). Currently, 23 IMP-type MβLs have been identified worldwide; the majority described in *P. aeruginosa* from European and Asian countries (accessed August 28, 2007, http://www.lahey.org/studies), but variants have been identified in a wide spectrum of bacterial species as well as numerous countries (73). The VIM enzymes resemble the IMP types with regard to their hydrolytic spectrum, but low amino acid homology exists between them (approximately 30–40%) (25). In 1997, the first enzyme of this family, VIM-1, was found in *P. aeruginosa* in Italy. Many of the eighteen VIM variants identified to date have been reported almost exclusively in *P. aeruginosa* (accessed August 28, 2007, http://www.lahey.org/studies). VIM-2, which shares 90% amino acid identity to that of VIM-1, is the most widespread VIM in terms of both host organism and geography. Since 2000, the metalloenzymes have shown a remarkable increase worldwide, not only in their prevalence but also in the overall number of enzymes (74,75).

Although they have disseminated globally, there have been only a few sporadic occurrences of MβLs in North America. A nosocomial outbreak of carbapenem-resistant *P. aeruginosa* in Canada resulted from an IMP-7 (76), and another study identified that 45% of the imipenem-nonsusceptible *P. aeruginosa* isolated from one central laboratory in Calgary harbored a MβL (77). We are aware of only three instances of metalloenzymes in the United States. Two reports described single *P. aeruginosa* isolates; one from Texas carrying a VIM-8 (78), the other in New Mexico producing an IMP-18 (79). The third was a nosocomial outbreak involving multiple *P. aeruginosa* isolates from Chicago hospitals that produced a VIM-2 (80).

The genes for VIM and IMP enzymes, like those for OXA-ESBLs, are transferable as most are found as gene cassettes located primarily on integrons, sometimes within transposons or on plasmids. Integrons are natural recombination systems that assemble series of acquired genes behind a single promoter, and this machinery enables resistance to spread horizontally (73). While the resistance cassettes carried on the MβL-containing integrons may vary, the beta-lactamase genes are often adjacent to aminoglycoside 6'-N acetyltransferase [aac(6'-1b)] determinants (81,82). A *P. aeruginosa* with this combination of cassettes is susceptible only to polymyxins, ciprofloxacin, and perhaps, aztreonam.

Pan-resistant strains (resistance to all antimicrobials tested except the polymyxins) of *P. aeruginosa* are a reality in some facilities (79,80,83,84). In an outbreak of *P. aeruginosa* in Belgium, pan-resistance was identified as a result of the convergence of AmpC overexpression, OprD loss and the upregulation of mexXY efflux system (which includes aminoglycosides and fluoroquinolones in its substrate spectrum) (84). In the outbreak of *P. aeruginosa* in Chicago, pan-resistance was identified in a subset of the isolates. All isolates carried a MβL enzyme (VIM-2) on an integron, along with two different aminoglycoside-modifying enzymes. While the majority of isolates remained susceptible to aztreonam (MβLs do not hydrolyze aztreonam), resistance was noted in two isolates that was likely the result of chromosomal AmpC hyperproduction (80).

Additionally, if MexAB-OprM is up-regulated by mutation, or if the isolates have topoisomerase or *ampD* mutations (resulting in AmpC cephalosporinase hyperproduction) then only susceptibility to the polymyxins remains. These examples illustrate the organisms' ability to accumulate numerous effective mechanisms in response to the multiple challenges they face surviving in the antimicrobial-rich hospital environment.

CONTROVERSIES ABOUT ANTIMICROBIAL THERAPY FOR *P. AERUGINOSA*

Antibiotic selection for treatment of *P. aeruginosa* may be problematic. Clinical efficacy does not always correlate with in vitro antibiotic susceptibility or in vivo studies in animals. There are few prospective, randomized clinical trials of therapeutic agents for *Pseudomonas* infections. Most studies that are published involve empiric therapy in febrile neutropenic patients. Strain differences, presence of a protective mucoid capsule, and the ability of the organism to develop resistance while on therapy complicate antibiotic selection.

There is an ongoing clinical debate over the role of combination antimicrobial therapy. Combination therapy had been considered the mainstay of therapy for many years, but this is based on limited data. Much of the support for combination therapy emanated from the study of Hilf et al. (85). In his prospective observational study of 200 consecutive patients with *P. aeruginosa* bacteremia, combination therapy was found to be significantly better than monotherapy in improving outcome (85). Mortality was significantly higher in patients given monotherapy (47%) than in patients given combination therapy (27%). It should be noted that the most common combination used was piperacillin or ticarcillin combined with tobramycin or gentamicin. The monotherapy group was dominated by patients given an aminoglycoside alone. Few patients received cephalosporins, aztreonam, carbapenems or quinolones.

More recently, a prospective observational study from Israel evaluated monotherapy versus beta-lactam-aminoglycoside combination therapy for Gram-negative bacteremia (86). 16% of the 2165 patients in the study had *P. aeruginosa*. Thirty-four percent (21/61) of the patients with *P. aeruginosa* bacteremia died on beta-lactam monotherapy while 28% (11/39) patients died after receipt of combination therapy. This corresponded to an odds ratio of 0.7, with 95% confidence intervals of 0.3–1.8.

To definitively show that combination therapy is superior to monotherapy would require a randomized controlled trial of several hundred patients. It is highly unlikely that such a study will be performed in the near future. Combinations of beta-lactams and quinolones are increasingly used but clinical data to support this is sparse. Based on demonstration of in vitro synergy between antipseudomonal beta-lactam antibiotics and aminoglycosides, combined with the development of resistance with monotherapy, we continue to recommend combination antibiotic therapy for serious pseudomonal infections.

Double beta-lactam therapy is not recommended. Although the data are limited, it has proved inferior to the beta-lactam-aminoglycoside combination in animal models (87). One study in humans showed emergence of resistance in 40% of cases (2/5) in one series of *P. aeruginosa* infection treated with double beta-lactams (88).

Dosing of antimicrobial agents in therapy of serious *Pseudomonas* infections should be aggressive. For ciprofloxacin, an intravenous dose of 400 mg every 8 hr is recommended instead of standard 400 mg every 12 hr (89). In the case of levofloxacin, we suggest 750 mg per day rather than 500 mg per day for serious pseudomonal infections (90). For beta-lactams, the rate of bactericidal activity of beta-lactams does not increase substantially once concentrations exceed four times the MIC (91). Beta-lactams other than the carbapenems do not exhibit a postantibiotic effect against *P. aeruginosa* (92). High concentrations do not kill *P. aeruginosa* any faster than lower concentrations, and bacterial regrowth begins immediately after serum and tissue levels fall below the MIC. The duration of time that serum levels exceed the MIC is the pharmacokinetic parameter that best correlates with in vivo efficacy of the beta-lactams (93). Continuous or prolonged infusion of antipseudomonal beta-lactams is therefore theoretically attractive. At this time, this approach remains to be validated in large clinical studies.

Aminoglycosides, even when in combination therapy, should be dosed once daily when used against *P. aeruginosa*. Aminoglycosides exhibit concentration-dependent bactericidal activity, and also produce prolonged post-antibiotic effects, supporting the practice of once daily dosing. Dosing tobramycin or gentamicin at 5 to 7 mg/kg/day, and amikacin 15 mg/kg/day, are recommended (94). It is not clear whether aminoglycosides need to be continued for the full treatment course, as toxicity correlates with duration of therapy. When aminoglycosides are used in combination with beta-lactam antibiotics, we would discontinue aminoglycosides within one week if possible.

ALTERNATIVE THERAPIES

Due to the complex interplay of mutational and acquired resistance mechanisms previously discussed, occasional *P. aeruginosa* isolates arise that are resistant to all commercially available antibiotics, other than colistin/polymyxin B. The polymyxins were originally isolated from *Bacillus* spp.: polymyxin B from *B. polymyxa* in 1947, and colistin (also known as polymyxin E) from *B. colistinus* in 1950. The polymyxins act primarily on the bacterial cell wall, leading to rapid permeability changes in the cytoplasmic membrane; therefore, entry into the cell is not necessary. They may also have anti-endotoxin activity (95,96). Concerns arose regarding adverse effects (e.g., nephrotoxicity and neurotoxicity) with their use, and as a result the polymyxins were abandoned in favor of newer, safer anti-microbials. The increasing frequency of multidrug-resistant *P. aeruginosa* isolates causing life-threatening infections has resulted in a re-evaluation of the potential therapeutic indication for the parenteral use of polymyxins (97,98), usually colistin in North American medical centers.

Against pathogens from the SENTRY Antimicrobial Surveillance Program, polymyxin B and colistin exhibited excellent potency against *P. aeruginosa*, demonstrating a nearly identical in vitro spectrum of activity. The minimum inhibitory concentration that inhibited 90% of isolates [MIC_{90}] was $\leq 2\,\mu g/mL$ for both compounds (99). In vitro studies suggest that use of colistin as part of combination therapy may result in greater killing of *P. aeruginosa* than monotherapy, even when the strains are resistant to the individual antibiotics. Combinations investigated have included colistin plus rifampin and amikacin (100), colistin plus ceftazidime, colistin plus aztreonam, colistin plus meropenem, and colistin plus ciprofloxacin (101). In vitro time-kill studies have shown bactericidal activity by combinations of polymyxin B with rifampin and/or imipenem (102). However, there is little published clinical data, and the clinical usefulness of these combinations is still to be determined. However, in critically ill patients, we believe that combination therapy with colistin may be prudent.

Most pharmacokinetic studies with colistin were performed more than 30 years ago using intramuscular administration of the drug. As such, modern pharmacokinetic data for the polymyxins is lacking. The current recommended dosings of colistin are the following: creatinine clearance $\geq 80\,mL/min$: 2.5 mg/kg every 12 hr; creatinine clearance 30 to 80 mL/min: loading dose of 3 mg/kg on day 1 then 1.25 to 1.9 mg/kg every 12 hr; and creatinine clearance $< 30\,mL/min$: loading dose of 3 mg/kg on day 1 then 1.25 mg/kg every 12 hr (97).

There is no data from randomized controlled trials to effectively evaluate the safety and efficacy of the polymyxins in treating Gram-negative bacteria resistant to other antibiotics. The increasing prevalence of MDR *P. aeruginosa* (19,20) has led to the accumulation of reports on the polymyxins' clinical use borne out of necessity. These typically involve critically ill patients where the polymyxins are used as salvage therapy.

In a study from Brazil, 59 patients with MDR *P. aeruginosa* and *Acinetobacter* strains were treated using intravenous colistin (103). In patients with normal renal function, initial doses were 2.5 to 5 mg/kg/day, divided into two or three doses, up to a maximum of 300 mg daily. A range of infections were treated, including pneumonia, urinary tract infections, bacteremias, central nervous system infections, peritonitis, catheter-related infections, and otitis media. Overall, colistin treatment resulted in a positive clinical outcome in 58% of patients, although pneumonias had a poorer response rate (25%).

One clinical trial examined the effectiveness of colistin in the treatment of acute respiratory exacerbations in 53 cystic fibrosis patients with chronic *P. aeruginosa* colonization. They found intravenous colistin to be an effective treatment and showed that the combination of colistin with an antipseudomonal agent (azlocillin, piperacillin, aztreonam, ceftazidime, imipenem, or ciprofloxacin) was more effective than colistin monotherapy (104).

More recent pharmacodynamic studies in *P. aeruginosa* isolates from cystic fibrosis suggest that colistin doses higher than 2 to 3 mg/kg every 12 hr may be required for effective therapy (105). In a study of 12 patients with cystic fibrosis, 160 mg three times per day was found to be safe (106). Despite their reintroduction into clinical practice, concern revolving around the poly-myxins' reputation for toxicity, including nephrotoxicity and neurotoxicity, still remains.

SUMMARY

The body of knowledge regarding antibiotic resistance in *P. aeruginosa* has grown tremendously in recent years. *P. aeruginosa* possesses a wide array of tools for circumventing the activity of current antimicrobials. The complex interplay of numerous combinations of resistance mechanisms at their disposal can potentially result in comprehensive resistance to every antipseudomonal agent available. As antimicrobial resistance rates continue to evolve towards an increasing prevalence of strains with resistance to not only single agents, but to multiple antibiotics, clinicians are faced with fewer and fewer therapeutic options. Prudent use of currently available drugs and an emphasis on infection control measures must be combined with the development of newer drugs if we want to try to retain agents with activity against these pathogens.

REFERENCES

1. Stratton CW. *Pseudomonas aeruginosa* revisited. Infection Control Hosp Epidemiol 1990; 11:101–4.
2. Pollack M. *Pseudomonas aeruginosa*. In: Mandell GL, Bennett JE, Dolin R, eds. Principles and Practice of Infections Diseases. Philadelphia: Churchill Livingstone, 2000:2310–35.
3. Donskey CJ. Antibiotic regimens and intestinal colonization with antibiotic-resistant Gram-negative bacilli. Clin Infect Dis 2006; 43(Suppl. 2):S62–9.
4. Olson B, Weinstein RA, Nathan C, et al. Epidemiology of Endemic *Pseudomonas aeruginosa*: why infection control efforts have failed. J Infect Dis 1984; 150:808–16.
5. Neu HC. The role of *Pseudomonas aeruginosa* in infections. J Antimicrob Chemother 1983; 11:1–15.
6. Rello J, Jubert P. Evaluation of outcome for intubated patients with pneumonia due to *Pseudomonas aeruginosa*. Clin Infect Dis 1996; 23:973–8.
7. Doig P, Todd T. Role of pili in adhesion of *Pseudomonas aeruginosa* to human respiratory epithelial cells. Infect Immun 1988; 56:1641–6.
8. Nicas TI, Bradley J, Lochner JE, et al. The role of exoenzyme S in infections with *Pseudomonas aeruginosa*. J Infect Dis 1985; 152:716–21.
9. Kipnis E, Sawa T, Wiener-Kronish J. Targeting mechanisms of *Pseudomonas aeruginosa* pathogenesis. Med Mal Infect 2006; 36:78–91.
10. Costerton JW, Stewart PS, Greenberg EP. Bacterial biofilms: a common cause of persistent infections. Science 1999; 284:1318–22.
11. Richards MJ, Edwards JR, Culver DH, et al. Nosocomial infections in medical intensive care units in the United States. Crit Care Med 1999; 27:887–92.
12. Govan JR, Deretic V. Microbial pathogenesis in cystic fibrosis: mucoid *Pseudomonas aeruginosa* and *Burkholderia cepacia*. Microbiol Rev 1996; 60:539–74.
13. Drenkard E, Ausubel FM. *Pseudomonas* biofilm formation and antibiotic resistance are linked to phenotypic variation. Nature 2002; 416:695–6.
14. Gaynes R, Edwards JR. National Nosocomial Infections Surveillance System. Overview of nosocomial infections caused by Gram-negative bacilli. Clin Infect Dis 2005; 41:848–54.
15. Neuhauser MM, Weinstein RA, Rydman R, et al. Antibiotic resistance among Gram-negative bacilli in US intensive care units: implications for fluoroquinolone use. JAMA 2003; 289:885–8.

16. National Nosocomial Infections Surveillance System. National Nosocomial Infections Surveillance (NNIS) System Report, data summary from January 1992 through June 2004, issued October 2004. Am J Infect Control 2004; 32:470–85.
17. Obritsch MD, Fish DN, MacLaren R, et al. National surveillance of antimicrobial resistance in *Pseudomonas aeruginosa* isolates obtained from intensive care unit patients from 1993 to 2002. Antimicrob Agents Chemother 2004; 48:4606–10.
18. Jones ME, Draghi DC, Thornsberry C, et al. Emerging resistance among bacterial pathogens in the intensive care unit—a European and North American Surveillance study (2000–2002). Ann Clin Microbiol Antimicrob 2004; 3:14.
19. D'Agata EM. Rapidly rising prevalence of nosocomial multidrug-resistant, Gram-negative bacilli: a 9-year surveillance study. Infect Control Hosp Epidemiol 2004; 25:842–6.
20. Karlowsky JA, Draghi DC, Jones HE, et al. Surveillance for antimicrobial susceptibility among clinical isolates of *Pseudomonas aeruginosa* and *Acinetobacter baumannii* from Hospitalized Patients in the United States, 1998 to 2001. Antimicrob Agents Chemother 2003; 47:1681–8.
21. Quinn JP, Dudek EJ, DiVincenzo CA, et al. Emergence of resistance to imipenem during therapy for *Pseudomonas aeruginosa* infections. J Infect Dis 1986; 154:289–94.
22. Fink MP, Torres-Viery C, Venkataraman L, et al. Treatment of severe pneumonia in hospitalized patients: results of a multicenter, randomized, double-blind trial comparing intravenous ciprofloxacin with imipenem-cilastatin. Antimicrob Agents Chemother 1999; 38:547–57.
23. Manian FA, Meyer L, Jenne J, et al. Loss of antimicrobial susceptibility in aerobic Gram-negative bacilli repeatedly isolated from patients in intensive-care-units. Infect Control Hosp Epidemiol 1996; 17:222–6.
24. Gould IM, Wise R. *Pseudomonas aeruginosa*: clinical manifestation and management. Lancet 1985; 2:1224–7.
25. Livermore DM. Multiple mechanisms of resistance in *Pseudomonas aeruginosa:* our worst nightmare? Clin Infect Dis 2002; 34:634–40.
26. Jacobsen KL, Cohen SH, Inclardi JF, et al. The relationship between antecedent antibiotic use resistance to extended-spectrum cephalosporin in group I beta-lactamase-producing organisms. Clin Infect Dis 1995; 21:1107–13.
27. Carmeli Y, Troillet N, Eliopoulos GM, et al. Emergence of antibiotic-resistant *Pseudomonas aeruginosa:* Comparison of risks associated with different antipseudomonal agents. Antimicrob Agents Chemother 1999; 43:1379–82.
28. Hancock RE, Speert DP. Antibiotic resistance in *Pseudomonas aeruginosa*: mechanisms and impact on treatment. Drug Resist Updat 2000; 3:247–55.
29. Li XZ, Zhang L, Poole K. Interplay between the MexA-MexB-OprM multidrug efflux system and the outer membrane barrier in the multiple antibiotic resistance of *Pseudomonas aeruginosa*. J Antimicrob Chemother 2000; 45:433–6.
30. Stover CK, Pham XQ, Erwin AL, et al. Complete genome sequence of *Pseudomonas aeruginosa* PA01, an opportunistic pathogen. Nature 2000; 46:959–64.
31. Livermore DM. The threat from the pink corner. Ann Med. 2003; 35:226–34.
32. Juan C, Macia MD, Gutierrez O, et al. Molecular mechanisms of beta-lactam resistance mediated by AmpC hyperproduction in *Pseudomonas aeruginosa* clinical strains. Antimicrob Agents Chemother 2005; 49:4733–8.
33. Hancock REW, Bellido F. Antibacterial in vitro activity of fourth generation cephalosporins. J Chemother 1995; 7(Suppl. 5):29–34.
34. Fung-Tomc JC, Dougherty YJ, deOrio FJ, et al. Activity of cefepime against ceftazidime-resistant Gram-negative bacteria. Antimicrob Agents Chemother 1989; 33:498–502.
35. Flamm RK, Weaver MK, Thornsberry C, et al. Factors associated with relative rates of antibiotic resistance in *Pseudomonas aeruginosa* isolates tested in clinical laboratories in the United States from 1999 to 2002. Antimicrob Agents Chemother 2004; 48:2431–36.
36. Karlowsky JA, Jones ME, Thornsberry C, et al. Stable antimicrobial susceptibility rates for clinical isolates of *Pseudomonas aeruginosa* from the 2001–2003 tracking resistance in the United States today surveillance studies. Clin Infect Dis 2005; 40 (Suppl. 2):S89–98.

37. Sader HS, Fritsche TR, Jones RN. Accuracy of three automated systems (MicroScan WalkAway, VITEK, and VITEK 2) for susceptibility testing of *Pseudomonas aeruginosa* against five broad-spectrum beta-lactam agents. J Clin Microbial 2006; 44:1101–4.

38. Hocquet D, Nordmann P, El Garch F, et al. Involvement of the MexXY-OporM efflux system in emergence of cefepime resistance in clinical strains of *Pseudomonas aeruginosa*. Antimicrob Agents Chemother 2006; 50:1347–51.

39. Chen HY, Livermore DM. In-vitro activity of biapenem, compared with imipenem and meropenem, against *Pseudomonas aeruginosa* strains and mutants with known resistance mechanisms. J Antimicrob Chemother 1994; 33:949–58.

40. Quinn JP, Studemeister AE, DiVencenzo CA, et al. Resistance to imipenem in *Pseudomonas aeruginosa*: Clinical experience and biochemical mechanisms. Rev Infect Dis 1988; 10:892–8.

41. Huang H, Hancock RE. Genetic definition of the substrate selectivity of outer membrane porin protein OprD of *Pseudomonas aeruginosa*. J Bacteriol 1993; 175: 7793–800.

42. Masuda N, Sakagawa E, Ohya S, et al. Substrate specificities of MexAB-OprM, MexCD-OprJ, and MexXY-oprM efflux pumps in *Pseudomonas aeruginosa*. Antimicrob Agents Chemother 2000; 44:3322–7.

43. Kohler T, Michea-Hamzehpour M, Epp SF, et al. Carbapenem activities against *Pseudomonas aeruginosa*: Respective contributions of OprD and efflux systems. Antimicrob Agents Chemother 1999; 43:524–7.

44. Yoshida H, Nakamura M, Bogaki M, et al. Proportion of DNA gyrase mutants among quinolone-resistant strains of *Pseudomonas aeruginosa*. Antimicrob Agents Chemother 1990; 34:1273–5.

45. Poole K, Krebes K, McNally C, et al. Multiple antibiotic resistance in *Pseudomonas aeruginosa*: evidence for involvement of an efflux operon. J Bacteriol 1993; 175:7363–72.

46. Le Thomas I, Couetdic G, Clermont O, et al. In vivo selection of a target/efflux double mutant of *Pseudomonas aeruginosa* by ciprofloxacin therapy. J Antimicrob Chemother 2001; 48:553–5.

47. Nakajima A, Sugimoto Y, Yoneyama H, et al. High-level fluoroquinolone resistance in *Pseudomonas aeruginosa* due to interplay of the MexAB-OprM efflux pump and the DNA gyrase mutation. Microbiol Immunol 2002; 46:391–5.

48. Cho, D., D. Lofland, J. Blais, K. et al. Prevalence of efflux pumps among clinical isolates of fluoroquinolone-resistant *Pseudomonas aeruginosa* (abstract F-1267). In: Program and abstracts of the 39th Interscience Conference on. Antimicrobial Agents and Chemotherapy (San Francisco). Washington DC: American Society for Microbiology, 1999.

49. Ma D, Cook DN, Herast JE, et al. Efflux pumps and drug resistance in Gram-negative bacteria. Trends Microbiol 1994; 2:489–93.

50. Kohler T, Epp SF, Curty LK, et al. Characterization of MexT, the regulator of the MexE-MexF-OprN multidrug efflux system of *Pseudomonas aeruginosa*. J Bacteriol 1999; 181:6300–5.

51. Robicsek A, Jacoby GA, Hooper DC. The worldwide emergence of plasmid-mediated quinolone resistance. Lancet Infect Dis 2006; 6:629–40.

52. Bryan LE, O'Hara K, Wong S. Lipopolysaccharide changes in impermeability-type aminoglycoside resistance in *Pseudomonas aeruginosa*. Antimicrob Agents Chemother 1984; 26:250–5.

53. Poole K. Aminoglycoside resistance in *Pseudomonas aeruginosa*. Antimicrob Agents Chemother. 2005; 49:479–87.

54. Lee A, Mao W, Warren MS, et al. Interplay between efflux pumps may provide either additive or multiplicative effects on drug resistance. J Bacteriol 2000; 182:3142–50.

55. Macia MD, Blanquer D, Togores B, et al. Hypermutation is a key factor in development of multiple-antimicrobial resistance in Pseudomonas aeruginosa strains causing chronic lung infections. Antimicrob Agents Chemother 2005; 49:3382–6.

56. Chopra I,.O'Neill AJ, Miller K. The role of mutators in the emergence of antibiotic-resistant bacteria. Drug Resist Updat 2003; 6:137–45.

57. Oliver A, Canton R, Campo P, et al. High frequency of hypermutable *Pseudomonas aeruginosa* in cystic fibrosis lung infection. Science 2000; 288:1251–4.
58. Oliver A, Levin BR, Juan C, et al. Hypermutation and the preexistence of antibiotic-resistant *Pseudomonas aeruginosa* mutants: implications for susceptibility testing and treatment of chronic infections. Antimicrob Agents Chemother 2004; 48:4226–33.
59. Blazquez J. Hypermutation as a factor contributing to the acquisition of antimicrobial resistance. Clin Infect Dis 2003; 37:1201–9.
60. Livermore DM. beta-Lactamases in laboratory and clinical resistance. Clin Microb Rev 1995; 8:557–84.
61. Nordmann P, Ronco E, Naas T, et al. Characterization of a novel beta-lactamase from *Pseudomonas aeruginosa*. Antimicrob Agents Chemother. 1993; 37:962–9.
62. Vahaboglu H, Ozturk R, Aygun G, et al. Widespread detection of PER-1-type extended-spectrum beta-lactamases among nosocomial *Acinetobacter* and *Pseudomonas aeruginosa* isolates in Turkey: a nationwide multicenter study. Antimicrob Agents Chemother 1997; 41:2265–9.
63. Kolayli F, Gacar G, Karadenizli A, et al. PER-1 is still widespread in Turkish hospitals among *Pseudomonas aeruginosa* and *Acinetobacter* spp. FEMS Microbiol Lett 2005; 249:241–5.
64. De Champs C, Chanal C, Sirot D, et al. Frequency and diversity of Class A extended-spectrum beta-lactamases in hospitals of the Auvergne, France: a 2 year prospective study. J Antimicrob Chemother 2004; 54:634–9.
65. Pagani L, Mantengoli E, Migliavacca R, et al. Multifocal detection of multidrug-resistant *Pseudomonas aeruginosa* producing the PER-1 extended-spectrum beta-lactamase in Northern Italy. J Clin Microbiol 2004; 42:2523–9.
66. Bauernfeind A, Stemplinger I, Jungwirth R, et al. Characterization of beta-lactamase gene blaPER-2, which encodes an extended-spectrum class A beta-lactamase. Antimicrob Agents Chemother 1996; 40:616–20.
67. Celenza G, Pellegrini C, Caccamo M, et al. Spread of bla(CTX-M-type) and bla(PER-2) beta-lactamase genes in clinical isolates from Bolivian hospitals. J Antimicrob Chemother 2006; 57:975–8.
68. Bradford PA. Extended-spectrum beta-lactamases in the 21st century: characterization, epidemiology, and detection of this important resistance threat. Clin Microbiol Rev 2001; 14:933–51.
69. Naas T, Nordmann P. OXA-type beta-lactamases. Curr Pharm Des 1999; 5:865–79.
70. Danel F, Hall LM, Duke B, et al. OXA-17, a further extended spectrum variant of OXA-10 beta-lactamase, isolated from *Pseudomonas aeruginosa*. Antimicrob Agents Chemother 1999; 43:1362–6.
71. Livermore DM, Woodford N. Carbapenemases: a problem in waiting? Curr Opin Microbiol 2000; 3:489–95.
72. Senda K, Arakawa Y, Nakashima K, et al. Multifocal outbreaks of metallo-beta-lactamase-producing *Pseudomonas aeruginosa* resistant to broad-spectrum beta-lactams, including carbapenems. Antimicrob Agents Chemother 1996; 40:349–53.
73. Walsh TR, Toleman MA, Poirel L, et al. Metallo-beta-lactamases: the quiet before the storm? Clin Microbiol Rev 2005; 18:306–25.
74. Jones RN, Biedenbach DJ, Sader HS, et al. Emerging epidemic of metallo-beta-lactamase-mediated resistances. Diagn Microbiol Infect Dis 2005; 51:77–84.
75. Fritsche TR, Sader HS, Toleman MA, et al. Emerging metallo-beta-lactamase-mediated resistances: a summary report from the worldwide SENTRY antimicrobial surveillance program. Clin Infect Dis 2005; (Suppl. 4) 41:S276–8.
76. Gibb AP, Tribuddharat C, Moore RC, et al. Nosocomial outbreak of carbapenem-resistant *Pseudomonas aeruginosa* with a new bla$_{IMP}$ allele, bla$_{IMP-7}$. Antimicrob Agents Chemother 2002; 46:255–8.
77. Pitout JD, Gregson DB, Poirel L, et al. Detection of *Pseudomonas aeruginosa* producing metallo-beta-lactamases in a large centralized laboratory. J Clin Microbiol 2005; 43:3129–35.

78. Toleman HA, Rolston K, Jones RN, et al. blaVIM-7, an evolutionarily distinct metallo-beta-lactamase in a *P. aeruginosa* isolate from the United States. Antimicrob Agents Chemother 2004; 48:329–32.

79. Hanson ND, Hossain A, Buck L, et al. First occurrence of a *Pseudomonas aeruginosa* isolate in the United States producing an IMP metallo-beta-lactamase, IMP-18. Antimicrob Agents Chemother 2006; 50:2272–3.

80. Lolans K, Queenan AM, Bush K, et al. First nosocomial outbreak of *Pseudomonas aeruginosa* producing an integron-borne metallo-beta-lactamase (VIM-2) in the United States. Antimicrob Agents Chemother 2005; 49:3538–40.

81. Lauretti L, Riccio MI, Mazzariol A, et al. Cloning and characterization of bla$_{VIM}$, a new integron-borne metallo-beta-lactamase gene from a *Pseudomonas aeruginosa* clinical isolate. Antimicrob Agents Chemother 1999; 43:1584–90.

82. Arakawa Y, Murakami M, Suzuki K, et al. A novel integron-like element carrying the metallo–beta-lactamase gene bla$_{IMP}$. Antimicrob Agents Chemother 1995; 39:1612–15.

83. Zavascki AP, Gaspareto PB, Martins AF, et al. Outbreak of carbapenem-resistant *Pseudomonas aeruginosa* producing SPM-1 metallo-{beta}-lactamase in a teaching hospital in southern Brazil. J Antimicrob Chemother 2005; 56:1148–51.

84. Deplano A, Denis O, Poirel L, et al. Molecular characterization of an epidemic clone of panantibiotic-resistant *Pseudomonas aeruginosa*. J Clin Microbiol 2005; 43:1198–204.

85. Hilf M, Yu VL, Sharp J, et al. Antibiotic therapy for *Pseudomonas aeruginosa* bacteremia: outcome correlations in a prospective study of 200 patients. Am J Med 1989; 87:540–6.

86. Leibovii L. Paul M. Poznanski O, et al. Monotherapy versus beta-lactam-aminoglycoside combination treatment for Gram-negative bacteremia: a prospective, observational study. Antimicrob Agents Chemother 1997; 41:1127–33.

87. Johnson DE, Thompson B. Efficacy of single–agent therapy with azlocillin, ticarcillin, and amikacin and beta-lactam/amikacin combinations for treatment of *Pseudomonas aeruginosa* bacteremia in granulocytopenic rats. Am J Med 1986; 80:53–8.

88. Winston DJ, Barnes RC, Ho WG, et al. Moxalactam plus piperacillin versus moxalactam plus amikacin in febrile granulocytopenic patients. Am J Med 1984; 77:442–50.

89. Echols RM. The selection of appropriate dosages for intravenous ciprofloxacin. J Antimicrob Chemother 1993; 31:783–7.

90. Kahn JB. Latest industry information on the safety profile of levofloxacin in the US. Chemotherapy. 2001; 47(Suppl. 3):32–7.

91. Craig WA, Ebert SC. Antimicrobial therapy in *Pseudomonas aeruginosa* infection. In: Baltch AL, Smith RP, eds. *Pseudomonas aeruginosa* Infections and Treatment. New York: Marcel Dekker, 1994:441–518.

92. Craig WA, Ebert SC. Killing and regrowth of bacteria in vitro: a review. Scand J Infect Dis 1990; 74(Suppl.):63–70.

93. DeRyke CA, Lee SY, Kuti JL, et al. Optimising dosing strategies of antibacterials utilising pharmacodynamic principles: impact on the development of resistance. Drugs 2006; 66:1–14.

94. Deamer RL, Dial LK. The evolution of aminoglycoside therapy: a single daily dose. Am Fam Physician 1996; 53:1782–6.

95. Cooperstock MS. Inactivation of endotoxin by polymyxin B. Antimicrob Agents Chemother 1974; 6:422–5.

96. Morrison DC, Jacobs DM. Inhibition of lipopolysaccharide-initiated activation of serum complement by polymyxin B. Infect Immun 1976; 13:298–301.

97. Evans ME, Feola DJ, Rapp RP. Polymyxin B sulfate and colistin: old antibiotics for emerging multiresistant Gram-negative bacteria. Ann Pharmacother 1999; 33:960–7.

98. Falagas ME, Kasiakou SK. Colistin: the revival of polymyxins for the management of multidrug-resistant gram-negative bacterial infections. Clin Infect Dis 2005; 40:1333–41.

99. Gales AC, Reis AO, Jones RN. Contemporary assessment of antimicrobial susceptibility testing methods for polymyxin B and colistin: review of available interpretative criteria and quality control guidelines. J Clin Microbiols 2001; 39:183–90.

100. Tascini C, Ferranti S, Messina F, et al. In vitro and in vivo synergistic activity of colistin, rifampin and amikacin against a multiresistant *Pseudomonas aeruginosa* isolate. Clin Microbiol Infect 2000; 6:690–1.
101. Rynn C, Wootton M, Bowker KE, et al. In vitro assessment of colistin's antipseudomonal antimicrobial interactions with other antibiotics. Clin Microbiol Infect 1999; 5:32–6.
102. Landman D, Bratu S, Alam M, et al. Citywide emergence of *Pseudomonas aeruginosa* strains with reduced susceptibility to polymyxin B. J Antimicrob Chemother 2005; 55:954–7.
103. Levin AS, Barone AA, Penco J, et al. Intravenous colistin as therapy for nosocomial infections caused by multidrug-resistant *Pseudomonas aeruginosa* and *Acinetobacter baumannii*. Clin Infect Dis 1999; 28:1008–11.
104. Conway SP, Pond MN, Watson A, et al. Intravenous colistin sulphomethate in acute respiratory exacerbations in adult patients with cystic fibrosis. Thorax 1997; 52:987–93
105. Li J, Turnidge J, Milne R, et al. In vitro Pharmacodynamic properties of colistin and colistin methanesulfatone against *Pseudomonas aeruginosa*. Antimicrob Agent Chemother 2001; 45:781–5.
106. Conway SP, Etherrington C, Munday J, et al. Safety and tolerability of bolus intravenous colistin in acute respiratory exacerbations in adults with cystic fibrosis. Ann Pharmacother 2000; 34:1238–42.

10 Problematic Beta-Lactamases: An Update

Marion S. Helfand
Infectious Diseases Section and Research Division, Louis Stokes Cleveland Department of Veterans Affairs Medical Center and the Case Western Reserve School of Medicine, Cleveland, Ohio, U.S.A.

Louis B. Rice
Louis Stokes Cleveland Department of Veterans Affairs Medical Center and the Case Western Reserve School of Medicine, Cleveland, Ohio, U.S.A.

INTRODUCTION

Long before beta-lactams were used in clinical practice, bacteria have exhibited resistance to these antibiotics. Especially in the Gram-negative bacteria, the production of beta-lactam hydrolyzing enzymes called beta-lactamases is an important cause of such resistance. In this chapter, we discuss general concepts about these resistance enzymes that have allowed them to propagate and evolve into formidable beta-lactam destroying adversaries, and suggest current treatment options.

WHAT IS A BETA-LACTAMASE?

Beta-lactamases are enzymes produced by the great majority of clinically important bacteria. In addition to their relatively well-known job of destroying antibiotics like penicillins, cephalosporins, and carbapenems, they probably also serve other cellular maintenance roles involving the bacterial cell wall. It is hypothesized that beta-lactamases are distant relatives of bacterial cell wall synthesis and cross-linking enzymes called penicillin-binding proteins, which are the actual targets of beta-lactam antibiotics that we use commonly in the clinical setting (1). In terms of antibiotic resistance, the production of beta-lactamases is most important in Gram-negative bacteria like *Escherichia coli*, *Klebsiella pneumoniae*, and *Pseudomonas aeruginosa*. However, some Gram-positive bacteria also produce beta-lactamases; e.g., penicillin resistance in *Staphylococcus aureus* is partly mediated by an enzyme called PC1, which the bacterium secretes into the surrounding environment.

Beta-lactamases come in two major types: serine and metallo-beta-lactamases. The serine beta-lactamases are further divided into groups according to how alike the proteins are via amino acid sequence identity [Ambler classification (2)] or according to a functional classification scheme by the type of beta-lactam they preferentially hydrolyze (oxacillin, other penicillins, advanced generation cephalosporins). The latter is known as the Bush-Jacoby-Medeiros classification (3). A comparison of the two classification systems is shown in Table 1.

The metallo beta-lactamases are also further subclassified according to key active site amino acids and whether the active site contains one or two Zn^{2+} ions. For the purposes of this chapter, we use the more streamlined Ambler classification scheme to discuss clinically important beta-lactamases.

TABLE 1 Comparison of Beta-Lactamase Classification Systems

Bush-Jacoby-Medeiros system	Major subgroups	Ambler system	Main attributes
Group 1 cephalosporinases	—	C (cephalosporinases)	Usually chromosomal; resistance to all beta-lactams except carbapenems; not inhibited by clavulanate, e.g., CMY-2
Group 2 penicillinases	2a	A (penicillinases)	Staphylococcal penicillinases, e.g., PC1
(clavulanic acid susceptible)	2b	A	Broad-spectrum – TEM-1, TEM-2, SHV-1
	2be	A	Extended-spectrum – TEM-3– ??, SHV-2
	2br	A	Inhibitor resistant TEM
	2c	A	Carbenicillin-hydrolyzing
	2e	A	Cephalosporinases inhibited by clavulanate, e.g., CTX-Ms
	2f	A	Carbapenemases inhibited by clavulanate, e.g., KPC-1,-2,-3.
	2d	D (oxacillin-hydrolyzing)	Cloxacillin-hydrolyzing (OXA)
Group 3 metallo- beta–lactamase	3a	B (metalloenzymes)	Zinc-dependent carbapenemases, e.g., IMPs and VIMs
	3b	B	
	3c	B	
Group 4		Not classified	Miscellaneous enzymes, most not yet sequenced

Abbreviations: CMY, active on cephamycins; CTX-M, active on cefotaxime, first isolated at Munich; IMP, active on imipenem; KPC, *Klebsiella pneumoniae* carbapenemase; OXA, active on oxacillin; PC1, from *Staphylococcus aureus* strain PC1; SHV, sulfhydryl reagent variable; VIM, Verona integron-encoded metallo-beta-lactamase.

Class A Beta-Lactamases

In the Ambler classification, the serine enzymes are subdivided into Classes A, C, and D. Clinically, the Class A enzymes were the first described. The first Class A beta-lactamase from a Gram-negative bacterium was the TEM beta-lactamase of *E. coli*, named for the patient from which it was isolated (4,5). Another well-known Class A beta-lactamase is the "sulfhydryl variant (of TEM)" SHV, which is found in *K. pneumoniae* (5,6). The Class A enzymes TEM and SHV can be found in the chromosomal DNA of their host bacteria, or on mobile genetic elements called plasmids, which bacteria can share freely with one another. This enhances the spread of resistance among different types of bacteria in both the hospital and general environment. The original or "wild type" TEM and SHV enzymes were highly suited to hydrolyzing penicillins, with active sites that accommodated the penicillins like a hand in a glove. In contrast to the penicillins, highly active third-generation cephalosporins possessed bulky side chains that precluded entry into the TEM active site. The widespread use of these "extended-spectrum" cephalosporins in the 1980s was associated with the appearance of the so-called "extended-spectrum beta-lactamases" (ESBLs) (7–10). Through DNA base pair mutations leading to replacement of highly critical active site amino acids in the resulting beta-lactamase proteins, TEM and SHV were turned into ESBLs, enzymes now highly effective at hydrolyzing bulky third generation cephalosporins, especially ceftazidime. The most common mutation leading to the ESBL-type of enzyme is a serine to glycine substitution at position 238 (11).

Figure 1 shows how the ESBL mutations open the active site, leading to greater rates of cephalosporin hydrolysis, causing antibiotic resistance. An interesting property, or phenotype, of these ESBLs was noted: despite their ability to hydrolyze our most potent antibiotics of the time, they were inhibited even more effectively than their progenitors by drugs like clavulanic acid and tazobactam. These inhibitor drugs had been developed specifically to target the wild-type TEM and SHV Class A type enzymes, and were designed to be given together with extended spectrum penicillins like amoxicillin, ampicillin, and piperacillin. This inhibitor-sensitive phenotype is being used in the clinical microbiology laboratory to detect ESBL production in *Enterobacteraciae* [reviewed in (12)].

More recently, newer class A beta-lactamases that preferentially hydrolyze cefotaxime, now designated CTX-Ms (for cefotaximases), are being found in *K. pneumoniae*, *E. coli*, typhoidal and nontyphoidal *Salmonella*, *Shigella*, *Citrobacter freundii*, *Enterobacter* spp., and *Serratia marcescens* (13–15). The first variant of these enzymes, appropriately named FEC-1, was isolated from the feces of a dog used in beta-lactam pharmaceutical studies in Japan in 1986 (16). CTX-M enzymes have been termed "born ESBLs" (attributed to Gabriel Gutkind) because no wild-type progenitor enzyme has been identified for the CTX-M family. They appear to be

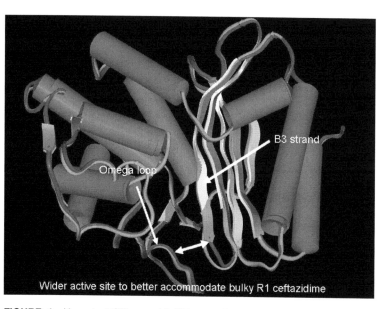

FIGURE 1 How do ESBLs work? This superimposed rendering of SHV-1 beta-lactamase of *Klebsiella pneumoniae* (*white loops*) and the common ESBL enzyme SHV-2 (*dark loops*), with a glycine → serine change at position 238 (*right tip of double arrow*), demonstrates the 2 Å widening of the active site due to movement of the B3 strand. This allows accommodation of the bulky R1 sidechains of third-generation cephalosporins like ceftazidime. The cylindrical structures represent alpha helices, the flat ribbon structures represent beta pleated sheets, and the remaining loops represent randomly coiled segments of the beta-lactamase proteins. *Abbreviations*: ESBL, extended-spectrum beta-lactamase; SHV, sulfhydryl reagent variable.

related to chromosomal beta-lactamases native to *Kluverya* spp. [reviewed in (17)]. In addition to their predilection for cefotaxime and ceftriaxone over ceftazidime, most of these enzymes also appear to favor tazobactam as an inhibitor over clavulanic acid.

Despite their activity against cephalosporins and penicillins, TEM and SHV ESBLs and CTX-M enzymes have not conferred resistance to carbapenems (ertapenem, imipenem, and meropenem). The carbapenems' "immunity" to ESBLs has been associated with clinical success, resulting in widespread concurrence that carbapenems represent optimal therapy for infections caused by ESBL-producing organisms. Unfortunately, *Klebsiella* strains are now being reported that produce a Class A enzyme, *Klebsiella pneumoniae* carbapenemase, or KPC [reviewed in (18)]. Several U.S. hospitals have reported intensive care unit outbreaks with multi-drug-resistant *Klebsiella* spp. Extremely high rates of mortality have been attributed to failures of carbapenems that were administered empirically for patients with sepsis syndromes. These *Klebsiella* strains were found to produce KPC. These strains were also resistant to beta-lactam–beta-lactamase inhibitor combinations like piperacillin-tazobactam, presumably due to concomitant loss of outer membrane proteins (OMPs) that prevented drug entry into the bacteria. To date three different KPC enzymes (KPC-1,-2,-3) have been described, some of which are encoded on plasmids. Perhaps due to plasmid transfer, KPC has already found its way into other clinically important bacteria like *Enterobacter* spp., *Citrobacter freundii*, *Salmonella enteriditis*, *E. coli*, and *K. oxytoca*. The emergence of these enzymes has been termed a "global sentinel event" [(19) and references therein].

Class C Beta-Lactamases

Class C beta-lactamases remain an important source of antimicrobial resistance in specific pathogens like *C. freundii*, *E. aerogenes* and *E. cloacae*, *Morganella morganii*, *Pseudomonas aeruginosa* (PSDA), and *Serratia marcescens*. In addition, plasmid-mediated AmpC enzymes have found their way into organisms such as *Klebsiella* spp., *E. coli*, and *Salmonella* spp., and may be mistakenly identified as ESBLs (20). Class C beta-lactamases are cephalosporinases by nature, due to their naturally larger active site that can more easily accommodate the bulky R1 sidechains of third-generation cephalosporins. The Class A beta-lactamase inhibitors, clavulanic acid, tazobactam, and sulbactam, are not clinically effective against the bacteria that produce Class C beta-lactamases. In general, beta-lactams such as carbapenems, monobactams such as aztreonam, and the advanced generation cephalosporin, cefepime, can be used to treat patients with Class C producers. Sometimes, bacteria will restrict entry of antibiotics through the loss of OMPs; coupled with Class C beta-lactamase production, this can lead to carbapenem and cefepime resistance.

The amount of beta-lactamase produced by a bacterium can influence the MIC and hence resistance or susceptibility to antibiotic reported by the clinical microbiology laboratory. This "expression effect" is especially important in the case of the Class C beta-lactamases. While nearly all bacteria produce Class C beta-lactamases, most are only produced at low levels. In *Citrobacter, Enterobacter, Pseudomonas*, and *Serratia*, however, Class C beta-lactamase production is regulated by a complex feedback mechanism that depends on the intracellular concentrations of small, cell-wall–derived peptides (21). During periods when bacteria are exposed to antibiotics, cell wall fragments accumulate and act to alter the conformation of a "repressor" molecule, called AmpR from the regulatory region in front of the gene that encodes the beta-lactamase. Complexing with specific cell wall breakdown products (N-acetyl-muramyl-tripeptide) changes AmpR from a repressor to an activator of AmpC expression. Thus there is increased expression or "induction" of resistance as the beta-lactamase gene is "de-repressed." Certain kinds of antibiotics are especially potent at causing this induction. They include: cefoxitin, imipenem, clavulanic acid, and ciprofloxacin. Resistance to beta-lactam antibiotics can thus develop while the patient is being treated with what was initially appropriate therapy. In a small fraction of the bacterial population, a cytosolic amidase enzyme, AmpD, responsible for recycling the cell wall peptides, may also be absent or function poorly due to mutations. Under persistent selective pressure, such strains may emerge as the predominant population, yielding high-level constitutive cephalosporin resistance. In clinical studies, treatment of *Enterobacter* infections with third generations cephalosporins has led to the emergence of constitutive resistance in a significant number of cases (22).

Class D Beta-Lactamases

The last group of serine beta-lactamases to consider are the Class D or oxacilli-nase (OXA) enzymes. These are found most commonly in *Pseudomonas* and *Acinetobacter* spp. Some examples have been found in which the active site has been chemically modified by the addition of bicarbonate to the ϵ-NH$_2$ group of a lysine side chain (so-called "carbamoylation"). Otherwise, these enzymes function similarly to the Class A and C enzymes. They are further grouped according to their function or the type of beta-lactam they hydrolyze most efficiently. For example, some of the OXA enzymes are best at hydrolyzing cephalosporins (OXA-11, OXA-14 to OXA-20); others preferentially hydrolyze carbapenems (OXA-23 to OXA-26, OXA-40, OXA-50, OXA-58, OXA-64 to OXA-66, OXA-68 to OXA-71). There are no simple point mutations that result in an expanded spectrum (ESBL) type like in the Class A enzymes. The number and hence clinical significance of these enzymes is growing, especially as their host bacteria, *P. aeruginosa* and *Acinetobacter baumanni,* become increasingly prevalent nosoco-mial pathogens.

Class B Beta-Lactamases

Metallo beta-lactamases (Class B Ambler designation) are typically identified in *Pseudomonas* and *Acinetobacter* isolates. They have become widely disseminated in Asia, South America, southern Europe, and parts of Canada, but remain rare in the United States with the exception of sporadic case reports. These beta-lacta-mases confer resistance to most beta-lactams including carbapenems. A minority are active against aztreonam, and they cannot be inhibited by our current clinical inhibitors. New methods to detect and report metallo-beta-lactamases are being developed and employed in the clinical microbiology laboratory. Class B enzymes are inhibited under conditions where their metal ions have been removed, e.g., by addition of a metal chelator like ethylene diamine tetraacetate or EDTA. Because the Class B enzymes are an unusual cause of beta-lactam resistance in U.S. hospitals, they are not discussed further in this chapter. The interested reader is referred to an excellent review by Walsh et al. (23).

HOW DO THEY WORK?

Bacterial beta-lactamases are enzymes. By definition, an enzyme is a protein that catalyzes a particular biochemical reaction. To catalyze a reaction, the enzyme has to act in a way to lower the amount of energy required to break and make chemical bonds in the small molecules on which it acts. In the case of the beta-lactamases, the enzyme orients the beta-lactam antibiotic in a precise manner in its active site to facilitate the breaking of the C–N bond in the four-membered beta-lactam ring. The enzyme relieves some of the strain in the beta-lactam ring during the bond breaking, thereby lowering the amount of energy required to break the C–N bond (about 290 kJ/mole). In this process, the beta-lactam molecule, with the lactam ring opened, becomes attached to a serine in the active site of the serine beta-lactamases in a process called acylation, or makes a transient complex with a Zn^{2+} ion in the case of the Class B metallo-beta-lactamases. The other aspect of catalysis is that the catalyst is not consumed or changed in the process of catalysis; thus the beta-lactamase must have a means of regenerating itself following the acylation step. Again, critically positioned amino acid side-chains, of which glutamate 166 is the most well known and important in the Class A enzymes, are present to facilitate the water-mediated hydrolysis of the acyl-enzyme complex, thereby freeing the enzyme to hydrolyze the next beta-lactam molecule. It should be noted that some beta-lactamases, like TEM and SHV of the Class A variety, can hydrolyze or "turn over" beta-lactams like ampicillin at the rate of 1000 to 2000 molecules per second, literally at a rate in which the overall turnover is simply limited by how rapidly new beta-lactam molecules can diffuse into the active site. Even ESBL beta-lactamases with modest turnover rates (1–2 molecules/sec) can confer resistance to third-generation cephalosporins (MICS ≥ 8 mcg/mL). When combined with reduced quantities of outer membrane channels in many Gram-negative bacteria, these ESBLs can lead to very high-level resistance, with the beta-lactamase enzyme akin to a sharpshooter, waiting patiently for the next unwitting beta-lactam to enter the periplasmic space.

HOW DO BETA-LACTAMASES CHANGE TO CONFER RESISTANCE?

Even single amino acid changes in a beta-lactamase can lead to clinically significant levels of beta-lactam resistance in many nosocomial pathogens. In fact, certain amino acid alterations are statistically more likely than others. Table 2 illustrates some examples of single base pair changes resulting in codon changes.

The expression of "foreign" proteins is also a consideration in resistance. For example, if a bacterium obtains a new beta-lactamase via plasmid exchange from another species of bacterium, the newly acquired DNA may contain codons that

TABLE 2 Single Base Pair Changes that Result in Amino Acid Changes in Beta-Lactamases

Beta-lactamase example	Amino acid	Changes to	Possible codon changes
SHV-2 (ESBL) or TEM-19	Glycine 238	Serine 238	GGT→AGT or GGC→AGC
TEM-3 (ESBL) (also has the G238S change)	Glutamate 104	Lysine 104	GAA→AAA or GAG→AAG
TEM-12 (ESBL)	Arginine 164	Serine 164	CGT→AGT or CGC→AGC
TEM-32 (inhibitor resistant, also has M182T change)	Methionine 69	Isoleucine 69	ATG→ATT, ATC or ATA

Abbreviations: ESBL, extended spectrum beta-lactamase; SHV, sulfhydryl reagent variable.

are not commonly used by the new host bacterium. Thus, the new host may not have sufficient amounts of specific tRNAs to fully incorporate certain amino acids into the new beta-lactamase. Codon changes within a bacterium may also result in lower levels of expression of the beta-lactamase protein. Once a new amino acid is introduced into the protein, the net effect may be to enhance or expand the enzyme's known activity, cause no change, or lead to instability or inactivity of the enzyme. Certain amino acid substitutions may produce different enzymatic phenotypes [such as the ESBL or the inhibitor resistant (IRT) beta-lactamase phenotypes] that contribute to clinical resistance. Some amino acid substitutions are accompanied by additional compensatory mutations, like the M182T mutation in TEM ESBLs and IRT enzymes, that serve to stabilize the protein structure, presumably against degradation by bacterial proteases. Table 2 shows the common amino acid substitutions that are associated with important resistance phenotypes. In general, for the ESBL cephalosporinases the amino acid substitutions at 104, 164, 179, 237, and 238 serve to increase the size of the active site cavity, thereby allowing better accommodation of the bulky cephalosporin R1 side chains (Fig. 1). One way this occurs is by outward movement of a part of the protein called the b3 strand. The b3 strand is a segment of the protein that folds in a characteristic way called "beta-pleating." This segment runs along one side of the enzyme active site; it contains a residue at position 237 whose backbone amide NH group forms an attractive electron-poor "hole" that serves to dock and stretch the C=O bond of the beta-lactam molecule, prior to C–N bond breaking. The active site can also be enlarged when mutations involve the Ω loop of the protein (amino acid regions 160–179, so named because of its resemblance to the Greek letter Ω). The Ω loop is an unstructured segment that contains the critical glutamate residue that is required for deacylation (regeneration) of the Class A beta-lactamases.

The Class C enzymes already have a larger active site, and thus are well prepared to hydrolyze the bulky third-generation cephalosporins. As such, they do not develop ESBL mutations to make them even better cephalosporinases. The GC1 enzyme of *Enterobacter cloacae* is one exception, in which the insertion of a tripeptide repeat in the Ω loop of the enzyme (A211-V212-R213) has led to increased activity against oxyimino cephalosporins (24).

The structural changes resulting in inhibitor resistance in Class A beta-lactamases are somewhat more subtle. In general, a major effect of mutations at positions 69, 130, 244, 275, and 276 is to decrease affinity of the enzyme for the inhibitor. Thus it requires more inhibitor to "knock out" the beta-lactamase. Mutations at these positions seem to lead to subtle and concerted changes in the position of other critical active site groups including the catalytic serine 70. Much research is still being devoted to understanding the structural basis of this resistance (25–29).

Carbapenem resistance remains a rare phenotype in Class A enzyme-producing bacteria. It has been noted that a single mutation at position 170 in the GES-1 beta-lactamase results in a carbapenemase phenotype (30) as well as cephamycin and inhibitor resistance. With KPC Class A carbapenemases, amino acids responsible for carbapenem resistance are still being determined. Compared to the classical TEM and SHV type beta-lactamases, the KPC enzymes have several amino acid substitutions, with a few in critical functional locations such as a proline at the 104 position (instead of the usual aspartate or glutamate). Instead of a disulfide bridge between amino acids 77 and 123, KPC has a disulfide bridge between the 69 and

237 positions. The 170 position is an asparagine in KPC, SHV, and TEM. KPC-1, KPC-2, and KPC-3 differ from one another by single amino acid changes. KPC-3 is the most broad spectrum and most catalytically efficient of the three enzymes and contains the mutations S174G, as in KPC-2, and an additional mutation, H272Y (19). It is speculated that the H272Y mutation influences an important interaction between R209 in the enzyme and the COO-group of the substrate (31). Structural studies are underway to determine which of these changes lead to the carbapenemase activity of this Class A beta-lactamase. In the CTX-M type cefotaximases, a glycine at position 240 and a proline at position 167 seem to be important in conferring substrate specificity towards cefotaxime and ceftriaxone, over ceftazidime (17). Again it is noted that these residues are part of the active site beta-sheet and Ω loop structures so critical in determining the size and shape of the active site.

HOW DO THEY SPREAD? GENETIC CONSIDERATIONS

Beta-lactamases are encoded by genes, and so the genetic structure of the regions surrounding the beta-lactamase genes is of considerable interest. Information about the genetic environment can give clues to the likely mobility of the gene, the extent to which it may be expressed, and to its origins and evolution. Unfortunately, the terminology surrounding genetic structures in bacteria is often arcane and difficult for the non-expert to follow. It is therefore worthwhile to start with a few definitions. A bacterial gene is a sequence of nucleotides that includes a promoter region (to get the RNA polymerase started), a ribosome-binding site (to get the tRNA started on protein synthesis), an open reading frame encoding a series of amino acids that make up the eventual protein, and a stop codon to tell the tRNA-ribosome complex to disassociate, completing the process of protein synthesis. A gene cassette is generally a ribosome binding site, open reading frame, and stop codon associated with a specific sequence that allows the gene to be incorporated into the integron by the integron's integrase. An integron is a "sink" for collecting stray gene cassettes. It contains a place for the cassette to enter and an integrase to facilitate entry. It also contains a promoter to facilitate transcription of the integrated gene cassettes. Since more than one gene cassette can be incorporated into an integron, expression of genes that are further from the promoter is less than those closer (it is never good to be last in line). By themselves, integrons are generally not mobile, but they may be incorporated into transposons or plasmids. Transposons are segments of DNA that contain genes that facilitate mobility of the segment between different replicons in the cell. They may be integrated into plasmids or into the chromosome. Plasmids are closed, circular, supercoiled segments of DNA that replicate independently of the chromosome. They may be transferable to other bacteria, and may integrate into the chromosome and use their transfer functions to facilitate chromosomal gene transfer.

Beta-lactamase-mediated resistance is often transferable between cells because the genes are encoded on transferable plasmids (32,33). These plasmids may encode many resistance phenotypes, and even several beta-lactamases. Confusion often arises about whether the beta-lactamase genes are encoded in integrons, or transposons, or plasmids, etc. In fact, it is pointless to make these distinctions, since in many cases all such statements will be true. It is perhaps best to think of this group of elements like a Russian doll (Fig. 2), in which progressively smaller dolls are placed inside larger versions. Any of the individual dolls may be missing, but usually several of the dolls are present. The end result is a

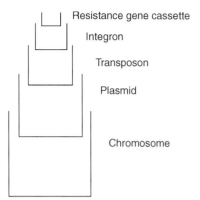

Resistance gene cassette

Integron

Transposon

Plasmid

Chromosome

FIGURE 2 Organization of resistance elements within the bacterial genome. One can think of a group of genetic resistance determinants like a Russian doll, in which progressively smaller dolls (gene cassettes, integrons, transposon, etc.) are placed inside larger versions. Any of the individual elements may be missing, but usually several are present.

highly mobile resistance phenotype that can spread rather quickly through bacterial populations.

Several beta-lactamase genes have been reported within integrons, including OXA-, CTX-M, and metallocarbapenemases, among others (34–36). The rapid spread of some beta-lactamases has been attributed to the incorporation of the genes into highly mobile plasmids.

WHICH ONES ARE CLINICALLY RELEVANT TODAY AND WHAT ANTIBIOTICS SHOULD WE USE TO TREAT?

Infectious disease practitioners rarely know the type of beta-lactamase present in a given bacterial isolate. In outbreaks such as the New York City KPC-producing *Klebsiella* outbreak, research laboratories may characterize the beta-lactamase more closely. Most clinical microbiology laboratories test for the presence of ESBLs in *Enterobacteraciae*, using the phenotypic tests currently recommended by the Clinical and Laboratory Standards Institute (CLSI) (37). If the ESBL phenotype is detected, the laboratory reports that the isolate is resistant to all cephalosporins, even if some of the cephalosporins show antibacterial activity in vitro. An astute practitioner can also guess at the type of beta-lactamase present in a given isolate by looking at the organism type and antibiogram. To date, other than avoiding third-generation cephalosporins when an ESBL producer is found (38–40), third-generation cephalosporins and quinolones when an AmpC producer is suspected (39,41), or using empiric colistin in a KPC-producing *Klebsiella* outbreak (42,43), knowledge of the type of beta-lactamase has had little impact in the day-to-day practice of infectious disease physicians. There is a growing body of evidence, however, that in severely ill patients, choosing the correct empiric antibiotic does have an impact on mortality [(40) and reviewed in (38)]. Hence rapid testing of clinical specimens to detect the presence of resistance determinants such as beta-lactamases is likely to be implemented as these tests are developed in the future. Currently, all such rapid testing is based on polymerase chain reaction (PCR) technology in one form or another. A major limitation of PCR-based assays is that they test for the presence of, rather than the expression of, beta-lactamase genes. Knowledge of the most important beta-lactamases that lead to antibiotic treatment failures is necessary to design appropriate PCR primer libraries to screen for these

TABLE 3 Suggested Antimicrobial Treatments for Beta-Lactamase Producing Organisms

Clinical syndrome	Microbiological considerations	Beta-lactamase resistance determinants	Empiric/specific antibiotic recommendations	Selected references
Nosocomial pneumonia	*Klebsiella* spp.	ESBLs like SHV-2; CTX-Ms	Carbapenems, beta-lactam–beta-lactamase inhibitor combinations (tazobactam), cefepime, fluoroquinolones, aminoglycosides	47,48
		KPC carbapenemases	Colistin, tetracyclines	
	PSDA	Amp Cs, OXA carbapenemases, VIM metallocarbapenemases	Carbapenems, beta-lactam–beta-lactamase inhibitor combinations, cefepime, fluoroquinolones, aminoglycosides	18,19,38
	Acinetobacter spp., *Enterobacter* spp.	TEM and SHV ESBLs, AmpC and ADC cephalosporinases, OXA carbapenemases	Carbapenems, beta-lactam–beta-lactamase inhibitor combinations (sulbactam, tazobactam), cefepime, fluoroquinolones, aminoglycosides	47
			Colistin, tetracyclines	
Bloodstream infections	*Klebsiella* spp.	ESBLs like SHV-2; CTX-M enzymes	Carbapenems, beta-lactam–beta-lactamase inhibitor combinations (tazobactam), cefepime, fluoroquinolones, aminoglycosides	38,49
		KPC carbapenemases	Colistin, tetracyclines	
Skin and soft tissue infections	*Enterobacteriacie*	ESBLs, AmpCs, CTX-Ms	Carbapenems, beta-lactam–beta-lactamase inhibitor combinations, cefepime, fluoroquinolones, aminoglycosides	17
		KPC	Colistin, tetracycline	
	PSDA	AmpC, OXAs, VIMs	See above	
	Acinetobacter spp.	AmpC, OXAs, VIMs	See above	
Uncomplicated urinary tract/GU infections	*Enterobacteriaciae* (including *Proteus* spp.)	ESBLs, AmpCs, KPC, CTX-Ms	See above	50
	PSDA	AmpC, OXAs, VIMs		
	Acinetobacter spp.	ESBLs, AmpCs,		

Abbreviations: ADC, *Acinetobacter*-derived cephalosporinase; AmpC, acts on ampicillin class C; CTX-M, active on cefotaxime, first isolated at Munich; ESBL, extended spectrum beta-lactamases; GU, genitourinary; KPC, *Klebsiella pneumoniae* carbapenemase; OXA, oxacillinase; PSDA, *Pseudomonas aeruginosa*; SHV, sulfhydryl reagent variable; TEM, named after the patient (Temoneira) providing the first sample; VIM, verona integron-encoded metallo-beta-lactamase.

clinically relevant enzymes like TEM and SHV ESBLs, AmpCs, CTX-Ms, OXAs, and metallo-beta-lactamases (IMP and VIM families).

Empiric treatment choices for specific infectious disease syndromes should take into account the potential presence of a beta-lactamase and patient epidemiology, as well as the unique resistance patterns present in the local clinical milieu. Some suggestions advocated by various infectious disease organizations and practitioners are listed in Table 3 (which in no way is meant to be comprehensive).

Importantly, once bacterial cultures are positive and the organism's resistance and susceptibility patterns are known, empiric therapy should be tailored to reflect these results. Too often, patients remain on broad-spectrum agents that risk unnecessary morbidities and even mortality when a narrow-spectrum antibiotic would have been sufficient.

WHICH ONES DO WE NEED TO LOOK OUT FOR IN THE FUTURE?

Metallo-beta-lactamases and KPC-producing *Enterobactericiae* are likely to increase in the United States in the future. Reports are already emerging regarding the spread of the KPC to Europe (44) and throughout other parts of the United States. VIM (a carbapenemase metallo-enzyme)-producing *P. aeruginosa* isolates are being reported sporadically, particularly in critically ill patients (45). VIM- and IMP (another metallo-carbapenemase)-producing isolates are being frequently identified in Calgary, Alberta, and other parts of Canada (46). Organisms producing KPC will show unusual resistance to carbapenems, beta-lactam–beta-lactamase inhibitors, and cephalosporins. They are often resistant to fluoroquinolones as well. *P. aeruginosa* with broad-spectrum resistance to beta-lactams should also be suspected to carry a metallo-beta-lactamase enzyme. If there is a suspicion of increasing resistance among particular isolates, it behooves astute infectious disease practitioners to investigate the precise cause of this resistance. Knowledge of the presence and prevalence of specific resistance mechanisms will inform infection control practices and empiric antibiotic choices.

CONCLUSIONS

Beta-lactam antibiotics arguably remain the safest and most effective antimicrobial agents used today. Unfortunately, beta-lactamases are, and will continue to be, formidable adversaries in the clinical arena when beta-lactams are used. Detailed knowledge of the epidemiology, microbiology, kinetic, and mechanistic details of their functioning, and genetic aspects of their dissemination, have already led to changes in clinical detection and treatment and infection control practices. In the future, as newer and more challenging enzymes emerge, this knowledge will be critical in the design of new beta-lactam antibiotics and beta-lactamase inhibitors, particularly for the Class B, C, and D enzymes. Rapid detection of resistance determinants in the clinical setting will allow for appropriate initial antibiotic use, thereby limiting the number of instances where potent broad-spectrum agents, such as carbapenems or colisitin, need to be administered. This will improve patient outcomes and limit the emergence of new resistance in the healthcare setting.

ACKNOWLEDGMENT

We acknowledge Ms. Magdalena Taracila for her assistance in preparing Figure 1.

REFERENCES

1. Massova I, Mobashery S. Kinship and diversification of bacterial penicillin-binding proteins and beta-lactamases. Antimicrob Agents Chemother 1998; 42:1–17.
2. Ambler RP. The structure of beta-lactamases. Philos Trans Royal Soc London B Biol Sci 1980; 289:321–31.
3. Bush K, Jacoby GA, Medeiros AA. A functional classification scheme for beta-lactamases and its correlation with molecular structure. Antimicrob Agents Chemother 1995; 39:1211–33.
4. Datta N, Kontomichalou P. Penicillinase synthesis controlled by infectious R factors in *Enterobacteriaciae*. Nature (London) 1965; 208.
5. Jacoby GA. Beta-lactamase nomenclature. Antimicrob Agents Chemother 2006; 50:1123–9.
6. Matthew M, Hedges RW, Smith JT. Types of beta-lactamase determined by plasmids in Gram-negative bacteria. J Bacteriol 1979; 138:657–62.
7. Kliebe C, Nies BA, Meyer JF, Tolxdorff-Neutzling RM, Wiedemann B. Evolution of plasmid-coded resistance to broad-spectrum cephalosporins. Antimicrob Agents Chemother 1985; 288:302–7.
8. Podbielski A, Schonling J, Melzer B, Warnatz K, Leusch H-G. Molecular characterization of a new plasmid-encoded SHV-type beta-lactamase (SHV-2 variant) conferring high-level cefotaxime resistance upon *Klebsiella pneumoniae*. J Gen Microbiol 1991; 137:569–78.
9. Sirot D, Sirot J, Labia R, et al. Transferable resistance to third-generation cephalosporins in clinical isolates of *Klebsiella pneumoniae*: identification of CTX-1, a novel beta-lactamase. J Antimicrob Chemother 1987; 20:323–34.
10. Sougakoff W, Goussard S, Courvalin P. The TEM-3 beta-lactamase, which hydrolyzes broad-spectrum cephalosporins, is derived from the TEM-2 penicillinase by two amino acid substitutions. FEMS Microbiol Lett 1988; 56:343–8.
11. www.lahey.org/studies/webt.asp (last accessed August 31, 2007).
12. Pfaller MA, Segreti J. Overview of the epidemiological profile and laboratory detection of extended-spectrum beta-lactamases. Clin Infect Dis 2006; 42:S153–63.
13. Kim J, Lim YM, Jeong YS, Seol SY. Occurrence of CTX-M-3, CTX-M-15, CTX-M-14, and CTX-M-9 extended-spectrum beta-lactamases in *Enterobacteriaceae* clinical isolates in Korea. Antimicrob Agents Chemother 2005; 49:1572–5.
14. Lartigue MF, Poirel L, Decousser JW, Nordmann P. Multidrug-resistant *Shigella sonnei* and *Salmonella enterica* Serotype typhimurium isolates producing CTX-M beta-lactamases as causes of community-acquired infection in France. Clin Infect Dis 2005; 40:1069–70.
15. Paterson DL, Hujer KM, Hujer AM, et al. Extended-spectrum beta-lactamases in *Klebsiella pneumoniae* bloodstream isolates from seven countries: dominance and widespread prevalence of SHV-and CTX-M-type beta-lactamases. Antimicrob Agents Chemother 2003; 47:3554–60.
16. Matsumoto Y, Ikeda F, Kamimura T, Yokota Y, Mine Y. Novel plasmid mediated B-lactamase from. *E. coli* that inactivates oxyimino-cephalosporins. Antimicrob Agents Chemother 1988; 32:1243–6.
17. Bonnet R. Growing group of extended-spectrum beta-lactamases: the CTX-M enzymes. Antimicrob Agents Chemother 2004; 48:1–14.
18. Bradford PA, Bratu S, Urban C, et al. Emergence of carbapenem-resistant *Klebsiella* species possessing the class A carbapenem-hydrolyzing KPC-2 and inhibitor-resistant TEM-30 beta-lactamases in New York City. Clin Infect Dis 2004; 39:55–60.
19. Woodford N, Tierno PMJ, Young K, et al. Outbreak of *Klebsiella pneumoniae* producing a new carbapenem-hydrolyzing class A beta-lactamase, KPC-3, in a New York Medical Center. Antimicrob Agents Chemother 2004; 48:4793–9.
20. Hanson ND. Amp-C beta-lactamases: what do we need to know for the future? J AntimicrobChemother 2003; 52:2–4.
21. Jacobs C, Frere J-M, Normark S. Cytosolic intermediates for cell wall biosynthesis and degradation control inducible beta-lactam resistance in Gram-negative bacteria. Cell 1997; 88:823–32.

22. Jacobs C, Joris B, Jamin M, et al. AmpD, essential for both beta-lactamase regulation and cell wall recycling, is a novel cytosolic N-acetylmuramyl-L-alanine amidase. Mol Microbiol 1995; 15:553–9.

23. Walsh TR, Toleman MA, Poirel L, Nordmann P. Metallo-beta-lactamases: the quiet before the storm? Clinical Microbiology Reviews 2005; 18:306–25.

24. Crichlow GV, Kuzin AP, Nukaga M, Mayama K, Sawai T, Knox JR. Structure of the extended-spectrum class C beta-lactamase of *Enterobacter cloacae* GC1, a natural mutant with a tandem tripeptide insertion. Biochemistry 1999; 38:10256–61.

25. Sun T, Bethel CR, Bonomo RA, Knox JR. Inhibitor-resistant class A beta-lactamases: consequences of the Ser130-to-Gly mutation seen in Apo and tazobactam structures of the SHV-1 variant. Biochemistry 2004; 43:14111–7.

26. Helfand MS, Bethel CR, Hujer AM, Hujer KM, Anderson VE, Bonomo RA. Understanding resistance to beta-lactams and beta-lactamase inhibitors in the SHV beta-lactamase: lessons from the mutagenesis of SER-130. J Biol Chem 2003; 278:52724–9.

27. Sulton D, Pagan-Rodriguez D, Zhou X, et al. Clavulanic acid inactivation of SHV-1 and the inhibitor-resistant S130G SHV-1 beta-lactamase. Insights into the mechanism of inhibition. J Biol Chem 2005; 280:35528–36.

28. Meroueh SO, Roblin P, Golemi D, et al. Molecular dynamics at the root of expansion of function in the M69L inhibitor resistant TEM beta-lactamase from *Escherichia coli.* J Am Chem Soc 2002; 124:9422–30.

29. Wang X, Minasov G, Shoichet BK. The structural bases of antibiotic resistance in the clinically derived mutant beta-lactamases TEM-30, TEM-32 and TEM-34. J Biol Chem 2002; 277:32149–56.

30. Wachino J-I, Doi Y, Yamane K, et al. Molecular characterization of a cephamycin-hydrolyzing and inhibitor-resistant class A beta-lactamase, GES-4, possessing a single G170S substitution in the omega loop. Antimicrob Agents Chemother 2004; 48:2905–10.

31. Alba J, Ishii Y, Thomson KS, Moland ES, Yamaguchi K. Kinetics study of KPC-3, a plasmid-encoded class A carbapenem-hydrolyzing beta-lactamase. Antimicrob Agents Chemother 2005; 49:4760–2.

32. Rice LB, Carias LL, Bonomo RA, Shlaes DM. Molecular genetics of resistance to both ceftazidime and beta-lactam-beta-lactamase inhibitor combinations in *Klebsiella pneumoniae* and in vivo response to beta-lactam therapy. J Infect Dis 1996; 173:151–8.

33. Rice LB, Willey SH, Papanicolaou GA, et al. Outbreak of ceftazidime resistance caused by extended-spectrum beta-lactamases at a Massachusetts chronic care facility. Antimicrob Agents Chemother 1990; 34:2193–9.

34. Lauretti L, Riccio ML, Mazzariol A, et al. Cloning and characterization of *bla*VIM, a new integron-borne metallo-beta-lactamase gene from a *Pseudomonas aeruginosa* clinical isolate. Antimicrob Agents Chemother 1999; 43:1584–90.

35. Poirel L, Gerome P, De Champs C, Stephanazzi J, Naas T, Nordmann P. Integron-located oxa-32 gene cassette encoding an extended-spectrum variant of OXA-2 beta-lactamase from *Pseudomonas aeruginosa.* Antimicrob Agents Chemother 2002; 46:566–9.

36. Sabate M, Navarro F, Miro E, et al. Novel complex sull-type integron in *Escherichia coli* carrying bla(CTX-M-9). Antimicrob Agents Chemother 2002; 46:2656–61.

37. CLSI. Performance standards for antimicrobial susceptibility testing 15th informational supplement M100-S15. Clin Lab Standards Inst 2005; 39.

38. Ramphal R, Ambrose PG. Extended-spectrum beta-lactamases and clinical outcomes: current data. Clin Infect Dis 2006; 42:S164–72.

39. Owens RC Jr, Rice L. Hospital-based strategies for combating resistance. Clin Infect Dis 2006; 42:S173–81.

40. Paterson DL, Ko WC, Von Gottberg A, et al. Outcome of cephalosporin treatment for serious infections due to apparently susceptible organisms producing extended-spectrum beta-lactamases: implications for the clinical microbiology laboratory. J Clin Microbiol 2001; 39:2206–12.

41. Goossens H, Grabein B. Prevalence and antimicrobial susceptibility data for extended-spectrum beta-lactamase and AmpC-producing *Enterobacteriaceae* from the MYSTIC Program in Europe and the United States (1997–2004). Diagn Microbiol Infect Dis 2005; 53:257–64.

42. Livermore DM. The impact of carbapenemases on antimicrobial development and therapy. Curr Opin Investig Drugs 2002; 3:218–24.

43. Bratu S, Tolaney P, Karumudi U, et al. Carbapenemase-producing *Klebsiella pneumoniae* in Brooklyn, NY: molecular epidemiology and in vitro activity of polymyxin B and other agents. J Antimicrob Chemother 2005; 56:128–32.

44. Naas T, Nordmann P, Vedel G, Poyart C. Plasmid-mediated carbapenem-hydrolyzing beta-lactamase KPC in a *Klebsiella pneumoniae* isolate from France. Antimicrob Agents Chemother 2005; 49:4423–4.

45. Lolans K, Queenan AM, Bush K, Sahud A, Quinn JP. First nosocomial outbreak of *Pseudomonas aeruginosa* producing an integron-borne metallo-beta-lactamase (VIM-2) in the United States. Antimicrob Agents Chemother 2005; 49:3538–40.

46. Laupland KB, Parkins MD, Church DL, et al. Population-based epidemiological study of infections caused by carbapenem-resistant *Pseudomonas aeruginosa* in the Calgary Health Region: importance of metallo-beta-lactamase (MBL)-producing strains. J Infect Dis 2005; 192:1606–12.

47. American Thoracic Society/Infectious Diseases Society of America. Guidelines for the management of adults with hospital-acquired, ventilator-associated, and healthcare-associated pneumonia. Am J Respir Crit Care Med 2005; 171:388–416.

48. Paterson DL, Ko WC, Von Gottberg A, et al. Antibiotic therapy for *Klebsiella pneumoniae* bacteremia: implications of production of extended-spectrum beta-lactamases. Clin Infect Dis 2004; 39:31–7.

49. Mermel LA, Farr BM, Sheretz RJ, et al. Guidelines for the management of intravascular catheter-related infections. Clin. Infect Dis 2001; 32:1249–72.

50. Naber KG, Bergman B, Bishop MC, et al. EAU guidelines for the management of urinary and male genital tract infections. Urinary Tract Infection (UTI) Working Group of the Health Care Office (HCO) of the European Association of Urology (EAU). Eur Urol 2001; 40:576–88.

11 | *Clostridium difficile* Infection: Overview and Update with a Focus on Antimicrobial Resistance as a Risk Factor

Robert C. Owens, Jr.
Department of Clinical Pharmacy Services, Division of Infectious Diseases, Maine Medical Center, Portland, Maine and the Department of Medicine, University of Vermont, College of Medicine, Burlington, Vermont, U.S.A.

August J. Valenti
Department of Hospital Epidemiology and Infection Prevention, Division of Infectious Diseases, Maine Medical Center, Portland, Maine and the Department of Medicine, University of Vermont, College of Medicine, Burlington, Vermont, U.S.A.

Mark H. Wilcox
Consultant, Clinical Director of Microbiology, Pathology Lead Infection Control Doctor, Leeds Teaching Hospitals NHS Trust, and Professor of Medical Microbiology, University of Leeds, Leeds, West Yorkshire, U.K.

INTRODUCTION

Early investigations of antibiotic-associated diarrhea (AAD) pointed toward staphylococci and *Candida albicans* as causes of this phenomenon (1). A face was finally put to the disease when in 1978, Bartlett et al. demonstrated that *Clostridium difficile* was the causative pathogen associated with antibiotic-associated pseudomembranous colitis (2). It was determined later that pseudomembranes were not apparent in all instances of the disease (in fact they are evident in less than half of the cases). Since its recognition, there has been an ebb and flow of reported outbreaks typically due to distinct strains of *C. difficile* that feature particular resistance patterns. One of the purposes of this chapter is to discuss what is known about risk factors for *C. difficile* infection (CDI), which includes the administration of antimicrobials that are relatively inactive (in vitro) against the infecting strain of *C. difficile* thus predisposing the patient to this unintended consequence of antimicrobial use. It is not possible to do this without gaining an appreciation for the advances in our understanding of the disease as well as discussing the prodigious changes noted in the pathogen itself and the disease it causes. CDI, in its mildest form, causes self-limiting diarrhea, which may respond solely to the discontinuation of the inciting antimicrobial(s). In its most severe forms, CDI causes significant diarrhea leading to fulminant, life-threatening disease (severe dehydration, sepsis, colonic perforation). Paradoxically, CDI may not present with diarrhea at all in some patients, but may be associated with ileus or toxic megacolon. Severe CDI may progress to colonic perforation, sepsis, and death. While severe cases are seen occasionally in all age groups, most occur in the elderly. It should be remembered that *C. difficile* is not the only cause of AAD (3).

A variety of other pathogens, such as *C. perfringens*, *S. aureus*, and *Klebsiella oxytoca*, to list a few, have also been implicated in AAD (3,4). *K. oxytoca* ADD can be distinguished from *C. difficile* based on the appearance of grossly bloody stools, although this is also a possible, but uncommon, presentation of CDI (4).

An increased incidence and severity of disease over the last decade have been documented (5–8). A number of outbreaks associated with severe manifestations of CDI have recently captured the attention of clinicians, epidemiologists, patients, and the media. Given the fact that CDI is primarily a healthcare-associated adverse event, occurring as an "unintended consequence" of antimicrobial use, regulatory and accrediting agencies as well as the consumer-driven public reporting movement can be expected to take action. In fact, two Canadian provinces (Quebec and Manitoba) have already required mandatory reporting of *C. difficile* (but not to the public) after being implicated in nearly 2,000 deaths (9). In England, every *C. difficile* laboratory-positive case occurring in hospitals now has to be reported centrally via a web-based system.

Again, the primary purpose of this chapter is to discuss the current evidence that establishes the role of antimicrobial resistance as a risk factor for CDI. In turn, a better understanding of this risk will hopefully translate into more judicious antimicrobial use and more research to define the role of antimicrobial resistance as a risk factor for CDI. As a part of the discussion, the many complexities of *C. difficile* as a pathogen and CDI are discussed to impart a better overall understanding to the practicing clinician. To round out the discussion, the management of routine cases of CDI, as well as recurrent, fulminant, and refractory CDI are discussed.

DIAGNOSIS OF CDI

In brief, the presenting features of CDI typically include watery diarrhea without the presence of visible blood in stool, fever, abdominal pain, cramping, diarrhea, and leukocytosis (10,11). In some cases, diarrhea is not a presenting feature of CDI, particularly when ileus or toxic megacolon is evident (11). CDI is typically limited to the colonic mucosa; however, a small number of cases have reported disease involving the distal small intestine (12). These cases of "*C. difficile* enteritis" were most commonly identified in patients following total colectomy. In more severe disease, radiographic studies of the abdomen can reveal a thickened colon wall, ascites, or colonic dilatation (typically indicating toxic megacolon). Computed tomography (CT) of the abdomen and pelvis may be helpful in severe cases of CDI to provide visual identification of potential complications and may be used to supplement the decision for surgical intervention. Colonoscopy usually reveals inflammation with or without the characteristic yellowish, often coalescing plaques or pseudomembranes. The presence of pseudomembranes typically reflects advanced disease and is not evident at all in many cases of CDI (1), although sigmoidoscopy may miss more proximal lesions. Histopathologic studies of biopsy specimens obtained at colonoscopy can show a spectrum of findings including acute nonspecific inflammation with or without crypt abscesses (13). In some cases, "volcano" lesions can be apparent, which indicate the eruption of exudate (consisting of neutrophils and fibrin) into the colonic lumen (14).

Laboratory testing for *C. difficile* toxins should only be ordered when CDI is suspected, since toxin positivity without clinical symptoms can indicate colonization with a toxigenic strain of *C. difficile*. However, the caveat here is that, especially in hospitalized patients who have a likelihood of current or recurrent exposure to antibiotics, CDI should be considered a possible cause of diarrhea. A laboratory diagnosis is usually made by determining the presence of toxins A and/or B in the stool. The most common test in use in the United States is the enzyme immunoassay (EIA) kit for toxins A and B (8). Kits that test for toxin A alone should not be used, as some strains that are pathogenic produce only functional toxin B, and indeed these may predominate within occasional institutions (16). To improve its sensitivity, we typically order a single test per day for three consecutive days (or less if the test returns positive). Once the test is positive, there is no need for further testing (e.g., there is no laboratory "test of cure") since the EIA test will remain positive in patients who have been clinically cured for months (15). The more resource-intensive cell culture cytotoxin assay is also used in some countries and is more sensitive and specific than EIA testing (17). Culture alone cannot be used to diagnose CDI because nontoxigenic strains of *C. difficile* are prevalent and do not cause disease. However, a renewed interest in culturing *C. difficile* is emerging in an effort to learn more about toxigenic strains, epidemiology, and antimicrobial susceptibility (18).

NEW VIRULENCE FACTORS DISCOVERED IN BI/NAP1 (THE EPIDEMIC STRAIN)

The first reports of BI/NAP1 strains causing severe CDI (although not known at the time) were from the University of Pittsburgh in 2000 (19–21). Circa 2002, in a small region in Quebec, Canada, nearly 2,000 fatalities related to CDI associated with outbreaks of this strain were reported, and healthcare facilities were besieged by the resultant media attention (9). Simultaneously, in the United States, several geographically dispersed hospitals were experiencing outbreaks with reportedly greater disease severity, which were investigated by the laboratories of Drs. Dale Gerding at the Hines Veterans Affairs Medical Center and Cliff McDonald at the Centers for Disease Control and Prevention (CDC) (22). Since that time, the isolate has spread rapidly to encompass all seven Provinces in Canada, most states in the United States, many parts of Europe, and, most recently, Japan (11,23).

Accelerated Toxin Production

BI/NAP1, similar to other strains of *C. difficile*, produces the two traditional toxins, toxin A and toxin B (24). Both toxin genes are typically harbored and expressed by toxigenic strains of *C. difficile* (but not always) (25). Both toxins are among the largest to be produced by bacteria (270–308 kDa) and are encoded on a region of the chromosome referred to as the pathogenicity locus (PaLoc) (26). Also located within the PaLoc are regulatory genes such as *tcdC*, which is a downstream negative regulator that modulates the expression of toxins A and B. Thus far, all BI/NAP1 strains contain an 18 base-pair deletion and/or a single base-pair deletion resulting in a frame shift in the *tcdC* gene that is thought to be responsible for the accelerated kinetics of toxin production (22,27). In vitro studies have demonstrated that BI/NAP1 strains produce 16- and 23-times more toxin A and B, respectively, compared with toxinotype 0 strains (note: categorically, toxinotype 0 strains include the most common clinically isolated strains of *C. difficile*) (28). Fawley et al. (29) advise caution in the interpretation of toxin production studies conducted in vitro in batch cultures, as the dynamics of *C. difficile* toxin production are complex and influenced by a variety of in vivo factors. Recent data using a gut model of CDI demonstrate that the BI/NAP1 strain produces toxins for longer periods in association with extended duration of germination compared with an earlier epidemic *C. difficile* strain (154).

Binary Toxin

BI/NAP1 strains also possess a previously uncommon binary toxin gene (noted to be present in 6% of a historical sample of clinical isolates) (22). The binary toxin is located outside of the PaLoc and, therefore, is not regulated by the *tcdC* gene. This binary toxin is similar to others such as the iota toxin that is produced by *C. perfringens*. Although patients infected with binary toxin-positive strains of *C. difficile* trended towards having greater disease severity, (20) toxin A- and B-negative but binary toxin-positive strains of *C. difficile* have been shown to be non-lethal in nonclinical a hampster model of infection, where 100% mortality following exposure to toxigenic toxin A and B positive *C. difficile* strains is normally seen (30). The exact role of the binary toxin in the pathogenesis of CDI remains unknown.

Nomenclature Harmonization

In addition to restriction endonuclease analysis (REA), polymerase chain reaction (PCR) ribotyping, and pulsed field gel electrophoresis (PFGE), strains can also be distinguished by toxinotyping studies. This particular epidemic strain is type BI (by REA typing), NAP1 (by PFGE), and ribotype 027 (by PCR). Most recently, a highly discriminatory DNA fingerprinting technique [multi-locus variable number of tandem repeat analysis (MLVA)] has been applied to 90 ribotype 027 strains, resulting in 23 sub-types (155). MLVA was far superior to PFGE for analyzing clusters of CDI cases, both within a single institution and between hospitals. Such studies offer the opportunity to better understand how strains spread within institutions. Toxinotyping studies examine subtle sequence variations in the PaLoc of the *C. difficile* strain. To date, at least 22 different toxinotypes have been reported (26). Typical, nonoutbreak clinical isolates of *C. difficile* belong to toxinotype 0. Toxinotype III, to which BI/NAP1 belongs, was previously rare, accounting for only 2% to 3% of historical clinical isolates (22). As a variety of methods have been deployed to characterize strains of *C. difficile*, in reflection of the various typing systems used in Europe and North America to distinguish the most recent epidemic strain, the remainder of this chapter will refer to it as BI/NAP1/027.

Spore Formation

C. difficile, like *Bacillus anthracis*, possesses an uncommon bacterial virulence factor in that it is capable of forming spores in response to an inhospitable environment or a nutrient-deprived milieu. Therefore, *C. difficile* is capable of surviving for long periods of time in the environment as well as potentially in sanctuaries within the gastrointestinal tract. This "persistence" is likely to be responsible for the unique transmission dynamics that facilitate this pathogen's spread and may play a role in persistent disease. Some genotypically distinct strains of *C. difficile* demonstrate a propensity for hypersporulating and are often associated with outbreaks (31). BI/NAP1/027, like other outbreak strains, has demonstrated the capacity to hypersporulate compared with other non-outbreak strains (32). Further study of sporulation characteristics, as well as the other identified putative virulence factors of this organism, is required to elucidate their role in the transmission of *C. difficile* and the pathogenesis of CDI.

RISK FACTORS AND PATHOGENESIS

Risk factors for acquiring CDI are complex and consist of exposure to toxigenic strains of the organism (33), prior use of any antimicrobial agent (34), duration of antimicrobial exposure (35), the degree of an antimicrobial's in vitro activity against *C. difficile* (36), exposure to gastric acid suppressants (37), poor host serum immunoglobulin (Ig) levels (38), poor colonic IgA production (39), advanced age (40), the presence of a feeding tube, and severity of underlying illness of the host (40). To clarify the issue of resistance as a risk factor, in this sense, does not refer to *C. difficile* possessing resistance to treatments such as metronidazole or vanco-mycin. Resistance as a risk factor refers to strains of *C. difficile* present in the colon that are resistant to antimicrobials the patient may be receiving or has recently received. It is hypothesized that antimicrobials may select for the overgrowth of *C. difficile* if the organisms are resistant to the antimicrobials being administered. It is probably not appreciated by most that *C. difficile* is actually inhibited by a number of antimicrobial agents at relatively low concentrations.

Importantly, CDI has been proposed to be at least a "three-hit" disease as postulated by Johnson and Gerding, and the sequence of the "hits" appears to be important (40). Patients are made susceptible to infection following exposure to drugs that alter the intestinal microbiota (the most common culprit is anti-microbials), which leads to the *first hit*, and if exposed to toxigenic strains of *C. difficile* (*second hit*) they may or may not develop CDI depending on the presence of another variable (*third hit*), chief among which are host-related immunity issues (increased age, inability to mount adequate antitoxin A IgG, and/or colonic IgA responses). For the purposes of discussion, risk factors can generally be broken down into *host* risks (first and third "hits") and *exposure* or *environmental* risks (second "hit").

HOST FACTORS
Antimicrobials

In the current theory of pathogenesis proposed by Drs. Johnson and Gerding (40), antimicrobial exposure [or any means that interfere with the complex intestinal flora such as antimicrobials, certain cancer chemotherapeutic agents, and perhaps antisecretory gastrointestinal drugs, especially proton pump inhibitors (PPIs), which do possess some activity against a limited number of organisms found in intestinal flora, such as *Helicobacter pylori*] leads to the first "hit." All antimicrobials have the potential to disrupt the host's colonization resistance (a defensive barrier comprised of commensal organisms in the gastrointestinal tract that protects the host from some colonizing or infecting pathogens). Once colonization resistance is disrupted, and the patient is exposed to toxigenic strains of *C. difficile*, the probability of *C. difficile* establishing itself in the intestinal flora is significantly elevated; however, this is a gross oversimplification of the complex bug–drug–host relationship (34). As mentioned, all antimicrobials disrupt the normal microbiota enough to allow for toxigenic strains of *C. difficile* to initiate disease; this actually includes exposure to the treatments themselves (oral vancomycin, metronidazole) (41,42). Variables that have been identified which may add to or augment risk for CDI, including prolonged exposure to the antimicrobial(s) (35) and exposure to antimicrobials lacking in vitro activity against the infecting strain of *C. difficile* (36). It is this risk factor that is discussed in more detail below.

Before we consider such issues, it is crucial to highlight a key issue that is often neglected in risk factor studies of CDI: exposure to *C. difficile*. This cannot be assumed to be equal for all patients included in risk factor studies, and indeed the epidemiology of CDI often includes clusters of cases that will potentially represent greater transmission risks for contacts (156). This phenomenon may mask or bias CDI risk factors, including antibiotic or other drug exposure, notably in the outbreak setting (which ironically is when many risk factor studies are carried out). Furthermore, antibiotic polypharmacy and duration of administration have often not been examined despite their potential to confound results (157).

Antimicrobial Resistance as a Risk Factor for CDI

As mentioned, the degree of antimicrobial activity exerted by the drug being administered to the patient regardless of reason (prophylaxis or treatment, whether appropriate or inappropriate) may play a substantial role in terms of whether or not the patient develops CDI. Exposure to antimicrobials possessing enough activity against *C. difficile* may sufficiently suppress the growth of *C. difficile* during or shortly after therapy, and so prevent CDI as an unintended consequence of antimicrobial therapy. Similarly, the patient could receive an antimicrobial lacking activity against *C. difficile*, creating an environment that is ideal for the overgrowth of *C. difficile*, potentially leading to CDI. Table 1 contains a list of antimicrobials possessing various degrees of in vitro activity against *C. difficile*. For explanation purposes, the scenarios above greatly oversimplify reality. Some flaws exist with this theory but it is in large part supported by a continually growing body of literature. This body of literature consists of in vitro susceptibility studies that have determined the activities of certain antimicrobials against the infecting strains of *C. difficile* isolates obtained from patients, typically collected in institutions that have experienced outbreaks. This occurred at two major time points in the United States, the first in the late 1980s and early 1990s and most recently from outbreaks that started in 2000 in North America. In addition, this body of literature includes risk factor ascertainment studies that have been conducted over the last two decades. The challenge in translating this theory from benchtop to bedside is several-fold. First, we do not culture *C. difficile* strains as a regular part of clinical practice and therefore we do not know susceptibilities in real time. Second, most antimicrobials have either poor or variable activity against *C. difficile*, making it difficult to avoid treatment of underlying infections with antimicrobials that lack activity against *C. difficile*. Third, the local epidemiology of *C. difficile* strains may change, with strains that are susceptible to a systemic antibiotic being replaced by resistant clones. And lastly, at least one example can be brought up that is not explained by the theory, which is the fact that ampicillin and penicillin have excellent in vitro activity against strains of *C. difficile* but they have been strongly implicated as causes of CDI in well-conducted studies (43,44). In addition to this, the current treatments themselves (metronidazole, oral vancomycin) may predispose patients to future episodes of CDI. Some of this can be explained by the complexity of CDI and factors related to it, such as the fact that the human IgG and IgA antitoxin A antibody response rates in individuals varies, and many other potential host and pathogen factors that are interwoven.

TABLE 1 Differences in Activity Between Antimicrobials Against Strains of Clostridium difficile

Antimicrobials with good activity against C. difficile (MIC50/MIC90)	Ref.	Antimicrobials with moderate or variable activity against C. difficile (MIC50/MIC90) moderate activity based on a low MIC50 but high MIC90[a]	Ref.	Antimicrobials with poor activity against C. difficile (MIC50/MIC90)	Ref.
Ampicillin (2.0/2.0)	44	Clindamycin (4/>128)	44	Cefotaxime (≥128)	148
Doripenem (1.0/2.0)	153	Erythromycin (<1/>128)	44	Cefoxitin (>64/>64)	47
OPT-80 (0.125/0.125)	153	Gatifloxacin →? (1.0/16)[b]	153	Ceftriaxone (≥256)	Not published
Linezolid (0.5/2.0)	149	Moxifloxacin →? (1.0/16)[b]	153	Cefuroxime (≥128)	148
Metronidazole (0.125/0.25)	153	Tetracycline (<1/32)	44	Ciprofloxacin (8/32)	150
Meropenem (2.0/2.0)	153			Levofloxacin (4/32)[b]	153
Nitazoxanide (0.06/0.125)	153			Trimethoprim-sulfamethoxazole (≥128/≥128)	148
Penicillin G (—/1.0)	151				
Piperacillin (—/16)	47				
Piperacillin/tazobactam (4/4)	152				
Ramoplanin (0.25/0.5)	153				
Rifalazil[c] (0.0075/0.03)	153				
Rifaximin[c] (0.0075/0.015)	153				
Tigecycline (0.125/0.25)	153				
Tinidazole (0.125/0.25)	153				
Tizoxanide (0.06/0.125)	153				
Vancomycin (1.0/1.0)	153				

Note: This table should be interpreted with caution as data were obtained using different isolates and numbers of isolates, reflecting different geographies and time periods. Only the Hecht study (151) includes strains that are of the recent epidemic type (BI/NAP1/027). **BOLD** text indicates that the antimicrobial is used to treat CDI (investigational or approved treatment).

[a] While some strains have very high MIC values to the drugs listed in this category, many strains, comparatively, are also quite susceptible, with very low MIC values. It is difficult to assign these drugs a category because of the variability they possess in terms of their activity against C. difficile.

[b] Indicates that MICs within the higher range (32–64 μg/mL) have been reported recently, although the MIC50/90 listed would suggest that these drugs are of moderate risk. The recent epidemic strains (BI/NAP1/027) possess elevated MIC values; thus, when used in a widespread manner, they are likely to provide a similar risk to that of higher risk drugs (those will higher MICs).

[c] Lowest MIC values tested, but (at least) 3% of isolates (likely to be far greater, as this appears to be an emerging resistance issue) also noted to possess high-level resistance (MIC values >256). Rifampin has similarly low MIC values (data not shown) as well as similar cross-resistance rates.

Abbreviations: CDI, Clostridium difficile infection; MIC, minimum inhibitory concentration.

Source: Adapted From Ref. 153.

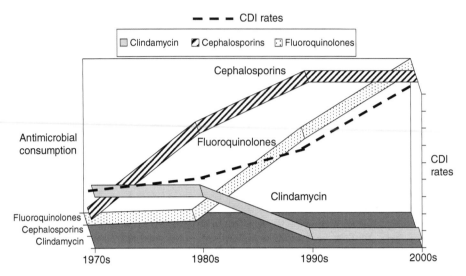

FIGURE 1 Popularity of antimicrobials by decade with superimposed rates of *Clostridium difficile* infection (CDI). *Source*: Courtesy of Robert C. Owens, Jr.

Figure 1 illustrates the popularity of specific antimicrobials/antimicrobial classes and the overall rates of CDI over a period of time from the 1970s through current times. Clindamycin gained notoriety in the late 1970s and 1980s as a "high risk" antimicrobial, in part, because it was the antimicrobial at the center of the discovery of *C. difficile* as the causative agent of pseudomembranous colitis, and because it was causally associated with CDI outbreaks in the 1980s and early 1990s. *C. difficile* strains isolated from those outbreaks belonged to the REA "J-type" epidemic strain and were universally resistant to clindamycin (36). Unlike other antibiotics, clindamycin is also known to persist in the cecal contents of hamsters at high concentrations for prolonged periods of time following the completion of dosing (45), potentially increasing the "susceptibility window" in patients treated with clindamycin who are ultimately exposed to clindamycin-resistant strains of *C. difficile* (e.g., REA type J-7 and J-9 strains). Because clindamycin has a so-called "prolonged" susceptibility window, rendering the recipient susceptible to infection with clindamycin-resistant strains of *C. difficile*, it is conceivable that this unique characteristic of clindamycin was responsible for the success in reducing CDI at institutions identified with REA J-type outbreak strains in the late 1980s (where clindamycin was restricted or removed from formulary) (46).

During the mid-to-late 1980s through 1990s, cephalosporins became popular choices (Fig. 1) for broad-spectrum therapy and the once-daily administration of ceftriaxone found a home (so to speak) with the widespread acceptance of outpatient parenteral antimicrobial therapy as institutions began to focus on reducing length of stay. *C. difficile* strains tested to date are universally resistant to the cephalosporins (Table 1), with most minimum inhibitory concentration (MIC) values exceeding the ranges tested (e.g., >64 μg/mL

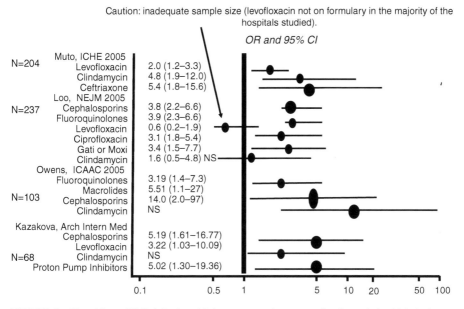

FIGURE 2   *Clostridium difficile* infection risk factor ascertainment studies for antimicrobials in the era of BI/NAP1/027. *Source*: Courtesy of Robert C. Owens, Jr. Adapted from Refs. 21, 27, 48, and 49.

and >256 µg/mL) (47). As the overall consumption of cephalosporins increased with the burgeoning market availability of later (third) generation cephalosporins and their favorable placement in the treatment of common infections such as community-acquired pneumonia and pyelonephritis, their use began to be associated with CDI in some of the only appropriately designed risk factor studies conducted prior to 2001 (43). Most recent studies continue to demonstrate that even with the new "epidemic" strain of *C. difficile*, cephalosporins possess the highest odds ratios, reinforcing their association with acquiring CDI, greater even than the fluoroquinolones that have captured most of the headlines for their "high risk" status as comparatively illustrated in Figure 2 (11,21,8–51).

   Most recently, the fluoroquinolones (along with cephalosporins) have been implicated in outbreaks where the BI/NAP1/027 strain of *C. difficile* has been identified. Unlike the parenteral cephalosporins where all but one are generically available, many of the fluoroquinolones that are used today are still marketed and are under patent protection. Consequently, there has been a series of potentially misleading claims concerning the relative propensity of different fluoroquinolones to induce CDI. Issues such as fluoroquinolones possessing anaerobic activity and/or those with hepatobiliary versus renal elimination being more likely to cause CDI have received particular attention (37,49,52–54).

   So, what do we know?… Well, prior to the emergence of BI/NAP1/027, fluoroquinolones were considered "low risk" antimicrobials for CDI. The collision of two important events has changed their risk category over the last 5 to 7 years.

First, the fluoroquinolones have emerged to become among the most commonly used inpatient and outpatient antimicrobials in adults in North America. Second, uniform resistance among BI/NAP1/027 strains to all fluoroquinolones has appeared (22). It should be noted, however, that epidemic *C. difficile* strains predating BI/NAP1/027 were also relatively resistant to fluoroquinolones (150). Several recent studies have demonstrated strong statistical associations between ALL fluoroquinolones (ciprofloxacin, gatifloxacin, levofloxacin, moxifloxacin) and CDI outbreaks (21,35,48,49,55,56). Because of minimal use, particularly in high-risk settings, gemifloxacin remains the only fluoquinolone not yet implicated in an outbreak. Interestingly, in most of these studies where there was a strong association between CDI and fluoroquinolone exposure, clindamycin was not consistently implicated as a risk factor (perhaps because it is used less frequently compared with previous decades and/or because BI/NAP1/027 strains are invariably susceptible to clindamycin) (27,48,49). Also of interest is the fact that the cephalosporins, in most cases, have been associated with higher relative risks of CDI than the fluoroquinolones in more recent outbreaks (21,49,55).

Partly in response to marketing campaigns, some institutions have gone as far as switching fluoroquinolones on their formularies to provide a simple answer to a complex problem. Based on this anti-anaerobic activity misconception, one hospital changed their formulary from moxifloxacin to levofloxacin (57). Following this formulary intervention, the CDI rates actually increased when the non–anti-anaerobic fluoroquinolone levofloxacin was re-instituted. Interestingly, as one would expect, it appeared that total antimicrobial consumption at this institution increased throughout the entire study period, providing a more realistic explanation for the continued increase in CDI rates. It must also be assumed that transmission of *C. difficile* was occurring more frequently than before the outbreak commenced. To their credit, the authors concluded: "Substituting use of one fluoroquinolone with use of another without also controlling the overall use of drugs from this class is unlikely to control outbreaks caused by the NAP1 strain of *C. difficile*" (57). Peak toxin production, germination, and proliferation were similar when *C. difficile* strains (including *C. difficile* ribotype 027) were exposed in a human gut model to moxifloxacin, levofloxacin, or ciprofloxacin. Early toxin production was seen after moxifloxacin exposure, possibly due to a moxifloxacin-resistant sub-population, or expansion of hetero-resistant cells under antibiotic selective conditions (158).

Two recent reports have further highlighted that early studies noting associations between fluoroquinolones and outbreaks of CDI may have missed increased transmission of, and thus exposure to, *C. difficile* in an institution or other antimicrobials as crucial risk factors explaining an increased incidence of cases. In both examples, CDI rates were controlled despite increases in fluoroquinolone use. In Montreal, CDI rates decreased in association with antimicrobial restriction of first (−21%), second (−93%), and third (−79%) cephalosporins, clindamycin (−87%), macrolides (−78%), and ciprofloxacin (−29%); usage of respiratory fluoroquinolones (predominantly moxifloxacin) and piperacilin tazobactam increased by +79% and +114%, respectively (159). Following an outbreak, Muto et al. (21) used a package of measures to first reduce the incidence of infection from peak levels, and then eventually to return to baseline rates of CDI. As well as multiple infection control measures, antimicrobial usage was altered, including an increase in moxifloxacin and ciprofloxacin prescribing (levofloxacin was removed from the formulary).

Separating specific antibiotics and antibiotic classes in terms of high, moderate, and low risk for *C. difficile* is exceedingly difficult. It should be remembered that exposure to any antibiotic carries the liability of increasing a patient's individual risk of developing CDI as an unintended consequence of its use (as properly identified in the product package inserts of all antibiotics). Thomas et al. (43) published a comprehensive systematic review of antimicrobial risk factor studies conducted prior to 2001. Of more than 600 studies considered, only two were found to be conducted in a manner that avoided serious threats to the validity of their findings. Threats included: inappropriate choice of control group, sample size, case selection, matching variables, inappropriate statistical analysis, among others. The vast majority of the studies were incapable of supporting their conclusions. The two valid studies incriminated cephalosporins, penicillins, and clindamycin as high-risk antimicrobials in studies conducted prior to the identification and widespread prevalence of the BI/NAP1/027 *C. difficile* strain.

Interestingly, recent observations and population-based studies suggest that factors other than antimicrobial exposure may also be responsible for this first "hit" (37). For example, 61% of patients who developed community-associated CDI did not receive antimicrobials within the previous 90 days prior to developing disease (37). Another recent study also demonstrated that 59% of patients who developed community-associated CDI also did not have documented antimicrobial exposure (58). In these studies where antimicrobial exposure appeared to be absent, PPI exposure has emerged as a risk factor in multivariable analyses.

So, in summary, data strongly suggest that the in vitro activity possessed by an antimicrobial can play a role in determining who develops CDI and who does not. However, due to the convoluted nature of CDI and the bug–drug–host trinity, it does not account for all aspects of an antimicobial's attributable risk to cause disease. The administration of antimicrobials possessing activity against the infecting strain of *C. difficile* does seem to suppress its growth and decrease the likelihood of infection. In contrast, the administration of antimicrobials lacking activity against the infecting strain of *C. difficile* appears to increase risk for disease. More research is needed to more fully elucidate this particular risk and, importantly, how we might be able to utilize this information to guide necessary antimicrobial use so as to minimize CDI risk. Antimicrobials listed in Table 1 illustrate the spectrum of their in vitro activities against *C. difficile*. The problem with the table is that the MIC values were determined in large part from different studies (different strain types and numbers of *C. difficile*, perhaps even using different testing methods). Despite this, drugs like linezolid, piperacillin, piperacillin/tazobactam, tigecycline, doripenem, and meropenem have been shown to have a high degree of activity against *C. difficile*, and for some of the antimicrobials listed, a strong inverse correlation exists in terms of use-versus-CDI rate. For moderate risk antimicrobials (e.g., respiratory fluoroquinolones, such as gatifloxacin, and moxifloxacin, whose anti-anaerobic activity imparts activity against some strains of *C. difficile*), antianaerobic activity in general, coupled with relatively poor activity against some *C. difficile* strains, including the recent epidemic strain BI/NAP1/027, may result in increased CDI risk. And finally, some antimicrobials such as the cephalosporins are uniformly poorly active against *C. difficile* and have been associated with outbreaks for three decades. However, transmission remains a key driver of outbreaks and should be an early focus for interventions to reduce CDI incidence.

Gastric Acid Suppression

The suppression of gastric acid can increase host susceptibility to a variety of infections. Dial and et al. (59) used cohort and case-control study designs to determine if exposure to PPIs was an independent risk factor for CDI. Multi-variable analyses conducted in each of the studies indicated significant adjusted odds ratios (95% confidence interval) of 2.1 (1.2–3.5) and 2.7 (1.4–5.2), identifying PPI exposure as a potential risk factor for CDI. The use of gastric acid suppressants has also been associated with the development of community-acquired CDI (37). Other investigations have implicated the use of PPIs as an independent risk factor for CDI in hospitalized patients (21,48,49,60,61), while others have not (35,62). One reason that PPIs may not be associated with risk in some studies is that antimicrobial use may be masking the PPI risk because of the strong statistical association for antimicrobials. Also, data confounding, which is inherent in retrospective studies, is likely to affect risk factor analyses. Thus, prospective studies are needed to resolve the issue of whether PPIs are truly associated with CDI, either directly or as a marker for other risk factors.

PPIs have been shown to cause diarrhea with or without specific histologic findings from biopsy specimens obtained during colonoscopy (forms of microscopic colitis such as lymphocytic and collagenous colitis) (63,64). And in some of these cases of collagenous colitis, pseudomembranes have been identified (65). Clinicians should be mindful of this as colitis caused by PPIs may interfere with, confuse, or delay the diagnosis of CDI.

Immune Response as a Risk Factor for CDI

Perhaps the most important host-related determinant in the development of CDI (after perturbations in the intestinal microbiota caused by antimicrobials or other drugs) is the ability to mount a sufficient Ig response to toxins produced by *C. difficile*. In a landmark study, those who failed to mount high serum antitoxin A IgG titers despite colonization with *C. difficile* were 48 times more likely to develop diarrhea than patients with an adequate immune response (133). The same workers went on to show that patients who had sub-optimal serum antitoxin A IgG responses were significantly more likely to experience recurrent CDI (66). In addition, a significant reduction in colonic mucosal IgA producing cells and macrophages is linked to recurrent CDI (39).

ENVIRONMENTAL RISKS

Since *C. difficile* is a spore-forming organism, it is not surprising that it is able to survive on inanimate surfaces for long periods of time (67). Admission to inpatient acute care facilities, long-term care facilities, and rehabilitation centers are consistently identified as risk factors for acquiring *C. difficile* since it is at these locations where most patients develop or are treated for CDI. Length of stay as well as proximity to symptomatic patients with CDI at these high-risk facilities increases the risk of acquiring toxigenic strains of *C. difficile* (156). This is not unique to *C. difficile*; placing patients in a room previously occupied by a patient with a drug-resistant organism (methicillin-resistant *S. aureus* or vancomycin-resistant enterococci, for instance) places the new tenant at risk for infection with the same organism (68). Likewise, it is known that as levels of environmental contamination rise, so does the prevalence of *C. difficile* found on the hands of healthcare workers (69). The risk of acquiring CDI during hospitalization is logically increased at dilapidated healthcare facilities, facilities with communal toilets and showers, institutions where cutbacks involving environmental services budgets and/or personnel have negatively impacted both the frequency and the extent of cleaning surfaces and equipment in patient rooms, and facilities where hand hygiene compliance is poor (159). Feeding tubes have been identified as risk factors for CDI (70), as they are surrogate markers for both increased contact with healthcare personnel and a means of delivering the organism directly from the environment into the gastrointestinal tract. The environment has proven a very important factor in the transmission dynamics of CDI, and interventions aimed at improving environmental cleaning must be implemented when an increased incidence of cases occurs (156).

PREVENTING AND MANAGING OUTBREAKS
Infection Control Interventions
One of the methods used to increase the yield of *C. difficile* from clinical samples when doing studies with this organism, particularly in asymptomatic carriers, is to use what is called the *alcohol shock procedure* (71). The bottom line is that *C. difficile* LOVES alcohol! Thus, perhaps AA (antibiotics anonymous) may be one of the most effective means to reduce CDI risk. While effective in its action against most pathogenic bacteria found in hospital settings, alcohol is ineffective against spore-forming organisms. In a recent study, between 18% and 60% of the initial inoculation of *C. difficile* spores on a contaminated hand could be readily transferred by a handshake after using commercially available alcohol gels (72). In contrast, the mechanical action of washing hands with running water and soap has proven effective in physically removing *C. difficile* from the hands of healthcare workers. While some anecdotally blame reliance on alcohol hand rubs for escalating *C. difficile* rates, a retrospective study did not support this notion (73). The CDC recommends handwashing using soap and running water rather than alcohol-based hand gels during outbreak situations and also recommends the use of contact precautions in all CDI patients (74). When caring for patients with CDI, washing hands with soap and running water should be done by healthcare workers to reduce the transmission of *C. difficile*. For all other patients, alcohol hand rubs should continue to be encouraged when there is no visible soiling of the hands.

Environmental Cleaning Interventions
Historically, *C. difficile*-associated epidemics have been attributed to specific strains, most of which have been shown to hypersporulate in contrast with their nonepidemic strain counterparts. It has been shown that the infamous United Kingdom outbreak strain (CD 001) is the "king of all spore producers." Notably, the most recent outbreak strain (CD BI/NAP1/027) also is considered

a hypersporulating strain when compared with typical *C. difficile* strains (31,32,75). For patients with CDI, fecal soiling of the environment occurs and, following exposure to air, spore forms of the organism predominate (77). A variety of cleaning agents are effective in killing the vegetative forms of the organism, but only chlorine-based disinfectants and high-concentration, vaporized hydrogen peroxide are sporicidal against *C. difficile* (78). Published data are lacking regarding the use of several expensive, commercially available combination products with sporicidal claims (chlorine-containing/surfactant detergent-containing products). Therefore, careful attention to the selection of hospital cleaning agents is necessary when attempting to impact rates of CDI (31,75,76,79).

Diluting concentrated sodium hypochlorite for use as a disinfecting solution to clean surfaces in patients' rooms has been shown to be effective in reducing environmental contamination of *C. difficile* and controlling CDI in high-rate facility units (79–82). Mayfield et al. (82) evaluated the effectiveness of sodium hypochlorite (5,000 ppm available chlorine), mixed fresh daily, versus quaternary ammonium environmental cleaning in patients' rooms for those with a positive *C. difficile* toxin test. In units where CDI rates exceeded three cases per 1,000 patient days, the use of sodium hypochlorite demonstrated a significant reduction in the rate of CDI. Interestingly, when the protocol was reversed and quaternary ammonium-based cleaning agents were reintroduced to those units, the rates returned to a high baseline (8.1 cases per 1,000 patient days). A follow-up evaluation revealed that an increase in CDI had occurred at the same institution from 3.9 cases per 1,000 patient days in 2001, to 5.8 cases per 1,000 patient days during the first six months of 2002 in the medical intensive care unit, and from 6.7 to 8 cases per 1,000 patient days in the bone marrow transplant unit over the same time period (80). Other investigations have demonstrated similar success when chlorine-based cleaning interventions were instituted (79,81). In one outbreak, sodium hypochlorite solutions at 500 parts per million (ppm) and 1,600 ppm decreased surface contamination by 79% and 98%, respectively (81). Similarly, Wilcox et al. (79) used 1,000 ppm available chlorine and showed, in a crossover study, that one of two wards had a significant reduction in incidence of CDI associated with hypochlorite cleaning. It is noteworthy that these two studies successfully used concentrations of bleach that were less than the concentrations used in some hospitals; e.g., 1,000 ppm vs. 5,000 ppm. Because sodium hypochlorite at higher concentrations can have damaging effects on equipment and other inanimate surfaces and may have deleterious effects in humans (respiratory reactions), it would be appealing to use lower concentrations, if possible. Currently, inexpensive bleach stabilizers that extend the potency of diluted bleach for longer than 30 days are available. This is attractive because adding stabilizers to diluted bleach is inexpensive, less resource intensive (eliminating the need to make fresh diluted bleach solutions daily), and, because the stabilizer does not contain surfactants (but does have detergent properties), a lower concentration can be used as a cleaning agent that does not provoke *C. difficile* sporulation (32). The use of higher concentrations could be reserved for outbreaks. The use of bleach is recommended by the CDC during outbreaks of CDI.

From an environmental control perspective, it is not only important to consider the choice of cleaning agents (e.g., proven sporicidal activity), but also to address the cleaning process itself. This means cleaning horizontal (high-touch) surfaces that commonly harbor *C. difficile* spores (e.g., bedrails, call buttons, telephones, floors) more often than upon terminal cleaning of the room. In Canada, a best practices document actually recommends twice daily cleanings in healthcare facilities. Due to staffing inadequacies faced by hospitals today, environmental services departments may have altered important cleaning practices unbeknownst to the infectious diseases experts within the facility. Failure to clean high-touch surfaces with the appropriate agent may lead to increased transmission within an institution. When faced with an outbreak (or even as a preventative measure), multidisciplinary discussions that include environmental services leadership should take place to determine what cleaning products are being used, what surfaces are being cleaned, and how often. "Bundled" approaches where resources are dedicated toward environmental cleaning, infection control, and programmatic antimicrobial stewardship interventions have been shown to be most effective in quelling outbreaks (49,80,83,84).

Hurdles (such as the reluctance to fund adequately staffed environmental services and/or infection control department) placed in the path of patient safety by nonclinicians in governmental or administrative roles had been encountered early in the battle against the epidemic *C. difficile* strain. A somewhat analogous situation led to a famous quotation during the Civil War in 1862. A dispatch sent by President Lincoln to Major-General George B. McClellan prompted by the Union general's unending list of feeble excuses for perpetually delaying a potentially war-ending intervention prompted the letter (abbreviated): *"My Dear Sir: ... you must act."* Indeed! A good example of government officials taking action occurred recently as a result, in part, of the BI/NAP1/027 strain of *C. difficile*-associated fatalities that received media attention in a relatively small region of Quebec, Canada. Ministry officials in Quebec subsequently directed 20 million dollars into hospital infection control resources and environmental infrastructure changes to combat CDI (85).

Since patients are often discharged to home following clinical improvement (but may remain symptomatic), it is advisable to recommend the bleaching of high-touch surfaces in the patient's environment (home bathrooms and other surfaces) as well as education regarding careful attention to hand hygiene. In addition, physicians' offices and outpatient surgical care centers, as part of the continuum of care, should be cognizant of the aforementioned vectors for transmission of *C. difficile* and how best to minimize transmission.

GENERAL MANAGEMENT PRINCIPLES OF CDI

Treatment algorithms used at our hospital and developed in collaboration with experts from North America and the United Kingdom (in light of the recent changes in CDI previously discussed and in the absence of national societal guidelines) are presented in Figures 4A and 4B (49). These guidelines were also co-developed in concert with local multidisciplinary opinion leaders, the guidelines were made accessible on the intranet, and were reproduced as order sets in our computerized physician order entry system in which the prescriber can order laboratory tests as well as the treatments to facilitate their use.

Some general principles of therapy should be outlined to preface any discussion of therapy for CDI. First, most references to vancomycin imply oral administration of the solution or capsule (or via retention enema where specified).

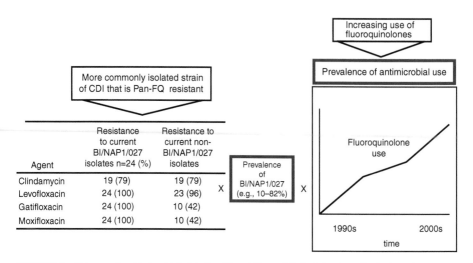

FIGURE 3 Drivers of antimicrobial risk for *Clostridium difficile* infection (CDI). This factors the appearance of resistant strains of *C. difficile*, the percentage of CDI cases caused by the strain expressing fluoroquinolone resistance, and the increasing amount of fluoroquinolones being used. Thus, an antimicrobial with a low odds ratio, if used frequently, will appear to be implicated to a greater extent in risk factor studies in contrast to a drug with a high odds ratio that is seldom used. This should be factored into the literature when evaluating studies and when formulating strategies to counter the escalating rates of CDI.

Intravenous vancomycin is ineffective for the treatment of CDI. Oral metronidazole is its preferred route of therapy, but unlike vancomycin, metronidazole can be administered intravenously for the therapy of CDI (although it has not been comparatively studied and failures have been noted) (15,86). To effectively navigate the following sections, therapy should be based on number of episodes of CDI the patient has had over the last six months, whether the patient has fulminant disease, and whether or not the gastrointestinal tract is functional or not. In addition to helping to guide appropriate therapy for CDI, knowledge of the previously mentioned information can facilitate early consultation of subspecialists such as infectious diseases, gastroenterology, and/or surgery.

The first step to managing a patient with suspected CDI is to implement optimal infection control precautions and place the patient into a private room if possible. We also switch from using alcohol hand rubs to handwashing with soap and water when caring for the identified potential CDI patient. Simultaneously, a *C. difficile* toxin test should be sent to the laboratory [we send a maximum of one per day, for three consecutive days (less if the test turns positive earlier) to increase the sensitivity of the EIA test], and to start empiric treatment according to our treatment algorithm while awaiting laboratory confirmation. It may be feasible in some centers that are not experiencing more severe forms of infection due to *C. difficile* to withhold therapy and "carefully watch and wait," as it has been shown that cessation of antibiotics alone is curative of CDI in approximately one quarter of patients with mild forms of disease. While we do not have the luxury of being in this position, as 69% of our isolates were of the BI/NAP1/027 strain when tested back in 2002 (22), some facilities may be able to carefully observe suspected patients with CDI without

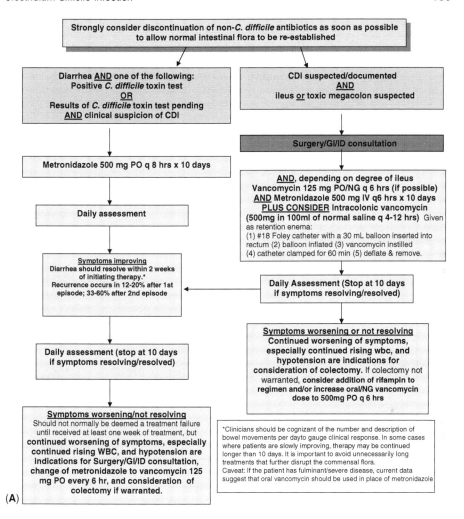

FIGURE 4A and **B** (A) *Clostridium difficile*-infection (CDI) in 1st or 2nd episode within 6 months. (*Continued*)

instituting empiric therapy, but those days, as mentioned, are limited. Once the *C. difficile* test is positive, there is no reason to send further samples to the laboratory as the patient is likely to have a positive test for a prolonged period of time following successful treatment. Thus, there is no such thing as a "test of cure" for *C. difficile* and no need for follow-up laboratory toxin testing. In addition, it is vitally necessary to re-evaluate the need for the offending anti-microbial agent or proton pump inhibitor (if the patient is still on therapy). For hospitals, this may be a function of education by the antimicrobial stewardship program, which hospitals are now encouraged to support (in part, for this very reason) (87). If the patient is receiving an antimicrobial for an underlying infection, its continued use must be carefully justified, potentially switched to an antimicrobial with reduced association with CDI, or otherwise discontinued. Because studies continue to report that antimicrobials are misused (e.g., given for

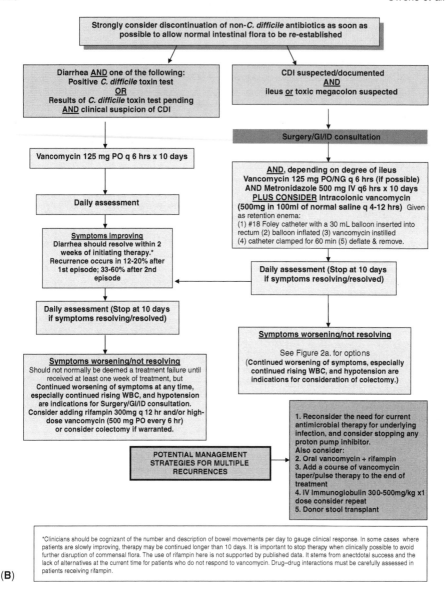

FIGURE 4A and **B** *(Continued)* **(B)** *Clostridium difficile*-infection (CDI) in ≥3rd episode within 6 months.

sinusitis without regard for duration of symptoms or issuing antibiotics to satisfy a patient's request rather than based on objective evaluation for actual infection) (88,89), it is not unreasonable to challenge the use of the antimicrobial and to promote short course therapy where indicated. A recent Cochrane review evaluated interventions to improve antibiotic prescribing practices among hospital inpatients (90); not surprisingly, they determined that programmatic strategies to improve antimicrobial use have been associated with significant reductions in CDI rates among other benefits.

There are several drugs that have been studied for the treatment of CDI, but only vancomycin is approved by the Food and Drug Administration (FDA) for this purpose. Because metronidazole has demonstrated equivalence, it has historically been adopted as the first-line drug for the treatment of CDI while oral vancomycin has been considered a second-line drug primarily due to cost. Teicoplanin (91), fusidic acid (92), and bacitracin (93,94) also have demonstrated efficacy similar to metronidazole or vancomycin.

THERAPY FOR 1ST OR 2ND EPISODES

For patients with 1st or 2nd episode of nonsevere CDI, and who have a functioning GI tract, up until now, metronidazole was recommended as first-line therapy (Fig. 4B). Data supporting this are derived from randomized comparative clinical trials with vancomycin recently compiled during a Cochrane systematic review (95), as well as in an informative review aptly titled "Metronidazole for *Clostridium difficile*-associated disease: is it okay for mom?" (96), a recent retrospective observational study of first recurrences that included infection with BI/NAP1/027 strains (97), and a recent study comparing metronidazole with nitazoxanide that demonstrated the latter was noninferior to metronidazole (98). However, two recent studies, one published (99), the other in abstract form from a randomized three-armed study, comparing tolevamer, vancomycin, and metronidazole, have demonstrated that vancomycin performs better for patients with severe disease. Therefore, guidelines will likely recommend that vancomycin is used preferably for patients with severe disease. Unfortunately, the definitions for severe disease, at least in the Zar paper (99), were very subjective. For example, the patients having mild/moderate versus severe disease had the same mean number of bowel movements per day. For first recurrences, guidelines have recommended retreatment with the same therapy used in the first episode (15). A recent study conducted during the Canadian outbreak with BI/NAP1/027 confirmed this approach is still viable. Regardless of whether metronidazole or vancomycin was used for the second episode cases, outcomes were similar (97). However, complication rates associated with recurrences were higher than that previously reported (97). A slightly delayed response has been observed with metronidazole with the mean number of days, with symptoms being 4.6 days compared with 3.0 days for vancomycin, but, ultimately, patients responded equally and experienced similar relapse rates (100). In most circumstances, metronidazole remains the drug of choice. Vancomycin is preferable when multiple episodes of CDI have been documented (see recurrent disease section), for severe CDI, or if intolerance to metronidazole exists. In vitro data have highlighted the potential poor efficacy of metronidazole in terms of cessation of toxin production by BI/NAP1/027. Furthermore, recent studies have highlighted inferior outcomes for metronidazole-treated cases of severe *C. difficile* BI/NAP1/027 infection.

A key problem is defining severe CDI prospectively. The three most frequently recognized risk factors for severe CDI are age, peak leukocytosis, and serum creatinine (6,27). However, age is too non-specific to be used as a predictor of severe CDI, and such observations are based on retrospective observations. No single parameter alone is highly predictive of severe CDI, with the possible exception of very high white blood cell count (WCC). Zar et al. (99) used a score based on age, WCC, temperature, albumin, endoscopy findings, and admission to the intensive care unit to define severe cases. Louie et al. (160) used number of stools, WCC, and abdominal pain to define severe CDI. Importantly, a definition of severe CDI based on number of diarrheal stools may suffer from difficulties in recording such episodes, especially in elderly patients with fecal incontinence. Furthermore, severe CDI may occasionally be characterized by ileus with no diarrhea. A prospectively validated severity score is needed. Until such time as this is available, clinicians need to be alert to the possibility of severe CDI. Possibilities to define severe CDI include any of the following: WCC >15, acutely rising serum creatinine (e.g., >50% increase above baseline), temperature > 38.5°C, or evidence of severe colitis (abdominal signs, radiology). The use of oral vancomycin is preferred to metronidazole. When oral vancomycin is used, evidence dictates that 125 mg administered every 6 hr is equivalent to 500 mg given every 6 hr in terms of efficacy (101), but costs significantly less. There also appears to be no value to adding rifampin to metronidazole for 1st episode cases of CDI (102). After the 1st episode of CDI, 15% to 30% of patients can expect to relapse, while if a second episode of CDI occurs, 33% to 60% of patients can expect to have a relapse (15).

In most parts of the world in vitro resistance among clinical isolates of *C. difficile* to either metronidazole or vancomycin have not been reported (103); therefore, the fear of in vitro resistance to metronidazole or vancomycin should not guide the selection of treatment. A small number of environmental isolates with elevated MICs to metronidazole and vancomycin has been reported (104) but validation by an outside laboratory has not occurred, and the clinical significance is unclear (as concentrations in stool, particularly for vancomycin, far exceed the MICs reported).

MANAGEMENT OF REFRACTORY CDI

For patients with refractory disease—those not responding at the day 4 to 6 evaluation point or who are worsening during treatment upon daily assessments—a few decisions need to be made. If markers for severe disease are present at any time during therapy (high WCC, increasing creatinine, ascites, obstruction, colonic perforation, toxic megacolon), surgical consultation is obligatory. Because of the high mortality associated with severe CDI, colectomy needs to be considered (105). Unfortunately, in one series of 67 patients undergoing colectomy for severe CDI, surgical morbidity was 81% and overall mortality was 48% (106).

If patients were originally started on oral metronidazole and are not responding (showing a reduction in the frequency of bowel movements) within 4 to 6 days, therapy can be changed to oral vancomycin. If vancomycin was the initial therapy (e.g., as in the case of recurrent disease), higher doses of vancomycin (500 mg 4 times daily) and/or combining vancomycin and rifampin may be tried. There are insufficient data to support the addition of rifampin; however, we have anecdotally had a number of successful outcomes by using this approach.

Intravenous Ig (IVIg) has been studied in a limited number of patients with refractory disease, but results have been mixed (107,108). The premise for therapy with IVIg is based on the fact that patients who develop severe disease and/or relapsing disease mount a poor antitoxin antibody response. Pooled IVIg may contain antitoxin A IgG. The largest study to date of IVIg was a retrospective, observational evaluation of 14 patients (107). Six of 14 patients responded clinically, and no relapse occurred within the timeframe reported. The doses used ranged from 150 to 400 mg/kg administered as a single-dose (one patient received a second dose). The median response time was 10 days. In another study, three of five patients treated with doses of IVIg between 300 and 500 mg/kg (with the most commonly used dose being 400 mg/kg) were deemed successes, with resolution occurring within 11 days (108). An upside to IVIg is that it may provide therapeutic option for patients with severe/relapsing disease where no other therapeutic options are available. Unfortunately, marginal efficacy, lack of data regarding the optimal dose, cost (~$1,500/dose for a 70 kg patient), and frequent shortages are significant disadvantages (109). That being said, there is enough data to recommend IVIg as an option at this point.

MANAGEMENT OF RECURRENT CDI

In the clinic it is difficult to determine if multiple episodes of CDI are due to re-infection with a new strain or relapses involving the original infecting strain of *C. difficile*. Vancomycin appears to be the drug of choice for multiply recurring cases of CDI (Fig. 4B) (110). One approach is to use vancomycin (125 mg 4 times daily) for 10 days followed by either pulse-dosed or tapered vancomycin regimens (110,111).

For endogenously recurring CDI, where spores may be the source of the problem (110,112), we favor a regimen of vancomycin administered in a pulsed fashion, 125 to 500 mg given as a single dose every 3 days for 2 to 3 weeks as described by McFarland (110). It is theorized that persistent spores revert to their vegetative state in the absence of a hostile environment (e.g., one that contains antimicrobials) where they regain susceptibility to the killing effects of the drug. Although higher-dose vancomycin (500 mg 4 times daily) is effective when given for 10 days to patients with recurrent CDI, it associated with higher recurrence rates than standard therapy followed by a pulsed or tapered vancomycin regimen (110). Higher-dose metronidazole was not effective at reducing future recurrences (and if used for longer periods of time may be associated with increased neurological adverse events) (110). The addition of rifampin to vancomycin has been reported to be effective in a small study of patients with recurrent CDI (113). We tend to use lower doses of rifampin (300 mg twice daily) than that studied (600 mg twice daily) for tolerability reasons (49). As always, the potential for drug interactions must be evaluated carefully prior to the addition of rifampin.

Donor stool transplantation has been shown to be remarkably effective in a small number of patients, and in a small number of our own cases (114–117). However, for obvious reasons that include the potential spread of other infections, this should currently be considered as a last resort and should involve some form of consent.

Adminstration of nontoxigenic strains of *C. difficile* has demonstrated efficacy in the classic hamster model of infection as well as in a limited number of patients (45,118). Toxigenic strains of *C. difficile* maintain their populations with a large fitness cost compared with nontoxigenic strains of *C. difficile*. There is demonstrable efficacy to this approach in animal studies. Nontoxigenic strains introduced into antibiotic-treated animals successfully compete with subsequently introduced toxigenic strains resulting in no mortality post-infection (45). This novel biopreventative strategy may indeed be one of the most promising and intriguing modalities currently being investigated. As of May 2007, nontoxigenic *C. difficile* (or NTX) has been given permission by the FDA to be studied in humans, pending a small study, required by the FDA.

Nonrecommended Strategies

A variety of management options with theoretical benefits, including probiotics, cholestyramine, and antiperistaltic agents, have gained popularity with some clinicians trying to manage recurrent and severe CDI. Unfortunately, data are insufficient to recommend these modalities or contradict their use. In addition, there is evidence of significant harm associated with their use [e.g., bacteremia/fungemia associated with probiotics, intraintestinal binding of vancomycin (and other drugs) by cholestyramine, toxic megacolon in association with loperamide use] (119–121). The efficacy of probiotics in patients with CDI remains to be a proven strategy, a position reinforced by a recent systematic review (122). Though historically at least two attempts to conduct meta-analyses have been tried to determine the efficacy of probiotics (123,124), this is not a statistically valid approach because study populations and designs/methods of the various small studies are so heterogeneous (patients, patient age groups, definitions of disease, lack of control for confounding, single organism vs. multi-organism preparations, some studies combined antimicrobial treatment with probiotics, others did not, duration of therapy) and introduction of author bias, that meta-analyses simply cannot be reliably performed or interpreted. These meta-analyses tend to have more in common with metaphysics. The one study evaluating *Saccharomyces boulardii* for the prevention of recurrent CDI demonstrated a slight benefit and has received the most attention (125); however, it did not result in approval from the FDA for this purpose (41). Moreover, an increasing body of literature has demonstrated the potential harm of probiotics when used in patients with CDI, chiefly in the form of bacteremias due to *Lactobacillus* sp. and fungemias due to *S. boulardii* in both immunocompetent and immunocompromised hosts (126–129).

A recent randomized, double-blind, placebo-controlled trial showed a beneficial effect of using a proprietary yogurt as prophylaxis in patients receiving antibiotics (161), but was fatally flawed because of several methodological issues. Crucially, only 7% of those screened for inclusion were recruited to the study, and controls received a milkshake as placebo, which may have increased the risk of diarrhea because of lactose intolerance (162). Thus, we do not recommend the use of probiotics for the prevention of CDI.

Similarly, anion-binding resins or adsorbants (cholestyramine, colestipol) have found their way into review articles as viable treatment options. These agents theoretically bind *C. difficile* toxins; however, a placebo-controlled trial demonstrated that colestipol was no more effective than placebo in reducing fecal excretion of *C. difficile* toxins (130). The potential for harm exists when these drugs are used, as they have been shown to bind to and reduce the biological activity of vancomycin (and a number of other drugs) (120,121). During our CDI outbreak, we witnessed an upsurge in the use of combined oral vancomycin and oral metronidazole combinations, *Lactobacillus* species-based probiotics, and cholestyramine (with or without anti-CDI antibiotics) (49). Because of their potential for harm with little or no benefit provided, we instituted locally specific, multidisciplinary developed (gastroenterology, infectious diseases, surgery, pharmacy), evidence-based guidelines, which were supplemented by prospective intervention and feedback provided by our antimicrobial stewardship program and our infection control colleagues (49). The result was statistically significant reductions in the use of the aforementioned potentially harmful regimens for CDI (51).

SPECIAL SITUATIONS
Fulminant Disease
Fulminant disease is marked by patients presenting with severe disease loosely defined by a constellation of the following: clinical markers such as a "toxic appearance," fever, admission to the intensive care unit, hypotension requiring vasopressors, laboratory findings of significant leukocytosis, lactate ≥ 5 mm, CT findings suggestive of free air in the abdomen (indicating perforation), colonic dilatation (indicating toxic megacolon), thickened colon wall, and/or ascites. In these patients, mortality rates attributable to CDI are high. In patients in whom these markers for severe disease are present, surgical consultation is urgently required to determine the need for urgent colectomy. In a recent retrospective evaluation of 165 patients with fulminant disease requiring intensive care unit admission, 53% ($n = 87$) died within 30 days of intensive care unit admission (38 of the 87 patients, 44%, actually died within 48 hr of admission to the intensive care unit) (104). Independent predictors of mortality included leukocytosis $\geq 50 \times 109$ (AOR, 18.6; 95% CI, 3.7–94.7), lactate ≥ 5 mm (AOR, 12.4; 95% CI, 2.4–63.7), age ≥ 75 years (AOR, 6.5; 95% CI, 1.7–24.3), immunosuppression (AOR, 7.9; 95% CI, 2.3–27.2), and shock requiring vasopressors (AOR, 3.4; 95% CI, 1.3–8.7). After correcting for confounding, patients benefited from emergency colectomy (AOR, 0.22; 95% CI, 0.07–0.67; $p = 0.0008$) over receiving medical therapy alone, particularly in those patients who were at least 65 years of age or older, immunocompetent, leukocytosis was $\geq 20 \times 109$, and lactate was between 2.2 and 4.9 mmol/L. Thus, surgical therapy is likely to be necessary and if medical therapy is to be tried, regimens as described in the following paragraph would be most appropriate. In addition, the use of IVIg may be warranted if the patient is not a surgical candidate and if disease is progressing despite recommended medical therapy. As mentioned, the data from Zar et al. (99) and the tolevamer registration trial seem to indicate that vancomycin should be used preferably over metronidazole for severe or fulminant disease.

CDI with a Non- or Partially-Functioning GI Tract
Not many choices are currently available for patients with a nonfunctional GI tract (Fig. 4A and 4B) and no randomized controlled trials have been conducted in this specific patient population. The best data come from an anectdotal 10 year experience at a single center (131). The goal is to get biologically active drug to a potentially walled-off site(s) of infection. This would include a regimen of intravenous metronidazole administered concurrently with vancomycin given orally or via nasogastric tube (if possible) and intracolonic vancomycin (if possible) (131). The treatment of CDI with intravenous metronidazole has not been rigorously studied and failures have been noted; therefore, this route alone is not optimal (86). Intracolonic vancomycin should be used with caution due to the friable state of the colonic mucosa, and surgical consultation is strongly advised in these patients. As these are treatment measures of last resort, colectomy should be considered if the patient continues to deteriorate during therapy.

PROPHYLAXIS

"Prophylaxis" with metronidazole or other anticlostridial treatments to prevent CDI in high-risk patients receiving antimicrobials for an underlying infection is unwarranted, as the very antibiotics that treat CDI are also capable of causing the disease (34,41,42). Moreover, the treatments themselves are only active against vegetative forms of C. *difficile* and have no effect on C. *difficile* spores; antimicrobials further disrupt the beneficial intestinal microbiota increasing the patient's susceptibility to CDI, and may select for other resistant organisms. Genuine methods for preventing disease, in the form of a vaccine, are under current investigation and are discussed later in this manuscript.

TREATMENT OF ASYMPTOMATIC CARRIERS

Like prophylaxis for CDI, the treatment of asymptomatic carriers is inappropriate and in all likelihood will increase the patient's chance of developing actual clinical disease (132). This is why it is important to only test patients' stools for toxin positivity in whom one suspects clinical disease. It is human nature to treat laboratory results rather than patients. Toxin test results should be used to supplement the diagnosis of CDI and not used to unilaterally define the presence of the bacterium. Patients who are toxin test positive, but lack clinical symptoms are most likely to be capable of mounting an adequate antitoxin A, IgG serum antibody response as described by Kyne et al. (66,133).

DRUGS BEING STUDIED FOR CDI

Rifaximin (Xifaxan®; Salix Pharmaceuticals, Morrisville, North Carolina, U.S.A.), a nonabsorbed semi-synthetic rifamycin derivative, is approved for use in traveler's diarrhea and is useful for hepatic encephalopathy. Unlike its analogues, rifampin and rifapentine, rifaximin is not well absorbed following oral administration. In fact, rifaximin is minimally absorbed (<0.4%) secondary to the addition of a benzimidazole ring. Rifaximin exerts its activity against susceptible strains by inhibiting the initiation of RNA synthesis secondary to its binding to RNA polymerase (134). Rifaximin does have good in vitro activity against C. *difficile*, with MIC values similar to rifampin; however, in vitro high-level resistance (MIC values >256 µg/mL) already exists to this compound (3% of strains tested in one series and occurred during therapy in another case series) (135,136). Because of documented resistance, coupled with a lack of clinical efficacy data, this drug should not be used for the treatment of CDI until its efficacy is confirmed in adequate trials and the clinical import of resistance to rifaximin is evaluated. In addition, because high-level resistance to this class of drugs exists already, and the number is said to be growing, its utility as monotherapy is all but over. Reports of the success of a small number of significant recurrent CDI patients (previously nearly dependent on continuous vancomycin treatment) treated with an active regimen (metronidazole or vancomycin), then followed by a two-week course of 800 mg/day (divided into 2–3 doses) of rifaximin was shown to be effective in seven of eight patients; however, high-level resistance occurred during therapy in one of the patients (136). Even if approval is granted by the FDA for CDI, with high-level resistance already reported, it will be difficult to imagine that this drug will be used as monotherapy.

Nitazoxanide (Alinia®; Romark Pharmaceuticals, Tampa, Florida, U.S.A.) is currently marketed for the treatment of a variety of parasitic diarrheal diseases. Nitazoxanide has in vitro activity against *C. difficile* and has recently been studied as a 500 mg twice daily regimen given for either 7 or 10 days versus metronidazole 250 mg 4 times daily for 10 days (98). This was a randomized, double-blind study in adult hospitalized patients, with between 36 and 40 patients in each of the 3 treatment arms. Response rates after 7 days of treatment and at 31 days after beginning treatment were 82.4, 57.6% for metronidazole; 90, 65.8% for nitazoxanide ×7 days; and 88.9, 74% for nitazoxanide ×10 days (98). In this relatively small study, nitazoxanide demonstrated noninferiority to metronidazole. The published analysis did not include an evaluation of the intent-to-treat population, which is important since ~23% of patients were excluded (32 patients) and may have influenced the outcome of the study. Importantly, the authors' state that, based on the results of the study, nitazoxanide may be useful for patients who fail to respond to metronidazole or patients in whom frequent recurrences occur. Clinicians need to be aware that this statement is not supported by the study results for two reasons: the study population was not representative of "metronidazole failures" and, second, it was not representative of a patient population with recurrent disease. The authors' view that nitazoxanide may be used to minimize the use of oral vancomycin, which they state should be used sparingly to minimize the selection of vancomycin-resistant bacteria, is misleading, as antimicrobials with anti-anaerobic activity (such as metronidazole), i.e., not only vancomycin, have been strongly linked to the selection of vancomycin-resistant enterococci in humans (98,137).

Tinidazole (Tindamax®; Mission Pharmacal, San Antonio, Texas, U.S.A.) is in the family of nitroimidizoles, like metronidazole. Tinidazole was approved by the FDA in 2004 for the treatment of trichomoniasis, giardiasis, and amebiasis. Tinidazole has been available in Europe for more than two decades. Similar to metronidazole, tinidazole exerts its activity by covalently binding to DNA, leading to the loss of helical structure, impaired template function, and strand breakage, consequently leading to cell death (138). Tinidazole is active in vitro against clinical isolates of *C. difficile* (139). Taste perversion, similar to metronidazole, is a common adverse event. Clinical studies evaluating the efficacy of tinidazole for the management of CDI are lacking, and, as such, this compound cannot be recommended for CDI at this time.

OPT-80, which has also been called PAR-101, and is likely to be named daxomicin, is an 18-membered macrolide compound with limited activity against intestinal flora, with good activity against *C. difficile*. This antibiotic was originally isolated from the fermentation broth of *Dactylsporangium aurantiacum*, subspecies *hamdenensis*. Phase III studies of OPT-80 are ongoing (140). Similar to other novel treatments for *C. difficile*, OPT-80 is minimally absorbed, demonstrates low MIC values against *C. difficile*, and has been shown to be effective in nonclinical models of CDI (141). Phase III studies are now under way and OPT-80 is now the furthest along of the CDI therapies.

Ramoplanin (Oscient Pharmaceuticals, Waltham, Massachusetts, U.S.A.) is in phase III development at the current time. Ramoplanin is an oral lipoglycodepsipeptide that has a mechanism of action similar to vancomycin. Ramoplanin demonstrated similar efficacy compared to vancomycin in the clindamycin-induced *C. difficile* infection model in hamsters (142). Interestingly, ramoplanin appeared to be superior to vancomycin in its effect against *C. difficile* spores and spore recrudescence ($p < 0.05$) in the in vitro gut model (142).

Tolevamer (Genzyme Corp., Cambridge, Massachusetts, U.S.A.) is a liquid polystyrene preparation that binds to *C. difficile* toxins A and B. The results of a randomized, double-blind, active-controlled phase II study in patients with mild to moderate CDI were recently reported (143). Two doses of tolevamer (3 g/day, 6 g/day) were evaluated against vancomycin (125 mg q 6 hr). Tolevamer 6 g/day, but not 3 g/day, demonstrated noninferiority to vancomycin, with a trend toward reduced recurrence in the high-dose tolevamer arm ($p = 0.05$) (143). Because tolevamer is not an antibiotic per se, commensal microbiota are not impacted and its therapeutic effect is purely due to toxin neutralization. Overall, tolevamer was well tolerated except for hypokalemia, which occurred in 23% of the tolevamer treated patients versus 7% of vancomycin recipients, ($p < 0.05$) (143). As a result of this study, a new liquid formulation of tolevamer that allows for higher doses to be administered and that contains potassium as a counter ion to minimize hypokalemia has been studied in a phase I trial (143). The most recent three-armed study involves tolevamer at a daily dose of 9 g/day, and is compared with oral vancomycin and oral metronidazole for the treatment of CDI (138). Data from one of two phase II studies demonstrated that tolevamer did not meet its endpoint of noninferiority against comparators (i.e., metronidazole and vancomycin), and therefore is not likely to be pursued (at least for monotherapy) (144,163).

Human Monolonal Antibodies (Medarex, Inc., Princeton, New Jersey, U.S.A.) against toxins A (MDX-066) and B (MDX-1388) have been evaluated in cell neutralization assays, the hamster h model of CDI, and have begun studies in humans. In the hamster model, a combination of both antitoxins A and B reduced mortality from 100% to 45% ($p < 0.0001$) (145). This treatment modality, if proven effective in humans, should offer either: (*i*) a monotherapy alternative to antimicrobials for the treatment of CDI that may be less likely to cause recurrent disease since colonization resistance is not disrupted; or (*ii*) the potential for use in combination with antimicrobials for fulminant CDI.

Toxoid Vaccine (Acambis Pharmaceuticals) has entered phase II trials. In a very small study of three patients with recurrent CDI (patients requiring 7–22 months of continuous vancomycin therapy), this parenterally administered *C. difficile* vaccine containing toxoid A and toxoid B was evaluated (146). Two of the three patients demonstrated increased IgG antitoxin A antibodies (3- and 4-fold increases), while an increased IgG antitoxin B antibody response was observed (20- and 50-fold) (146). All three patients were able to discontinue the use of vancomycin without further recurrence following vaccination.

SUMMARY

Since its original description in 1935, to its later proven association with disease and clindamycin administration in 1978, to periodic outbreaks around the world since that time, *C. difficile* has proven to be an evolutionary marvel that Darwin himself would be proud of. From outbreaks in the late 1980s and early 1990s due to the REA "J-type" strains demonstrating resistance to clindamycin and cephalosporins, to the REA "BI-type" *C. difficile* strains resistant to fluoroquinolones and cephalosporins, studies have implicated these antimicrobials as risks. There appears to be a strong association between antimicrobial resistance to *C. difficile* and the widespread use of the particular antimicrobial and the development of CDI. Further research should be focused on antimicrobial resistance as a risk factor for CDI, but this would require a paradigm shift; chiefly, more routine culturing of *C. difficile*. This would allow epidemiologic studies to help further delineate the role of antimicrobial resistance as a risk factor for CDI. Greater knowledge of this association would guide the selection of antimicrobial therapy for a patient's underlying infection that may also be at high risk for developing CDI.

The most recent epidemic strain of *C. difficile*, BI/NAP1/027, has been identified to possess relatively novel virulence characteristics. BI/NAP1/027 has the potential to hypersporulate, which in concert with cutbacks in health-care spending leading to reduced environmental services, nursing resources, and the decline of infrastructure, may explain its widespread dissemination. In contrast to other outbreak strains, certain virulence characteristics, such as increased toxin production, seem to provide rationale for more severe disease resulting in delayed response to traditional therapies, increased morbidity, and increased mortality.

If the greater morbidity and mortality have not captured the attention of healthcare systems, hospitals, and third party payers, the attributable costs associated with developing CDI should capture their attention. Lost revenue to healthcare systems due to extended lengths of stay, which in turn impedes patient flow; unoccupied beds in multiple-bed rooms; the imminent surge in pharmacy drug expenditures secondary to a predictable demand for a plethora of undoubtedly expensive drugs and biologics that will be trickling out of the pipeline; as well as the movement toward public reporting of infection due to *C. difficile* are also nonclinical incentives to become interested in CDI.

Hopefully it has been learned that it is too simplistic to assume that a basic change in an antimicrobial formulary or restricting a single antimicrobial will be successful in reducing CDI rates where BI/NAP1/027 strains are endemic. "Bundled" approaches—across the continuum of care—with strong administrative support for establishing formal antimicrobial stewardship programs in concert with infusing adequate resources into infection control, environmental services departments, and microbiology laboratories have been proven to make the greatest impact on reducing CDI rates.

From the clinician's perspective, using antimicrobials more judiciously (prescribing antimicrobials only when necessary; carefully monitoring completion of antimicrobials, with close observation in mild infections where antimicrobial use has not demonstrated a benefit; stopping antibiotics when infection is ruled out; using shortened courses of therapy when possible) is an achievable goal and one step toward reducing the risk of CDI. Initiating treatment for CDI early and closely monitoring the patient's clinical progress, washing hands with soap and water when specifically caring for CDI patients, and educating staff at the workplace and patients as they are discharged regarding proper cleaning and disinfection of the surrounding environment when dealing with this sporulating organism are likely to have an immediate impact. Finally, a host of treatments and preventative strategies are being investigated and may provide hope for reducing clinically frustrating recurrences as well as potentially life-threatening complications.

ACKNOWLEDGMENTS

We would like to express our deep gratitude to Drs. Dale Gerding and Tobi Karchmer and our internal *C. difficile* team of interested clinicians for their ongoing input into the treatment algorithm used at our hospital.

REFERENCES

1. Bartlett JG. Narrative review: the new epidemic of *Clostridium difficile*-associated enteric disease. Ann Intern Med 2006; 145(10):758–64.
2. Bartlett JG, Chang TW, Gurwith M, Gorbach SL, Onderdonk AB. Antibiotic-associated pseudomembranous colitis due to toxin-producing clostridia. N Engl J Med 1978; 298(10):531–4.
3. Asha NJ, Tompkins D, Wilcox MH. Comparative analysis of prevalence, risk factors, and molecular epidemiology of antibiotic-associated diarrhea due to *Clostridium difficile, Clostridium perfringens*, and *Staphylococcus aureus*. J Clin Microbiol 2006; 44(8):2785–91.
4. Hogenauer C, Langner C, Beubler E, et al. *Klebsiella oxytoca* as a causative organism of antibiotic-associated hemorrhagic colitis. N Engl J Med 2006; 355(23):2418–26.
5. McDonald LC, Owings M, Jernigan DB. *Clostridium difficile* infection in patients discharged from US short-stay hospitals, 1996–2003. Emerg Infect Dis 2006; 12(3):409–15.
6. Pepin J, Valiquette L, Alary ME, et al. *Clostridium difficile*-associated diarrhea in a region of Quebec from 1991 to 2003: a changing pattern of disease severity. CMAJ 2004; 171(5):466–72.
7. Wilcox MH, Freeman J. Epidemic *Clostridium difficile*. N Engl J Med 2006; 354(11):1199–203.
8. Nielsen ND, Layton BA, McDonald LC, Gerding DN, Liedtke LA, Strausbaugh LJ. Changing epidemiology of *Clostridium difficile*-associated disease: experience and perception of infectious diseases consultants. Infect Dis Clin Pract 2006; 14(5):296–302.
9. Eggertson L. Hospitals to report. *C. difficile* and MRSA. CMAJ 2007; 176(10):1402–3.
10. Wanahita A, Goldsmith EA, Marino BJ, Musher DM. *Clostridium difficile* infection in patients with unexplained leukocytosis. Am J Med 2003; 115(7):543–6.
11. Owens RC. *Clostridium difficile*-associated disease: changing epidemiology and implications for management. Drugs 2007; 67(4):487–502.
12. Freiler JF, Durning SJ, Ender PT. *Clostridium difficile* small bowel enteritis occurring after total colectomy. Clin Infect Dis 2001; 33(8):1429–31.
13. Nash SV, Bourgeault R, Sands M. Colonic disease associated with a positive assay for *Clostridium difficile* toxin: a retrospective study. J Clin Gastroenterol 1997; 25(2):476–9.
14. Mylonakis E, Ryan ET, Calderwood SB. *Clostridium difficile*–associated diarrhea: a review. Arch Intern Med 2001; 161(4):525–33.
15. Gerding DN, Johnson S, Peterson LR, Mulligan ME, Silva J Jr. *Clostridium difficile*-associated diarrhea and colitis. Infect Control Hosp Epidemiol 1995; 16(8):459–77.
16. Johnson S, Kent SA, O'Leary KJ, et al. Fatal pseudomembranous colitis associated with a variant *Clostridium difficile* strain not detected by toxin A immunoassay. Ann Intern Med 2001; 135(6):434–8.
17. Cloud J, Kelly CP. Update on *Clostridium difficile* associated disease. Curr Opin Gastroenterol 2007; 23(1):4–9.
18. Gerding DN. New definitions will help, but cultures are critical for resolving unanswered questions about *Clostridium difficile* 1. Infect Control Hosp Epidemiol 2007; 28(2):113–5.
19. Dallal RM, Harbrecht BG, Boujoukas AJ, et al. Fulminant *Clostridium difficile*: an underappreciated and increasing cause of death and complications. Ann Surg 2002; 235(3):363–72.
20. McEllistrem MC, Carman RJ, Gerding DN, Genheimer CW, Zheng L. A hospital outbreak of *Clostridium difficile* disease associated with isolates carrying binary toxin genes. Clin Infect Dis 2005; 40(2):265–72.
21. Muto CA, Pokrywka M, Shutt K, et al. A large outbreak of *Clostridium difficile*-associated disease with an unexpected proportion of deaths and colectomies at a teaching hospital following increased fluoroquinolone use. Infect Control Hosp Epidemiol 2005; 26(3):273–80.
22. McDonald LC, Killgore GE, Thompson A, et al. An epidemic, toxin gene-variant strain of *Clostridium difficile*. N Engl J Med 2005; 353(23):2433–41.

23. Eggertson L. Quebec strain of C. difficile in 7 provinces. CMAJ 2006; 174(5):607–8.
24. Giannasca PJ, Warny M. Active and passive immunization against *Clostridium difficile* diarrhea and colitis. Vaccine 2004; 22(7):848–56.
25. Alfa MJ, Kabani A, Lyerly D, et al. Characterization of a toxin A-negative, toxin B-positive strain of *Clostridium difficile* responsible for a nosocomial outbreak of *Clostridium difficile*-associated diarrhea. J Clin Microbiol 2000; 38(7):2706–14.
26. Voth DE, Ballard JD. *Clostridium difficile* toxins: mechanism of action and role in disease. Clin Microbiol Rev 2005; 18(2):247–63.
27. Loo VG, Poirier L, Miller MA, et al. A predominantly clonal multi-institutional outbreak of *Clostridium difficile*-associated diarrhea with high morbidity and mortality. N Engl J Med 2005; 353(23):2442–9.
28. Warny M, Pepin J, Fang A, et al. Toxin production by an emerging strain of *Clostridium difficile* associated with outbreaks of severe disease in North America and Europe. Lancet 2005; 366(9491):1079–84.
29. Freeman J, Fawley W, Baines S, Wilcox M. Measurement of toxin production by *Clostridium difficile*. Lancet 2006; 367(9515):982–3.
30. Barbut F, re D, Lalande V, et al. Clinical features of *Clostridium difficile*-associated diarrhoea due to binary toxin (actin-specific ADP-ribosyltransferase)-producing strains. J Med Microbiol 2005; 54(Pt. 2):181–5.
31. Wilcox MH, Fawley WN. Hospital disinfectants and spore formation by *Clostridium difficile*. Lancet 2000; 356(9238):1324.
32. Underwood S, Stephenson K, Fawley WN, et al. Effects of hospital cleaning agents on spore formation by N American and UK outbreak *Clostridium difficile* strains. 2005.
33. McFarland LV, Mulligan ME, Kwok RY, Stamm WE. Nosocomial acquisition of *Clostridium difficile* infection. N Engl J Med 1989; 320(4):204–10.
34. Bignardi GE. Risk factors for *Clostridium difficile* infection. J Hosp Infect 1998; 40(1):1–15.
35. Pepin J, Saheb N, Coulombe MA, et al. Emergence of fluoroquinolones as the predominant risk factor for *Clostridium difficile*-associated diarrhea: a cohort study during an epidemic in Quebec. Clin Infect Dis 2005; 41(9):1254–60.
36. Gerding DN. Clindamycin, cephalosporins, fluoroquinolones, and *Clostridium difficile*-associated diarrhea: this is an antimicrobial resistance problem. Clin Infect Dis 2004; 38(5):646–8.
37. Dial S, Delaney JA, Barkun AN, Suissa S. Use of gastric acid–suppressive agents and the risk of community-acquired *Clostridium difficile*-associated disease. JAMA 2005; 294(23):2989–95.
38. Mulligan ME, Miller SD, McFarland LV, Fung HC, Kwok RY. Elevated levels of serum immunoglobulins in asymptomatic carriers of *Clostridium difficile*. Clin Infect Dis 1993; 16(Suppl. 4):S239–44.
39. Johal SS, Lambert CP, Hammond J, James PD, Borriello SP, Mahida YR. Colonic IgA producing cells and macrophages are reduced in recurrent and non-recurrent *Clostridium difficile* associated diarrhoea. J Clin Pathol 2004; 57(9):973–9.
40. Johnson S, Gerding DN. *Clostridium difficile*-associated diarrhea. Clin Infect Dis 1998; 26(5):1027–34.
41. Bartlett JG. New drugs for *Clostridium difficile* infection. Clin Infect Dis 2006; 43(4):428–31.
42. Bingley PJ, Harding GM. *Clostridium difficile* colitis following treatment with metronidazole and vancomycin. Postgrad Med J 1987; 63(745):993–4.
43. Thomas C, Stevenson M, Riley TV. Antibiotics and hospital-acquired *Clostridium difficile*-associated diarrhoea: a systematic review. J Antimicrob Chemother 2003; 51(6):1339–50.
44. Clabots CR, Shanholtzer CJ, Peterson LR, Gerding DN. In vitro activity of efrotomycin, ciprofloxacin, and six other antimicrobials against *Clostridium difficile*. Diagn Microbiol Infect Dis 1987; 6(1):49–52.
45. Sambol SP, Merrigan MM, Tang JK, Johnson S, Gerding DN. Colonization for the prevention of *Clostridium difficile* disease in hamsters. J Infect Dis 2002; 186(12):1781–9.

46. Climo MW, Israel DS, Wong ES, Williams D, Coudron P, Markowitz SM. Hospital-wide restriction of clindamycin: effect on the incidence of *Clostridium difficile*-associated diarrhea and cost. Ann Intern Med 1998; 128(12 Pt. 1):989–95.
47. Pankuch GA, Jacobs MR, Appelbaum PC. Susceptibilities of 428 Gram-positive and - negative anaerobic bacteria to Bay y3118 compared with their susceptibilities to ciprofloxacin, clindamycin, metronidazole, piperacillin, piperacillin-tazobactam, and cefoxitin. Antimicrob Agents Chemother 1993; 37(8):1649–54.
48. Kazakova SV, Ware K, Baughman B, et al. A hospital outbreak of diarrhea due to an emerging epidemic strain of *Clostridium difficile*. Arch Intern Med 2006; 166(22):2518–24.
49. Owens RC. *Clostridium difficile*-associated disease: an emerging threat to patient safety: insights from the Society of Infectious Diseases Pharmacists. Pharmacotherapy 2006; 26(3):299–311.
50. Owens RC Jr. Optimizing formulary choices of the fluoroquinolones. Manag Care Interface 2005; Suppl:7–8, 12.
51. Owens RC Jr, Loew B, Soni S, Suissa S. Impact of interventions on non-evidence based treatment strategies during an outbreak of *Clostridium difficile*-associated disease due to BI/NAP1. (Abstract 687). In: Program and abstracts of the 44th Annual Infectious Diseases Society of America, Toronto, Ontario, CA. 2006:60.
52. Mohr J. Outbreak of *Clostridium difficile* infection and gatifloxacin use in a long-term care facility. Clin Infect Dis 2004; 39(6):875–6.
53. Owens RC Jr, Ambrose PG. Antimicrobial safety: focus on fluoroquinolones. Clin Infect Dis 2005; 41(Suppl. 2):S144–57.
54. Gaynes R, Rimland D, Killum E, et al. Outbreak of *Clostridium difficile* infection in a long-term care facility: association with gatifloxacin use. Clin Infect Dis 2004; 38(5):640–5.
55. McCusker ME, Harris AD, Perencevich E, Roghmann MC. Fluoroquinolone use and *Clostridium difficile*-associated diarrhea. Emerg Infect Dis 2003; 9(6):730–3.
56. Dhalla IA, Mamdani MM, Simor AE, Kopp A, Rochon PA, Juurlink DN. Are broad-spectrum fluoroquinolones more likely to cause *Clostridium difficile*-associated disease? Antimicrob Agents Chemother 2006; 50(9):3216–9.
57. Biller P, Shank B, Lind L, et al. Moxifloxacin therapy as a risk factor for *Clostridium difficile*-associated disease during an outbreak: attempts to control a new epidemic strain. J Infect Control Hosp Epidemiol 2007; 28(2):198–201.
58. Kutty P, Benoit S, Woods C, et al. Emerging *Clostridium difficile*-associated disease in the community and the role of non-antimicrobial risk factors. (Abstr. LB-28). 2006:242.
59. Dial S, Alrasadi K, Manoukian C, Huang A, Menzies D. Risk of *Clostridium difficile* diarrhea among hospital inpatients prescribed proton pump inhibitors: cohort and case-control studies. CMAJ 2004; 171(1):33–8.
60. Al-Tureihi FI, Hassoun A, Wolf-Klein G, Isenberg H. Albumin, length of stay, and proton pump inhibitors: key factors in *Clostridium difficile*-associated disease in nursing home patients. J Am Med Dir Assoc 2005; 6(2):105–8.
61. Cunningham R, Dale B, Undy B, Gaunt N. Proton pump inhibitors as a risk factor for *Clostridium difficile* diarrhoea. J Hosp Infect 2003; 54(3):243–5.
62. Lowe DO, Mamdani MM, Kopp A, Low DE, Juurlink DN. Proton pump inhibitors and hospitalization for *Clostridium difficile*-associated disease: a population-based study. Clin Infect Dis 2006; 43(10):1272–6.
63. Rammer M, Kirchgatterer A, Hobling W, Knoflach P. Lansoprazole-associated collagenous colitis: a case report. Z Gastroenterol 2005; 43(7):657–60.
64. Thomson RD, Lestina LS, Bensen SP, Toor A, Maheshwari Y, Ratcliffe NR. Lansoprazole-associated microscopic colitis: a case series. Am J Gastroenterol 2002; 97(11):2908–13.
65. Yuan S, Reyes V, Bronner MP. Pseudomembranous collagenous colitis. Am J Surg Pathol 2003; 27(10):1375–9.
66. Kyne L, Warny M, Qamar A, Kelly CP. Association between antibody response to toxin A and protection against recurrent *Clostridium difficile* diarrhoea. Lancet 2001; 357(9251):189–93.

67. Kim KH, Fekety R, Batts DH, et al. Isolation of *Clostridium difficile* from the environment and contacts of patients with antibiotic-associated colitis. J Infect Dis 1981; 143(1):42–50.
68. Huang SS, Datta R, Platt R. Risk of acquiring antibiotic-resistant bacteria from prior room occupants. Arch Intern Med 2006; 166(18):1945–51.
69. Samore MH, Venkataraman L, DeGirolami PC, Arbeit RD, Karchmer AW. Clinical and molecular epidemiology of sporadic and clustered cases of nosocomial *Clostridium difficile* diarrhea. Am J Med 1996; 100(1):32–40.
70. Bliss DZ, Johnson S, Savik K, Clabots CR, Willard K, Gerding DN. Acquisition of *Clostridium difficile* and *Clostridium difficile*-associated diarrhea in hospitalized patients receiving tube feeding. Ann Intern Med 1998; 129(12):1012–9.
71. Clabots CR, Gerding SJ, Olson MM, Peterson LR, Gerding DN. Detection of asymptomatic *Clostridium difficile* carriage by an alcohol shock procedure. J Clin Microbiol 1989; 27(10):2386–7.
72. Leischner J, Johnson S, Sambol S, Parada J, Gerding DN. Effect of alcohol hand gels and chlorhexidine hand wash in removing spores of *Clostridium difficile* from hands. (Abstract KB-29) In: Program and Abstracts of the 45th Annual Interscience Conference on Antimicrobial Agents and Chemotherapy. Washington, D.C., December 2005.
73. Boyce JM, Ligi C, Kohan C, Dumigan D, Havill NL. Lack of association between the increased incidence of *Clostridium difficile*-associated disease and the increasing use of alcohol-based hand rubs. Infect Control Hosp Epidemiol 2006; 27(5):479–83.
74. Information About a New Strain of *Clostridium Difficile*, 2005. (Accessed August 21, 2006, at http://www.cdc.gov/ncidod/dhqp/id_CdiffFAQ_newstrain.html)
75. Wilcox MH. Cleaning up *Clostridium difficile* infection. Lancet 1996; 348(9030):767–8.
76. Underwood S, Stephenson K, Fawley WN, et al. Effects of hospital cleaning agents on spore formation by N American and UK outbreak *Clostridium difficile* strains. (Abstract LB-28). In: Program and abstracts of the 45th Annual Interscience Conference on Antimicrobial Agents and Chemotherapy, Washington, DC, December 16–19, 2005. Washington, DC: American Society for Microbiology, 2005.
77. Wilcox MH, Fawley WN, Parnell P. Value of lysozyme agar incorporation and alkaline thioglycollate exposure for the environmental recovery of *Clostridium difficile*. J Hosp Infect 2000; 44(1):65–9.
78. Rutala WA, Weber DJ. Uses of inorganic hypochlorite (bleach) in health-care facilities. Clin Microbiol Rev 1997; 10(4):597–610.
79. Wilcox MH, Fawley WN, Wigglesworth N, Parnell P, Verity P, Freeman J. Detergent versus hypochlorite cleaning and *Clostridium difficile* infection. J Hosp Infect 2004; 56(4):331.
80. Apisarnthanarak A, Zack JE, Mayfield JL, et al. Effectiveness of environmental and infection control programs to reduce transmission of *Clostridium difficile*. Clin Infect Dis 2004; 39(4):601–2.
81. Kaatz GW, Gitlin SD, Schaberg DR, et al. Acquisition of *Clostridium difficile* from the hospital environment. Am J Epidemiol 1988; 127(6):1289–94.
82. Mayfield JL, Leet T, Miller J, Mundy LM. Environmental control to reduce transmission of *Clostridium difficile*. Clin Infect Dis 2000; 31(4):995–1000.
83. Davey P, Brown E, Fenelon L, et al. Systematic review of antimicrobial drug prescribing in hospitals. Emerg Infect Dis 2006; 12(2):211–6.
84. Valenti AJ. The role of infection control and hospital epidemiology in the optimization of antibiotic use. In: Owens RCJr, Ambrose PG, Nightingale CH, eds. Antibiotic Optimization: Concepts and Strategies in Clinical Practice. 1st ed. New York: Marcel Dekker, 2005:209–59.
85. Eggertson L. Quebec puts up 20 million dollars for. *C. difficile* fight 1. CMAJ 2005; 172(5):622.
86. Friedenberg F, Fernandez A, Kaul V, Niami P, Levine GM. Intravenous metronidazole for the treatment of *Clostridium difficile* colitis. Dis Colon Rectum 2001; 44(8):1176–80.
87. Dellit TH, Owens RC, McGowan JE Jr, et al. Infectious diseases society of america and the society for healthcare epidemiology of america guidelines for developing an

institutional program to enhance antimicrobial stewardship. Clin Infect Dis 2007; 44(2):159–77.

88. Palmer DA, Bauchner H. Parents' and physicians' views on antibiotics. Pediatrics 1997; 99(6):E6.

89. Watson RL, Dowell SF, Jayaraman M, Keyserling H, Kolczak M, Schwartz B. Antimicrobial use for pediatric upper respiratory infections: reported practice, actual practice, and parent beliefs. Pediatrics 1999; 104(6):1251–7.

90. Davey P, Brown E, Fenelon L, et al. Interventions to improve antibiotic prescribing practices for hospital inpatients. Cochrane Database Syst Rev 2005; (4):CD003543.

91. de LF, Nicolin R, Rinaldi E, et al. Prospective study of oral teicoplanin versus oral vancomycin for therapy of pseudomembranous colitis and *Clostridium difficile*-associated diarrhea. Antimicrob Agents Chemother 1992; 36(10):2192–6.

92. Wullt M, Odenholt I. A double-blind randomized controlled trial of fusidic acid and metronidazole for treatment of an initial episode of *Clostridium difficile*-associated diarrhoea. J Antimicrob Chemother 2004; 54(1):211–16.

93. Dudley MN, McLaughlin JC, Carrington G, Frick J, Nightingale CH, Quintiliani R. Oral bacitracin vs vancomycin therapy for *Clostridium difficile*-induced diarrhea. A randomized double-blind trial. Arch Intern Med 1986; 146(6):1101–4.

94. Young GP, Ward PB, Bayley N, et al. Antibiotic-associated colitis due to *Clostridium difficile*: double-blind comparison of vancomycin with bacitracin. Gastroenterology 1985; 89(5):1038–45.

95. Bricker E, Garg R, Nelson R, Loza A, Novak T, Hansen J. Antibiotic treatment for *Clostridium difficile*-associated diarrhea in adults. Cochrane Database Syst Rev 2005; (1):CD004610.

96. Gerding DN. Metronidazole for *Clostridium difficile*-associated disease: is it okay for mom? Clin Infect Dis 2005; 40(11):1598–600.

97. Pepin J, Routhier S, Gagnon S, Brazeau I. Management and outcomes of a first recurrence of *Clostridium difficile*-associated disease in Quebec, Canada. Clin Infect Dis 2006; 42(6):758–64.

98. Musher DM, Logan N, Hamill RJ, et al. Nitazoxanide for the treatment of *Clostridium difficile* colitis. Clin Infect Dis 2006; 43(4):421–7.

99. Zar FA, Bakkanagari SR, Moorthi KA, et al. A comparison of vancomycin and metronidazole for the treatment of *Clostridium difficile*-associated diarrhea, stratified by disease severity. Clin Infect Dis 2007; 45:302–7.

100. Wilcox MH, Howe R. Diarrhoea caused by *Clostridium difficile*: response time for treatment with metronidazole and vancomycin. J Antimicrob Chemother 1995; 36(4):673–9.

101. Fekety R, Silva J, Kauffman C, Buggy B, Deery HG. Treatment of antibiotic-associated *Clostridium difficile* colitis with oral vancomycin: comparison of two dosage regimens. Am J Med 1989; 86(1):15–9.

102. Lagrotteria D, Holmes S, Smieja M, Smaill F, Lee C. Prospective, randomized inpatient study of oral metronidazole versus oral metronidazole and rifampin for treatment of primary episode of *Clostridium difficile*-associated diarrhea. Clin Infect Dis 2006; 43(5):547–52.

103. Freeman J, Stott J, Baines SD, Fawley WN, Wilcox MH. Surveillance for resistance to metronidazole and vancomycin in genotypically distinct and UK epidemic *Clostridium difficile* isolates in a large teaching hospital. J Antimicrob Chemother 2005; 56(5):988–9.

104. Pelaez T, Alcala L, Alonso R, Rodriguez-Creixems M, Garcia-Lechuz JM, Bouza E. Reassessment of *Clostridium difficile* susceptibility to metronidazole and vancomycin. Antimicrob Agents Chemother 2002; 46(6):1647–50.

105. Lamontagne F, Labbe AC, Haeck O, et al. Impact of emergency colectomy on survival of patients with fulminant *Clostridium difficile* colitis during an epidemic caused by a hypervirulent strain. Ann Surg 2007; 245(2):267–72.

106. Longo WE, Mazuski JE, Virgo KS, Lee P, Bahadursingh AN, Johnson FE. Outcome after colectomy for *Clostridium difficile* colitis. Dis Colon Rectum 2004; 47(10):1620–6.

107. McPherson S, Rees CJ, Ellis R, Soo S, Panter SJ. Intravenous immunoglobulin for the treatment of severe, refractory, and recurrent *Clostridium difficile* diarrhea. Dis Colon Rectum 2006; 49(5):640–5.

108. Wilcox MH. Descriptive study of intravenous immunoglobulin for the treatment of recurrent *Clostridium difficile* diarrhoea. J Antimicrob Chemother 2004; 53(5):882–4.
109. Thorpe CM, Gorbach SL. Update on *Clostridium difficile*. Curr Treat Options Gastroenterol 2006; 9(3):265–71.
110. McFarland LV, Elmer GW, Surawicz CM. Breaking the cycle: treatment strategies for 163 cases of recurrent *Clostridium difficile* disease. Am J Gastroenterol 2002; 97(7):1769–75.
111. McFarland LV. Alternative treatments for *Clostridium difficile* disease: what really works? J Med Microbiol 2005; 54(Pt. 2):101–11.
112. Tedesco FJ, Gordon D, Fortson WC. Approach to patients with multiple relapses of antibiotic-associated pseudomembranous colitis. Am J Gastroenterol 1985; 80(11):867–8.
113. Buggy BP, Fekety R, Silva J Jr. Therapy of relapsing *Clostridium difficile*-associated diarrhea and colitis with the combination of vancomycin and rifampin. J Clin Gastroenterol 1987; 9(2):155–9.
114. Aas J, Gessert CE, Bakken JS. Recurrent *Clostridium difficile* colitis: case series involving 18 patients treated with donor stool administered via a nasogastric tube. Clin Infect Dis 2003; 36(5):580–5.
115. Liacouras CA, Piccoli DA. Whole-bowel irrigation as an adjunct to the treatment of chronic, relapsing *Clostridium difficile* colitis. J Clin Gastroenterol 1996; 22(3):186–9.
116. Persky SE, Brandt LJ. Treatment of recurrent *Clostridium difficile*-associated diarrhea by administration of donated stool directly through a colonoscope. Am J Gastroenterol 2000; 95(11):3283–5.
117. Tvede M, Rask-Madsen J. Bacteriotherapy for chronic relapsing *Clostridium difficile* diarrhoea in six patients. Lancet 1989; 1(8648):1156–60.
118. Seal D, Borriello SP, Barclay F, Welch A, Piper M, Bonnycastle M. Treatment of relapsing *Clostridium difficile* diarrhoea by administration of a non-toxigenic strain. Eur J Clin Microbiol 1987; 6(1):51–3.
119. Nakai A, Nishikata M, Matsuyama K, Ichikawa M. Drug interaction between simvastatin and cholestyramine in vitro and in vivo. Biol Pharm Bull 1996; 19(9):1231–3.
120. Taylor NS, Bartlett JG. Binding of *Clostridium difficile* cytotoxin and vancomycin by anion-exchange resins. J Infect Dis 1980; 141(1):92–7.
121. Wilcox MH. Treatment of *Clostridium difficile* infection. J Antimicrob Chemother 1998; 41(Suppl. C):41–6.
122. Dendukuri N, Costa V, McGregor M, Brophy JM. Probiotic therapy for the prevention and treatment of *Clostridium difficile*-associated diarrhea: a systematic review. CMAJ 2005; 173(2):167–70.
123. D'Souza AL, Rajkumar C, Cooke J, Bulpitt CJ. Probiotics in prevention of antibiotic associated diarrhoea: meta-analysis. BMJ 2002; 324(7350):1361.
124. McFarland LV. Meta-analysis of probiotics for the prevention of antibiotic associated diarrhea and the treatment of *Clostridium difficile* disease. Am J Gastroenterol 2006; 101(4):812–22.
125. McFarland LV, Surawicz CM, Greenberg RN, et al. A randomized placebo-controlled trial of *Saccharomyces boulardii* in combination with standard antibiotics for *Clostridium difficile* disease. JAMA 1994; 271(24):1913–18.
126. Salminen MK, Rautelin H, Tynkkynen S, et al. *Lactobacillus* bacteremia, clinical significance, and patient outcome, with special focus on probiotic *L. rhamnosus* GG. Clin Infect Dis 2004; 38(1):62–9.
127. Lherm T, Monet C, Nougiere B, et al. Seven cases of fungemia with *Saccharomyces boulardii* in critically ill patients. Intensive Care Med 2002; 28(6):797–801.
128. Enache-Angoulvant A, Hennequin C. Invasive *Saccharomyces* infection: a comprehensive review. Clin Infect Dis 2005; 41(11):1559–68.
129. Cassone M, Serra P, Mondello F, et al. Outbreak of *Saccharomyces cerevisiae* subtype *boulardii* fungemia in patients neighboring those treated with a probiotic preparation of the organism. J Clin Microbiol 2003; 41(11):5340–3.
130. Mogg GA, George RH, Youngs D, et al. Randomized controlled trial of colestipol in antibiotic-associated colitis. Br J Surg 1982; 69(3):137–9.

131. Olson MM, Shanholtzer CJ, Lee JT Jr, Gerding DN. Ten years of prospective *Clostridium difficile*-associated disease surveillance and treatment at the Minneapolis VA Medical Center, 1982–1991. Infect Control Hosp Epidemiol 1994; 15(6):371–81.

132. Johnson S, Homann SR, Bettin KM, et al. Treatment of asymptomatic *Clostridium difficile* carriers (fecal excretors) with vancomycin or metronidazole. A randomized, placebo-controlled trial. Ann Intern Med 1992; 117(4):297–302.

133. Kyne L, Warny M, Qamar A, Kelly CP. Asymptomatic carriage of *Clostridium difficile* and serum levels of IgG antibody against toxin A. N Engl J Med 2000; 342(6):390–7.

134. Gerard L, Garey KW, Dupont HL. Rifaximin: a nonabsorbable rifamycin antibiotic for use in nonsystemic gastrointestinal infections. Expert Rev Anti Infect Ther 2005; 3(2):201–11.

135. Gerding DN, Johnson S, Osmolski JR, Sambol SP. In vitro activity of ramoplanin, rifalazil, rifaximin, metronidazole, and vancomycin against 110 unique toxigenic *Clostridium difficile* clinical isolates. (Abstract E-1439). 2005:171.

136. Johnson S, Schriever C, Galang M, Kelly CP, Gerding DN. Interruption of recurrent *Clostridium difficile*-associated diarrhea episodes by serial therapy with vancomycin and rifaximin. Clin Infect Dis 2007; 44(6):846–8.

137. Donskey CJ, Chowdhry TK, Hecker MT, et al. Effect of antibiotic therapy on the density of vancomycin-resistant enterococci in the stool of colonized patients. N Engl J Med 2000; 343(26):1925–32.

138. Jodlowski TZ, Oehler R, Kam LW, Melnychuk I. Emerging therapies in the treatment of *Clostridium difficile*-associated disease. Ann Pharmacother 2006; 40(12):2164–9.

139. Citron DM, Tyrrell KL, Warren YA, Fernandez H, Merriam CV, Goldstein EJ. In vitro activities of tinidazole and metronidazole against *Clostridium difficile*, *Prevotella bivia* and *Bacteroides fragilis*. Anaerobe 2005; 11(6):315–17.

140. Louie TJ. Treatment of first recurrences of *Clostridium difficile*-associated disease: waiting for new treatment options. Clin Infect Dis 2006; 42(6):765–7.

141. Ackermann G, Loffler B, Adler D, Rodloff AC. In vitro activity of OPT-80 against *Clostridium difficile*. Antimicrob Agents Chemother 2004; 48(6):2280–2.

142. Freeman J, Baines SD, Jabes D, Wilcox MH. Comparison of the efficacy of ramoplanin and vancomycin in both in vitro and in vivo models of clindamycin-induced *Clostridium difficile* infection. J Antimicrob Chemother 2005; 56(4):717–25.

143. Louie TJ, Peppe J, Watt CK, et al. Tolevamer, a novel nonantibiotic polymer, compared with vancomycin in the treatment of mild to moderately severe *Clostridium difficile*-associated diarrhea. Clin Infect Dis 2006; 43(4):411–20.

144. Owens RC Jr., Valenti AJ. *Clostridium difficule*-associated disease in the new millenium: "The Perfect Storm" has arrived. Infect Dis Clin Practice 2007; 15(5):299–315.

145. Babcock GJ, Broering TJ, Hernandez HJ, et al. Human monoclonal antibodies directed against toxins A and B prevent *Clostridium difficile*-induced mortality in hamsters. Infect Immun 2006; 74(11):6339–47.

146. Sougioultzis S, Kyne L, Drudy D, et al. *Clostridium difficile* toxoid vaccine in recurrent. *C. difficile*-associated diarrhea. Gastroenterology 2005; 128(3):764–70.

147. McCaig LF, Besser RE, Hughes JM. Trends in antimicrobial prescribing rates for children and adolescents. JAMA 2002; 287(23):3096–102.

148. Ensminger PW, Counter FT, Thomas LJ, Lubbehusen PP. Susceptibility, resistance development, and synergy of antimicrobial combinations against *Clostridium difficile*. Curr Microbiol 1982; 7:59–62.

149. Pelaez T, Alonso R, Perez C, Alcala L, Cuevas O, Bouza E. In vitro activity of linezolid against *Clostridium difficile* 1. Antimicrob Agents Chemother 2002; 46(5):1617–18.

150. Wilcox MH, Fawley W, Freeman J, Brayson J. In vitro activity of new generation fluoroquinolones against genotypically distinct and indistinguishable *Clostridium difficile* isolates. J Antimicrob Chemother 2000; 46(4):551–6.

151. Dzink J, Bartlett JG. In vitro susceptibility of *Clostridium difficile* isolates from patients with antibiotic-associated diarrhea or colitis. Antimicrob Agents Chemother 1980; 17(4):695–8.

152. Nord CE. In vitro activity of quinolones and other antimicrobial agents against anaerobic bacteria. Clin Infect Dis 1996; 23(Suppl. 1):S15–18.

153. Hecht DW, Galang MA, Sambol SP, Osmolski JR, Johnson S, Gerding DN. In vitro activities of 15 antimicrobial agents against 110 toxigenic *Clostridium difficile* clinical isolates collected from 1983 to 2004. Antimicrob Agents Chemother 2007; 51:2716–9.

154. Freeman J, Baines SD, Saxton K, Wilcox MH. Effect of metronidazole on growth and toxin production by epidemic *Clostridium difficile* PCR ribotypes 001 and 027 in a human gut model. J Antimicrob Chemother 2007; 60:83–91.

155. Harmanus C, van den Berg R, Fawley W, et al. Use of highly discriminatory fingerprinting to analyse epidemic *Clostridium difficile* ribotype 027 isolates. 47th Interscience Conference on Antimicrobial Agents and Chemotherapy, Chicago, 2007. Abstract K-424.

156. Dubberke ER, Reske KA, Olsen MA, et al. Evaluation of *Clostridium difficile*-associated disease pressure as a risk factor for *C. difficile*-associated disease. Arch Intern Med 2007; 167:1092–7.

157. Wilcox MH, Freeman J. Epidemic *Clostridium difficile*. N Engl J Med 2006; 354:1199–203.

158. Saxton K, Baines SD, Freeman J, Wilcox MH. Effects of exposure of *Clostridium difficile* 027 to fluoroquinolones in a human gut model: 47th Interscience Conference on Antimicrobial Agents and Chemotherapy, Chicago, 2007. Abstract B-824.

159. Fawley WN, Wilcox MH. Molecular epidemiology of endemic *Clostridium difficile* infection. Epidemiol Infect 2001; 126:343–50.

160. Louie T, Gerson M, Grimard D, et al. Results of a phase III trial comparing tolevamer, vancomycin and metronidazole in patients with *Clostridium difficile* associated diarrhea. ICAAC 2007. Abstract LB 3826.

161. Hickson M, D'Souza AL, Muthu N, et al. Use of probiotic *Lactobacillus* preparation to prevent diarrhoea associated with antibiotics: randomised, 2007, double blind placebo controlled trial. BMJ 2007; 335:80.

162. Wilcox MH, Sandoe JA. Results of study of probiotic yoghurt drink to prevent antibiotic-associated diarrhoea are not widely applicable. BMJ 2007. http://www.bmj.com/cgi/eletters/335/7610/80 (last accessed October 2007).

163. Louie T, Gerson M, Grimard D, et al. Results of a phase III trial comparing tolevamer, vancomycin and metronidazole in patients with *Clostridium difficile* associated diarrhea. ICAAC 2007. Abstract LB 3826.

Emerging Resistance Among *Candida* Species: Trends and Treatment Considerations for Candidemia

Ingi Lee
Division of Infectious Diseases, Hospital of the University of Pennsylvania, Philadelphia, Pennsylvania, U.S.A.

Theoklis Zaoutis
Department of Pediatrics and Epidemiology, University of Pennsylvania School of Medicine, and Division of Infectious Diseases, The Children's Hospital of Philadelphia, Philadelphia, Pennsylvania, U.S.A.

BACKGROUND

Fungal infections first became recognized as an important cause of human disease in the 1980s, particularly among immunocompromised patients. Over the past two decades, there has been a significant increase in their incidence (1,2). This increase has mirrored the increase in vulnerable patient populations, including bone marrow transplant recipients, solid organ transplant recipients, patients undergoing abdominal surgery, patients with malignancy undergoing chemotherapy, and patients treated with various immunosuppressant medications, as well as an increase in the use of broad-spectrum antibiotics (3).

The most common invasive fungal infections are secondary to *Candida*, *Cryptococcus*, and *Aspergillus* species. Of these, *Candida* species are the most commonly encountered in the healthcare setting and have been associated with significant morbidity and mortality. Interestingly, there has been a shift in the epidemiology of candidemia, with a decrease in *C. albicans* and an increase in non-*C. albicans* species, particularly *C. glabrata* (4). This emergence is notable given that *C. glabrata*, unlike *C. albicans*, is often associated with fluconazole resistance. Therefore, this has had important implications on the clinical management of candidemia.

This chapter discusses the impact of candidemia, including its spectrum of disease, the notable shift in epidemiology, resistance trends, morbidity and mortality costs, identifiable risk factors, diagnosis and susceptibility testing, and treatment options, with a focus on the emergence of more resistant *Candida* species, particularly *C. glabrata*.

SPECTRUM OF DISEASE

Candida species are ubiquitous yeast found not only in the environment, but as a normal colonizer of human skin and gastrointestinal tracts. Human infections are primarily thought to occur when there is disruption of normal skin or mucosal surfaces. However, studies utilizing restriction enzyme analysis have also found identical *Candida* species strains isolated in hospitalized patients and environmental surfaces, suggesting that horizontal transmission may occur as well (5,6).

Candida species are responsible for a spectrum of diseases including mucocutaneous candidiasis; cutaneous candidiasis; and invasive candidiasis, particularly candidemia. Although there are over a hundred different *Candida* species, >95% of clinical infections are attributable to the following five species: *C. albicans, C. glabrata, C. parapsilosis, C. tropicalis,* and *C. krusei* (3,7). *C. albicans* is responsible for >90% of mucosal and cutaneous infections (8). Invasive candidiasis, most often candidemia, can be secondary to any *Candida* species. In the United States, approximately half of the cases of candidemia are secondary to *C. albicans* followed by *C. glabrata,* which comprises 20–24% of the cases (3,7). The remaining small percentage of candidemia can be attributable to other species including *C. guilliermondii, C. lusitaniae, C. dubliniensis,* and *C. rugosa.*

EPIDEMIOLOGY

Similar to the increase in invasive fungal infections, invasive candidiasis, particularly candidemia, has also increased over the past two decades. The National Nosocomial Infection Surveillance System (NNIS) of the Centers for Disease Control and Prevention (CDC) reported that, during the 1980s, rates of candidemia increased between 219% and 487% (9). Recent studies suggest that the incidence may have leveled off at 22 to 29 infections per 100,000 U.S. population per year (3). *Candida* species are now recognized as the fourth most common cause of healthcare-associated bloodstream infections, accounting for 8% to 10% of all cases (7).

Candidemia was historically found in intensive care unit (ICU) patients. However, a study by Trick and colleagues reported that from 1989 to 1999, there was a decrease in candidemia among ICU patients, attributable to an overall decrease in *C. albicans* isolates (4). There appears to be a shift of candidemia from ICU patients to generalized hospitalized patients as well as outpatients. Hajjeh and colleagues used population-based surveillance of candidemia in Baltimore, Maryland, and Connecticut to report that only 36% of candidemia occurred in the ICU while approximately 28% occurred in the community setting (10).

Along with a shift in the patient population, there has also been a shift in the species responsible for candidemia. In the 1980s, most candidemia in the United States was secondary to *C. albicans.* However, the incidence has decreased and it now accounts for approximately half the cases (4,7,11). Along with a decrease in *C. albicans,* there has been a notable increase in certain non-*C. albicans* isolates. Trick and colleagues reported in the 1990s that *C. glabrata* was the only species that increased significantly among ICU patients (4). It is now the second most common cause of candidemia in the United States (4).

The incidence of candidemia due to *C. glabrata* varies geographically, ranging anywhere from 12% to 37% throughout the nine U.S. Bureau of the Census Regions (12). Interestingly, fluconazole resistance patterns do not clearly correspond with increased incidence. For example, a study by Pfaller and colleagues reported that the highest rates of *C. glabrata* bloodstream infections occurred in New England (37.3%) where 70% of these isolates were fluconazole-susceptible and 30% were fluconazole dose-dependent susceptible. Meanwhile, the South Atlantic, which had one of the lowest rates of candidemia (15.5%), was comprised of 55% fluconazole-susceptible and 45% fluconazole dose-dependent susceptible or resistant isolates (12).

There is also worldwide geographic variability in candidemia. Although *C. albicans* is the most common cause of candidemia worldwide, the incidence of *C. glabrata* varies, ranging from 4% to 7% in Latin America up to 20% to 24% in the United States (3,13). Differing from the United States, *C. parapsilosis* is the second most common *Candida* species reported in Asia and Europe, accounting for 12% to 17% of the isolates, while *C. tropicalis* is the second most common *Candida* species found in Latin America (8,13).

RISK FACTORS FOR CANDIDEMIA

Because of the complications associated with candidemia, researchers have investigated potential risk factors, which could be used to develop and implement preventive measures or to identify high-risk patients who might benefit from prophylactic or empiric antifungal treatment. Classic risk factors, including host- and healthcare-related factors, for candidemia are well known (38–41). Host-related factors include malignancy with chemotherapy, solid organ transplantation, hematopoietic stem cell transplantation, human immunodeficiency virus (HIV) infection, neutropenia, end-stage renal disease (ESRD) requiring hemodialysis (HD), cirrhosis, and colonization with *Candida* species. Healthcare-related factors include abdominal surgery, use of central venous catheters (CVCs), exposure to broad-spectrum antibiotics, corticosteroid use, ICU stay, and use of total parenteral nutrition (TPN).

Because many hospitalized patients, particularly those in the ICU, typically have one or more of the above described risk factors, risk stratification strategies have been designed to better target patients who might benefit from antifungal prophylaxis or empiric treatment (42,43). For example, Leon and colleagues developed a "*Candida* score," which includes the following variables: surgery, multifocal colonization, TPN, and severe sepsis. They determined that a "*Candida* score" threshold of 2.5 had a sensitivity of 81% and a specificity of 74% (42). Those with scores >2.5 also had a 7.75-fold greater risk for developing candidemia (42). Further validation, however, is required before these risk stratification strategies become part of standard care.

OUTCOMES OF CANDIDEMIA: MORBIDITY AND MORTALITY

Candida species are recognized as important causes of healthcare-associated infections and are associated with significant morbidity and mortality. Patients with candidemia have 10 to 30 day excess lengths of hospital stay compared to age-, sex-, and diagnosis-related group-matched controls (32). Candidemia is also associated with significant costs totaling more than $1 billion per year (33). Approximately 85% appear to be attributable to this increased length of stay (32).

Candidemia appears to be an independent risk factor for death. Patients with candidemia have a crude mortality risk ranging from 46% to 75%, an attributable mortality risk ranging from 7% to 49%, and are at twice the risk for in-hospital mortality compared to patients with bloodstream infections secondary to non-*Candida* species (3,30,34,35).

Despite the introduction of several new antifungal agents, there has not been a significant decrease in mortality rates among patients with candidemia over the past two decades. The consistently high mortality rates are attributed to inappropriate treatment of candidemia. This includes delays in treatment, an inappropriate choice or dose of antifungal agent, inappropriate duration of treatment, or no treatment at all (3,34,36,37).

A few recent studies have impressed the importance of initiating antifungal therapy in a timely manner. A retrospective cohort study by Morrell and colleagues reported that independent risk factors for in-hospital mortality include higher

APACHE II scores (adjusted OR 1.24; 95% CI 1.18–1.31), prior antibiotic treatment (adjusted OR 4.05; 95% CI 2.14–7.65), and initiation of antifungal treatment ≥ 12 hours after drawing a positive blood culture (adjusted OR 2.09; 95% CI 1.53–2.84) (37). Garey and colleagues performed a multi-center retrospective cohort study and found that there was a time-dependent increase in mortality rates. Among patients with bloodstream infections due to *Candida* species, mortality rates ranged from 15% for those who received antifungal treatment on day 0 (when blood cultures were drawn) up to 40% for those who received antifungal treatment after day 3 ($p = .0009$) (36). As part of their subgroup analysis, they reported mortality rates by *Candida* species. They found that those patients with *C. glabrata* had higher mortality rates as compared to those with bloodstream infections due to other *Candida* species. It is unclear whether this was related to the increased severity of illness in patients with *C. glabrata* or whether this was due to inappropriate treatment. Traditional fluconazole dosing is often ineffective in treating *C. glabrata*, which can be fluconazole dose-dependent susceptible or resistant. Therefore, perhaps the patients with *C. glabrata* isolates took longer to be placed on appropriate treatment. This cannot be confirmed, however, since susceptibility testing was not performed in this study.

Appropriate duration of therapy is also crucial in the treatment of candidemia. A study by Morgan and colleagues performed in Connecticut and Baltimore reported that patients with candidemia who received adequate treatment, defined as ≥ 7 days of antifungal treatment, had lower attributable mortality rates (11% in Connecticut; 16% in Baltimore and Baltimore County) than those who received <7 days of treatment (31% in Connecticut; 41% in Baltimore and Baltimore County) (34). In total, these studies suggest that similar to bacteremias, starting the appropriate antifungal treatment early in the course of candidemia and continuing it for adequate lengths of time are important in decreasing mortality rates.

ANTIFUNGAL RESISTANCE IN *C. GLABRATA*

Among *Candida* species, *C. glabrata* has become recognized as an emerging infection not only because of its increasing incidence, but also because it is often associated with antifungal resistance. Unlike *C. albicans*, which is almost universally fluconazole-susceptible, *C. glabrata* is often fluconazole dose-dependent susceptible or resistant as defined by the Clinical Laboratory Standards Institute (CLSI) (14). The increase in fluconazole dose-dependent susceptible and resistant isolates has had important treatment implications.

Fluconazole, which was first introduced in 1990, has the following mechanism of action. It inhibits the fungal cytochrome P-450 dependent enzyme, 14-α-demethylase, which converts lanosterol to ergosterol, an important component of fungal cell membranes. A decrease in ergosterol synthesis coupled with an accumulation of intermediary byproducts results in fungal cell membrane disruption and death. Hypothetically, fluconazole resistance in *C. glabrata* could be due to several different mechanisms. Point mutations could occur in the *ERG11* gene, which encodes 14-α-demethylase, thereby altering its binding to fluconazole. Prior fluconazole use could also upregulate the expression of the *ERG11* gene, resulting in more 14-α-demethylase compared to the available fluconazole. Lastly, resistance could occur via efflux pumps. Of these possible resistance mechanisms, PCR studies have suggested that the upregulation of efflux pumps, specifically those of the ATP-binding cassette transporter family, plays an integral role (15,16).

Patients with fluconazole-resistant *C. glabrata* may have cross-resistance to other triazoles including voriconazole (17–19). *C. glabrata* may also be associated with resistance to other antifungal agents. Krogh-Madsen and colleagues reported increasing minimum inhibitory concentrations (MICs) to amphotericin B and caspofungin in an ICU patient who had persistently positive *C. glabrata* blood cultures (20).

ANTIFUNGAL RESISTANCE IN NON-*C. ALBICANS*, NON-*C. GLABRATA* ISOLATES

Other *Candida* species responsible for candidemia are also associated with antifungal resistance. *C. krusei* is inherently fluconazole-resistant due to differences in its 14-α-demethylase (21). It has been reported to have decreased susceptibilities to amphotericin B and flucytosine as well (10,22). Despite its fluconazole resistance, unlike *C. glabrata*, it is often voriconazole susceptible.

C. parapsilosis and *C. guilliermondii* have been reported to have increased MICs to echinocandins compared to other *Candida* species (23,24). A study by Mora-Duarte and colleagues reported that caspofungin was as effective as amphotericin B in the treatment of invasive candidiasis (25). However, five of the nine treatment failures in the caspofungin arm had *C. parapsilosis* bloodstream infections. Therefore, there is concern that patients with invasive *C. parapsilosis* infections who are treated with caspofungin may develop resistance and experience clinical failures.

There is also concern that *C. lusitaniae* may be less susceptible to amphotericin B with clinical failures noted in the literature (26,27). However, recent reports suggest that this may occur less frequently than once thought (28,29). A study by Pfaller and colleagues reported that 98% of their *C. lusitaniae* isolates were amphotericin B-susceptible, similar to the percentages observed for *C. albicans* (28).

Uncommon causes of candidemia such as *C. guilliermondii* have also been reported to have decreased susceptibilities to amphotericin B and fluconazole (30,31). Another species, *C. rugosa*, has been reported to have decreased susceptibility to amphotericin B (28).

RISK FACTORS FOR *C. GLABRATA* BLOODSTREAM INFECTIONS

Despite the emergence of bloodstream infections due to *C. glabrata*, only a few studies have evaluated the risk factors for this infection. None of these studies performed susceptibility testing to differentiate between fluconazole-susceptible and fluconazole dose-dependent susceptible or resistant isolates. The possible association between fluconazole and the emergence *C. glabrata* has been mentioned in the literature. As previously mentioned, prior fluconazole use could result in resistance endogenously by upregulating drug efflux pumps, or exogenously by providing selective pressure, decreasing *C. albicans* colonization in the skin or gastrointestinal tract, and allowing colonization with more resistant *Candida* species.

Studies of oncology patients seem to most strongly support this association. Abi-Said and colleagues performed a retrospective review of all cases of hematogeneous candidiasis, defined as episodes of candidemia and acute disseminated candidiasis, which occurred at a single cancer center from 1988 to 1992. They found that fluconazole prophylaxis was more common in *C. glabrata* ($n = 53$; adjusted OR 5.08; 95% CI 2.32–11.11) and *C. krusei* ($n = 20$; adjusted OR 27.07; 95% CI 9.23–79.36) infections than those attributable to other *Candida* species (11).

Other *C. glabrata* risk factors included the absence of CVCs (adjusted OR 2.45; 95% CI 1.11–5.38) and the absence of broad-spectrum antibiotics (adjusted OR 2.16; 95% CI 1.04–4.48). Bodey and colleagues compared bloodstream infections due to *C. glabrata* to *C. albicans* that occurred at the same cancer center from 1993 to 1999. They reported that *C. glabrata* isolates (n =116) were more likely in patients with hematologic malignancies (adjusted OR 2.3; CI 1.1–4.5), higher APACHE II scores (adjusted OR 2.6; CI 1.3–5.1), and those who had received fluconazole prophylaxis (adjusted OR 11; CI 4.9–23) (44).

Although strong associations have been found between prior fluconazole use and *C. glabrata* in oncology patients, these associations have not been supported among generalized patients. Several ecologic studies, including reports from Iceland and Switzerland, reported significant increases in fluconazole use over a 10+ year period, but did not find any change in the incidence of *C. glabrata* (45,46). Lin and colleagues performed a retrospective case-case-control study to evaluate antimicrobial risk factors for *C. glabrata* (n = 56) and *C. krusei* (n = 4). Multivariate analysis demonstrated that independent risk factors for bloodstream infections due to *C. glabrata* and *C. krusei* included prior use of piperacillin/tazobactam (adjusted OR 4.15; 95% CI 1.04–16.50) and vancomycin (adjusted OR 6.48; 95% CI 2.2–19.13) (47). Fluconazole was not found to be a risk factor in either bi- or multivariable analyses (adjusted OR 1.81; 95% CI 0.48–6.92) (47). The researchers hypothesized that perhaps vancomycin and piperacillin/tazobactam altered patient skin and gastrointestinal flora more significantly than fluconazole, thereby allowing colonization with resistant organisms including resistant *Candida* species.

In total, the above studies seem to suggest that the emergence of bloodstream infections due to *C. glabrata* may be more complicated than pure selective pressure from increased fluconazole use. Other factors including age, geographic location, broad-spectrum antibiotic use, CVCs, ICU stay, and TPN use may also play important roles. There is evidence to support a possible association between age and geographic variability on *C. glabrata* infections. Studies have shown that bloodstream infections due to *C. glabrata* increase in incidence with age. The SENTRY Antimicrobial Surveillance program reported that among patients with candidemia, the prevalence of *C. glabrata* ranged from 3% in patients ≤ 1 year of age up to 23% in patients ≥ 65 years of age (48). There is also geographic variability of candidemia both in the United States and worldwide, as was mentioned previously.

DIAGNOSIS AND SUSCEPTIBILITY TESTING

Candidemia is diagnosed using blood cultures. Despite the improvements in blood culture systems, candidemia often takes longer to diagnose and is more difficult to isolate than most bacteremias.

Once yeast is cultured from blood, various methods are used to identify the specific *Candida* species. Many laboratories utilize the biochemical tests of the API-20C strip. Other methods that can assist in identifying the particular species include the germ tube tests, the ChromAGAR test, and the *C. albicans* peptide nucleic acid fluorescence in situ hybridization (PNA FISH) test. The germ tube test is performed by placing a pure culture of an unknown yeast in serum. If the test is positive, germ tube formation will become apparent within a few hours. The ChromAGAR test differentiates between *C. albicans*, *C. krusei*, and *C. tropicalis* using distinctive colors associated with these species. The newest FDA approved test is PNA FISH, which differentiates between *C. albicans*, which accounts for approximately 50% candidemia and is almost always fluconazole-susceptible, and other non-*C. albicans* species. A study by Rigby and colleagues reported that the PNA FISH test has a sensitivity and specificity of 100% and is able to correctly identify *C. albicans* within 2.5 hours of a blood culture positive for yeast (50).

Antifungal susceptibility testing has also gained importance. CLSI defines clinically useful MIC breakpoints using broth dilution and disk diffusion testing for fluconazole, itraconazole, voriconazole, and flucytosine (14). Breakpoints for fluconazole are as follows: isolates with MICs $\leq 8\,\mu g/mL$ are designated susceptible (S); those with MICs between 16 and $32\,\mu g/mL$ are designated dose-dependent susceptible (S-DD) and treatment with either higher doses of fluconazole or a different antifungal agent is recommended; and those isolates with MICs $\geq 64\,\mu g/mL$ are designated resistant (R) since fluconazole does not inhibit *C. glabrata* growth in vitro (14). Susceptibility patterns for itraconazole (S: MIC $\leq 0.125\,\mu g/mL$; S-DD: MIC 0.25–$0.5\,\mu g/mL$; R: $\geq 1\,\mu g/mL$), voriconazole (S: MIC $\leq 1\,\mu g/mL$; S-DD $2\,\mu g/mL$; R: $\geq 4\,\mu g/mL$), and flucytosine (S: MIC $\leq 4\,\mu g/mL$; intermediate (I): MIC 8–$16\,\mu g/mL$; R: MIC $\geq 32\,\mu g/mL$) are listed here as well.

MIC breakpoints for posaconazole and echinocandins are currently unavailable, but under development. Lastly, it has been difficult to establish MIC breakpoints for amphotericin B given its narrow range of MICs.

TREATMENT OF CANDIDEMIA

Any blood culture positive for *Candida* species should be treated as a serious infection and appropriate treatment should be initiated in a timely manner, including instituting antifungal therapy and removing all indwelling percutaneous catheters (23). Empiric treatment of candidemia has often involved initiating the antifungal agent, fluconazole, given its comparable efficacy and improved tolerability in comparison to amphotericin B (51). Fluconazole is also available both in an oral as well as an intravenous form.

However, the emergence of fluconazole-resistant species including *C. glabrata* has resulted in important treatment implications, and the choice of early antifungal treatment has become much more complicated. Although there are no definitive recommendations as to what antifungal treatment to start once yeast is identified from blood cultures, experts advocate tailoring early treatment to the patient and suspected pathogens. For example, caspofungin or amphotericin B should be considered in patients with a higher severity of illness or hemodynamic instability, and when there is a high suspicion for infection with *C. glabrata* or *C. krusei* (23,52,53). The use of amphotericin B may be limited by its nephrotoxicity and the widespread use of caspofungin may be hindered by its increased costs.

Once blood culture results, including identification of *Candida* species and susceptibility testing, are finalized, antifungal therapy can be appropriately modified. If there is no evidence for end-organ involvement, the patient should receive at least 2 weeks of appropriate antifungal therapy.

EMPIRIC ANTIFUNGAL THERAPY

Empiric antifungal therapy should be considered in neutropenic patients who remain febrile despite being on broad-spectrum antibacterial therapy for 4–7 days (23). Several antifungal agents, including amphotericin B, fluconazole, itraconazole, and voriconazole, have been utilized in this setting. Antifungal agents that have activity against not only yeast, but also molds, are preferable. Fluconazole does not have activity against *Aspergillus* species. Therefore, according to the Infectious Diseases Society of America guidelines, fluconazole should be considered in a select group of patients who have not received prior azole prophylaxis and are at low risk for infection with aspergillosis and azole-resistant *Candida* species (23).

ANTIFUNGAL PROPHYLAXIS

Given the high morbidity and mortality costs associated with candidemia, it is important to implement preventive measures. Zaoutis and colleagues calculated that one life could be saved, for every ten children or seven adults in whom candidemia could be prevented (35).

Three basic interventions that are crucial in decreasing the rates of candidemia include improving hand hygiene measures, following appropriate insertion and care of central catheters, and advocating for judicious use of antibiotics (8). These measures should be optimized before considering antifungal prophylaxis.

There is evidence supporting the use of antifungal prophylaxis in certain patient populations, including neutropenic patients and liver transplant recipients. Patients with prolonged neutropenia, including those undergoing intensive chemotherapy or bone marrow transplantation, are at higher risk for invasive candidiasis and mold infections. Antifungal therapy should be considered in high risk patients and, if given, should extend at least through the neutropenic period (23). In solid organ transplantation, liver transplant recipients, particularly those with identified risk factors (renal insufficiency, retransplantation, fungal colonization, choledochojejunostomy, and numerous intraoperative blood transfusions), are at higher risk for invasive candidiasis (23,54). A randomized, double-blinded, placebo-controlled study demonstrated that liver transplant recipients who received fluconazole prophylaxis have significantly decreased rates of superficial (4% vs. 28%; $p<.001$) as well as invasive infection (6% vs. 23%; $p<.001$) (55). However, in this study, fluconazole was less effective in preventing infections due to *C. glabrata*.

There are limited data on the use of antifungal prophylaxis in non-neutropenic critically ill patients. Cruciani and colleagues performed a meta-analysis of nine studies, evaluating the utility of antifungal prophylaxis in non-neutropenic, trauma, and surgical ICU patients. They reported that prophylaxis with ketoconazole or fluconazole was associated with significant reductions in candidemia (RR 0.3; 95% CI 0.10–0.82), candidemia attributable mortality (RR 0.25; 95% CI 0.08–0.80), and overall mortality (RR 0.6; 95% CI 0.45–0.81). However, the meta-analysis was limited by significant differences in the definitions of outcomes in each of the studies (55). Further studies are still needed to clarify the role of prophylaxis in this population.

SUMMARY

In summary, candidemia continues to be an important cause of healthcare-associated infections and, despite the introduction of various antifungal treatments, it remains a significant cause of morbidity and mortality. There has been an important shift in the epidemiology of candidemia with a decrease in bloodstream infections due to *C. albicans* and an increase in *C. glabrata*, which is often associated with fluconazole resistance. Other causes of a minority of candidemia, including *C. krusei*, *C. parapsilosis*, *C. lusitaniae*, *C. guilliermondii*, and *C. rugosa*, have also been associated with antifungal resistance. Given the emergence of antifungal resistance, as well as studies suggesting the importance of initiating appropriate antifungal treatment in a timely manner, quickly diagnosing and performing susceptibility testing of these pathogens has become crucial. The treatment of candidemia has also become more challenging, with agents other than fluconazole being considered as primary options.

REFERENCES

1. Martin GS, Eaton S, Moss M. The epidemiology of sepsis in the United States from 1979 through 2000. N Engl J Med 2003; 348:1546–54.
2. Wisplinghoff H, Tallent B, Seifert H, Wenzel RP, Edmond MB. Nosocomial bloodstream infections in US hospitals: analysis of 24,179 cases from a prospective nationwide surveillance study. Clin Infect Dis 2004; 39:309–17.
3. Pfaller M, Diekema D. Epidemiology of invasive candidiasis: a persistent public health problem. Clin Microbiol Rev 2007; 20:133–63.
4. Trick W, Fridkin S, Edwards J, et al. Secular trend of hospital-acquired candidemia among intensive care unit patients in the United States during 1989–1999. Clin Infect Dis 2002; 35:627–30.
5. Pfaller M. Nosocomial candidiasis: emerging species, reservoirs, and modes of transmission. Clin Infect Dis 1996; 22 (Suppl. 2):S89–94.
6. Vazquez J, Sanchez V, Dmuchowski C, et al. Nosocomial acquisition of *Candida albicans*: an epidemiologic study. J Infect Dis 1993; 168:195–201.
7. Wisplinghoff H, Bischoff T, Tallent S, et al. Nosocomial bloodstream infections in U.S. hospitals: analysis of 24,179 cases from a prospective nationwide surveillance study. Clin Infect Dis 2004; 39:309–17.
8. Pfaller M, Pappas P, Wingard J. Invasive fungal pathogens: current epidemiological trends. Clin Infect Dis 2006; 43:S3–14.
9. Banerjee S, Emori T, Culver D, et al. Secular trends in nosocomial primary bloodstream infections in the United States, 1980–1989. National Nosocomial Infections Surveillance System. Am J Med 1991; 91(3B):86S–9.
10. Hajjeh R, Sofair A, Harrison L, et al. Incidence of bloodstream infections due to *Candida* species and in vitro susceptibilities of isolates collected from 1998 to 2000 in a population-based active surveillance program. J Clin Microbiol 2004; 42:1519–27.
11. Abi-Said D, Anaissie E, Uzun O, et al. The epidemiology of hematogenous candidiasis caused by different *Candida* species. Clin Infect Dis 1997; 24:1122–8.
12. Pfaller M, Messer S, Boyken L, et al. Variation in susceptibility of bloodstream isolates of *Candida glabrata* to fluconazole according to patient age and geographic location. J Clin Microbiol 2003; 41:2176–9.
13. Pfaller M, Diekema D, I.F.S.P. Group. Twelve years of fluconazole in clinical practice: global trends in species distribution and fluconazole susceptibility of bloodstream isolates of Candida. Clin Microbiol Infect 2004; 10S:11–23.
14. National Committee for Clinical Laboratory Standards. 2004. Methods for antifungal disk diffusion susceptibility testing of yeasts: approved guideline, M44-A. National Committee for Clinical Laboratory Standards, Wayne, PA.
15. Sanguinetti M, Posteraro B, Fiori B, et al. Mechanisms of azole resistance in clinical isolates of Candida glabrata collected during a hospital survey of antifungal resistance. Antimicrob Agents Chemother 2005: 49:668–79.
16. Posteraro B, Tumbarello M, La Sorda M, et al. Azole resistance of *Candida glabrata* in a case of recurrent fungemia. J Clin Microbiol 2006; 44:3046–7.
17. Borst A, Raimer M, Warnock D, et al. Rapid acquisition of stable azole resistance by *Candida glabrata* isolates obtained before the clinical introduction of fluconazole. Antimicrob Agents Chemother 2005; 49:783–7.

18. Magill S, Shields C, Sears C, et al. Triazole cross-resistance among *Candida* spp.: case report, occurrence among bloodstream isolates, and implications for antifungal therapy. J Clin Microbiol 2006; 44:529–35.
19. Panackal A, Gribskov J, Staab J, et al. Clinical significance of azole antifungal drug cross-resistance in *Candida glabrata*. J Clin Microbiol 2006; 44:1740–3.
20. Krogh-Madsen M, Arendrup M, Heslet L, et al. Amphotericin B and caspofungin resistance in *Candida glabrata* isolates recovered from a critically ill patient. Clin Infect Dis 2006; 42:938–44.
21. Orozco A, Higginbotham L, Hitchcock C, et al. Mechanism of fluconazole resistance in Candida krusei. Antimicrob Agents Chemother 1998; 42:2645–9.
22. Antoniadou A, Torres H, Lewis RT, et al. Candidemia in a tertiary care cancer center: in vitro susceptibility and its association with outcome of initial antifungal therapy. Medicine 2003; 82:309–21.
23. Pappas P, Rex J, Sobel J, et al. Guidelines for treatment of candidiasis. Clin Infect Dis 2004; 38:161–89.
24. Barchiesi F, Spreghini E, Tomassetti S, et al. Effects of caspofungin against *Candida guilliermondii* and *Candida parapsilosis*. Antimicrob Agents Chemother 2006; 50:2719–27.
25. Mora-Duarte J, Betts R, Rotstein C, et al. Comparison of caspofungin and amphotericin B for invasive candidiasis. N Engl J Med 2002; 347:2020–9.
26. Minari A, Hachem R, Raad I. *Candida lusitaniae*: a cause of breakthrough fungemia in cancer patients. Clin Infect Dis 2001; 32:186–90.
27. Guinet R, Chanas J, Goullier A, et al. Fatal septicemia due to amphotericin B-resistant *Candida lusitaniae*. J Clin Microbiol 1983; 18:443–4.
28. Pfaller M, Diekema D, Messer S, et al. In vitro activities of voriconazole, posaconazole, and four licensed systemic antifungal agents against *Candida* species infrequently isolated from blood. J Clin Microbiol 2003; 41:78–83.
29. Favel A, Michel-Nguyen A, Datry A, et al. Susceptibility of clinical isolates of *Candida lusitaniae* to five systemic antifungal agents. J Antimicrob Chemother 2004; 53:526–9.
30. Pfaller M, Diekema D, Mendez M, et al. *Candida guilliermondii*, an opportunistic fungal pathogen with decreased susceptibility to fluconazole: geographic and temporal trends from the ARTEMIS DISK Antifungal Surveillance Program. J Clin Microbiol 2006; 44:3551–6.
31. Vasquez J, Lundstrom T, Dembrey L, et al. Invasive *Candida guilliermondii* infection: in vitro susceptibility studies and molecular analysis. Bone Marrow Transplant 1995; 16:849–53.
32. Rentz A, Halpern M, Bowden R. The impact of candidemia on length of hospital stay, outcome, and overall cost of illness. Clin Infect Dis 1998; 27:781–8.
33. Miller L, Edwards J, Hajjeh R. Estimating the cost of nosocomial candidemia in the United States. Clin Infect Dis 2001; 32:1110.
34. Morgan J, Meltzer M, Plikaytis B, et al. Excess mortality, hospital stay, and cost due to candidemia: a case-control study using data from population-based candidemia surveillance. Infect Control Hospital Epidemiol 2005; 26:540–7.
35. Zaoutis T, Argon J, Chu J, et al. The epidemiology and attributable outcomes of candidemia in adults and children hospitalized in the United States: a propensity analysis. Clin Infect Dis 2005; 41:1232–9.
36. Garey K, Rege M, Pai M, et al. Time to initiation of fluconazole therapy impacts mortality in patients with candidemia: a multi-institutional study. Clin Infect Dis 2006; 43:25–31.
37. Morrell M, Frazer V, Kollef M. Delaying the empiric treatment of *Candida* bloodstream infection until positive blood culture results are obtained: a potential risk factor for hospital mortality. Antimicrob Agents Chemother 2005; 49:3640–5.
38. Wenzel R. Nosocomial candidemia: risk factors and attributable mortality. Clin Infect Dis 1995; 20:1531–4.
39. Wey S, Mori M, Pfaller M, et al. Risk factors for hospital-acquired candidemia: a matched case-control study. Arch Int Med 1989; 149:2349–53.
40. Pagano L, Antinori A, Ammassari A, et al. Retrospective study of candidemia in patients with hematological malignancies. Clinical features, risk factors, and outcome of 76 episodes. Eur J Haematol 1999; 63:77–85.

41. Karabinis A, Hill C, Leclercq B, et al. Risk factors for candidemia in cancer patients: a case-control study. J Clin Microbiol 1988; 26:429–32.
42. Leon C, Ruiz-Santana S, Saavedra P, et al. A bedside scoring system ("Candida score") for early antifungal treatment in nonneutropenic critically ill patients with *Candida* colonization. Crit Care Med 2006; 34:730–7.
43. Wenzel R, Gennings C. Bloodstream infections due to *Candida* species in the intensive care unit: identifying especially high-risk patients to determine prevention strategies. Clin Infect Dis 2005; 41:S389–93.
44. Bodey G, Mardani M, Hanna H, et al. Epidemiology of *Candida glabrata* and *Candida albicans* fungemia in immunocompromised patients with cancer. Am J Med 2002; 112:380–5.
45. Asmundsdottir L, Erlendsdottir H, Gottfredsson M. Increasing incidence of candidemia: results from a 20-year nationwide study in Iceland. J Clin Microbiol 2002; 40:3489–92.
46. Marchetti O, Bille J, Fluckiger U, et al. Epidemiology of candidemia in Swiss tertiary care hospitals: secular trends, 1991–2000. Clin Infect Dis 2004; 38:311–20.
47. Lin M, Carmeli Y, Zumsteg J, et al. Prior antimicrobial therapy and risk for hospital-acquired *Candida glabrata* and *Candida krusei* fungemia: a case-case-control study. Antimicrob Agents Chemother 2005; 49:4555–60.
48. Pfaller M, Diekema DJ, Jones R, et al. Trends in antifungal susceptibility of *Candida* spp. isolated from pediatric and adult patients with bloodstream infections: SENTRY antimicrobial surveillance program, 1997 to 2000. J Clin Microbiol 2002; 40:852–6.
49. Pappas P. Invasive candidiasis. Infect Dis Clin North Am 2006; 20(3):654–9.
50. Rigby S, Procop G, Haase G, et al. Fluorescence in situ hybridization with peptide nucleic acid probes for rapid identification of *Candida albicans* directly from blood cultures bottles. J Clin Microbiol 2002; 40:2182–6.
51. Rex J, Bennett J, Sugar A. A randomized trial comparing fluconazole with amphotericin B for the treatment of candidemia in patients without neutropenia. Candidemia Study Group and the National Institute. N Engl J Med 1994; 331:1325–30.
52. Spellberg B, Filler S, Edwards J. Current treatment strategies for disseminated candidiasis. Clin Infect Dis 2006; 42:244–51.
53. Alexander B, Ashley E, Reller L, Reed S, et al. Cost savings with implementation of PNA FISH testing for identification of *Candida albicans* in blood cultures. Diag Microbiol Infect Dis 2006; 54:277–82.
54. Collins L, Samore M, Roberts M, et al. Risk factors for invasive fungal infections complicating orthotopic liver transplantation. J Infect Dis 1994; 170:644–52.
55. Winston D, Pakrasi A, Busuttil R. Prophylactic fluconazole in liver transplant recipients. Ann Int Med 1999; 131:729–37.
56. Cruciani M, de Lalla F, Mengoli C. Prophylaxis of *Candida* infections in adult trauma and surgical intensive care patients: a systematic review and meta-analysis. Int Care Med 2005; 31:1479–87.

13 Early Appropriate Empiric Therapy and Antimicrobial De-Escalation

James M. Hollands, Scott T. Micek, and Peggy S. McKinnon
Department of Pharmacy, Barnes-Jewish Hospital, Saint Louis, Missouri, U.S.A.

Marin H. Kollef
Pulmonary and Critical Care Division, Washington University School of Medicine, Saint Louis, Missouri, U.S.A.

INTRODUCTION

Bacterial resistance to antibiotics creates a therapeutic challenge to clinicians when treating patients with a known or suspected infection. Increasing rates of resistance lead many clinicians to empirically treat patients with multiple broad-spectrum antibiotics, which can perpetuate the cycle of increasing resistance and create an economic burden to society (see Chapter 4). Conversely, inappropriate initial therapy, defined as a regimen that lacks in vitro activity against an isolated organism, can lead to treatment failures that have negative patient outcomes.

De-escalation therapy is a treatment strategy that attempts to provide appropriate initial antimicrobial therapy to reduce the risk of negative patient outcomes and avoid the consequences of excessive or unnecessary antibiotic administration. Avoiding unnecessary use of antibiotics can help minimize the development of resistance, as detailed in other chapters in this book. This chapter explains why it is beneficial to initiate broad-spectrum empiric coverage and then tailor the regimen based on culture and sensitivity results.

FACTORS IMPACTING EMPIRIC ANTIBIOTIC SELECTION

To provide an empiric regimen with an adequate spectrum of activity, one must appreciate (*i*) the likely pathogens causing a variety of nosocomial infections, (*ii*) local pathogen distribution and resistance patterns, and (*iii*) patient-specific risk factors for resistance. Ideally, administration of appropriately broad-spectrum empiric antimicrobial therapy is based on consideration of all of these factors and each are examined in the following section.

Data from the National Nosocomial Infections Surveillance (NNIS) outlines the most frequent infections in participating acute care general hospitals in the United States. This surveillance network was established in 1970 and initially reported only hospital-wide infection rates; however, since 1986 the network has reported intensive care unit (ICU) infection rates as well. In the 2000 report, it was noted that device-related infection predominated; 83% of nosocomial pneumonia episodes were associated with mechanical ventilation, 97% of urinary tract infections (UTIs) occurred in catheterized patients, and 87% of primary bloodstream infections (BSIs) occurred in patients with a central line (1). The most recent publication of the NNIS data reports pathogen distribution by site of infection and compared data from 1975 to 2003. Data from the 2000 report (2), summarized for years 1989 to 1998, is also included for comparison in Table 1.

In patients with pneumonia, Gram-negative aerobes remain the most frequently reported pathogen associated with pneumonia (65.9%); however, *Staphylococcus aureus* (27.8%) was the most frequently reported single species. In patients with primary BSIs, coagulase-negative staphylococci (42.9%) has remained the most common pathogen reported and *S. aureus* (14.3%) was reported as frequently as enterococci (14.5%). In patients with UTIs, *Escherichia coli* (26%) was the most frequently reported isolate; however, *Pseudomonas aeruginosa* comprised 16.3% of reported isolates, increasing from 10.6% in the 1989 to 1998 data. In surgical site infections (SSIs), the proportion of isolates that were Gram-negative decreased significantly during the past two decades. Gram-positive pathogens are now more commonly associated with both BSI and SSI, while Gram-negative aerobes predominate in pneumonia and UTI (1,3).

Perhaps the most noteworthy trend was the increase in *Acinetobacter* sp. isolated in UTIs, pneumonias, and SSIs. While overall numbers of isolates of *Acinetobacter* are still relatively small ($\sim 2.0\%$), the percentage increase is quite significant. These authors comment that the reduction in infections due to *E. coli* and subsequent increase in *Acinetobacter* sp. suggest that antimicrobial use has had a significant impact on which pathogens are isolated from a site of hospital-acquired infection.

Also disconcerting was that for each of the antibiotic-pathogen combinations tested, there was a significant increase in resistance between study periods. Most impressive were trends in carbapenem- and cephalosporin-resistant *P. aeruginosa*, and *Acinetobacter* sp. Rates of imipenem- and amikacin-resistant *Acinetobacter* isolates are approaching 20% and have been steadily increasing since 1990. The intrinsically multidrug-resistant (MDR) nature of this organism makes these trends particularly worrisome, as many isolates lack effective treatment options and represent a serious public health concern (1). Lastly, 2003 rates of third generation cephalosporin-resistance in *E. coli* (6.4%) and *K. pneumoniae* (14.2%) provide estimates of the presence of extended-spectrum beta-lactamase (ESBL)- producing, often MDR, bacteria, again with very limited treatment options in ICUs in the United States.

The prevalence of MDR pathogens varies by patient population, hospital, and type of ICU, which underscores the need for local surveillance data. MDR pathogens are more commonly isolated from patients with severe, chronic underlying disease, for example those with risk factors for healthcare-associated pneumonia (HCAP) and patients with late-onset hospital-acquired pneumonia (HAP) or ventilator-associated pneumonia (VAP). Risk factors for VAP caused by potentially antibiotic-resistant bacteria were investigated in 135 mechanically ventilated patients (4). The duration of ventilation before the onset of VAP and prior antibiotic use (within 15 days prior to developing VAP) were both significant risk factors associated with VAP caused by antibiotic-resistant pathogens. Early-onset VAP (pneumonia occurring within 5 days of hospitalization) in patients who had not received prior antibiotic therapy tended to be caused by susceptible bacteria. Late-onset VAP (5 days or more), in patients who had previously received antibiotics, was generally caused by MDR pathogens such as *P. aeruginosa*, *Acinetobacter baumannii*, *Stenotrophomonas maltophilia*, and methicillin-resistant *S. aureus* (MRSA). The authors concluded that this study provided evidence for

Early Appropriate Empiric Therapy and Antimicrobial De-Escalation

TABLE 1 Relative Percentage by Site of Infection of Pathogens Associated with Nosocomial Infection, National Nosocomial Infections Surveillance System, 1975, 1989–1998, and 2003

Pathogen	PNEU			BSI			SSI			UTI		
Year	1975	1989–1998	2003	1975	1989–1998	2003	1975	1989–1998	2003	1975	1989–1998	2003
n	4,018	65,056	4,365	1,054	50,091	2,351	7,848	22,043	2,984	16,434	47,502	4,109
Coag-negative staphylococci	2.6	2.5	1.8	10.3	39.3	42.9	7.4	13.5	15.9	3.2	3.1	4.9
Staphylococcus aureus	13.4	16.8	27.8	16.5	10.7	14.3	18.5	12.6	22.5	1.9	1.6	3.6
Pseudomonas aeruginosa	9.6	16.1	18.1	4.8	3	3.4	4.7	9.2	9.5	9.3	10.6	16.3
Enterococcus spp.	3	1.9	1.3	8.1	10.3	14.5	11.9	14.5	13.9	14.2	13.8	17.4
Enterobacter spp.	9.6	10.7	10	6	4.2	4.4	4.6	8.8	9	4.7	5.7	6.9
Escherichia coli	11.8	4.4	5	15	2.9	3.3	17.6	7.1	6.5	33.5	18.2	26
Klebsiella pneumoniae	8.4	6.5	7.2	4.5	2.9	4.2	2.7	3.5	3	4.6	6.1	9.8
Serratia marcescens	2.2	—	4.7	2.6	—	2.3	0.5	—	2	1.4	—	1.6
Acinetobacter sp.	1.5	—	6.9	1.8	—	2.4	0.5	—	2.1	0.6	—	1.6
Other	37.9	37.1	17.3	30.4	21.8	8.2	31.6	26	15.6	26.6	25.6	11.9
Candida albicans	—	4	—	—	4.9	—	—	4.8	—	—	15.3	—

Abbreviations: BSI, blood stream infection; PNEU, pneumonia; SSI, surgical site infection; UTI, urinary tract infection; —, not reported.

the need for a more rational approach to selecting initial empiric antibiotic therapy before culture results were available in patients with VAP in order to reduce resistance selection.

The recent American Thoracic Society (ATS)/Infectious Diseases Society of America (IDSA) guidelines (5), however, point out that patients with early-onset HAP who have received prior antibiotics or who have had prior hospitalization within the past 90 days are also at greater risk for colonization and infection with MDR pathogens and should be treated similar to patients with late-onset HAP or VAP (Table 2).

When patients at risk for infection with MDR pathogens are identified, empiric therapy should be initiated with agents that are known to be effective against these organisms. Trouillet et al. found that 57% of 135 consecutive episodes were caused by "potentially resistant" organisms (4). According to logistic regression analysis, three variables predicted potentially drug-resistant bacterial etiology for VAP: duration of mechanical ventilation, 7 days or more [odds ratio (OR), 6.0]; prior antibiotic use (OR, 13.5); and prior use of broad-spectrum drugs (third generation cephalosporin, fluoroquinolone, and/or a carbapenem) (OR, 4.1).

The converse of this is also true. Some patients (those who develop an infection within 5 days of hospitalization, those without recent antibiotic exposure, and those without hospitalization in the past 3 months) are at low risk of infection by resistant organisms. In that subset, adequate initial selection should be a more narrow-spectrum regimen to target usual community-acquired organisms in addition to some Enterobacteriaceae and *S. aureus* (6).

It is important to recognize that resistance rates may be highly variable among countries, institutions and specific ICUs. Dramatic differences in antimicrobial resistance exist within individual hospitals and may depend on both antimicrobial use and infection control practices (7). Furthermore, even within an institution, ICU susceptibility rates may vary between ICUs, creating serious implications for empiric antibiotic selection strategies. The types of pathogens associated with episodes of VAP in ICUs, along with their antibiotic susceptibility profiles, were shown to be highly variable across four treatment centers, three in

TABLE 2 Risk Factors for Multidrug-Resistant Pathogens Causing Hospital-Acquired Pneumonia, HCAP, and Ventilator-Associated Pneumonia

---

Antimicrobial therapy in the preceding 90 days
Current hospitalization of 5 days or more
High frequency of antibiotic resistance in the community or in
  the specific hospital unit
Presence of risk factors for HCAP:
    Hospitalization for 2 days or more in the preceding 90 days
    Residence in a nursing home or extended care facility
    Home infusion therapy (including antibiotics)
    Chronic dialysis within 30 days
    Home wound care
    Family member with multidrug-resistant pathogen
Immunosuppressive disease and/or therapy

Abbreviation: HCAP, healthcare-associated pneumonia.
Source: Adapted from Ref. 5.

Spain and one in France (8). This retrospective multicenter study compared microorganisms documented by quantitative cultures from bronchoscopic samples from three different institutions in Spain, and then these observations were compared with the findings reported by Trouillet et al. in Paris (4). Significant variations in etiologies ($p < 0.05$) were found in all of the microorganisms isolated from VAP episodes across three Spanish treatment sites when compared with the site in Paris. One study objective was to evaluate whether a classification of etiologies of VAP, based on the number of ventilator days and previous antimicrobial use, might contribute to establishing generalized guidelines for empiric therapy; however, the variation among sites led the authors to conclude that instead of following general recommendations, antimicrobial prescribing practices for VAP should be individualized based on up-to-date information of the pattern of MDR isolates from each institution.

Within one institution, Namias et al. described highly variable rates of susceptibility to a number of problem pathogens in their trauma, surgical, and medical ICUs and found that while *Acinetobacter* sp. susceptibility rates to imipenem were low in the surgical ICU, susceptibility was very good in the trauma ICU (9). A different trend was reported for ceftazidime-resistant *P. aeruginosa*, with highest susceptibility in the trauma and surgical ICUs and lowest in the medical ICU. These data suggest that consensus guidelines for antimicrobial therapy will need to be modified at the local level (for example, according to county, city, hospital, and ICU) to take into account local patterns of antimicrobial resistance. In addition, it is helpful to appreciate ICU specific resistance rates of certain Gram-negative pathogens such as ESBL-producing *K. pneumonia* or *E. coli*, fluoroquinolone-resistant *P. aeruginosa*, or carbapenem-resistant *A. baumannii*. When risk of these pathogens is identified, empiric therapy must be tailored accordingly. Clinicians must be aware of the prevailing bacterial pathogens in their hospitals, their associated antimicrobial susceptibilities, and patient risk factors for infection. Furthermore, hospitals need to develop systems for reporting patterns of antimicrobial susceptibility in individual hospital areas or units and must update antibiotic policies regularly to allow for optimal therapy based on current resistance trends.

In addition to regional variance, there are numerous patient-specific factors that impact the risk of isolation of a resistant pathogen. Therefore, the choice of empiric antibiotic agents should be based on local patterns of antimicrobial susceptibility, and must also take into account patient-specific characteristics that may influence risk of infection with a resistant pathogen. Patients of particular concern are those at risk for VAP caused by *S. aureus* and *P. aeruginosa* due to the high frequency with which they cause VAP, their resistance to numerous antibiotics, and their associated high mortality rates (10–13). Historically, infections caused by MRSA have occurred primarily among hospitalized patients and/or among patients with extensive hospitalization history and other predisposing risk factors like indwelling catheters, past antimicrobial use, decubitus ulcers, postoperative surgical wound, or treatment with enteral feedings or dialysis. Risk factors for VAP caused by methicillin-sensitive *S. aureus* include younger age, traumatic coma, and neurosurgical problems (14), while risk factors for VAP due to MRSA include COPD, longer duration of mechanical ventilation, prior antibiotic therapy, and prior steroid treatment (11). In VAP, resistant staphylococcal infections are typically seen only in late-onset VAP. Recently, however, there has been an emergence of MRSA strains containing important virulence factors and toxins such as the Panton-Valentine leukocidin gene, associated with invasive, necrotic skin infections and severe necrotizing pneumonia. Although most described cases have been community–acquired, and these strains have been frequently termed "community acquired" MRSA, nosocomial acquisition of these strains has been described, underlining that these strains may also be hospital–acquired (15,16).

Patients at risk for VAP caused by *P. aeruginosa* include those with concurrent use of corticosteroids, prior use of antibiotics, and structural lung disease (5,17). Patients with cystic fibrosis frequently experience infection with MDR isolates of *P. aeruginosa* and frequently have several isolates with different susceptibility patterns. In addition, innately resistant organisms such as *Burkholderia cepacia* complex, *S. maltophilia,* and *Achromobacter (Alcaligenes) xylosoxidans* are becoming more prevalent in these patients (18). In addition to underlying comorbid conditions, the presence of invasive devices, such as endotracheal tubes, intravascular catheters, and urinary catheters, also may encourage infection with resistant pathogens. Risk factors for ESBL-producing organisms have been evaluated and include residence in a long-term care facility, duration of stay in the hospital or ICU, and prior exposure cephalosporin antibiotics, particularly ceftazidime and ceftriaxone (19,20). Consideration must be given to antibiotic therapies a patient has recently received (within the past 90 days), as these may promote infection with a resistant pathogen. Furthermore, it is recommended to avoid the same antimicrobial class a patient has been previously exposed to, if possible (5). Finally, outbreaks of antibiotic-resistant bacterial infection may render the usual empiric antibiotic selections ineffective. Consideration of current resistance trends is essential to effectively prescribing antibiotics within the ICU (21).

DIAGNOSIS, MICROBIOLOGY ISSUES, AND INITIAL SOURCE CONTROL

To make the most accurate microbiologic diagnosis of an infection, infected body materials must be obtained before the administration of antimicrobial therapy. In doing so, the possibility of false-negative culture results is reduced, the likelihood of detecting a pathogen via Gram stain is improved, and the confidence from which clinicians make treatment decisions, particularly de-escalation of therapy, is increased.

The cornerstone of microbiologic confirmation is positive blood cultures. Recommended procedure for obtaining blood cultures involves obtaining a pair of blood cultures, ideally from peripheral sites after the initial elevation in temperature, followed by a second pair within the next 24 hr (22). Blood cultures should not be obtained alone, as they are only positive in approximately one-third of patients, particularly those with severe sepsis (23–25). Therefore, it is also important to obtain samples from the suspected site of infection, if possible.

Much of the literature regarding antimicrobial de-escalation is based on the microbiologic diagnosis via bronchoscopic or nonbronchoscopic techniques and subsequent treatment of VAP. At the present time, bronchoscopic sampling of the lower airways, using either a bronchoalveolar lavage (BAL) or protected specimen brush (PSB), is accepted as the most accurate method of establishing a microbiologic diagnosis of VAP, short of direct tissue examination. Quantitative cultures should be performed on the bronchoscopic specimens, with thresholds of 10,000 colony forming units (cfu)/mL for BAL specimens and 1000 cfu/mL for PSB samples being indicators of VAP (5,26). Invasive lower respiratory tract sampling via BAL or PSB for the diagnosis of VAP does not appear to reduce patient mortality (27,28).

However, when compared to noninvasive diagnostic methods, bronchoscopy significantly increases the likelihood of narrowing the spectrum of antibiotic therapy based on positive findings or can be employed to stop antibiotics sooner, possibly within 72 hr if the culture result is negative without the influence of a recently altered antimicrobial regimen (5,27,29).

Invasive diagnostic techniques should be employed to microbiologically confirm infections from other sources. Intra-abdominal infection requires sampling of the anatomical site of origin via percutaneous aspirations under sterile technique or direct surgical observation with acquisition of the culture material directly from the infected site (30,31). Cultures from drain sites are not considered diagnostic of intra-abdominal infections (32). Patients experiencing diarrhea should have one stool sample evaluated for *Clostridium difficile* toxin and other enteric pathogens if appropriate exposure or travel history exists. If the first *C. difficile* specimen is negative, an additional sample should be evaluated (22). Urine should also be obtained for culture for urinalysis with microscopy to determine of the presence of pyuria. When indicated, pus expressed from an implanted catheter site should be sent for Gram stain and culture. In patients with an unexplained altered consciousness or focal neurological signs, lumbar puncture should be performed and cerebral spinal fluid should be evaluated by cytology, Gram stain, and culture.

In circumstances where identifying the site of infection has proven not to be straightforward, an exhaustive systematic workup for possible noninfectious causes of the clinically manifested systemic inflammatory response syndrome should be undertaken. These may include surgery or trauma, venous thrombosis or hematoma, myocardial infarction, pancreatitis, transplant rejection, acute adrenal insufficiency, thyroid storm, malignancy, and others (33).

In summary, aggressive diagnostic practices allow for better diagnostic information that may provide grounds for more rapid de-escalation of antimicrobial therapy and should ultimately reduce antibiotic selection pressure, limit the emergence of drug-resistant bacterial strains, and in due course decrease the likelihood of treating future patients with inappropriate therapy.

IMPORTANCE OF EARLY APPROPRIATE THERAPY

Therapy should be initiated with an appropriately broad-spectrum regimen to cover all likely pathogens and narrow coverage once a pathogen is identified. This can ensure that appropriate antimicrobials are started as early as possible, improving patient outcomes. The American Thoracic Society and Infectious Diseases Society of America define inappropriate antimicrobial therapy as "the use of antibiotics with poor or no in vitro activity against the identified microorganisms causing infection at the tissue site of infection" (5). The influence of early appropriate therapy on patient outcomes has been evaluated in a variety of infections; however, this topic has been most extensively studied in infections in ICU patients, specifically HAP/VAP, sepsis and BSI.

General ICU Infections

Kollef and colleagues prospectively studied two thousand ICU patients to evaluate outcomes associated with inappropriate antimicrobial treatment of infections (34). Of these, 655 patients were diagnosed with an infection at some point during their hospital stay, with 8.5% receiving inappropriate initial antimicrobial therapy. The administration of inappropriate therapy was associated with increased ICU lengths of stay (10.2 ± 10.2 days vs. 7.1 ± 8.2 days) and the development of severe sepsis (40.2% vs. 24.1%, $p < 0.001$). Inappropriate antimicrobial therapy was also found to be an independent predictor for hospital mortality [adjusted OR, 4.26; 95% confidence interval (CI), 3.35–5.44; $p < 0.001$].

Multi-Drug Resistant Organisms

Patients in the ICU are at risk for developing infections with MDR organisms and the impact of appropriate initial antimicrobial therapy in these infections is a topic that has recently received attention. Hyle et al. retrospectively identified 187 patients at two hospitals who were infected with ESBL-producing Enterobacteriaceae (35). There was a trend toward higher hospital mortality in patients receiving inappropriate initial antimicrobial therapy compared to patients with appropriate antimicrobial therapy (21.4% vs. 10.7%; OR, 2.28; 95% CI, 0.92–6.24; $p = 0.06$). Multivariate analyses revealed that inappropriate therapy was an independent risk factor for mortality in patients with nonurinary ESBL infections (adjusted OR, 10.04; 95% CI, 1.90–52.96). Similarly, the initial antimicrobial therapies of 286 patients with antibiotic-resistant Gram-negative bacteremia were retrospectively assessed to determine the influence on 30-day mortality (36). Appropriate initial therapy, defined by the authors as therapy initiated within 24 hr of blood culture collection that was active against the causative organism, was started in 135 patients (47.2%). The 30-day mortality rate was 27.4% in the patients receiving appropriate therapy compared with 38.4% in patients who did not receive appropriate therapy ($p = 0.049$). A multivariate analysis indicated that inappropriate initial antibiotic therapy was associated with increased mortality in patients with high-risk source (i.e., lung, peritoneum, or unknown source) of bacteremia (OR, 3.64; 95% CI, 1.13–11.72; $p = 0.03$), but not in patients with other, low-risk sources of bacteremia (OR 1.08; 95% CI, 0.28–4.18; $p = 0.91$). The authors concluded that inappropriate initial antibiotic therapy was associated with worse outcomes in patients with antibiotic-resistant Gram-negative bacteremia and MDR infections were risk factors for inappropriate initial antimicrobial therapy.

Ventilator-Associated or Hospital-Acquired Pneumonia

One of the most studied ICU infections in evaluating appropriate empiric therapy is VAP/HAP. Alvarez-Lerma and colleagues conducted one of the first trials evaluating empiric antimicrobials for the treatment of ICU-acquired pneumonia (37). The appropriateness of antibiotics was assessed in 430 cases, with 146 patients (34%) receiving inappropriate coverage. Patients who did not receive appropriate antibiotics had significantly higher rates of shock (28.8% vs. 17.1%, $p < 0.005$) and attributable mortality (24.7% vs. 16.2%, $p = 0.0385$) compared to patients who were administered appropriate antibiotics. Similarly, Luna et al. assessed the appropriateness of antibiotic therapy and the impact on mortality in bronchoscopically-proven VAP (38). The mortality rate in patients who received appropriate antibiotics was 38% compared with 91% in patients not receiving adequate therapy ($p < 0.001$). The mortality rate remained the same for patients initially treated with inappropriate therapy even if their therapy was modified to cover the causative organism after culture results were obtained. This underscores the importance of ensuring empiric antimicrobial therapy is appropriate.

A trial performed by Kollef et al. prospectively evaluated the empiric antibiotic therapy in patients that had a BAL performed for suspected VAP (39). In this prospective, observational study, the empiric therapies of 60 patients with positive mini-BAL cultures for clinically suspected VAP were evaluated. Patients who were not administered appropriate antibiotics had a significantly higher hospital mortality rate than patients who were appropriately covered initially (60.8% vs. 33.3%, $p < 0.001$). Inappropriate initial therapy (adjusted OR, 3.28; 95% CI, 2.12–5.06; $p = 0.006$) and having an immunocompromised state both were risk factors independently associated with hospital mortality, as determined by logistic regression analysis. Likewise, in a retrospective analysis of patients developing VAP in their medical-surgical ICU, Dupont and colleagues found that hospital mortality was higher (47.3% vs. 60.7%; OR = 1.72; 95% CI, 0.81–3.7) and ICU length of stay was longer (29 ± 25 days vs. 17 ± 11 days, $p = 0.01$) in patients who received inappropriate antibiotics than patients whose empiric coverage was appropriate (40).

Sepsis

Another ICU-related condition that is frequently studied in the analysis of appropriate initial antibiotic therapy is sepsis. In a prospective cohort study by Garnacho-Montero et al., 270 patients were identified with documented sepsis and had cultures available for analysis (41). Empiric antibiotics were appropriate in 224 (83%) of these patients. A multivariate analysis revealed that inappropriate empiric antibiotics in patients with nonsurgical sepsis was one of the predictors of in-hospital mortality (OR, 8.14; 95% CI, 1.98–33.5) and adequate empiric antimicrobial therapy had a protective effect in surgical sepsis (OR, 0.37; 95% CI, 0.18–0.77) and urologic sepsis (OR, 0.14; 95% CI, 0.05–0.41). More supporting evidence for the importance of appropriate initial antimicrobial therapy in sepsis was provided by Harbarth et al. (42). Using a multicenter database of 1342 patients with severe sepsis or septic shock enrolled in a separate double-blind, placebo-controlled phase 3 trial evaluating the experimental medication, lenercept, the empiric antimicrobial choice of 904 patients with microbiologically confirmed sepsis was assessed. Inappropriate initial antimicrobial therapy was administered in 211 (23%) patients. Twenty-eight day mortality was significantly higher in patients who received inappropriate therapy compared to patients receiving appropriate therapy (39% vs. 24%, $p < 0.001$). Results were similar regardless of whether they were randomized to the placebo group (38% mortality with inappropriate therapy vs. 25% with appropriate therapy, $p = 0.01$) or lenercept group (40% vs. 24%, $p = 0.001$). After performing a multivariate analysis, the authors concluded that inappropriate initial antimicrobial therapy was independently associated with increased mortality (OR 1.8; 95% CI, 1.2–2.6). Micek and colleagues performed a prospective observational cohort study to identify potential risk factors for hospital mortality in patients with severe sepsis (43). Data from 102 patients with severe sepsis treated with drotrecogin alfa (activated) were analyzed. A multivariate analysis indicated that administration of inappropriate initial antimicrobial treatment was independently associated with hospital mortality (OR 15.5, 95% CI, 6.78–35.6), as were vasopressin administration and number of acquired organ-system derangements, providing more supporting evidence for the importance of adequate initial antimicrobial therapy in patients with sepsis.

Bloodstream Infections

Many trials have evaluated outcomes associated with inappropriate treatment of bloodstream infections (44–47). An observational prospective cohort trial was conducted by Leibovici and others to determine the impact that appropriate antimicrobial therapy had on survival in patients with BSIs (44). BSI were identified in 3440 patients, of which 37% did not receive appropriate empiric therapy. The mortality rate was significantly higher in these patients when compared to patients receiving appropriate therapy (34% vs. 20%, respectively; $p = 0.0001$; OR, 2.1; 95% CI, 1.8–2.4). This mortality benefit held true for all subgroups in the stratified analysis, except for patients with infections caused by streptococci other than *Streptococcus* gr. A and *Streptococcus pneumoniae* and hypothermic patients, in which there was no difference in mortality. Likewise, Ibrahim and colleagues also performed a prospective, observational cohort study with one of the study objectives being to assess the impact that appropriate antimicrobial therapy had on clinical outcomes in ICU patients with BSIs (45). During the two-year study period, 4913 patients were prospectively followed, with 492 patients (10%) developing a bloodstream infection and thus included in the analysis. Similar to other trials, 30% of patients did not receive appropriate empiric therapy. Once again, inappropriate initial antimicrobial therapy was associated with a higher hospital mortality rate when compared to patients who received appropriate treatment (61.9% vs. 28.4%, $p < 0.001$; relative risk, 2.18; 95% CI, 1.77–2.69). Results have been consistent when BSIs caused by individual organisms have been studied, including *P. aeruginosa* (46) and *S. aureus* (47).

Table 3 lists the details of these trials assessing the impact of inappropriate initial antimicrobial therapy.

DE-ESCALATION

Modification of an initial, appropriately broad-spectrum antibiotic regimen using a de-escalation strategy should occur based on the results of the patient's clinical response and microbiologic testing. Based on the de-escalation strategy, modification of the initial antibiotic regimen should include decreasing the number and/or spectrum of antibiotics, if possible based on culture and sensitivity results, shortening the duration of therapy in patients with uncomplicated infections who are demonstrating signs of clinical improvement, or discontinuing antibiotics altogether in patients who have a noninfectious etiology identified for the patient's signs and symptoms (Fig. 1). Since the causative organism is frequently unknown when starting empiric antibiotics, combination therapy can increase the likelihood that the organism is being appropriately treated (46,48). However, once the cause has been identified, many infections in nonimmunocompromised hosts can be treated safely with a single agent (46,49).

INSTITUTION-SPECIFIC PROTOCOLS AND GUIDELINES

Antibiotic practice guidelines or protocols, particularly for the treatment of VAP, have emerged as a potentially effective means of both avoiding unnecessary antibiotic administration and limiting the course of therapy without compromising patient outcomes. Ibrahim et al. conducted a pre-/post-protocol study that evaluated a clinical guideline for clinically-diagnosed VAP employing the goals of de-escalation therapy and promoted a 7-day course of antimicrobial therapy in

TABLE 3 Details of Several Trials Assessing the Impact of Inappropriate Initial Antimicrobial Therapy

	Trial design	n	Study details	Mortality (%) Appropriate therapy	Mortality (%) Inappropriate therapy	Statistics
General ICU infections						
Kollef et al. 1999 (34)	Prospective, observational cohort trial	655	Medical and surgical ICU pts with ICU-associated infections	17.7	42.0	RR, 2.37; 95% CI, 1.83–3.08; $p < 0.001$
MDR organisms						
Hyle et al. 2005 (35)	Retrospective cohort study	187	ESBL-producing Enterobacteriaceae	10.7	21.4	OR, 2.28; 95% CI, 0.92–6.24; $p = 0.06$
Kang et al. 2005 (36)	Retrospective cohort study	286	Hospitalized pts with antibiotic-resistant Gram-negative bacteremia	27.4	38.4	$p = 0.049$
HAP/VAP						
Alvarez-Lerma et al. 1996 (37)	Prospective, multi-centered observational trial	430	Medical and surgical ICU pts in 30 Spanish hospitals	16.2[a]	24.7[a]	$p = 0.0385$
Luna et al. 1997 (38)	Prospective, observational cohort trial	132	Medical-surgical ICU pts with bronchoscopically-proven VAP	38	91	$p < 0.001$
Kollef et al. 1998 (39)	Prospective, observational cohort trial	60	Positive mini-BAL cultures for clinically suspected VAP	33.3	60.8	$p < 0.001$
Dupont et al. 2001 (40)	Retrospective cohort study	111	VAP diagnosed on clinical and microbiological data. Antibiotic therapy started after distal bronchial sampling was obtained	47.3	60.7	OR = 1.72, 95% CI 0.81–3.7
Sepsis						
Garnacho-Montero et al. 2003 (41)	Prospective cohort study	270	Medical-surgical ICU pts	—	—	Inappropriate empiric therapy in "nonsurgical sepsis", OR, 8.14; 95% CI 1.98–33.5
Harbarth et al. 2003 (42)	Retrospective, subgroup analysis of a prospective, multi-national trial	904	Pts with severe sepsis or septic shock enrolled in a phase 3 trial for lenercept	24	39	$p < 0.001$[b]

(Continued)

TABLE 3 Details of Several Trials Assessing the Impact of Inappropriate Initial Antimicrobial Therapy (*Continued*)

	Trial design	n	Study details	Mortality (%) Appropriate therapy	Mortality (%) Inappropriate therapy	Statistics
Sepsis						
Micek et al. 2005 (43)	Prospective, observational cohort trial	102	ICU pts treated with drotrecogin alfa (activated)	—	—	OR, 15.5; 95% CI 6.78–35.6
BSI						
Leibovici et al. 1998 (44)	Prospective, observational cohort trial	2,158	Hospitalized pts with BSIs	20	34	p = 0.0001
Ibrahim et al. 2000 (45)	Prospective, observational cohort trial	492	Medical and surgical ICU pts	28.4	61.9	RR, 2.18; 95% CI, 1.77–2.69; p < 0.001
Micek et al. 2005 (46)	Retrospective cohort trial	305	Hospitalized pts with *Pseudomonas aeruginosa* bacteremia	17.8	30.7	p = 0.018
Lodise et al. 2003 (47)	Retrospective cohort trial	167	Hospitalized pts with *Staphylococcus aureus* bacteremia	19.3	33.3	p = 0.05

[a]Comparison of appropriate empiric antibiotic therapy vs. changing to appropriate therapy after culture results.
[b]Significant difference seen whether pts enrolled in placebo or lenercept group.
Abbreviations: BAL, bronchoalveolar lavage; BSI, blood stream infection; CI, confidence interval; ESBL, extended-spectrum beta-lactamase; HAP, hospital-acquired pneumonia; ICU, intensive care unit; OR, odds ratio; pts, patients; RR, relative risk; VAP, ventilator-associated pneumonia; —, not reported.

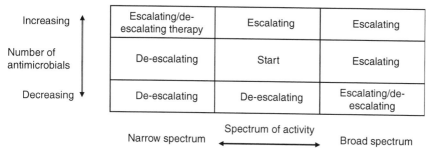

FIGURE 1 De-escalating therapy by decreasing the number or spectrum of activity of antimicrobials.

responding patients with uncomplicated VAP (i.e., absence of empyema or secondary bacteremia) (48). Therapy was initiated with a predetermined broad-spectrum regimen that would cover greater than 90% of the likely pathogens. The de-escalation guideline incorporated in this trial dictated that antibiotic treatment had to be modified via two modalities: (*i*) narrowing the spectrum of therapy 24 to 48 hr into treatment based on the availability of culture results and the patient's clinical course and (*ii*) subsequent recommendation of a 7-day course of therapy. Use of antibiotic treatment beyond 7 days was only encouraged for patients with clinical parameters that remained abnormal or consistent with persistent infection. Prior to implementation of the protocol, 48% of patients with VAP were administered appropriate therapy compared with 94% in the post-protocol period. Upon implementation of the clinical guideline, 98% of patients had 1 or 2 antibiotics discontinued by 48 hr of treatment. The duration of treatment was significantly shorter during the post-protocol period compared with the pre-protocol period (8.6 ± 5.1 days vs. 14.8 ± 8.1 days, $p < 0.001$). Additionally, there were fewer secondary infections due to antibiotic resistant organisms during the clinical guideline phase. No differences in clinical outcome measures, including in-hospital mortality or ICU and hospital lengths of stay, were observed. Similarly, Micek and colleagues evaluated a formalized discontinuation policy of antimicrobials in patients with clinically-diagnosed VAP (50). Patients randomized to the discontinuation group were monitored during the weekday by a clinical pharmacist who made recommendations to stop one or more antibiotics if a noninfectious etiology for pulmonary infiltrates was identified or if all of the following criteria were met: (*i*) temperature $<38.3°C$, (*ii*) white blood cell count $<10 \times 10^3$ or decreased 25% from peak value, (*iii*) improvement or lack of progression on chest x-ray, (*iv*) absence of purulent sputum, and (*v*) PaO2:FiO2 ratio >250. Eighty-nine percent of patients in the discontinuation group had at least one antibiotic discontinued within 48 hr of recommendation. The overall duration of treatment was significantly shorter in the discontinuation group compared to standard therapy (6.0 ± 4.9 days vs. 8.0 ± 5.6 days, $p = 0.001$). No differences were observed with respect to in-hospital mortality, ICU and hospital length of stay, the duration of mechanical ventilation, or the acquisition of a second episode of VAP.

SHORTER COURSES OF ANTIMICROBIAL THERAPY

Several groups of investigators have demonstrated that shorter courses of therapy for VAP can be efficacious while potentially reducing the emergence of antimicrobial resistance. This premise is based on a study conducted by Denneson et al. in which the clinical and microbiological response to appropriate antimicrobial therapy for VAP was evaluated over a 14-day period (51). To characterize the infectious process, the investigators serially recorded patients' clinical (maximum daily temperature, PaO2:FiO2 ratio, peripheral white blood cell count) and microbiologic response (the results of semi-quantitative cultures of endotracheal aspirates). Resolution of all clinical and microbiologic parameters occurred a mean (median) of 9 (8) days into appropriate antimicrobial therapy. Importantly though, after 7 days of antibiotic therapy, newly isolated, potentially antibiotic-resistant bacteria such as *S. aureus* and *P. aeruginosa* were cultured in over half of the patients. This finding might have been of some consequence in that 66% patients who had a recurrent episode of VAP were infected with pathogens resistant to antibiotics used to treat the first infection.

Singh and colleagues attempted to reduce the emergence of resistance by limiting the number of antibiotics and duration of antibiotic therapy in patients having a low likelihood of VAP, as indicated by a clinical pulmonary infection score (CPIS) ≤ 6 (52). Patients with the clinical diagnosis of VAP (not uniformly diagnosed via quantitative cultures of BAL or PSB) but with CPIS ≤ 6 were randomized to conventional therapy determined by the treating physician or to ciprofloxacin monotherapy. Per study protocol, patients in the ciprofloxacin monotherapy group had treatment discontinued on day 3 if the CPIS remained ≤ 6, whereas therapy was permitted to continue in the conventional therapy group. Patients in the ciprofloxacin monotherapy group had significantly shorter courses of antibiotic therapy (3 days vs. 10 days; $p = 0.0001$), significantly less development of antimicrobial resistance or subsequent super-infection (15% vs. 35%; $p = 0.017$), and shorter ICU lengths of stay (median 4 days vs. 9 days; $p = 0.04$), with a slight trend to improvement in 30-day all cause mortality (13% vs. 31%; $p = 0.06$). This indicates that empiric therapy can be safely discontinued after three days in patients with a low likelihood of pneumonia.

Antibiotic management of bronchoscopically-confirmed, uncomplicated VAP treated initially with appropriate therapy should be limited to a short duration. Chastre et al. conducted a randomized, double-blind, multicenter, noninferiority trial comparing an 8-day course of treatment with a 15-day course in patients who had received appropriate therapy for a bronchoscopically-confirmed VAP (53). Patients receiving 8 days of therapy had a mortality rate of 18.8% compared with 17.2% in the 15-day group, an absolute difference of 1.6% (90% CI, 3.7 to 6.9), which indicated noninferiority. Overall, pulmonary infection recurrence, the number of mechanical ventilator-free days, and the ICU length of stay did not differ between groups. Patients in the 8-day group had a significantly greater number of antibiotic-free days at day 28, and had less frequent isolation of antibiotic-resistant pathogens when recurrent infection was diagnosed.

The individual theories of de-escalation are combined into a diagram in Figure 2.

CLINICAL APPLICATIONS: HOW TO IMPLEMENT A DE-ESCALATION STRATEGY

As outlined, the concept of provision of initially broad-spectrum antibiotic therapy with secondary de-escalation is highly attractive. The benefits of early appropriate therapy may be realized in a majority of patients, while de-escalation provides a

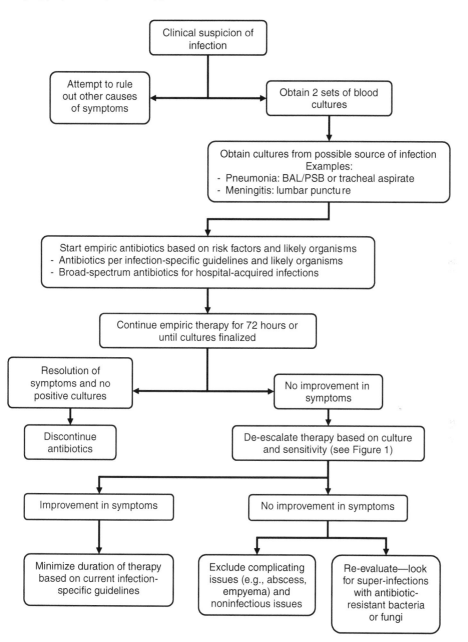

FIGURE 2 Approach to de-escalation. *Abbreviations*: BAL, bronchoalveolar lavage; PSB, protected specimen brush.

means to reduce unnecessary antibiotic exposure and secondary development of bacterial resistance. Discussion of this practice would be remiss to neglect the practical considerations of implementing such a program and consideration of the potential barriers to effective implementation that exist.

A more "traditional" approach to antibiotic therapy, and one taught for years in many medical schools, would be to start with minimal coverage of likely pathogens, and expand coverage only if a resistant pathogen is isolated. Likewise, widespread recognition of increasing antibiotic resistance has prompted many institutions to employ various antibiotic restriction strategies (54–58). Many centers have developed antibiotic restriction policies to restrict access to broad-spectrum antibiotics as first-line therapy or have an antibiotic approval process cumbersome enough to discourage use of these agents. In dealing with critically ill patients, however, it is essential that these policies allow for permissive empiric prescribing of broad-spectrum agents for patients at risk of infection due to resistant pathogens. The high cost of antibiotic therapy is a frequent reason cited for restricting expensive, broad-spectrum antibiotics; however, consideration of the total cost of care versus drug cost alone reveals that length of hospital stay and clinical failures are far greater cost components of the total cost of care. Interventions to improve efficacy and reduce length of stay have been shown to reduce total cost of infection management (59).

A definitive diagnosis of infection is necessary to optimally employ a strategy employing de-escalation. Recognition that not everything that looks like infection is truly infection emphasizes the need for obtaining appropriate specimens for microbiologic and diagnostic testing. In VAP, for example, use of an invasive diagnostic approach, such as BAL, allows the clinician to be confident in the diagnosis of pneumonia. Antibiotics may then be safely discontinued in patients not meeting strict criteria for pneumonia. Unfortunately, in many clinical institutions, bronchoscopy is not immediately available, especially in the evenings, potentially reducing the utility of this tool in some settings. Controversy still exists around the best diagnostic approaches for HAP and VAP; however, it seems that when implementing a de-escalation strategy, clinicians are comfortable transitioning patients to narrow-spectrum agents when more information is available. In addition, a negative tracheal aspirate in a patient without a recent change in antibiotics is useful as it carries a strong negative predictive value and should lead to a search for alternative sources of fever (5).

Barriers to de-escalation include lack of physician acceptance, lack of objective measures demonstrating clinical improvement, and the potentially confounding impact of concomitant infections or other disease states on patient status. One of the most difficult scenarios is in a patient initially demonstrating signs of infection in which cultures are never positive (whether or not influenced by prior antibiotics) who subsequently has improved on the broad-spectrum regimen. It is then necessary to re-evaluate therapy and assess what is absent in the isolation of pathogens. If MRSA therapy had been initiated, but MRSA has not been isolated despite adequate diagnostic techniques, it is reasonable to consider discontinuation of this therapy. Similarly, if combination therapy was initiated secondary to suspicion of *P. aeruginosa* and it is not isolated, streamlining to monotherapy may be appropriate. Finally, if an initially suspected diagnosis leads to the use of broad-spectrum antibiotics, cultures do not prove helpful, and the patient is clinically not responding, an alternative diagnosis must be sought. This problematic scenario highlights the importance of performing adequate diagnostic testing at the onset of suspicion of infection.

One problem identified has been the lack of continuity of care in academic teaching centers where house staff and attending staff physicians rotate on a monthly or, in some centers, on a weekly basis. One practitioner may be reluctant to make a change in antibiotics started by another, without a clear appreciation of the initial rationale behind the therapy. A number of different strategies may be useful to assist in the daily assessment and de-escalation strategies. ICUs with clinical pharmacists have found that the constant presence of this one team member can provide a continuum of care and tracking mechanism to provide accountability for the necessity of antibiotics prescribed (50,61).

Another approach capitalizes on the ability of computer-assisted tracking of antibiotic prescribing. Evans et al. evaluated the use of a computerized anti-infective-management program in the shock trauma unit of Latter Day Saints Hospital (62). Physicians who followed the recommendation of the automated anti-infective program significantly reduced the number of days their patients received antimicrobial treatment in the ICU setting without any obvious detrimental consequences. Automated and nonautomated antimicrobial guidelines have been used to reduce the overall use of antibiotics and to limit the use of inadequate antimicrobial treatment, both of which could affect the development of resistance (63–65). Similar interventions could be developed for the ICU setting to reduce antibiotic misuse and overuse, decrease inadequate or ineffective antimicrobial treatment, and help curtail the problem of antimicrobial resistance (66).

CONCLUSION

Use of early, risk-directed, frequently broad-spectrum therapy can provide reduction in antibiotic exposure only when combined with diligent de-escalation and use of appropriately short course antibiotic therapy. It must be emphasized that continued use of unnecessarily broad-spectrum regimens for excessively prolonged durations of therapy will inevitably lead to antibiotic resistance. At the time of implementation of a de-escalation strategy, clinicians must embrace the need for daily assessment and active intervention to reduce the use of antimicrobials that are no longer proven to be necessary. Without resources available to ensure such follow-up, the risks of prolonged use of broad-spectrum antibiotics must be acknowledged and carefully considered.

REFERENCES

1. Gaynes R, Edwards JR. National Nosocomial Infections Surveillance System. Overview of nosocomial infections caused by Gram-negative bacilli. Clin Infect Dis 2005; 41:848–54.
2. National Nosocomial Infections Surveillance (NNIS) system report, data summary from January 1992–April 2000, issued June 2000. Am J Infect Control 2000; 28:429–48.
3. Richards MJ, Edwards JR, Culver DH, et al. Nosocomial infections in combined medical-surgical intensive care units in the United States. Infect Control Hosp Epidemiol 2000; 21:510–5.
4. Trouillet J-L, Chastre J, Vuagnat A, et al. Ventilator-associated pneumonia caused by potentially drug-resistant bacteria. Am J Respir Crit Care Med 1998; 157:531–9.
5. American Thoracic Society: Guidelines for the Management of Adults with Hospital-acquired, Ventilator-associated, and Healthcare-associated Pneumonia. Am J Respir Crit Care Med 2005; 171:388–416.
6. Vidaur L, Sirgo G, Rodriguez AH, et al. Clinical approach to the patient with suspected ventilator-associated pneumonia. Respir Care 2005; 50:965–74.

7. Babcock HM, Zack JE, Garrison T, et al. Ventilator-associated pneumonia in a multi-hospital system: differences in microbiology by location. Infect Control Hosp Epidemiol 2003; 24:853–8.
8. Rello J, Sa-Borges M, Correa H, et al. Variations in etiology of ventilator-associated pneumonia across four treatment sites. Am J Respir Crit Care Med 1999; 160:608–13.
9. Namias N, Samiian L, Nino D, et al. Incidence and susceptibility of pathogenic bacteria vary between intensive care units within a single hospital: implications for empiric antibiotic strategies. J Trauma 2000; 49:638–45.
10. Crouch Brewer S, Wunderink RG, Jones CB, et al. Ventilator-associated pneumonia due to *Pseudomonas aeruginosa*. Chest 1996; 109:1019–29.
11. Rello J, Torres A, Ricart M, et al. Ventilator-associated pneumonia by *Staphylococcus aureus*. Comparison of methicillin-resistant and methicillin-sensitive episodes. Am J Respir Crit Care Med 1994; 150:1545–9.
12. Combes A, Luyt CE, Fagon JY, et al. Impact of methicillin resistance on outcome of *Staphylococcus aureus* ventilator-associated pneumonia. Am J Respir Crit Care Med 2004; 170:786–92.
13. Cosgrove SE, Qi Y, Kaye KS, et al. The impact of methicillin resistance in Staphylococcus aureus bacteremia on patient outcomes: mortality, length of stay, and hospital charges. Infect Control Hosp Epidemiol 2005; 26:166–74.
14. Rello J, Quintana E, Ausina V, Puzo C, Net A, Prats G. Risk factors for *Staphylococcus aureus* nosocomial pneumonia in critically ill patients. Am Rev Respir Dis 1990; 142:1320–4.
15. Francis JS, Doherty MC, Lopatin U, et al. Severe community-onset pneumonia in healthy adults caused by methicillin-resistant *Staphylococcus aureus* carrying the Panton-Valentine Leukocidin genes. Clin Infect Dis 2005; 40:100–7.
16. Micek ST, Dunne WM, Kollef MH. Pleuropulmonary complications of Panton-Valentine leukocidin-positive community-acquired methicillin-resistant *Staphylococcus aureus*: importance of treatment with antimicrobials inhibiting exotoxin production. Chest 2005; 128:2732–8.
17. Rello J, Ausina V, Ricart M, et al. Risk Factors for infection by *Pseudomonas aeruginosa* in patients with ventilator-associated pneumonia. Intensive Care Med 1994; 20:193–8.
18. Conway SP, Brownlee KG, Denton M, et al. Antibiotic treatment of multidrug-resistant organisms in cystic fibrosis. Am J Respir Med 2003; 2:321–32.
19. Schiappa DA, Hayden MK, Matushek MG, et al. Ceftazidime-resistant *Klebsiella pneumoniae* and *Escherichia coli* bloodstream infection: a case-control and molecular epidemiologic investigation. J Infect Dis 1996; 174:529–36.
20. Lautenbach E, Patel JB, Bilker WB, Edelstein PH, Fishman NO. Extended-spectrum beta-lactamase-producing *Escherichia coil* and *Klebsiella pneumoniae*: risk factors for infection and impact of resistance on outcomes. Clin Infect Dis 2001; 32:1162–71.
21. Paterson DL, Rice LB. Empirical antibiotic choice for the seriously ill patient: are minimization of selection of resistant organisms and maximization of individual outcome mutually exclusive? Clin Infect Dis 2003; 36:1006–12.
22. O'Grady NP, Barie PS, Bartlett JG, et al. Practice guidelines for evaluating new fever in critically ill adult patients. Clin Infect Dis 1998; 26:1042–59.
23. Bernard GR, Vincent J-L, Laterre PF, et al. Efficacy and safety of recombinant human activated protein C for severe sepsis. N Engl J Med 2001; 344:699–709.
24. Annane D, Sebille V, Charpentier C, et al. Effect of treatment with low doses of hydrocortisone and fludrocortisone on mortality in patients with septic shock. JAMA 2002; 288:862–71.
25. Warren BL, Eid A, Singer P, et al. High-dose antithrombin III in severe sepsis: a randomized controlled trial. JAMA 2001; 286:1869–78.
26. Baselski VS, El-Torky M, Coalson JJ, et al. The standardization of criteria for processing and interpreting laboratory specimens in patients with suspected ventilator-associated pneumonia. Chest 1992; 102:571S–9S.
27. Shorr AF, Sherner JH, Jackson WM, et al. Invasive approaches to the diagnosis of ventilator-associated pneumonia: a meta-analysis. Crit Care Med 2005; 33:46–53.

28. Rello J, Vidaur L, Sandiumenge A, et al. De-escalation therapy in ventilator-associated pneumonia. Crit Care Med 2004; 2183–90.
29. Kollef MH, Kollef KE. Antibiotic utilization and outcomes for patients with clinically suspected ventilator-associated pneumonia and negative quantitative BAL cultures results. Chest 2005; 128:2706–13.
30. Evans HL, Raymond DP, Pelletier SJ, et al. Diagnosis of intra-abdominal infection in the critically ill patient. Curr Opin Crit Care 2001; 7:117–21.
31. Solomkin JS, Mazuski JE, Baron EJ, et al. Guidelines for the selection of anti-infective agents for complicated intra-abdominal infections. Clin Infect Dis 2003; 37:997–1005.
32. Calandra T, Cohen J. The international sepsis consensus conference on definitions of infection in the intensive care unit. Crit Care Med 2005; 33:1538–48.
33. Llewelyn M, Cohen J. Diagnosis of infection in sepsis. Int Care Med 2001; 27(Suppl): S10–32.
34. Kollef MH, Sherman G, Ward S, Fraser VJ. Inadequate antimicrobial treatment of infections: a risk factor for hospital mortality among critically ill patients. Chest 1999; 115:462–74.
35. Hyle EP, Lipworth AD, Zaoutix TE, et al. Impact of inadequate initial antimicrobial therapy on mortality in infections due to extended-spectrum beta-lactamase-producing Enterobacteriaceae: variability by site of infection. Arch Intern Med 2005; 165:1375–80.
36. Kang CI, Kim SH, Park WB, et al. Bloodstream infections caused by antibiotic-resistant Gram-negative bacilli: risk factors for mortality and impact of inappropriate initial antimicrobial therapy on outcome. Antimicrob Agents Chemother 2005; 49:760–6.
37. Alvarez-Lerma F. Modification of empiric antibiotic treatment in patients with pneumonia acquired in the intensive care unit. ICU-Acquired Pneumonia Study Group. Intensive Care Med 1996; 22:387–94.
38. Luna CM, Vujacich P, Niederman MS, et al. Impact of BAL data on the therapy and outcome of ventilator-associated pneumonia. Chest 1997; 111:676–85.
39. Kollef MH, Ward S. The influence of mini-BAL cultures on patient outcomes: implications for the antibiotic management of ventilator-associated pneumonia. Chest 1998; 113:412–20.
40. Dupont H, Mentec H, Sollet JP, et al. Impact of appropriateness of initial antibiotic therapy on the outcome of ventilator-associated pneumonia. Intensive Care Med 2001; 27:355–62.
41. Garnacho-Montero J, Garcia-Garmendia JL, Barrero-Almodovar A, et al. Impact of adequate empical antibiotic therapy on the outcome of patients admitted to the intensive care unit with sepsis. Crit Care Med 2003: 31:2742–51.
42. Harbarth S, Garbino J, Pugin J, et al. Inappropriate initial antimicrobial therapy and its effect on survival in a clinical trial of immunomodulating therapy for severe sepsis. Am J Med 2003; 115:529–35.
43. Micek ST, Isakow W, Shannon W, et al. Predictors of hospital mortality for patients with severe sepsis treated with drotrecogin alfa (activated). Pharmacotherapy 2005; 25:26–34.
44. Leibovici L, Shraga I, Drucker M, et al. The benefit of appropriate empirical antibiotic treatment in patients with bloodstream infection. J Intern Med 1998; 244:379–86.
45. Ibrahim EH, Sherman G, Ward S, et al. The influence of inadequate antimicrobial treatment of bloodstream infections on patient outcomes in the ICU setting. Chest 2000; 118:146–55.
46. Micek ST, Lloyd AE, Ritchie DJ, et al. *Pseudomonas aeruginosa* bloodstream infection: importance of appropriate initial antimicrobial treatment. Antimicrob Agents Chemother 2005; 49:1306–11.
47. Lodise TP, McKinnon PS, Swiderski L, et al. Outcomes analysis of delayed antibiotic treatment for hospital-acquired *Staphylococcus aureus* bacteremia. Clin Infect Dis 2003; 36:1418–23.
48. Ibrahim EH, Ward S, Sherman G, et al. Experience with a clinical guideline for the treatment of ventilator-associated pneumonia. Crit Care Med 2001; 29:1109–15.
49. Leibovici L, Paul M, Poznanski O, et al. Monotherapy versus beta-lactum-aminoglycoside combination treatment for Gram-negative bacteremia: a prospective, observational study. Antimicrob Agents Chemother 1997; 41:1127–33.

50. Micek ST, Ward S, Fraser VJ, et al. A randomized controlled trial of an antibiotic discontinuation policy for clinically suspected ventilator-associated pneumonia. Chest 2004; 125:1791–9.
51. Dennesen PJW, van der Ven AJ, Kessels AGH, et al. Resolution of infectious parameters after antimicrobial therapy in patients with ventilator-associated pneumonia. Am J Respir Crit Care Med 2001; 163:1371–5.
52. Singh N, Rogers P, Atwood CW, et al. Short course empiric antibiotic therapy for pulmonary infiltrates in the intensive care unit: a proposed solution for indiscriminate antibiotic prescription. Am J Respir Crit Care Med 2000; 162:505–11.
53. Chastre J, Wolff M, Fagon JY, et al. Comparison of 15 vs. 8 days of antibiotic therapy for ventilator-associated pneumonia in adults: a randomized trial. JAMA 2003; 290:2588–98.
54. Himmelberg CJ, Pleasants RA, Weber DJ, et al. Use of antimicrobial drugs in adults before and after removal of a restriction policy. Am J Hosp Pharm 1991; 48:1220–7.
55. Thomas AR, Cieslak PR, Strausbaugh LJ, et al. Effectiveness of pharmacy policies designed to limit inappropriate vancomycin use: a population-based assessment. Infect Control Hosp Epidemiol 2002; 23:683–8.
56. Erbay A, Colpan A, Bodur H, et al. Evaluation of antibiotic use in a hospital with an antibiotic restriction policy. Int J Antimicrob Agents 2003; 21:308–12.
57. Bassetti M, Di Biagio A, Rebesco B, et al. Impact of an antimicrobial formulary and restriction policy in the largest hospital in Italy. Int J Antimicrob Agents 2000; 16:295–9.
58. Vlahovic-Palcevski V, Morovic M, Palcevski G. Antibiotic utilization at the university hospital after introducing an antibiotic policy. Eur J Clin Pharmacol 2000; 56:97–101.
59. Shah NP, Reddy P, Paladino JA, et al. Direct medical costs associated with using vancomycin in methicillin-resistant *Staphylococcus aureus* infections: an economic model. Curr Med Res Opin 2004; 20:779–90.
60. Paladino JA. Economics of antibiotic use policies. Pharmacotherapy 2004; 12:232S–8S.
61. Papadopoulos J, Rebuck JA, Lober C, et al. The critical care pharmacist: an essential intensive care practitioner. Pharmacotherapy 2002; 22:1484–8.
62. Evans RS, Classen DC, Pestotnik SL, et al. Improving empiric antibiotic selection using computer decision support. Arch Intern Med 1994; 154:878–84.
63. Pestotnik SL, Classen DC, Evans RS, et al. Implementing antibiotic practice guidelines through computer-assisted decision support: clinical and financial outcomes. Ann Intern Med 1996; 124:884–90.
64. Evans RS, Pestotnik SL, Classen DC, et al. A computer-assisted management program for antibiotics and other antiinfective agents. N Engl J Med 1998; 338:232–8.
65. Leibovici L, Gitelman V, Yehezkelli Y, et al. Improving empirical antibiotic treatment: prospective, nonintervention testing of a decision support system. J Intern Med 1997; 242:395–400.
66. Yates RR. New intervention strategies for reducing antibiotic resistance. Chest 1999; 115:24S–7S.

Antimicrobial Cycling Programs

Bernard C. Camins and Victoria J. Fraser
*Division of Infectious Diseases, Washington University School of Medicine,
Saint Louis, Missouri, U.S.A.*

INTRODUCTION

Because of increasing antimicrobial resistance in hospitals, antimicrobial cycling programs have been introduced in an effort to decrease rates of antimicrobial resistance (1–4). By limiting the exposure of bacteria to a certain class of antimicrobials, the development of resistance to the same class of antimicrobials may be delayed or avoided. Unfortunately, despite several studies having been reported in the literature (5–19), it is still unclear if antimicrobial cycling prevents the development of resistance. Aside from conflicting study results, the variability in the study design and the duration of each antimicrobial cycle has made comparisons of the studies difficult. The majority of published studies also relied on clinical culture results instead of surveillance culture results for assessing outcomes. Clinical culture results may not accurately reflect the development of resistance among bacterial pathogens since they only represent a small minority of bacteria within a patient population. Mathematical modeling studies have also favored antimicrobial mixing strategies over antimicrobial cycling (20,21). Finally, because of increasing fluoroquinolone resistance among Gram-negative bacilli (22,23), there may not be enough feasible cycling regimens available to provide the antimicrobial heterogeneity necessary for an effective antimicrobial cycling program.

This chapter first covers the nomenclature and definitions used in antimicrobial cycling programs. This is followed by a discussion of the different studies on antibiotic cycling published in the literature, beginning with the accidental discovery of the effects of antimicrobial switching made by Gerding et al. (5). This chapter also considers the utility and feasibility of future antimicrobial cycling programs. Overall, the reader will see that there are insufficient data to support the use of antimicrobial cycling as a method to combat antimicrobial resistance.

DEFINITIONS

Antimicrobial cycling in the strictest sense of the word has been described as the "deliberate, scheduled removal and substitution of specific antimicrobials or classes of antimicrobials within an institutional environment (either hospital-wide or confined to specific units) to avoid or reverse the development of antimicrobial resistance" (3). Brown and Nathwani described cycling or rotation of antimicrobials as the scheduled substitution of a class of antibiotics (or a specific member of a class) with a different class (or a specific member of that class) that exhibits a comparable spectrum of activity (24). Yet another term that has been used to describe antimicrobial cycling is *proactive switching*, since a predetermined protocol or antimicrobial use schedule is planned prior to the development or appearance of antimicrobial resistance (25). Most authors also emphasize that reintroduction of one original antibiotic class must occur regardless of the number of substitutions (usually three or four) for the cycling definition to be met (3,24,26). If this strict definition is followed then there are limited data on the efficacy of antimicrobial cycling as a method to decrease antimicrobial resistance (3,24).

In contrast to true antimicrobial cycling, *reactive switching* is a single substitution of an antibicromial agent or class as empiric therapy in reaction to increased antimicrobial resistance (25). Although the precursors of the true antimicrobial cycling studies were actually reactive switching studies, they are also discussed in this chapter because they provide some insight into the impact of changing antimicrobial prescribing practices and they have guided investigators in designing more sophisticated future trials (5,7,8,27). More complex and well-defined reactive switching studies were also reported in the literature but because a return to the original class of antimicrobials was not included, these studies still cannot really be considered as true antimicrobial cycling studies (9,28). As for *true* antimicrobial cycling studies, there have only been six well-designed trials published in the literature (14–19).

ANTIMICROBIAL CYCLING PROGRAMS REPORTED IN THE LITERATURE

Antimicrobial cycling has potential as a method to decrease antimicrobial resistance rates because of its theoretical ease of implementation. In reality, 100% compliance with the cycling regimen is extremely difficult to achieve. In the published trials of antimicrobial cycling, as much as 50% of antimicrobial use was "off cycle" because of concerns over resistance, allergies, medication side effects, and use of antimicrobials in accordance with national guidelines (15,29,30). Possibly as a consequence of poor adherence to antimicrobial cycling regimens, antimicrobial cycling studies have produced conflicting results.

The duration of each cycling period as well as the cycled antimicrobial agents have not been standardized and so the duration of cycling periods differs among many of the studies. Furthermore, although data from the Centers for Disease Control and Prevention's (CDC) National Nosocomial Infections Surveillance (NNIS) system show increased antimicrobial resistance in both Gram-positive and Gram-negative pathogens in hospitals, particularly intensive care units (ICUs), the majority of the studies on antimicrobial cycling have involved empiric therapy for Gram-negative infections (31,32). To date, published antimicrobial cycling studies have been limited to single institutions. Only two studies included two or more ICUs (17,19).

The idea of antimicrobial switching or substitution as a strategy to prevent antimicrobial resistance was first observed by Gerding et al. at the Minneapolis Veteran's Administration Medical Center (VAMC) (5). This group noticed that resistance to gentamicin among Gram-negative bacilli decreased from 12% to 6.4% ($p < 0.001$) after gentamicin use was substituted with amikacin at their hospital. When gentamicin was reintroduced 26 months later, the resistance rate increased again by 2.8% (6.4–9.2%; $p < 0.001$). A similar intervention was performed at the Houston VAMC. Amikacin was substituted for gentamicin and a reduction in gentamicin resistance was seen (14–9.2%; $p < 0.001$) (5,7). The difference in this study is that, at the time gentamicin was reintroduced, the amikacin resistance rates had already increased to 4% from a baseline of 2.4% ($p < 0.001$) (7). Another example of successful reactive switching was demonstrated by Quale and his colleagues. In this study, the use of third-generation cephalosporins, vancomycin and clindamycin, was restricted in favor of beta-lactam/beta-lactamase inhibitor combinations for empiric therapy in the treatment of Gram-negative infections. This intervention resulted in a statistically significant decrease in the vancomycin-resistant enterococcus colonization rate among patients from 47% to 15% (33).

Kollef et al. conducted one of the first trials on proactive antimicrobial switching. They instituted a program in the cardiothoracic surgery ICU in which ceftazidime, the standard empiric therapy for hospital-acquired Gram-negative infections, was replaced by ciprofloxacin empiric therapy. This study was initiated in anticipation of increasing resistance rates as opposed to initiating a cycling program in response to increasing antimicrobial resistance. Their intervention resulted in a statistically significant decline in the incidence of ventilator-associated pneumonia (VAP) due to resistant Gram-negative bacilli (4.0–0.9%; $p < 0.001$). Although not statistically significant, there were also declines in the incidence of bacteremia (1.7–0.3%) and mortality (1.7–0.6%) due to resistant Gram-negative bacilli (8).

Other investigators have since followed suit with studies that included more than two antimicrobial regimens. Dominguez et al. conducted a more sophisticated switching study over a 19-month period. Four classes of antimicrobials, (*i*) ceftazidime with vancomycin, (*ii*) imipenem alone, (*iii*) aztreonam with cefazolin, and (*iv*) ciprofloxacin with clindamycin, were consecutively selected as the recommended regimen for treatment of febrile neutropenia. Although the duration of each regimen was not standardized, each one lasted for at least 4 months. Infection rates and antimicrobial resistance among clinical isolates were chosen as study endpoints. This was a small pilot study and ultimately only 271 patients were enrolled during the study period. There was no difference in efficacy among the chosen antimicrobial regimens and no increase in antimicrobial resistance rates was observed. Surveillance cultures were not obtained in these patients and data analysis was only limited to clinical isolates (9).

Hughes et al. performed a prospective cohort study in a surgical ICU over two years. This switching study included a year-long baseline period followed by four 3-month periods of scheduled changes in empiric antimicrobial regimens. A return to the original antimicrobial regimen also did not occur in this study. The authors reported a decrease in the incidences in both antimicrobial-resistant Gram-negative infections (7.7 infections/100 admissions vs. 2.5 infections/100 admissions; $p < 0.0001$) and antimicrobial-resistant Gram-positive infections (14.6 infections/100 admissions vs. 7.8 infections/100 admissions; $p < 0.001$). They also reported a decrease in infection-related mortality (9.6 deaths/100 admissions vs. 2.9 deaths/100 admissions; $p < 0.001$) but their definition of mortality has come into question (28). Infection-related mortality is very difficult to tease out in an ICU patient population since there are comorbid illnesses that can contribute to mortality (34). Furthermore, significant changes in infection control policies, such as the introduction of alcohol-based hand rubs and the establishment of an antimicrobial surveillance team, could have accounted for a reduction in the rates of infection.

One of the earliest true antimicrobial cycling studies that included two or more antimicrobial classes was conducted by Moss et al. in the pediatric ICU. Three antimicrobial regimens at 3-month intervals were all cycled at least once over an 18-month period. Surveillance cultures from the patient's nasopharynx and stool were performed at least twice a month. Although the results of this trial were inconclusive, the authors determined that antimicrobial cycling may be a safe and viable strategy in reducing antimicrobial resistance rates and that further studies were warranted (12). Investigators in the Netherlands then followed with another true antimicrobial cycling program using a fluoroquinolone (levofloxacin in cycles 1 and 3) and beta-lactams (cefpirome in cycle 2 and piperacillin-tazobactam in cycle 4) over four 4-month intervals. Both respiratory and rectal cultures were collected on admission to and discharge from the ICU and weekly while in the ICU. These weekly surveillance cultures significantly improved the methodology compared to previous studies. The primary endpoint was the acquisition of Gram-negative bacteria resistant to the antimicrobial of choice during that cycling period. Despite a very high rate of overall compliance with the protocol (95.6%), a 24% increase in overall antimicrobial use was seen from cycle 1 to cycle 4. They also discovered that even though antimicrobial resistance to beta-lactams and fluoroquinolones occur through different mechanisms, exposure to one class of antimicrobials still resulted in resistance to the other class of antimicrobials. Withdrawal of the previous class of antimicrobials also did not result in a decrease in resistance as they sought to prove (15).

Warren et al. performed an antimicrobial cycling study in the medical ICU (MICU) at Barnes-Jewish Hospital. Surveillance rectal swab cultures were performed on all patients admitted to the MICU for >48 hr to determine acquisition of resistance. A five-month period served as a baseline and the cycling study was conducted over a 24-month period. Although this study was conducted as a multi-center study, only the results from this study site have been published. Four different antimicrobial classes were introduced at four-month intervals (4th-generation cephalosporins, fluoroquinolones, extended-spectrum penicillin/beta-lactamase inhibitors, and carbapenems). The program did not result in a significant decrease in the actual acquisition of resistant Gram-negative bacteria as cultured from stool. Despite an increase in antimicrobial resistance among isolates of *P. aeruginosa* and Enterobacteriaceae hospital-wide during the study period, the rates of antimicrobial resistance among the MICU patients remained stable despite increased colonization pressure in the hospital. Just as in other studies, only a 48% compliance rate with the cycled antimicrobial regimen was achieved (Fig. 1). No change in patient-related outcomes such as VAP incidence rates, bloodstream infection rates, and mortality rates were seen during the cycling periods (14,29).

Damas et al. also conducted an antimicrobial cycling program in Belgium. Three cycling regimens lasting 8 months each were tested in three mixed population ICUs. Routine respiratory and urine cultures were collected from patients on admission and twice weekly. Stool surveillance cultures, however, were not obtained, which is one of this study's limitations, since the stool is a reservoir for resistant Gram-negative bacilli, and development of resistance may have gone undetected in this study population. Although no significant increase in the global antimicrobial resistance was observed, resistance to the cycled antimicrobial regimen was observed during the same cycling period (19).

The two latest published studies on antimicrobial cycling have much-improved study designs. Both studies included an evaluation of an antimicrobial mixing intervention. During the mixing intervention, each patient who met the inclusion criteria for antimicrobial treatment was assigned to receive a different antimicrobial regimen as opposed to receiving the same antimicrobial regimen during the antimicrobial cycling intervention. In the first study, empiric treatment

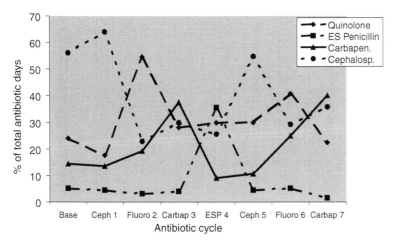

FIGURE 1 Compliance with the preferred antimicrobial cycling regimen in the medical intensive care unit at Barnes-Jewish Hospital during the 24-month intervention period. *Abbreviations*: Ceph, cephalosporin: cefipime; Fluoro, fluroquinolone: ciprofloxacin; Carbap, carbapenem: imipenem; ESP, extended spectrum penicillin: piperacillin-tazobactam. *Source*: Adapted from Ref. 14.

for suspected *Pseudomonas* infections was either accomplished through a typical antimicrobial cycling or a mixing program in two ICUs. The antimicrobial cycling program included four cycling regimens that were cycled over four one-month periods while the mixing program used the same order of antimicrobial classes as the cycling regimens but these were prescribed consecutively for each patient who met the entry criteria. Surveillance cultures were obtained from the patients' oropharynx, respiratory tract, and the rectum three times a week. Even though compliance rates for empiric coverage for suspected *Pseudomonas* infections were never higher than 45%, this study produced some interesting results. There was a trend towards a higher proportion of patients acquiring *Pseudomonas* isolates resistant to ceftazidime, imipenem, and meropenem during the mixing protocol compared to the cycling periods. There was even a significantly higher proportion of patients who acquired a *Pseudomonas* isolate resistant to cefepime during the mixing period compared to the cycling period (9% vs. 3%). No differences in the development of resistant Gram-negative bacterial infections and overall mortality between the two periods were noted, since this study was not powered to look at differences in these outcomes (17). This study suggests that antimicrobial cycling may be more effective in preventing the acquisition of resistant *Pseudomonas* than the mixing strategy. This finding contradicts what has been predicted by mathematical models (20). Unfortunately, there are several limitations to this study. Compliance with the preferred regimens was low, which could explain the inferiority of the mixing regimen. The duration of each cycling regimen (1 month) was also shorter than what is recommended by most experts (3–4 months). This last limitation would have biased the study in favor of the mixing study so this limitation does not explain the study findings.

The final study was also conducted in Spain by Sandiumenge and colleagues. The study protocol consisted of four different antimicrobial use strategies. In the initial 10 months, therapy for VAP was selected based on patient-specific risk factors such as the length of ICU stay and previous antimicrobial therapy. Use of any antimicrobial was allowed as long as it was appropriate. This patient-specific treatment period was followed by a two-year period in which two different antimicrobial cycling strategies were implemented. During the first twelve months, three different antimicrobial regimens were alternated as preferred treatment for VAP (prioritization cycle). The same antimicrobial cycling regimens were each restricted from being used over 4-month periods during the subsequent twelve months (restriction cycles). The period including the last ten months was known as the mixing period in which each antimicrobial regimen was consecutively assigned to each patient requiring treatment for VAP. Surveillance cultures were not performed in this study. The authors determined that maximal antimicrobial heterogeneity was achieved by both the patient-specific therapy and mixing periods but not during the antimicrobial cycling periods. High homogeneity (i.e., antimicrobial cycling periods) was associated with increased risks for isolation of carbapenems-resistant *Acinetobacter baumanii* and extended spectrum beta-lactamase (ESBL)-producing Enterobacteriaceae from clinical cultures. This study also has several limitations. As in previous studies, surveillance cultures were not performed. The use of a sequential intervention study design cannot control for temporal confounders such as seasonal variations and their effect on antimicrobial prescribing practices. And finally, infection control policies were also altered during the study period, which may account for the results observed in this study (18).

MATHEMATICAL MODELING STUDIES DO NOT FAVOR THE ANTIMICROBIAL CYCLING METHOD

The theoretical advantages of antimicrobial cycling are attractive since such a program is potentially easier to implement than other forms of antimicrobial control programs. However, as Sandiumenge and colleagues reported, antimicrobial mixing led to increased antimicrobial heterogeneity and this in turn decreases antimicrobial pressure (18). Mathematical modeling studies simulating the development of antimicrobial resistance in the hospital setting also support this finding. Bonhoeffer et al. simulated situations in which antimicrobials were either cycled, mixed (administration of each antimicrobial class to equal proportion of patients), or given in combination (21). Their model suggested that antimicrobial mixing or antimicrobial combination regimens would be superior to antimicrobial cycling programs regardless of the duration of the cycling periods. Bergstrom et al. also reported that the antimicrobial mixing strategy model was superior to antimicrobial cycling at reducing antimicrobial resistance using a stochastic model simulating the prevention of colonization of multi-drug resistant bacteria in the ICU setting (20).

INCREASED RESISTANCE TO SOME ANTIMICROBIAL CLASSES MAY MAKE ANTIMICROBIAL CYCLING IMPRACTICAL

Since antimicrobial cycling requires that different antimicrobial classes be initiated as empiric therapy, it is important that the antimicrobial cycling regimens be as structurally and mechanistically different as possible. In previous studies, fluoroquinolones were by themselves used as a cycling regimen. But because of increased resistance among Gram-negative bacteria to this antimicrobial class, fluoroquinolones can no longer be used alone for empiric treatment of serious infections (35). The current American Thoracic Society-Infectious Diseases Society of America (ATS-IDSA) guidelines for empiric treatment of VAP recommend the use of a carbapenems, an extended-spectrum penicillin/beta-lactamase inhibitor combination, or a 4th-generation cephalosporin in combination with a fluoroquinolone or an aminoglycoside (23). This recommendation was made to increase the likelihood that appropriate empiric therapy will be initially delivered to a critically ill patient even before culture and susceptibility results are available. With these new recommendations, all cycling regimens may only consist of beta-lactam antimicrobials leading to greater risks for development of cross-resistance. Unfortunately, there are no new non-beta-lactam antimicrobials under development that can be prescribed as empiric treatment for VAP as part of an antimicrobial cycling program.

CONCLUSIONS

Although some studies on antimicrobial cycling have shown some benefit, most published studies have failed to show any benefit from antimicrobial cycling. Some studies have even shown that antimicrobial cycling may even lead to an increase in overall antimicrobial usage. Physicians' adherence to only the use of the cycled antimicrobial was also erratic and this may have altered the results of some of the studies (14,15,17). Novel antimicrobial resistance mechanisms that emerge during one cycling period may persist during the following cycling period, reducing the efficacy of future antimicrobial cycling regimens. The simultaneous implementation of other infection-control interventions has also made the interpretation of antimicrobial cycling studies difficult (18,28). Antimicrobial mixing strategies may be promising alternatives as demonstrated by mathematical modeling studies (20,21) and one clinical trial (18), but this method still needs to be carefully evaluated. Based on the data currently available in the literature, a definitive opinion on the efficacy of antimicrobial cycling programs cannot be made at this time. Increasing rates of fluoroquinolone resistance among Gram-negative bacilli will likely make future antimicrobial cycling studies that include fluoroquinolone use as a single agent impractical and perhaps unethical. Alternative methods to control antimicrobial resistance, such as programs that promote antimicrobial streamlining, are currently being reported in the literature and may prove to be more effective in reducing antimicrobial resistance rates in the ICU setting than antimicrobial cycling programs (36–38).

REFERENCES

1. John JF Jr. Antibiotic cycling: is it ready for prime time? Infect Control Hosp Epidemiol 2000; 21:9–11.
2. McGowan JE Jr. Strategies for study of the role of cycling on antimicrobial use and resistance. Infect Control Hosp Epidemiol 2000; 21:S36–43.
3. Fridkin SK. Routine cycling of antimicrobial agents as an infection-control measure. Clin Infect Dis 2003; 36:1438–44.
4. Kollef MH. Is there a role for antibiotic cycling in the intensive care unit? Crit Care Med 2001; 29:N135–42.
5. Gerding DN, Larson TA. Aminoglycoside resistance in Gram-negative bacilli during increased amikacin use. Comparison of experience in 14 United States hospitals with

experience in the Minneapolis Veterans Administration Medical Center. Am J Med 1985; 79:1–7.

6. Gerding DN, Larson TA, Hughes RA, Weiler M, Shanholtzer C, Peterson LR. Amino-glycoside resistance and aminoglycoside usage: ten years of experience in one hospital. Antimicrob Agents Chemother 1991; 35:1284–90.

7. Young EJ, Sewell CM, Koza MA, Clarridge JE. Antibiotic resistance patterns during aminoglycoside restriction. Am J Med Sci 1985; 290:223–7.

8. Kollef MH, Vlasnik J, Sharpless L, Pasque C, Murphy D, Fraser V. Scheduled change of antibiotic classes: a strategy to decrease the incidence of ventilator-associated pneumonia. Am J Respir Crit Care Med 1997; 156:1040–8.

9. Dominguez EA, Smith TL, Reed E, Sanders CC, Sanders WE Jr. A pilot study of antibiotic cycling in a hematology-oncology unit. Infect Control Hosp Epidemiol 2000; 21:S4–8.

10. Gruson D, Hilbert G, Vargas F, et al. Rotation and restricted use of antibiotics in a medical intensive care unit. Impact on the incidence of ventilator-associated pneumonia caused by antibiotic-resistant Gram-negative bacteria. Am J Respir Crit Care Med 2000; 162:837–43.

11. Raymond DP, Pelletier SJ, Crabtree TD, et al. Impact of a rotating empiric antibiotic schedule on infectious mortality in an intensive care unit. Crit Care Med 2001; 29:1101–8.

12. Moss WJ, Beers MC, Johnson E et al. Pilot study of antibiotic cycling in a pediatric intensive care unit. Crit Care Med 2002; 30:1877–82.

13. Gruson D, Hilbert G, Vargas F, et al. Strategy of antibiotic rotation: long-term effect on incidence and susceptibilities of Gram-negative bacilli responsible for ventilator-associated pneumonia. Crit Care Med 2003; 31:1908–14.

14. Warren DK, Hill HA, Merz LR, et al. Cycling empirical antimicrobial agents to prevent emergence of antimicrobial-resistant Gram-negative bacteria among intensive care unit patients. Crit Care Med 2004; 32:2450–56.

15. van Loon HJ, Vriens MR, Fluit AC et al. Antibiotic rotation and development of Gram-negative antibiotic resistance. Am J Respir Crit Care Med 2005; 171:480–7.

16. Bruno-Murtha LA, Brusch J, Bor D, Li W, Zucker D. A pilot study of antibiotic cycling in the community hospital setting. Infect Control Hosp Epidemiol 2005; 26:81–7.

17. Martinez JA, Nicolas JM, Marco F, et al. Comparison of antimicrobial cycling and mixing strategies in two medical intensive care units. Crit Care Med 2006; 34: 329–36.

18. Sandiumenge A, Diaz E, Rodriguez A, et al. Impact of diversity of antibiotic use on the development of antimicrobial resistance. J Antimicrob Chemother 2006; 57:1197–204.

19. Damas P, Canivet JL, Ledoux D, et al. Selection of resistance during sequential use of preferential antibiotic classes. Intensive Care Med 2006; 32:67–74.

20. Bergstrom CT, Lo M, Lipsitch M. Ecological theory suggests that antimicrobial cycling will not reduce antimicrobial resistance in hospitals. Proc Natl Acad Sci USA 2004; 101:13285–90.

21. Bonhoeffer S, Lipsitch M, Levin BR. Evaluating treatment protocols to prevent anti-biotic resistance. Proc Natl Acad Sci USA 1997; 94:12106–11.

22. Neuhauser MM, Weinstein RA, Rydman R, Danziger LH, Karam G, Quinn JP. Antibiotic resistance among Gram-negative bacilli in US intensive care units: implica-tions for fluoroquinolone use. JAMA 2003; 289:885–8.

23. Guidelines for the management of adults with hospital-acquired, ventilator-associated, and healthcare-associated pneumonia. Am J Respir Crit Care Med 2005; 171:388–416.

24. Brown EM, Nathwani D. Antibiotic cycling or rotation: a systematic review of the evidence of efficacy. J Antimicrob Chemother 2005; 55:6–9.

25. Bergstrom CT, Lipsitch M, McGowan JE Jr. Nomenclature and methods for studies of antimicrobial switching (cycling). 2004. (Unpublished work)

26. Masterton RG. Antibiotic cycling: more than it might seem? J Antimicrob Chemother 2005; 55:1–5.

27. Quale J, Landman D, Saurina G, Atwood E, DiTore V, Patel K. Manipulation of a hospital antimicrobial formulary to control an outbreak of vancomycin-resistant enterococci. Clin Infect Dis 1996; 23:1020–5.
28. Hughes MG, Evans HL, Chong TW, et al. Effect of an intensive care unit rotating empiric antibiotic schedule on the development of hospital-acquired infections on the non-intensive care unit ward. Crit Care Med 2004; 32:53–60.
29. Merz LR, Warren DK, Kollef MH, Fraser VJ. Effects of an antibiotic cycling program on antibiotic prescribing practices in an intensive care unit. Antimicrob Agents Chemother 2004; 48:2861–5.
30. Warren DK, Hill HA, Merz LR, et al. Cycling empirical antimicrobial agents to prevent emergence of antimicrobial-resistant Gram-negative bacteria among intensive care unit patients. Crit Care Med 2004; 32:2450–6.
31. National Nosocomial Infections Surveillance (NNIS) System Report, data summary from January 1992 through June 2003, issued August 2003. Am J Infect Control 2003; 31:481–98.
32. National Nosocomial Infections Surveillance (NNIS) System Report, data summary from January 1992 through June 2004, issued October 2004. Am J Infect Control 2004; 32:470–85.
33. Quale J, Landman D, Saurina G, Atwood E, DiTore V, Patel K. Manipulation of a hospital antimicrobial formulary to control an outbreak of vancomycin-resistant enterococci. Clin Infect Dis 1996; 23:1020–5.
34. Allegranzi B, Gottin L, Bonora S, Zanoni L, Ischia S, Concia E. Antibiotic rotation in intensive care units: its usefulness should be demonstrated without pitfalls. Crit Care Med 2002; 30:2170–1.
35. Neuhauser MM, Weinstein RA, Rydman R, Danziger LH, Karam G, Quinn JP. Antibiotic resistance among Gram-negative bacilli in US intensive care units: implications for fluoroquinolone use. JAMA 2003; 289:885–8.
36. Micek ST, Shah RA, Kollef MH. Management of severe sepsis: integration of multiple pharmacologic interventions. Pharmacotherapy 2003; 23:1486–96.
37. Micek ST, Heuring TJ, Hollands JM, Shah RA, Kollef MH. Optimizing antibiotic treatment for ventilator-associated pneumonia. Pharmacotherapy 2006; 26:204–13.
38. varez-Lerma F, Alvarez B, Luque P, et al. Empiric broad-spectrum antibiotic therapy of nosocomial pneumonia in the intensive care unit: a prospective observational study. Crit Care 2006; 10:R78.

15 Antimicrobial Stewardship: Rationale for and Practical Considerations of Programmatic Institutional Efforts to Optimize Antimicrobial Use

Robert C. Owens, Jr.
Department of Clinical Pharmacy Services, Division of Infectious Diseases, Maine Medical Center, Portland, Maine and the Department of Medicine, University of Vermont, Burlington, Vermont, U.S.A.

INTRODUCTION

From time immemorial, an epic struggle for survival has existed. For pathogenic bacteria, the day-to-day skirmishes on the microscopic battlefield against mammalian species occurred virtually unopposed for thousands of years. The only means for mammalian defense was the host's evolving immune system that was substantial enough to prevent their extinction. A mere 70 years ago, the tide shifted, with the advent of antibacterial weapons that initially included the sulfa drugs and penicillin. The fruits of Gerhard Domagk's, Alexander Fleming's, and other countless unsung investigators' efforts soon paid off on a different battlefield, those of World War II, where countless human lives were saved. Reinforcements soon followed, and by 1957, representatives from the tetracycline, macrolide, aminoglycoside, glycopeptide, polymyxin, and antistaphylococcal penicillin families filled the quiver and were available for clinical use. With all of the so-called "easily exploitable" binding sites discovered, from this point forward with rare exception, the pipeline trickled out various "me too" compounds that would rarely overcome resistance mechanisms but did offer some notable benefits in terms of improved safety and offered competitive pricing. Nonetheless, we find ourselves already retreating only about 70 years into the battle. And this time, reinforcements are unlikely to be provided soon, particularly for multiple-drug resistant (MDR) Gram-negative pathogens. Why is this? Several reasons are to blame. One is mentioned above (all of the exploitable "easy" bacterial target sites have been discovered). Another chief reason is that larger pharmaceutical companies responsible for the development of most of our current antimicrobial arsenal have severed ties with antimicrobial discovery and development (1) because chronic medications for indications including male pattern baldness and erectile dysfunction are far more profitable. The declining state of affairs regarding antimicrobial development is discussed further in Chapter 3.

So what are we left to do? Figure 1 depicts the complex and interrelated issues contributing to the development, maintenance, and spread of resistance in and outside of healthcare settings (2), as well as broad-based interventions intended to neutralize the threats. It also shows the collaborative nature of antimicrobial stewardship programs (ASPs) with infection control programs (ICPs). While other chapters in this book address some of the potential solutions mentioned in the table, this chapter focuses on one of the mentioned strategies, that is the development of a prospective,

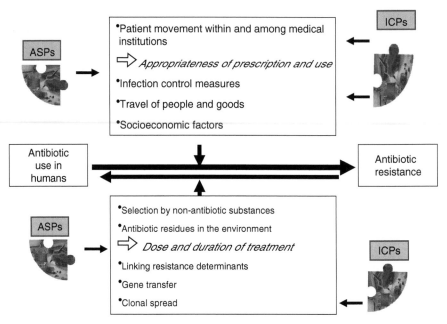

FIGURE 1 Factors contributing to antimicrobial resistance are complex and extend beyond antimicrobial use in humans. Also depicted are potential countermeasures and the collaborative "synergy" between ASPs and ICPs. *Abbreviations*: ASP, antimicrobial stewardship program; ICP, infection control program. *Source*: Adapted from Ref. 2.

formalized, programmatic strategy to ensure that antimicrobials are used appropriately (primarily) in healthcare settings. These programs are referred to as ASPs. So, what is antimicrobial stewardship? As Dr. Dale Gerding stated, "good antimicrobial steward-ship is the optimal selection, dose, and duration of an antimicrobial that results in the best clinical outcome for the treatment or prevention of infection, with minimal toxicity to the patient and minimal impact on subsequent resistance" (3). The consequences of unnecessary antimicrobial use extend beyond contributing to escalating rates of antimicrobial resistance. Unnecessary antimicrobial exposure can lead to avoidable harms to patients (4–7). Additionally, *Clostridium difficile* infection (CDI) is almost exclusively associated with the administration of antimicrobials (whether being used appropriately or inappropriately) (7–9). While antimicrobials have been shown to be overused in many studies (thus providing opportunities for better antimicrobial stewardship), it should be remembered that antimicrobials are necessary and life-saving drugs. When engaging in antimicrobial stewardship initiatives, one has to be careful not to reduce antimicrobial use to a point where needed therapy is delayed or omitted altogether. As Dr. Gerding pointed out in an editorial, "they (antimicrobials) are not cigarettes or cocaine: they are highly valuable life-saving therapeutic agents that have been designed to benefit mankind by being used" (3). This chapter reinforces why the judicious use of antimicrobials is essential in slowing the steady nationwide increase in antimicrobial resistance, the implementation (including potential barriers) of ASPs, and discuss the collaborative nature of ASPs with other key departments [e.g., ICPs, the clinical microbiology laboratory, information support (IS) services].

HISTORICAL PERSPECTIVE AND UNIQUE CHALLENGES RELATED TO ANTIMICROBIAL USE

Before we discuss ASPs, it is important to address some of the unique attributes of antimicrobials and their use. Antimicrobials have been termed "societal" drugs (10). Why? Because prescribing an antihypertensive to a patient with hypertension, for example, only impacts the patient for whom the drug is prescribed. Conversely, an antimicrobial administered to that same patient has an opportunity to impact not only that person, but countless others. Since antimicrobial resistance has the potential to develop during antimicrobial therapy in that patient (if not dosed correctly, if given for too long, if not taken as instructed, or even if all of these variables are optimized), the resultant resistant organism has the opportunity to be spread to persons who have never been exposed to that antimicrobial. Thus, the use and misuse of these resources have "societal consequences" and is why optimizing their use is important at the patient, institutional, and national/international level. An illustrative case exemplified this issue for us recently. An individual (Patient A) with a history of recurrent urinary tract infections (UTIs) due to *Escherichia coli* (required near-continuous antimicrobial use for a period of 5 years, all the while becoming increasingly resistant) was seen again as an outpatient for the recurrent UTIs. Culture, susceptibility, and additional testing [polymerase chain reaction (PCR)] by a reputable microbiology laboratory (our ASP had arranged for the additional testing due to the increasingly limited oral treatment options) determined that the *E. coli* strain harbored a CTX-M extended spectrum beta-lactamase (ESBL). The sister (Patient B) of patient A was admitted to the hospital for sepsis shortly after her sister's (Patient A) outpatient office visit. The *E. coli* isolated from the bloodstream of Patient B was later determined to be the same *E. coli* strain that was isolated from the urine of Patient A by pulsed-field gel electrophoresis (PFGE) of the two isolates (Karen Lolans and John Quinn, personal communication). Patient B, who had not been exposed to the antimicrobials that selected for the MDR ESBL-producing *E. coli*, died a few days after admission to the hospital as a result of the organism. Thus, antimicrobials are indeed societal drugs with consequences.

For therapeutic classes of drugs that are associated with increased complexity and/or posses a narrow margin between patient safety and the desired therapeutic outcome (e.g., cancer chemotherapy), only certain prescribers with specialty training (oncologists) routinely order these drugs. The complexity of antimicrobial use has increased over time, requiring the integration and synthesis of numerous and sometimes intricate data sources and variables. Virtually all clinicians with prescribing privileges order antimicrobials with varying degrees of frequency, from optometrists and podiatrists to infectious diseases (ID) physicians (and everyone in between). Although most clinicians feel that they understand enough about antimicrobials to use them properly, a plethora of studies have demonstrated that this is simply untrue (11–14). Optimizing antimicrobial use requires that the prescriber have adequate knowledge of general medicine, ID, microbiology, pharmacokinetics-pharmacodynamics (PK-PD), basic epidemiology, and common sense. Training programs often do not adequately equip the future or current prescriber with these basic underpinnings, as evidenced in one study by the fact that upper-level residents were no more knowledgeable about antimicrobial use than first-year residents (15).

So where do prescribers learn about antimicrobials? As a teacher of a wide variety of healthcare professionals, from medical students, residents, fellows, attendings, and allied health professionals, it is clear (at least to me) that medical school and allied health curricula need to be strengthened and to focus on critical thinking skills to match the increasing complexity of antimicrobial therapy. A major component of ASPs is the provision of education; thus, for clinicians practicing at institutions with ASPs, they have an opportunity to learn from the interactions with the ASP team members. Another provider of "education" is the pharmaceutical industry. This is not meant to have a negative connotation, as the pharmaceutical industry can be a sponsor of valid antimicrobial educational efforts when provided in the form of unrestricted educational grants that support institutionally aligned initiatives (e.g., grand rounds), but only when done by unbiased and reputable speakers.

This interaction, however, is not always a beneficial one to the prescriber or the patient. Because treatment decisions often occur in the context of uncertainty, this "uncertainty" is often exploitable. A clinician's deficiency in knowledge and/or confidence with the complexities of antimicrobial prescribing increases their susceptibility to the biased interpretations of clinical studies and information provided by some pharmaceutical representatives. Furthermore, patients are also susceptible to the direct-to-consumer advertisement that shows abundantly exuberant couples with herpes infections running hand-in-hand up and down a tropical beach after receiving an antiviral medication, for example. One has to remember that the intention of many pharmaceutical industry-based efforts is clear, to sell more drug by exploiting the conditions (the uncertainty) in which many antimicrobial prescriptions are issued, and to increase patient demand. These pressures and exploitations are not new, as Jawetz in 1956 eluded to several important points that are still as germane today as the day they were published: "he (the prescriber) is under great pressure to prescribe the 'newest', 'best', 'broadest' antibiotic preparation, prescribe it for any complaint whatever, quickly, and preferably without worrying too much about specific etiologic diagnosis or proper indication of the drug" (16). Jawetz goes on to describe the pharmaceutical representative and their role in influencing prescribing habits:

> He (the representative) is well briefed and of considerable persuasion. He desires to help the doctor, to clarify his ideas regarding a certain drug, and to lead him out of the bewildering jungle of confusing trade names and conflicting claims. He points out convincingly that the antibiotic manufactured by the company he represents is safe, effective, and will serve the doctor well in all circumstances. If he is successful, his soothing talk will make the physician remember a single antibiotic trade name and prescribe it freely. With the availability of a multitude of specific, effective drugs, many physicians are plagued by the question: "have I really done everything possible for the patient? Have I given him every drug that could possibly benefit him?" The medical representative restores the physician's peace of mind and resolves his conflict. He urges him to prescribe whenever in doubt, reassures him that the drug he sells usually helps, never harms. Thus, quantities of antibiotics are prescribed for the sake of the physician's psyche rather than the patient's infection. ... The pressures on the physician (and his sometimes weak resistance) have been described in some detail because they are among the factors responsible for the enormous abuse of antibiotics. It is a safe guess that not more than 5 to 10 percent of the hundreds of tons of antibiotics produced every year are employed on the proper clinical indication. Does this waste harm anything more than the patient's pocketbook? (16)

Again, this prophetic review article published in 1956 by famed microbiologist Dr. Ernest Jawetz points to relevant issues that face us still today in both inpatient and outpatient settings. It underscores the need for formalized programs that evaluate antimicrobial use in institutional settings where 50% to 75% of patients receive prophylactic or therapeutic antimicrobials and where studies have demonstrated that up to 50% of this use is inappropriate. One of the primary goals of an ASP is to provide education through feedback to prescribers regarding antimicrobial use, which will decrease the clinician's susceptibility to alternative means of potentially biased education provided by pharmaceutical representatives.

Although some have thrown in the towel, others have invested great time and care into ensuring that clinicians use antimicrobials more judiciously. For instance, McGowan and Finland demonstrated reduced antimicrobial use associated with antimicrobial restrictions that encouraged interactions between prescribers and clinicians with expertise in antimicrobial use in mid-1960s through the 1970s (17). In the late 1970s and 1980s, a formal program at Hartford Hospital that included an ID physician (Richard Quintiliani) and clinical pharmacists formed the first prospective audit and feedback ASP (18). Concepts introduced by this group included transitional therapy and streamlining (now referred to as "de-escalation"). In the late 1990s and into the new millennium, Drs. Fishman and Paterson in conjunction with clinical pharmacists with training in ID instituted large formalized programs using prior authorization as their core antimicrobial stewardship strategy (11–13). Building on the strategy initiated by Quintiliani et al., Fraser et al. (19) conducted a randomized controlled trial evaluating the prospective audit with intervention and feedback core strategy in the late 1990s, demonstrating that antimicrobial use could be significantly reduced without negatively impacting clinical outcomes. Stemming from this study, an institutionally supported clinical program was implemented using similar methods at the same hospital (20,21). In addition, this methodology was adopted by others at smaller hospitals, proving that this strategy was customizable and generalizable to other smaller facilities (22).

RATIONALE FOR OPTIMIZING ANTIMICROBIAL USE AND IMPLEMENTING ASPs
Antimicrobial Resistance
Resistance can occur during therapy and be witnessed by the prescribing clinician in a hospital setting, but this is relatively uncommon. More commonly, when resistance occurs during therapy it is not detected because the patient is either not serially cultured at the site of infection due to practical issues or, as is true in many cases, the clinical outcome is positive and carriage of the resistant organism may not be of importance until the patient later presents with an infection that is caused by the resistant organism (23–28). As a result, many clinical guidelines for the treatment of infections incorporate taking a good antimicrobial history from the patient to determine previous relevant antimicrobial exposure in order to increase the probability of prescribing empiric therapy that is active against the suspected causative pathogens (29–31). Again, because the prescriber might be distanced between the use of the antibiotic and the event (resistance development), they may not be as interested in antimicrobial resistance as they should be. This is an important consideration in optimizing empiric antimicrobial therapy that is discussed in more detail later, as well as an important concept that ASPs can incorporate into educational interactions with prescribers.

It should be recognized that all antimicrobials differ with respect to their inherent potential to provoke resistance (32). For example, clear resistance development occurred among staphylococci in a bacteremia and endocarditis trial that compared daptomycin to vancomycin (33). More daptomycin-resistant staphylococcal strains were actually created following daptomycin exposure in a single trial than have been identified among staphylococci to vancomycin in more than three decades of use (33). In this trial, resistance to daptomycin was clinically significant, as patients who developed resistant isolates had longer durations of bacteremia compared with patients who did not develop resistance during therapy (33). Moreover, the potential for developing resistance differs depending on the organism as well. For example, it is easier to create linezolid-resistant enterococci than it is to create linezolid-resistant staphylococci in the laboratory (34,35). This has turned out to be true in the clinic as well, where large surveillance studies have reported linezolid-resistant staphylococci are very rare (0 of 5442) after 7 years of use, and rare (but more commonly found) among enterococci (9 of 1343 strains) (34,35). Thus, when targeting initiatives that may potentially result in the decreased use of certain antimicrobials, one's expectations of reduced resistance as an outcome measure should be tempered by the specific "bug–drug" relationship that is being considered. If resistance reduction is going to be an expectation of the implementation of an ASP or a new initiative, the specific bug–drug relationships should be researched before it is placed in the business proposal (discussed later) or prior to considering new initiatives for an established program (36).

Data also show that, in order to study the relationship between antimicrobial use and resistance, well-designed studies that are typically resource intensive are required. However, the relationship between antimicrobial exposure and resistance has been delineated by data derived from in vitro investigations, ecological studies that correlate drug exposure with resistance, controlled trials in which patients with prior antimicrobial exposure were more likely to be colonized or infected with antimicrobial-resistant bacteria, as well as prospective studies in which drug use was associated with the development of resistant flora (37–40). A recent study examined the relationship between antimicrobial exposure and the subsequent development of resistance by obtaining pre-therapy rectal swabs, at the end of treatment, and 2 weeks after treatment (40). Fifteen of 156 patients (12.2%) who were exposed to piperacillin/tazobactam developed piperacillin/tazobactam-resistant enterobacteriaceae during therapy (40). Levy and colleagues also developed a biologic model that showed a clear relationship between antimicrobial use and the selection of resistance in humans (38). Therefore, regardless of whether the use of an antimicrobial is deemed appropriate or inappropriate, antimicrobial resistance can be a consequence. Therefore, reducing the incremental selective pressure caused by the prescribing of unnecessary antimicrobial use, including treatment durations that are longer than necessary, has been shown to reduce antimicrobial resistance (11,12,32,41). Specific interventions conducted by ASPs that result in a reduction in inappropriate and unnecessarily long antimicrobial therapy are discussed later.

Patient Safety

In another vein, antimicrobials, whether being used appropriately or inappropriately, have the potential for causing serious harm to patients in the form of adverse events. Some examples of harms are QT interval prolongation leading to potentially life-threatening arrhythmias (e.g., macrolides, ketolides, azole antifungals, fluoroquinolones), metabolic liability in the form of cytochrome P450 3A4 inhibition leading to serious drug interactions that may result in rhabdomyolysis or other serious adverse events (e.g., azoles, macrolides, ketolides), Stevens-Johnson syndrome (e.g., trimethaprim/sulfamethoxazole), nephrotoxicity (e.g., aminoglycosides, amphotericin b), and life-threatening hypersensitivity reactions (e.g., beta-lactams) (5–7); all antimicrobials are associated with CDI (8). Disturbingly, the rate and severity of CDI is increasing and the emergence of a new toxin gene variant strain of *C. difficile* appears to be responsible for epidemics (9,42–44). A recent study showed that one in five patients admitted to the intensive care unit (ICU) with CDI were receiving antimicrobials without any evidence of infection (45). Unnecessary antimicrobial use has been shown to be responsible for some of these life-threatening adverse events; therefore, programs that provide oversight of antimicrobials to minimize their unnecessary use can be viewed as an extension of patient safety efforts by healthcare facilities. A recent systematic review of ASPs by the Cochrane Group concluded ASPs are beneficial strategies to reduce the impact of CDI (46). The best approach to improve patient safety by reducing the potential for CDI is through the multidisciplinary approach of ASP interventions in concert with infection control and environmental cleaning interventions (9,47–49). In summary, the potential harm caused by the unnecessary use of antimicrobials should incentivize even the most temerarious clinicians to not casually prescribe antimicrobials in the absence of documented or suspected infection, as there are indeed quantifiable risks associated with their use (44).

Cost

In 2005, systemic anti-infectives accounted for the largest percentage of the pharmacy's drug expenditures in nonfederal hospitals in the United States (50). This figure was up 7% from 2004, demonstrating that expenditures nationally continue to rise. A proportion of these expenditures are attributable to unnecessary usage. For example, one of the common interventions performed by ASPs is the identification of redundant antimicrobial therapy (20,21,51). In addition to increasing the risk of side effects, medical errors, and resistance, unnecessary antimicrobial use in the form of redundant therapy is a waste of money! Therefore, it is not a surprise that ASPs have demonstrated that they are financially self-supporting. Further savings can be realized when looking beyond the "silo" mentality, which places costs involved in the management of infections (e.g., variable costs: pharmacy, radiographic imaging studies, laboratory studies; and fixed costs: daily hospitalization or "hotel" costs) into "buckets" or "silos." When considering the overall healthcare costs of treating a documented infection, it is well established that the cost of antimicrobials is small in the overall context of the treatment of that infection. In addition, infections caused by resistant organisms cost more than infections caused by susceptible organisms, primarily because resistant organisms result in excess, often not reimbursed, length of stay (52,53). Several well-conducted studies have demonstrated this is true for infections caused by both Gram-positive and Gram-negative pathogens (52,53). This is discussed in greater detail in Chapter 1 in this book, and how an ASP may impact overall healthcare costs is discussed later in this chapter. Once again, a collaborative approach involving a program that reduces unnecessary selective pressure for developing resistance and may assist with reducing the length of hospitalization for patients with infections due to resistant organisms (e.g., ASPs) and programs that prevent the horizontal transmission of resistant pathogens and may aid in the early recognition of patients harboring resistant pathogens (e.g., ICPs) are truly complementary. With the reality of a new environment for healthcare facilities today with public reporting of infections, increased regulatory attention, and pay-for-performance initiatives, the collaborative efforts provided by ASPs and ICPs have an increasing role more than ever to address resistance, patient safety, and costs.

One has to simply remember that regardless of purchase cost, the most expensive antimicrobial is the one that does not work. Formularies need to be stocked with the most effective treatment options for this reason. Less effective treatment choices that might cost fewer dollars per day may result in excess hidden costs (e.g., longer length of stay, managing side effects, clinical failures that result in additional antimicrobials to attempt to cure the patient's infection). ASPs play a role in reducing both direct and visible costs as well as the potential to reduce indirect costs.

INFECTIOUS DISEASES SOCIETY OF AMERICA (IDSA) AND THE SOCIETY FOR HEALTHCARE EPIDEMIOLOGY OF AMERICA (SHEA): GUIDELINES FOR DEVELOPING AN INSTITUTIONAL PROGRAM TO ENHANCE ANTIMICROBIAL STEWARDSHIP

In 2007, the IDSA and SHEA jointly published guidelines for the development of programs to enhance antimicrobial stewardship in the institutional setting (54). These guidelines were endorsed by multiple societies and organizations that share the common interest of antimicrobial stewardship, each from a different perspective and constituency that include the Society of Infectious Diseases Pharmacists, the Alliance for the Prudent Use of Antimicrobials, the Centers for Disease Control and Prevention (CDC), and the World Health Organization.

These guidelines provide the metrics for developing a customized program and may serve as an organizational/societal endorsed document to facilitate discussions with administrators and key individuals whose support are needed to start up a program. Various elements of these guidelines are discussed throughout the rest of this chapter. It is important to note that in addition to these guidelines, other countries have also realized the benefits of formalized institutional approaches to optimizing antimicrobial use and have invested resources into creating formalized institutional-based programs, some making it a national priority, particularly in the United Kingdom, some countries in Europe, as well as in the Far East (55–60).

PROGRAMS TO OPTIMIZE ANTIMICROBIAL USE

A variety of studies have evaluated the impact of interventions on antimicrobial use in healthcare systems. These studies have been conducted using a wide range of strategies and interventions (often bundled), methodologies, interventions, and outcome measures (cost, antimicrobial consumption, appropriateness of use, patient safety, and, less frequently, resistance). Over time, two core ASP strategies have evolved that include prior authorization (or "front-end" programs, where antimicrobials are made accessible only through an approval process) and pro-spective audit with intervention and feedback (also known as a "back-end" program, where antimicrobial use is reviewed after antimicrobial therapy has been ordered and recommendations are made as to their appropriateness in terms of selection, dose, route, and duration), as illustrated in Figure 2.

The prospective audit and feedback strategy entails obtaining a daily (or every-other-day for smaller hospitals) list of patients receiving antimicrobials and visually identifying patients in whom interventions are necessary. Because the list is comprehensive yet succinctly constructed, patients can be screened efficiently. For example, our list contains demographic information; certain laboratory values (e.g., serum creatinine, blood culture, and susceptibility data); dietary data; all antimicrobials being received, including their dose, interval, route, start date, who ordered them, and if it is restricted; and the name of the person authorizing their use. This list, of course, can be customized according to the institution's preference and, because it required resources from the IS or information technology (IT) departments, accounting for these resources should be considered in the early phases of developing the program.

From the aforementioned list, determining interventions such as pharmaco-dynamic dosage adjustment, streamlining/de-escalation and identification of redundant therapy based on culture and susceptibility results, parenteral-to-oral conversions, drug interaction identification, guideline/protocol compliance, and recommendation of more cost-effective treatments, as examples, can be performed. Typically, the list serves as a starting point where the potential intervention is identified, and further information is sought out to solidify the intervention (e.g., further information retrieved from the computer, medical record, or by discussing the case with the team/prescriber). Figure 3 shows the types of interventions that can be conducted in relationship to the timing of antimicrobial therapy, and an example of workflow is provided in Figure 4. Recommendations are provided to the prescriber in either written form or by direct conversation. Written forms (Fig. 5) of communication usually take place on nonpermanent forms placed in the patient's medical record that are removed at discharge. This allows flexibility in what can be communicated and allows the ASP team member to convey educational messages effectively and to provide citations or references as to why the intervention is being recommended. The benefits of this type of program are its customizability to smaller- (22) or larger-sized healthcare facilities (19,32), it avoids taking away the prescriber's autonomy, which also increases productive "educational" dialogue, and it circumvents the potential for delays in initiating timely antimicrobial therapy since the antimicrobial is already prescribed. The downside is that recommendations are optional, although there are ways to correct repeated unaccepted recommendations by communicating with either the department chief or an institutional committee (e.g., Medical Executive Committee, Pharmacy and Therapeutics Committee, Patient Safety Committee). Our program at Maine Medical Center has employed this primary strategy for over six years (19–21), and others have operated for longer periods of time (41).

The second chief strategy is a *preauthorization* or front-end program, where most antimicrobials are restricted to an approval process (Fig. 2). Here, a team member carries a pager or telephone and receives approval requests for restricted antimicrobials. At the time of interaction, the antimicrobial is either justified or approved, or an alternative recommendation is given. The University of Pennsylvania (12,61), The University of Pittsburgh (62), and others (63) have used this as their primary strategy for a number of years. The benefits of this strategy include the ability to funnel most initial orders for antimicrobials through experts versed

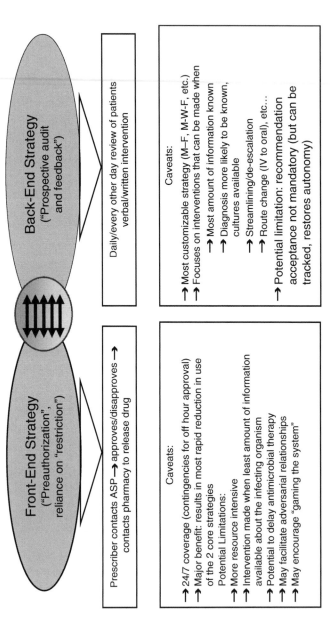

FIGURE 2 Antimicrobial stewardship program (ASP) core strategies. *Source:* Courtesy of Robert C. Owens, Jr.

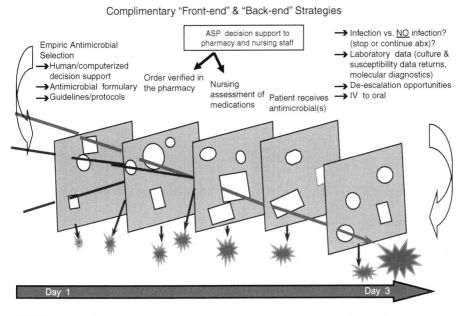

Complimentary "Front-end" & "Back-end" Strategies

FIGURE 3 Visual representation of when interventions may occur depending on the core strategy chosen and supplemental strategies selected. *Abbreviation*: ASP, antimicrobial stewardship program. *Source*: Courtesy of Robert C. Owens, Jr.

in antimicrobial therapy, and these programs have typically demonstrated immediate and significant cost savings (11,12,17,63). The potential downsides to this strategy include: the loss of prescriptive autonomy that may lead to "gaming the system" (64) and the fostering of potentially adversarial relationships (if not properly implemented with buy-in from important and opinionated prescribers); the potential for delaying initial therapy; time- and resource-intensive and usually 7 days per week with contingency plans for night coverage; and decisions are made when the least amount of information is known about the actual infection [culture and susceptibility results are not available for 2–3 days (Fig. 3); the quality of information relayed to the ASP team member by prescriber can be variable (65)]. These core strategies reflect formalized, active interventional programs that are the only types of programs that have demonstrated an impact on the quantity and quality of antimicrobial use (66).

In reality, although ASPs may lean toward one of the two primary strategies, overlap often exists (Fig. 2). For example, our program, while relying primarily on prospective audit and feedback, does incorporate a limited number of antimicrobials that require approval (21). A variety of supplemental strategies can be selected to complement the core strategy (e.g., transitional therapy programs, PK-PD dosing strategies, use of computerized decision support to supplement human decision support, and others that are discussed in greater detail later in this chapter). One of the most valuable aspects of an ASP is the assignment of institutionwide responsibility for overseeing the use of antimicrobials. Although in moderate-sized hospitals or larger, an ID physician consultation service, ID pharmacist, and infection control department are often present and coexist or collaborate on specific areas of interest, responsibility at the institutional level for

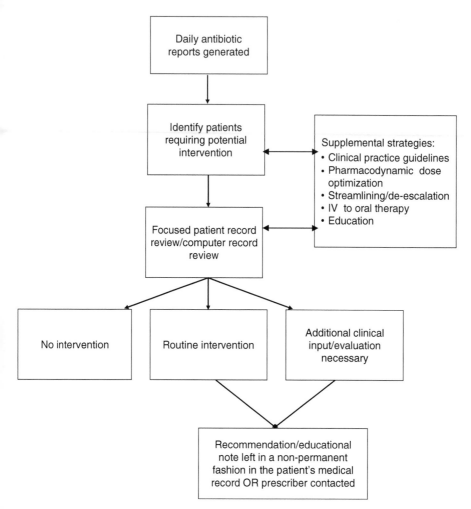

FIGURE 4 Prospective audit and feedback program workflow diagram. *Source*: Courtesy of Robert C. Owens, Jr.

antimicrobial stewardship is usually not assigned. An administratively supported ASP aligns resources from the various specialties listed above and assigns responsibility to them with remuneration. If additional resources are needed, they must be provided in order to be successful. Healthcare systems may hire an ID physician and ID pharmacist to cover a group of smaller hospitals within the system.

Realizing that institutions vary in size and type of specialty services offered, the ASP should be customized accordingly. ASPs provide a responsible and accountable source of antimicrobial oversight, whether in formulary management, facilitating the development of institutional guidelines for antimicrobial use, or working with the clinical microbiology laboratory to optimize susceptibility testing and reporting. The following sections discuss issues related to selecting a core

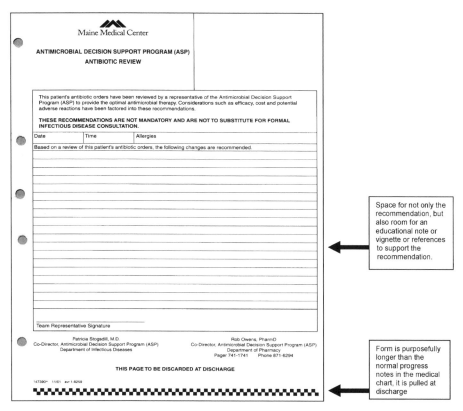

FIGURE 5 Example of a written intervention form (a 2-part carbonless form; one is left in the medical record and one is taken with the team member). *Source*: Courtesy of Robert C. Owens, Jr.

interventional strategy (strengths and weaknesses of each), supplemental strategies that are used in concert regardless of core strategy chosen (and examples), core members involved, potential barriers to implementation, and outcome and process measures to measure the ongoing impact of the program. An effective ASP is financially self-supporting and is aligned with patient safety goals (19–22,41, 67–69). For these reasons, there should be no excuse for an institution to not have a formal program dedicated toward improving the quality of antimicrobial use.

Team Members

The IDSA/SHEA guidelines for developing ASPs strongly recommend that these programs are directed or codirected by the two core team members (an ID physician and an ID-trained pharmacist), both receiving remuneration for their time (54). The pharmacist should have formal training in ID or be knowledgeable in the appropriate use of antimicrobials, with training being made available to maintain competency. Other team members would optimally include a dedicated computer IS specialist, microbiologist, and an infection control practitioner/hospital epidemiologist. Figure 6 illustrates an optimal schematic for collaboration and partnership that is used at our institution and was adapted from previous

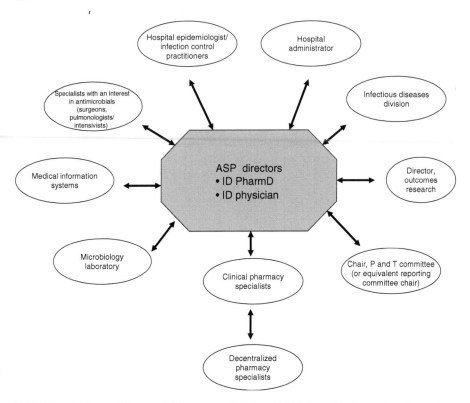

FIGURE 6 Antimicrobial stewardship program (ASP) multidisciplinary involvement and core team members. *Source*: Courtesy of Robert C. Owens, Jr.

models (11). Although not specifically recommended by the guidelines, but strongly believed by the author, is the inclusion of specialists with a strong interest in the use of antimicrobials (e.g., some surgeons, intensivists/pulmonologists). Administrative and committee support (e.g., Pharmacy and Therapeutics Committee) is critical. The particular interventional philosophy, as well as responsibilities, remuneration, and reporting measures, should be discussed in advance of implementation so that expectations and resources can be addressed. Effective communication between the ASP and administration and an appropriate committee should be maintained to facilitate dialogue over time as the healthcare environment continues to change.

SELECT LITERATURE REVIEW OF ACTIVE INTERVENTIONAL STUDIES TO IMPROVE THE USE OF ANTIMICROBIALS
Prospective Audit and Feedback Strategy
Fraser and colleagues (19) designed a prospective randomized controlled study of interventions for targeted antimicrobials in hospitalized patients. The team included a part-time ID physician and a PharmD with antimicrobial expertise. The intervention group ($n = 141$) received suggestions (written or verbally), whereas the control group did not ($n = 111$). Controlling for severity of illness between groups, outcomes were similar with respect to clinical and microbiological

response to therapy, adverse events, inpatient mortality, and readmission rates. Interventions included change to oral therapy (31%), regimen or dosing changes (42%), stopping therapy (10%), ordering additional laboratory tests (18%), and 85% of the suggestions were instituted. Multiple logistic regression models identified randomization of the intervention group as the sole predictor of lower antimicrobial expenditures. A conservative annualized reduction in antimicrobial expenditures of $97,500 was realized. The intervention group also showed a trend toward reduced mean length of stay compared to control (20 vs. 24 days, respectively). Fifty percent of patients receiving targeted regimens had their treatment refined on the third day of therapy, resulting in narrower spectrum therapy and lower antimicrobial costs; most importantly, reducing antimicrobial use did not adversely impact patient outcomes. This study was later used as a platform to implement an ASP that is more robust in terms of the types of activities and numbers of patients served by the program. The team currently includes a part-time ID physician (2 hr/day, 5 days/wk) and a full-time ID PharmD. Close collaboration exists with the Department of Epidemiology and Infection Prevention, the ID Division, the Pharmacy, Administration, the Patient Safety Officer, and the Pharmacy and Therapeutics Committee.

Srinivasan and colleagues studied the impact of an antimicrobial management program on antimicrobial expenditures at Johns Hopkins Hospital, a 1000-bed teaching facility. Prior to the introduction of a comprehensive ASP, the hospital utilized a closed formulary system and employed prior approval requirements on a number of antimicrobials. The ASP consisted of a hospital-funded ID physician, ID PharmD, and data analyst. The team concurrently reviewed antimicrobial therapy in all areas of the hospital except pediatrics and oncology. Their interventions included a survey, use of institution-specific guidelines, concurrent antimicrobial review, and educational sessions. A "knowledge, attitude, and beliefs" survey was used to determine awareness of antimicrobial use and resistance and sense deficiencies in knowledge that could lead to targeted education among house staff (15). Interestingly, only 18% viewed the program as an obstacle to patient care and 70% wanted additional feedback on antimicrobial choices. Hospital guidelines were published and updated annually. Antimicrobial therapy interventions occurred prior to culture and susceptibility results being available only when actively solicited or when called for prior authorization of an antimicrobial agent. For all others, interventions were suggested at the time the microbiological data became available. Compliance with suggested recommendations by the ASP was 79%. Costs for antimicrobial agents for the covered areas decreased by 6.4% the first year and 2.2% the second year. Assuming a steady inflation rate of 4.5%, savings translated to $224,753 and $413,998 for fiscal years 2002 and 2003.

Bantar and colleagues demonstrated the impact of their ASP's interventional program on antimicrobial use, cost savings, and antimicrobial resistance (70). The ASP consisted of an ID physician, two pharmacists, a microbiologist and laboratory technologist, an internal medicine physician, and a computer systems analyst. During the 6-month period, four consecutive intervention strategies were unveiled. During the first 6 months, an optional antibiotic order form (ID diagnosis, pertinent epidemiological data) was introduced and baseline data were collected (i.e., bacterial resistance, antibiotic use, prescribing practice, nosocomial infection, and crude mortality rates). In the second period, an "initial intervention" period consisted of transforming the optional order form to a compulsory form and providing feedback to clinicians based on a review of the data collected in the first period. In the third period, called the "education" period, clinicians were verbally engaged with each new antimicrobial order by members of the multidisciplinary team. The fourth or "active control" period was similar to the third period but prescriptions were modified by the ASP team member if necessary. During the four periods, no antimicrobial agent was restricted. To estimate the rates of use of a particular drug in relation to other drugs, an index was calculated (e.g., rate of cefepime use to that for third-generation cephalosporins—ceftriaxone and ceftazidime—equaled cefepime/consumption of ceftriaxone and ceftazidime × 100). Consumption data were measured in defined daily doses (DDD). The program periods were associated with declining cost savings as time advanced (periods II, III, and IV were associated with a reduction of $261,955, $57,245, and $12,881, respectively). Comparing antibiotic order forms from period one (voluntary form and preintervention, $n = 450$) with period four (mandatory form with active intervention, $n = 349$) an increase in microbiologically based treatment intent (27% vs. 62.8%, respectively, $p < 0.0001$) was noted. Twenty-seven percent of the period IV antibiotic order forms were intervened upon by the team. Of the interventions, either the dose or duration (not specified) was reduced in 11.5%, 86.1% were associated with cost reduction, and 47% involved streamlining therapy to a narrower choice. In terms of impact on nosocomial infection, length of hospitalization, and mortality, only length of stay was impacted significantly ($p = 0.04$). The increased rate of cefepime use relative to third-generation cephalosporins was associated with declining third-generation cephalosporin resistance rates among *Proteus mirabilis* and *Enterobacter cloacae* but not to *E. coli* and *Klebsiella pneumoniae*. The increased rate of aminopenicillin/sulbactam use relative to the third-generation cephalosporins in conjunction with a sustained reduction in vancomycin use was associated with a reduction in methicillin-resistant *Staphylococcus aureus* (MRSA) rates. In addition, *Pseudomonas aeruginosa* resistance rates to carbapenems declined to 0%. This was strongly associated with the reduction in carbapenem consumption over time.

This particular study is different than others in that it used a staggered approach to implementation. Although the cost reduction appeared to dwindle significantly with each newly introduced period, one cannot ignore the cumulative impact on cost. In addition, the final period offers a comprehensive mechanism for long-standing success and also serves as a template to introduce other initiatives as deemed necessary. Part of the success related to reduction in resistance rates noted by this program is related to the high rate of carbapenem and ceftriaxone use and the "seldom" ordered cefepime and aminopenicillin/sulbactam in conjunction with the types of problem pathogens noted at their hospital (e.g., ampC phenotypes and carbapenem-resistant *P. aeruginosa*). Penicillin-based inhibitor combinations and cefepime have been noted to more often "favorably" impact the environment in contrast to high usage rates of carbapenem and third-generation cephalosporin (32,71,72).

Another study demonstrated the impact of a multidisciplinary ASP using a blend of interventions including minimal formulary restrictions, comprehensive education (direct communication, antibiograms, peer feedback every 6 months), rounding with medical teams, and introduction of guidelines (appropriate initial empiric therapy, transitional therapy, duration of therapy) (68). All adult patients admitted to the medicine service were consecutively evaluated prior to the introduction of the program ($n = 500$ patients) and post-implementation. Using

DDD data and hospital expenditure data, they showed a 36% reduction in overall antimicrobial use ($p < 0.001$), intravenous antimicrobial use (46%, $p < 0.01$), and overall expenditures (53%, $p = 0.001$), all without compromising the quality of patient care (determined by inpatient survival, clinical improvement/cure, duration of hospitalization, and readmission rates within 30 days). These benefits were sustained for the 4-year period evaluated.

Carling and colleagues (41) evaluated their ASP over a 7-year time period. Their ASP consists of a physician (one-quarter time support) and PharmD (full-time support), both with specialty training in ID. Antimicrobial consumption was measured by using DDD/1000 patient days for targeted antimicrobial agents. This program operates 8 hr/day and 5 days/wk, and during this time, new orders are typically evaluated within 4 hr of their entry. Orders falling outside of the 8-hr day are reviewed as a priority the next time the PharmD is on duty. Informal written notes are generated when the team identifies a problematic regimen and is then placed in the patient's chart. "Academic detailing" occurs as well between the PharmD and the prescribing clinicians to supplement the written recommendations. They evaluated their impact on vancomycin-resistant enterococci (VRE), MRSA, and *C. difficile* disease by means of internal benchmarking as well as externally benchmarking themselves with similarly matched hospitals within the National Nosocomial Infections Surveillance System. A 22% reduction in parenteral broad-spectrum antibiotics occurred ($p < 0.0001$) during a time where they observed a 15% increase in the acuity of their patient population over the 7-year time period. Reductions in nosocomial infections caused by *C. difficile* ($p = 0.002$) and resistant enterobacteriaceae ($p = 0.02$) were reported. MRSA rates remained unaffected.

A description of a smaller hospital (120-bed community hospital) successfully implementing an ASP using a prospective audit and feedback strategy was published (22). The ASP involved an ID specialist physician and a clinical pharmacist as well as representatives from infection control and the microbiology laboratory. The ID physician was involved approximately 8–12 hr/wk. Antimicrobial therapy was reviewed 3 days a week in patients receiving targeted drugs or prolonged durations of therapy. Recommendations were conveyed using a form that was temporarily placed in the patient's chart and by telephone if necessary. During the first year, 488 recommendations were made with a 69% acceptance rate, and antimicrobial expenditures were reduced by 19%, saving an estimated $177,000. Common interventions were discontinuation of redundant antimicrobial therapy, discontinuation of treatment due to inappropriate use or excessive duration, transition from intravenous to oral therapy, and substitution or addition of an antibiotic to the regimen.

Preauthorization Strategy

White and colleagues (63) implemented an ASP, restricting the use of antimicrobials based on cost and/or spectra of activity. A 24 hr/day, 7 day/wk on-call system was established via dedicated pager that clinicians would call to receive approval for restricted agents. In their quasi-experimental study, patients in the pre-implementation period were similar to the post-implementation period patients in terms of severity of illness. Outcome measures that were not statistically significant between groups were survival ($p = 0.49$), infection-related length of stay for bacteremia ($p > 0.05$), and, importantly, time to administration of the antimicrobial ($p > 0.05$). Benefits noted in the post-ASP group included improved susceptibilities to a number of bug–drug pairings primarily involving nonfermenting Gram-negative rods and enterobacteriaceae, a significant reduction in the use of a number of broad-spectrum agents, and a significant reduction in annualized antimicrobial costs ($803,910) and costs per patient day ($18 to $14.4).

A variety of well-conducted studies at the University of Pennsylvania over the last two decades have contributed to our current knowledge of ASPs in general (11). Gross and colleagues (12) initially employed a dedicated beeper schedule for weekdays during normal business hours that was covered by an antimicrobial management team (AMT) member (an ID PharmD or ID MD). Second year ID fellows covered evenings and weekends. At night, restricted drugs were released pending a next-morning follow-up. Taking advantage of their existing program, they evaluated interventions performed by the ID fellows versus those made by the ID PharmD and/or ID ASP attending. They concluded that interventions performed by the veteran ASP team members (ID PharmD and/or ID MD) were more cost effective and resulted in narrower-spectrum therapy compared with those made by ID fellows. Based on the results of their study, the ID fellows have been more fully incorporated into their ASP and work with the PharmD and ID attending more directly. With regard to intranet/internet resources, they also have published their list of restricted antimicrobials and guidelines on a website that can be accessed, at least in part, by outside institutions (www.uphs.upenn.edu/bugdrug). In addition to the preauthorization method for active interventions, they also work closely with the hospital epidemiologist, are involved in establishing guidelines for antimicrobial use and dosing, are proactively involved in the antimicrobial formulary and work closely with the Pharmacy and Therapeutics Committee, provide education, and continuously evaluate antimicrobial consumption trends (11).

Potential Barriers

The literature is helpful to point out pitfalls that some have experienced. Delays in the approval for a necessary antimicrobial agent can be detrimental to critically ill patients in need of initial broad-spectrum antimicrobial therapy. White and colleagues showed no delay in the administration of antimicrobial agents prior to and after the introduction of their program; however, approval times and time to antibiotic administration must be monitored as a process measure (63). The perception of "threatened autonomy" can be a significant impediment to the efficacy of the program. In the study by LaRocco and colleagues (22), and in our experience (21), using the prospective audit and feedback strategy with few "restricted" antimicrobials promotes education at the point of intervention, neutralizing negative emotions. Thus, regardless of approach, constant communication with frontline prescribers and education are vital. The concept of "gaming the system" cannot be ignored and is a function of human nature. For example, one program reported an outbreak of nosocomial infection following the introduction of their ASP (64). A 30% relative increase in documentation of infection in the medical record occurred (incidence of infection increased from 11 to 14.3 per 1000 patient care days, $p < 0.05$) (64). After further investigation into this counterintuitive finding, the outbreak was termed a "pseudo-outbreak." Clinicians were required to document infection in the medical record in order to justify antimicrobial use; thus, more clinicians were documenting infections in an attempt to use particular restricted antimicrobials. The perception that ASPs are solely financially driven can also be an impediment. However, the IDSA/SHEA guidelines and other authorities endorse these programs not based on the potential for cost savings, but as a means to improve patient safety and to reduce the selective pressure exerted by unnecessary antimicrobial use that facilitates the evolution of antimicrobial resistance. Typically as a side effect of interventions to optimize antimicrobial use to improve efficacy and reduce resistance, cost saving is observed, which financially justifies the program. Administrators need to be cognizant of this when helping to develop ASPs. Program funding can be a barrier for some institutions, but as mentioned in SHEA/IDSA guidelines and as numerous studies in the area of ASPs point out, ASPs typically pay for themselves as a side effect of their existence.

The Business Proposal

When putting a proposal together for an ASP, one needs to consider the aforementioned discussion regarding the core strategy that will be employed, as this will determine the type of resources necessary. At minimum, a part-time or full-time physician (with ID training) and an ID-trained pharmacist are necessary and must be in the budget. In addition to these individuals, an IS/IT specialist must be budgeted to assist with developing daily reports, assisting with intranet site/ website directives, outcomes and process goal measurement, or explore your computer system for opportunities to build in decision support options as described in other sections of this chapter and in Chapter 16. All of the resources should be requested up front, as continually going back to administration for additional resources is typically not well received. List the goals and objectives for the program. Make sure they are clearly stated. Know the audience for the proposal. For example, if it is the chief financial officer, the economic goals should be listed first among the list of the goals. Consider that the proposal may be reviewed by a committee and know who may be on that committee. If the committee includes the patient safety administrator or other clinician administrators, consider placing goals that include those involving patient safety and other clinical endpoints such as reduction in inappropriate antimicrobial use at the top of the list. State the relevant expertise of the ASP team members; this obviously gives confidence to those in charge of the funding source if the key team members have expertise in this area. Do not be overly descriptive; keep the proposal generic and succinct. Bold certain key words (or the reader in their own mind will bold words for you), particularly if the proposal is long. Keep the proposal simple and its goals accomplishable. The program needs to deliver what is stated in the proposal, so make it a "mission possible," or in other words, do what you state you are going to do. Have a "power paragraph" in which key points are summarized and key words are bolded. Describe what you want the person in charge of funding the program to know the most about this effort. Have someone proof the proposal, particularly someone who is knowledgeable about ASPs.

Make sure you are plugged into a visible reporting source, such as the Pharmacy and Therapeutics Committee (which sends its minutes and reports to the Medical Executive Committee). One needs to report to this group or other designated, highly visible groups periodically (we report to the Pharmacy and Therapeutics Committee every six months, for example). This keeps your efforts visible so your colleagues and administrators see what the return on investment is. I would like to thank Ron Small at Wake Forest University, who is now an administrator but used to be the director of pharmacy and who helped establish funding for their ASP a number of years ago for advice on this section.

In our first year, we stated we would create a formulary pocket guide, begin the prospective audit with feedback interventions, and incorporate supplemental strategies such as focusing on optimal dosing based on PK-PD principles, reducing unnecessary combination (redundant) therapy, and focus on transitional therapy. After our initial success, we rolled in other supplemental strategies and became innovative by evaluating high-cost antimicrobials for opportunities in contracting or looking for efficient ways of administering other antimicrobials.

SUPPLEMENTAL STRATEGIES

The IDSA/SHEA guidelines for developing ASPs suggest several supplemental strategies that are listed in Table 1. These strategies can be used, regardless of core ASP strategy selected, and some are discussed in more detail below.

Formulary Management and Interventions

A survey of teaching hospitals suggests that 80% limit prescriber access to antibiotics using a variety of mechanisms (73). Formulary restriction is the most direct way to influence antimicrobial use and is central to the primary *preauthorization* ASP strategy. Most hospitals, regardless of having an ASP, will employ this strategy by limiting access to the numbers of drugs within a class. Limiting the number of available antimicrobials within a class is a passive intervention strategy, enforcement through ASPs using either *preauthorization* or *prospective audit and feedback* strategies shifts this to an active intervention. This method can be used effectively by either primary strategy. Working closely with the Pharmacy and Therapeutics Committee is de rigueur. A strong leader and a good working relationship is needed of the Pharmacy and Therapeutics Committee Chairman. Because the pharmacy is often viewed by some as a "candy shop," the committee chairman must support the ASP.

Careful selection of drugs within a class involves an in-depth analysis of not only the basics (efficacy, safety, and cost), but should include an evaluation of resistance, evoking potential where possible, and a pharmacodynamic evaluation of the drug. A benefit of having an ASP allows this process to be centralized and by working closely with the Pharmacy and Therapeutics Committee, helps to establish an optimal formulary stocked with the best drugs for the given institution. The cost evaluation should extend beyond purchase prices, although leveraging

TABLE 1 Supplemental Strategies

Education
Guidelines and clinical pathways
Combination therapy
Streamlining/de-escalation
Antimicrobial order forms/order sets
Conversion from parenteral to oral therapy
Computerized decision support

contracts is a useful tool (74). Importantly, the overall cost of care should be considered when evaluating an antimicrobial but this is not always done due to the compartmentalization of costs within an institution (also referred to as the "silo" mentality). For example, although 8- to 10- fold more expensive than intravenous vancomycin in purchase cost, the use of oral linezolid has been shown to decrease the length of stay and improve discharge dynamics for patients with MRSA infections (75–78). This is particularly financially appealing for institutions operating at maximal census (because bed costs far outweigh drug costs) and with high rates of MRSA, not to mention from the infection control perspective of reduced transmission dynamics when length of stay is shortened, and most important from the patient's perspective of being home rather than hospitalized. In our institution, our ASP working with the care coordination and infection control departments has taken advantage of efficiently transitioning the patient, once clinically stable, to an oral MRSA therapy such as linezolid and in some cases minocycline. This serves the purpose of reducing the barrier to discharge posed by home intravenous therapy arrangement or skilled nursing facility placement if solely for administering intravenous vancomycin (20).

Practical, evidence-based examples exist of preferentially replacing drugs with increased resistance evoking potential (e.g., ceftazidime) with a member of the same class, but that have demonstrated a reduced ability to select for resistance (e.g., cefepime) (21,32,70,79). For hospitals still characterized by high third-generation cephalosporin use, a number of studies have demonstrated that their replacement with cefepime or piperacillin/tazobactam are effective strategies (particularly in concert with infection control intervention) to minimize the selective pressure that facilitates the appearance of problematic beta-lactamases (e.g., AmpC enzymes, ESBLs) and VRE (32,80–82). As mentioned previously, not all drugs are created equal with regard to their potential to select for antimicrobial resistance, as exemplified by the contrast between vancomycin and daptomycin. Nuances related to the propensity for the antimicrobial to become resistant to the pathogens of interest within a particular institution's patient population should be considered from a formulary perspective, and monitoring the drug's susceptibility performance in a perpetual manner is an important component of an ASP working directly with the hospital epidemiologist and the clinical microbiology laboratory (83).

Finally, where an antimicrobial may fit into order sets and guidelines, as well as how its use will be monitored completes a comprehensive evaluation of how the antimicrobial will be most effectively utilized within the institution. With regard to following up on an antimicrobial's utilization in the institution, the support of the Pharmacy and Therapeutics Committee is vital as it provides a mechanism to report back inappropriate use of the drug and has the power (in many places) to be an effective countermeasure to correct inappropriate use by intervening.

The ASPs involvement in the antimicrobial formulary is not limited to drug evaluations, but also should periodically work with the pharmacy to evaluate pricing contracts, which can be complicated and may fluctuate. Having someone with expertise in antimicrobials working with the pharmacy buyer can greatly improve the institutional purchase costs and ensure competitive pricing is being received by the hospital/healthcare system. Also, frequent communication with the pharmacy buyer has been a requisite over the last several years due to antimicrobial shortages. Preparing for shortages when advanced notice is given can be helpful to maintain par levels of necessary drugs and to provide insight into alternative drugs that will likely be used in their place, and communicating these shortages with alternatives to the prescribers can be facilitated by the ASP. In fact, due to an ongoing nationwide shortage of piperacillin/tazobactam that has periodically challenged our institution, we developed a product that can be easily substituted. The combination product (cefepime combined with metronidazole in the same minibag) can be given as a single administered product due to their stability and compatibility in combination, is administered on average less than two times per day (cefepime and metronidazole can be given every 12 hr for most infections), and is approximately 30% less expensive than piperacillin/tazobactam (84). Because we have an institutionally supported ASP, we were able to creatively dedicate resources to an idea that is both beneficial to patients and cost-effective.

Combination Therapy vs. Redundant Therapy

Whether or not combination therapy is useful has been the subject of great debate for decades for certain infections but not for others. The answer depends on the context of the question. The proposed rationale for combination therapy includes (*i*) an additive or synergistic interaction, (*ii*) to broaden the activity of an empiric regimen to include resistant organisms (with the intention of "getting it right" up front), and (*iii*) to prevent the emergence of resistance (85). So when is combination therapy useful? Combination therapy is of proven benefit for infections involving the human immunodeficiency virus and tuberculosis.

An Additive or Synergistic Interaction

With regard to so-called "synergy," the only clinically well-proven example is for enterococcal endocarditis (an anti-enterococcal cell wall-active drug plus an aminoglycoside) (86). Additionally, "synergy," although not well-proven clinically, has been employed in patients with pulmonary exacerbations of cystic fibrosis (CF) for Gram-negative-directed therapy (87). In this example, synergy studies are sent out and performed on isolates collected from the CF patient to determine the best combination of drugs to use. This is a relatively unique therapeutic situation, as the organisms are typically pan-resistant and the premise for using "synergistic" combinations is to lower the overall minimum inhibitory concentration (MIC). Since the goal of this treatment is to reduce the burden of the infecting organisms because eradication of the organisms is typically not possible and the host is different, this type of synergy cannot be extrapolated to non-CF patients who develop pneumonia. For MDR nonfermenting Gram-negative bacilli, the concurrent use of antimicrobials such as the polymyxins (which act as "detergents" on the bacterial cell wall) may restore activity back to antimicrobials that test resistant by standard in vitro susceptibility testing methods (88). This is an example of "synergy" but has not been well-described outside of the laboratory (e.g., clinically). For Gram-negative organisms with higher MIC values than traditional therapies (typically *P. aeruginosa*), initial combination therapy results in more rapid reduction in the inoculum size, as demonstrated in nonclinical models of infection that mimic human infection (89–91). These studies are particularly useful as it is not ethical to conduct them in humans (e.g., randomize patients to the group receiving known lower antimicrobial exposures where it has been established that the amplification of resistant subpopulations occurs readily and also in whom it is not possible to gain consent to perform serial biopsies of lung tissue specimens during therapy for examination of organism counts). Therefore, brief use of combinations directed toward higher MIC pathogens, such as *P. aeruginosa*, in tissue sites of infection, makes sense based on the findings of these nonclinical models of infection. In some respects, this is already endorsed by the American Thoracic Society (ATS) and the IDSA guidelines for the treatment of healthcare facility-acquired pneumonia (HCAP), ventilator-associated pneumonia (VAP), and hospital-acquired pneumonia (HAP) (29). If *P. aeruginosa* is identified as the causative pathogen, combination therapy is recommended with an antipseudomonal beta-lactam plus an aminoglycoside (high-dose, extended interval dosing), where the aminoglycoside is recommended to be used for 5 days and then is discontinued while the beta-lactam is continued for the duration of therapy.

The addition of rifampin to a cell wall-active drug for device-related infections caused by staphylococci is not based on standard definitions of synergy, but is often referred to as a "synergistic interaction"; however, it stems from the premise that beta-lactams and glycopeptides are most active against rapidly dividing organisms and rifampin is added adjunctively for its activity against populations of bacteria that are in stationary growth phase (92,93). Beta-lactams and glycopeptides are most active against rapidly dividing organisms, and since infections involving foreign material offer bacteria the perfect milieu for entering stationary growth phase (a nondividing state), the addition of rifampin is therapeutically beneficial (92,93).

To Broaden the Activity of an Empiric Regimen to Include Resistant Organisms

In the modern sense of being beneficial, "combination therapy" for the purpose of broadening treatment to cover MDR pathogens for certain infections (e.g., pneumonia and sepsis) has been shown to reduce mortality. In this sense, combination therapy is endorsed by recent guidelines by the ATS and the IDSA for the treatment of HCAP, HAP, and VAP (29), and by the IDSA/SHEA antimicrobial stewardship guidelines (54). A growing body of literature exists supporting combination therapy for the purpose of broadening therapy in order to "get it right up front," resulting in decreased mortality (14,85,94,95). In many healthcare facilities, MDR Gram-negative organisms may be the cause of sepsis or pneumonia in elderly patients transferred from long-term care facilities, particularly those with reduced activity of daily living (or ADL) score and who have received previous antimicrobial therapy, and patients who acquire pneumonia as a result of extended length of hospitalization with previous antimicrobial exposure (96). Because empiric treatment with a single Gram-negative-directed antimicrobial has been shown to increase the likelihood of inadequate therapy (the organism eventually cultured on day 3 is resistant to the treatment selected by the clinician), regardless if the patient is changed to a drug that "gets it right" on day 3, the mortality rates remains higher than if the original empiric treatment therapy contained an antimicrobial that was active against the infecting pathogen.

Combination therapy directed toward specific pathogens once the culture and susceptibility data are known (and not meeting the criteria above) has not been shown to be of any benefit. In fact, it has been called a medical error by some (51). In the sense that it increases the probability of side effects, may increase the probability of resistance, and definitely increases drug costs without benefit, combination therapy when the pathogen is known is not justifiable. A systematic review conducted evaluated 64 trials involving more than 7500 patients demonstrated no difference in mortality for infections involving Gram-negative pathogens. In addition, patients treated with monotherapy regimens had significantly improved clinical and microbiological outcomes compared with those treated with combination therapy regimens (97). Furthermore, monotherapy regimens were associated with fewer side effects, particularly nephrotoxicity, primarily due to aminoglycosides (97). In this systematic review, the subgroup involving infections due to *P. aeruginosa* did not appear to benefit from combination therapy (97). The HAP/VAP/HCAP guidelines from the ATS and IDSA recommend a combination regimen for the empiric therapy of these infections, and if Gram-negative organisms other than *P. aeruginosa* are isolated, that combination therapy should be de-escalated to monotherapy. If *P. aeruginosa* is isolated, clinicians have an option to continue combination therapy with an aminoglycoside for a total of 5 days, then the aminoglycoside should be discontinued and monotherapy continued for the remainder of therapy. It is in this capacity that the prospective audit with feedback ASP can be very useful. Several studies have demonstrated the benefit of promoting broad therapy for HAP/VAP/HCAP, followed by de-escalation of therapy once culture and susceptibility results return. This is reviewed more completely elsewhere (98) and in Chapter 13. In brief, patients with VAP were evaluated in a randomized controlled trial of antimicrobial de-escalation (99). Patients with pneumonia who received broad-spectrum empiric therapy in the ICU had therapy de-escalated by the ICU-based clinical pharmacist (99). This study demonstrated a significant reduction in unnecessary antimicrobial use (approximately 300 antibiotic days). Again, de-escalation interventions reduce unnecessary (redundant) Gram-negative therapy for the treatment of pneumonia as well as other infections. Common "redundant" therapy regimens that we see frequently involve a carbapenem plus clindamycin or metronidazole (in situations where CDI is not involved) and beta-lactamase inhibitor combinations plus clindamycin or metronidazole. This duplication of anti-anaerobic therapy is unnecessary and contributes to increased cost, significant collateral damage to the intestinal microbiota, and an increased probability of potential superinfections (e.g., VRE, CDI, fungemia).

Pharmacodynamic Dose Optimization

Dose optimization interventions are likely to be one of the most common interventions from an ASP. Although formerly viewed as a means to efficiently trim excess drug exposure secondary to renal dysfunction, the modern application of pharmacodynamic principles is important in order to maximize drug exposure for organisms with elevated MICs, patients with excess body mass indices, and for closed-space or otherwise difficult-to-penetrate sites of infection (e.g., meningitis, endocarditis, pneumonia, bone and joint infections). A recent paper provides a more in-depth review of the subject and serves as a primer for all ASPs incorporating optimal dosing strategies (100). Although we approached our program with the thought that may patients would receive downward dose adjustments for renal impairment, what we found was a significant proportion of patients required increased drug exposure (20,21). Other examples of pharmacodynamic dose-optimization include regimens intended to treat higher MIC pathogens more effectively such as extended or "prolonged" infusion of short half-life beta-lactams (e.g., piperacillin/tazobactam, cefepime, meropenem), and extended-interval aminoglycoside dosing. At Albany Medical Center, choosing this option has become as simple as filling out a brief form or checking a box. This is discussed further in

Chapter 13, and a review paper by the same authors (101). A clinical study of the efficacy of extended infusions of piperacillin/tazobactam demonstrated that this particular drug, when administered in a pharmacodynamically optimized fashion, was associated with reduced mortality rates compared with intermittently infused piperacillin/tazobactam in patients with elevated APACHE II scores ≥ 17 (102).

As previously mentioned, we have exploited the fact that metronidazole, with its prolonged half-life ($\sim$10 hr) and active metabolite, can be given every 12 hr instead of every 6 or 8 hr for non-*C. difficile*, non–central nervous system infections. Moreover, as mentioned, we created a clinical program that integrates cefepime and metronidazole into a single administration product that can be infused twice daily, mimicking the spectrum of activity provided by piperacillin/tazobactam (84). The benefits are numerous: increased heterogeneous antimicrobial use (as the use of piperacillin/tazobactam had steadily been increasing, creating less diversity in antimicrobial use); it saves nursing time (if the combination was to be ordered traditionally, 4 administrations per day would be required; by combining it into one bag for infusion, the number of infusions by nursing staff is cut by half); in some cases, it has better activity against certain enterobacteriaceae such as *Serratia marcescens, Enterobacter* spp. (AmpC phenotypes); and through a thorough cost minimization analysis using regimens that were based on the renal function of patients actually receiving the two regimens and employing sensitivity analyses considering group purchasing organization contract pricing, we save 33% each day metropime is used in place of piperacillin/tazobactam.

Educational Efforts
Development and dissemination of pertinent information is the first step in any process leading to change. Early attempts at influencing prescribing behaviors relied heavily upon educational efforts—it was simplistically believed that the reason physicians frequently inappropriately prescribed antibiotics was that they were "therapeutically undereducated" (103). The assumption was that misuse of antibiotics was more often the result of insufficient information rather than inappropriate behavior.

Over the years that we have taught antibiotic principles and specifics of therapy at our hospital, we have been impressed by the intense interest both physicians-in-training and established practitioners have in learning more about antibiotics. But equally as impressive is the "laissez-faire" and even fatalistic attitude toward retaining and applying lessons learned in these educational sessions. Without direct application to current patients, prescribers often refer to antibiotics as "alphabet soup" and "impossible to understand." These impressions are supported in the literature. Although a supplemental cornerstone to any ASP, educational efforts when applied alone are the least effective, and certainly the shortest lasting, way to impact prescribing behaviors. Active intervention that is supplemented by education is a synergistic method for changing behavior, as mentioned previously.

Computer-Assisted Decision Support Programs
Direct computerized physician order entry (CPOE) is rapidly becoming the standard of care, and has been adopted as one of the Leapfrog initiatives to avoid medication errors and improve the quality of care (20). Computer-assisted decision

support programs have been designed to provide real-time integrated patient and institutional data including culture and susceptibility results, laboratory measures of organ function, allergy history, drug interactions, as well as cumulative or customized location-specific antibiogram data, and cost information. They provide therapeutic choices for clinicians and allow for the incorporation of clinical judgment by overriding suggestions. Autonomy is preserved while insuring that important variables in the choice of antimicrobial therapy are considered. This topic is covered in depth by Pestotnik in this book.

Almost all published data on the effect of computer-assisted decision support programs on antibiotic use are from researchers at the LDS Hospital in Salt Lake City, Utah. This approach has been associated with reductions in antibiotic doses, inappropriate orders, costs, treatment duration, and associated ADEs (104–106). This degree of computer sophistication is not universally available but has been made available through a variety of commercial systems (107,108). We have used our own CPOE system to design a logic-based algorithm to optimize the treatment of pneumonia (as discussed later). A recent randomized control trial of clinical decision support on the appropriateness of antimicrobial prescribing demonstrated improved appropriateness of use and reduced overall use of anti-microbials for respiratory tract infections (109). In this rural outpatient setting, handheld personal digital assistants (PDAs) and paper forms of decision support supplemented the prescribing decision and choice of therapy. Although patient-specific data had to be entered into the PDA, it provided a logic-based recommendation that was measurably useful in the prescribing process.

Adaptation of Locally Customized Published Guidelines

National guidelines put forth by the IDSA and SHEA (and other organizations) are available for a variety of infections, providing evidence-based diagnosis and prevention and treatment discussions, and are useful to construct clinical pathways, which can be customized locally. In addition, for some infections (CDI) where significant time has passed since the publication of national guidelines and where the disease process has changed significantly, an institution should have a mechanism to develop evidence-based guidelines. Evidence suggests that guidelines are often not followed and do not result in practice changes, an observation that has been personally made by years of clinical practice and through studies that have demonstrated lack of adherence to guidelines (96,110–112). The treatment of uncomplicated acute bacterial cystitis and acute pyelonephritis in women is a straightforward guideline published by the IDSA in 1999 (113). With regard to therapy for these infections, trimethaprim/sulfamethoxazole is recommended to be used so long as E. coli resistance rates do not exceed a threshold value, in which case ciprofloxacin is recommended. Realizing resistance rates vary according to geographic location, there would be expected to be variability in the use of these therapies depending on regional resistance trends. In the study by Taur and colleagues (111), the guidelines did not impact the use of trimethaprim/sulfa-methoxazole; in fact, the second-line therapy (ciprofloxacin) increased in use across all geographies for these indications, controlling for a wide range of variables that might influence the use of the two treatments. Unfortunately, 8 years later we find ourselves in a predicament where resistance rates to ciprofloxacin among strains of E. coli now exceeds that of trimethaprim/sulfamethoxazole resistance in many geographies. An editorial to this study emphasized that once guidelines are published, there should be more effort and additional funding to translate their recommendations into practice. Moreover, Mol and colleagues (112) evaluated guidelines for the treatment of lower respiratory tract infections, sepsis, and UTIs in a 1-year observational study with an adherence rate of 79%, 53%, and 40%, respectively. In another study, national guidelines for multiple infection types were customized to localized susceptibility patterns and introduced in a hospital (114). They were developed in concert with key opinion leaders within the institution that were also the end users of the guidelines, giving a sense of ownership to the prescribers, and were distributed in both paper and electronic format. In the second phase of this study, academic detailing was introduced (which was similar to a prospective audit with feedback core strategy where clinicians were given feedback based on their prescribing habits in group or individual sessions). Using interrupted time-series analysis with segmented regression, the changes in prescribing habits were significant (86% compliance). The investigators incorporated key elements that resulted in success, the guidelines were developed in a multidisciplinary fashion, giving ownership to those involved, and the guidelines were widely accessible to prescribers via paper and electronic formats. This is one of the few quasi-experimental (before-and-after) studies to employ the appropriate statistical technique to evaluate the results of their study (time series analysis). To this end, ASPs provide a mechanism to identify infections in need of guidelines, develop locally customized guidelines in conjunction with potential end-users of such guidelines, facilitate the development of mechanisms to educate and make using the guidelines easy (through human decision support, developing order forms, developing CPOE "order sets" with IS resources, making the guidelines as accessible as possible by using both paper and electronic means), and, finally, they provide a mechanism for determining adherence to guidelines and uncovering reasons why guidelines are not used so that they can be addressed. In addition, if determining outcomes in these quasi-experimental studies, ASPs should use interrupted time-series analysis to assess the impact of their interventions (need appropriate statistical resources to do so) so that administrators and department chiefs can see the impact of this type of intervention on antimicrobial use.

Another example from our hospital: in 2006, we were faced with (like many institutions) opportunities to improve quality/performance indicators associated with community-acquired pneumonia (CAP) such as improving the timing of antimicrobial administration for this indication in patients admitted in the ED and for direct admissions, as well as improving the quality of antimicrobial use (e.g., ensuring the administration of an antipseudomonal agent if risk factors existed). These were also included as "pay-for-performance" indicators by the Centers for Medicare and Medicade Services (CMS) which the hospital administration was concerned about (as expected). In an effort to improve compliance with these "core measures," we worked with the IS department to develop a decision support mechanism that not only was aimed at improving compliance with these core measures, but also at optimizing antimicrobial use in patients being admitted with pneumonia in general (not just CAP, but also HCAP). The clinicians would type in "pneumonia" to access the order set. This would provide access to the order set, where the clinician would answer six questions electronically through the use of drop-down menus: (*i*) Where the patient was admitted from? (home, long-term care facility, transfer from outside healthcare facility); (*ii*) Where the patient will be admitted to? (ward, ICU); (*iii*) Are risk factors for MRSA present? (drop-down menu lists these risks); (*iv*) Are risk factors for *P. aeruginosa* present?

(drop-down menu lists these risks); (*v*) Does the patient have a beta-lactam allergy?; and (*vi*) Has the patient already received a stat dose (of adequate antimicrobials)? Based on the responses to these questions, the list of antimicrobials provided directly below these questions (all on a single screen on the computer), which were all initially available to order, became unavailable to order (only appropriate treatment choices were available to order and the boxes to the left of the antimicrobial were checked for the prescriber). So, for example, the patient is admitted to the ward with the diagnosis of pneumonia, has risk for both MRSA (previously known to be colonized with MRSA) and *P. aeruginosa* (e.g., structural lung disease), does not have a beta-lactam allergy, and a stat dose of antimicrobials has not been administered, then the boxes next to cefepime, azithromycin, and vancomycin are checked for stat doses of each and for routinely scheduled doses for each. The ability to customize the dose is offered again on that same screen (without having to exit the order set) making it a one-step process (Fig. 7). Compliance with core measures was evaluated by our performance improvement department and before the decision support order set was implemented in January 2007, compliance was between 60% and 90% for several months. After the implementation from February through July 2007, adherence to core measures upon audits was 100% for every month following implementation. Reasons we feel this was successful were (*i*) that the decision support–based order set was easy to use (provided "one-stop shopping:" all of the questions, drugs,

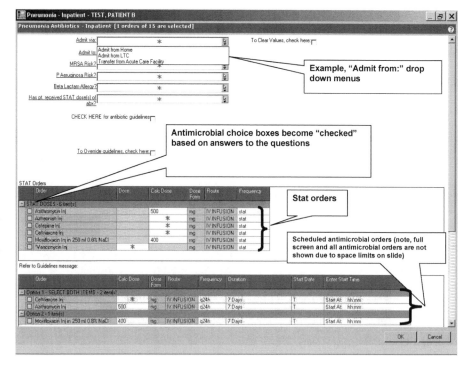

FIGURE 7   Example of computerized decision support designed to facilitate guidelines for the treatment of pneumonia.

and doses were on one page and easy to visualize) for the prescriber, (*ii*) it offered the flexibility to exit the order set at any time if the patient did not "fit" the order set for some reason and a typed-in box allowed us to capture the reason why the prescriber exited the order set (allowing us to keep this a fluid order set and modify it as we progressed), and (*iii*) feedback was provided to clinicians showing prescribers the effect they had on compliance. A collateral benefit of this order set was that it allowed for electronic documentation of risk (e.g., *P. aeruginosa*, MRSA) for auditors and coding personnel, which was previously poor and difficult to find in the medical record in many cases.

Another example facilitating guideline occurred as a result of an outbreak of CDI in 2002–2003. In collaboration with the department of hospital epidemiology and infection prevention who determined that the rates of CDI were escalating, we began to assemble CDI management guidelines in the absence of updated national guidelines (last published in 1995). Being one of the first identified institutions in North America with a hypervirulent strain of *C. difficile* (8,44), now known as BI/NAP1/027, we saw the clinical and prescribing impact almost immediately (115). We used the data obtained from obtained from Dr. Gerding's laboratory regarding our isolates to galvanize an effort between hospital epidemiology, infection prevention department, the departments of gastroenterology, surgery, and environmental services (and again ID and pharmacy were represented by the ASP), to standardize the management of CDI in the absence of updated guidelines (8). Prior to guidelines, we were observing combinations of oral metronidazole plus oral vancomycin, therapy in first case episodes lasting more than 4 weeks in some cases, the use of nonevidence-based treatments such as cholestyramine and probiotics. We coordinated a collective effort to develop treatment guidelines that were published locally on the intranet and we conducted educational interventions with our prospective audit and feedback ASP (8,9). We evaluated the impact of a bundled approach of multidisciplinary guidelines, creating an order set in our CPOE system, and daily audit and feedback strategies on nonevidence-based (and potentially harmful) prescribing cholestyramine, probiotics, and oral vancomycin plus oral metronidazole combination therapy using a quasi-experimental study design (115). We demonstrated a significant reduction in the prescribing habits previously mentioned despite a continuing escalation of CDI rates (115).

Parenteral-to-Oral Interventions/Optimizing Length of Stay

Oral therapy for the treatment of ID has become a cornerstone of therapy for a variety of reasons that are mostly well known to prescribers today. Certain antimicrobials have near complete bioavailability, such as older drugs like minocycline, doxycycline, trimethaprim/sulfamethoxazole, cephalexin, to fluoroquinolones, linezolid, and antifungals like fluconazole and voriconazole. In most cases, oral therapy options are less expensive than parenteral antimicrobials (with the exception of linezolid). The value of an oral medication extends far beyond the fact that they are less expensive than their parenteral counterparts. For example, once a hospitalized patient is clinically stable and able to take oral medications, it is in the patient's best interest to be transitioned to their home even though they may still require antimicrobial treatment, since continued hospitalization results in risks for developing a new MDR infection, CDI, and if on precautions, suffer from preventable adverse events (9,116). With near complete bioavailability, oral therapy has been shown to be as effective as parenteral therapy, which makes sense, as the organism has no idea whether the antimicrobial was administered by vein or via the gastrointestinal tract. Certain infections are less amenable to oral therapy, such as meningitis and endocarditis, for example. However, even for these infections it is not clear that parenteral therapy is necessary, depending on the antimicrobial and on the organisms, as studies have demonstrated that oral fluoroquinolones are as effective as traditional parenteral therapy for meningitis (117). From the standpoint of an ASP, transitional therapy is a fundamental supplemental intervention that most incorporate regardless of the primary core strategy selected. When we began our program, we illustrated the *who, what, when, why, where* approach in a program titled: "Let's Go PO" in the form of a poster campaign. An example of our original poster is shown in Figure 8. The results clearly demonstrated significant increases in oral use for targeted drugs that were used as markers for parenteral to oral conversion (ciprofloxacin, moxifloxacin, and fluconazole) (21).

Most of the incremental costs associated with developing an infection during hospitalization are due to the added length of stay it causes. The impact on length of hospitalization is even greater if the organism is antimicrobial-resistant (52,53,118). Because hospital length of stay is a primary driver of hospital expenditures, strategies to minimize length of stay can provide a substantial return on investment in resources (21,53). Traditionally, there has not been an oral alternative for moderate to severe infections for MRSA infections, establishing a paradigm of parenteral therapy (primarily involving vancomycin). With linezolid being approved nearly 7 years ago, it is the second most studied anti-MRSA drug in our arsenal; thus, for its approved indications, there is a high level of confidence regarding its efficacy. Although it is expensive (compared with other oral antimicrobials), its expense is relative. Linezolid is not more expensive than the "room and board" costs of a single day of hospitalization (77). Because of the prevalence of MRSA infections, reducing length of hospitalization for these patients would result in a significant unclogging of the current log-jammed patient flow debacle some hospitals are experiencing. The use of linezolid had resulted in shortened length of hospitalization compared with vancomycin in a variety of studies, primarily because of its availability in an oral dosing form (75,76,119,120). One study examined this issue; investigators evaluated all hospitalized patients receiving vancomycin for MRSA or MRSE infections (75). They revealed that 58% of patients qualified for a switch to oral therapy, and 53% of those patients qualified for early discharge (75). This resulted in 3.3 days of reduced length of hospitalization per patient, and 181 days annually (75). Our ASP developed a program focusing on evaluating patients with MRSA infections working directly with the care-coordination department. A knowledgeable care coordination and/or social services department can navigate the reimbursement methods (e.g., third-party payers, indigent care programs sponsored by the pharmaceutical industry), which is vital to its successful implementation. Involvement of the ASP can ensure appropriate utilization of the drug and provide continuity across the diversity of potential prescribers. Supporting the shortened length of stay paradigm are the number of published studies that have demonstrated that patients with MRSA infections treated with linezolid have shorter length of stays than those patients treated with vancomycin in comparative registration trials.

In order to improve the potential for success of this program, prior to implementation, an exigent amount of time was invested in developing consensus among our ID, surgical, administrators, care coordination, and pharmacy

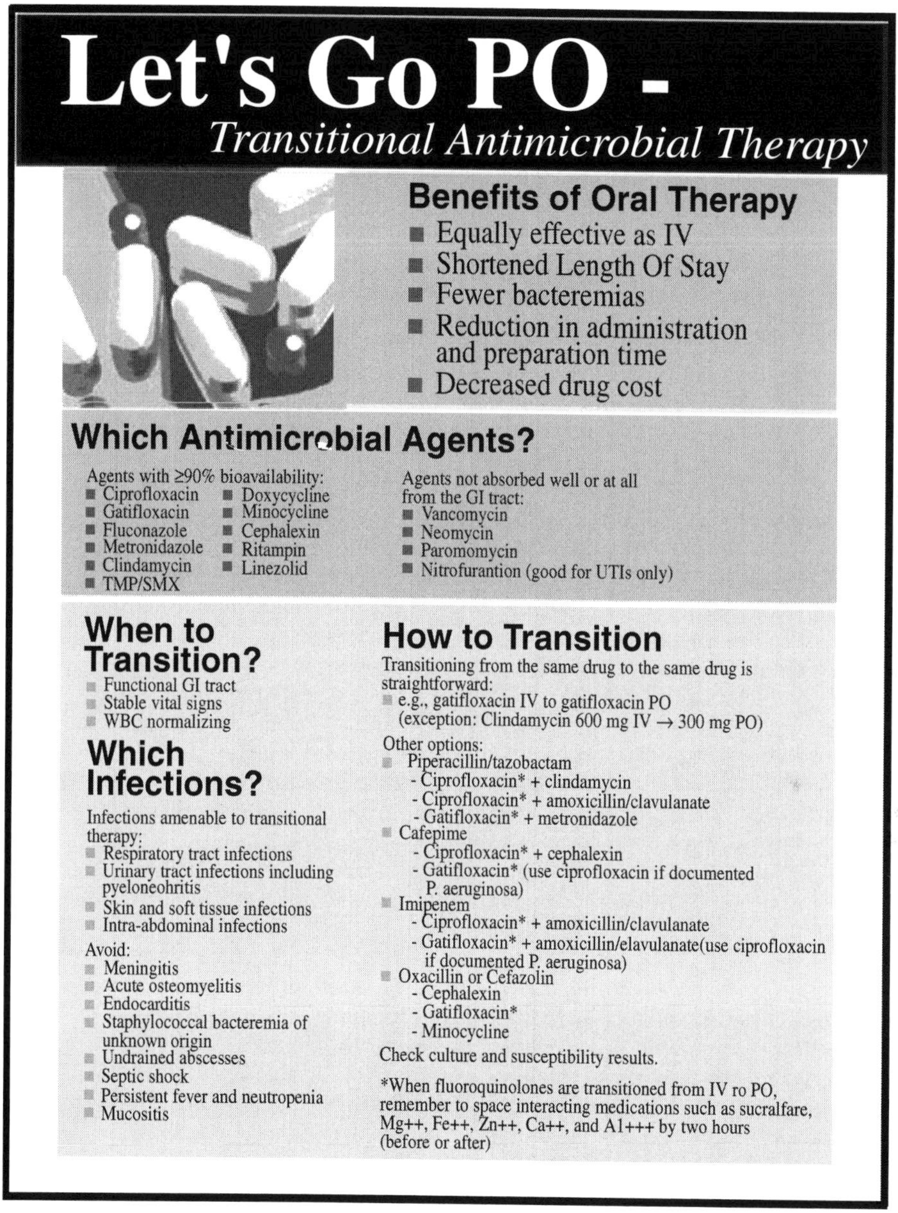

Let's Go PO -
Transitional Antimicrobial Therapy

Benefits of Oral Therapy
- Equally effective as IV
- Shortened Length Of Stay
- Fewer bacteremias
- Reduction in administration and preparation time
- Decreased drug cost

Which Antimicrobial Agents?

Agents with ≥90% bioavailability:
- Ciprofloxacin
- Gatifloxacin
- Fluconazole
- Metronidazole
- Clindamycin
- TMP/SMX
- Doxycycline
- Minocycline
- Cephalexin
- Ritampin
- Linezolid

Agents not absorbed well or at all from the GI tract:
- Vancomycin
- Neomycin
- Paromomycin
- Nitrofurantion (good for UTIs only)

When to Transition?
- Functional GI tract
- Stable vital signs
- WBC normalizing

Which Infections?

Infections amenable to transitional therapy:
- Respiratory tract infections
- Urinary tract infections including pyeloneohritis
- Skin and soft tissue infections
- Intra-abdominal infections

Avoid:
- Meningitis
- Acute osteomyelitis
- Endocarditis
- Staphylococcal bacteremia of unknown origin
- Undrained abscesses
- Septic shock
- Persistent fever and neutropenia
- Mucositis

How to Transition

Transitioning from the same drug to the same drug is straightforward:
- e.g., gatifloxacin IV to gatifloxacin PO
  (exception: Clindamycin 600 mg IV → 300 mg PO)

Other options:
- Piperacillin/tazobactam
  - Ciprofloxacin* + clindamycin
  - Ciprofloxacin* + amoxicillin/clavulanate
  - Gatifloxacin* + metronidazole
- Cafepime
  - Ciprofloxacin* + cephalexin
  - Gatifloxacin* (use ciprofloxacin if documented P. aeruginosa)
- Imipenem
  - Ciprofloxacin* + amoxicillin/clavulanate
  - Gatifloxacin* + amoxicillin/elavulanate(use ciprofloxacin if documented P. aeruginosa)
- Oxacillin or Cefazolin
  - Cephalexin
  - Gatifloxacin*
  - Minocycline

Check culture and susceptibility results.

*When fluoroquinolones are transitioned from IV ro PO, remember to space interacting medications such as sucralfare, Mg++, Fe++, Zn++, Ca++, and Al+++ by two hours (before or after)

FIGURE 8 Example of a hospital-wide poster campaign to facilitate oral therapy when and where appropriate (some of the specific antimicrobial examples are dated, as this was our original poster used in 2001, but the concepts remain the same). *Source*: Courtesy of Robert C. Owens, Jr.

colleagues. In addition, since some of our discharges were to skilled nursing facilities or long-term care facilities, we invested time in discussing reimbursement strategies with them as well as discussing with them that the linezolid's cost was going to be incurred for only a defined, short period of time and this was not a chronic medication. Coupled with the fact that Medicare patients qualify for a higher reimbursement rate if they have been on intravenous therapy within the last 14 days of hospitalization, barriers to accepting patients upon transfer from the hospital to long-term care facilities diminished. Outcomes measured are readmission rates, linezolid susceptibility monitoring, and days of length of stay avoided. The ASP's role in this process was to again quarterback this initiative and coordinate the consensus process, education, and outcome measurement.

ROLE OF THE ASP AND THE SUPPLEMENTAL STEWARDSHIP STRATEGIES

Because HAP, VAP, and HCAP provide another good example of the important role of the ASP in the aforementioned supplemental strategies, it will be used to provide a perspective. In other words, national guidelines exist for the treatment of HAP, VAP, and HCAP. Realizing that numerous published studies have demonstrated that guidelines are not adhered to (and from our own experience we realized this), despite the fact that much effort, time, and resources are invested into them. The *first step* was for the ASP to "convene the experts." In this case, we tagged onto an ongoing HAP, VAP, and HCAP prevention initiative and a therapeutic HAP, VAP, and HCAP initiative. Key team members included pulmonologists, surgeons, ID and pharmacy represented by the ASP team, a microbiology laboratory representative, a performance improvement department representative, respiratory therapists, and nursing leadership (because this was also a VAP prevention initiative). The *second step* was to customize the national treatment guidelines to locally applicable guidelines that involved five different areas, including: establishing the diagnosis/developing a definition; empiric therapy strategy based on ICU-specific antibiogram data; developing a targeted therapy strategy once the pathogen returns; developing criteria for oral therapy (optional for this disease state); and establishing an agreed-upon definition for the duration of therapy.

So while establishing a working definition for the various types of pneumonia (VAP being important for the reason that it was being tracked for state reporting purposes), we proceeded to simultaneously develop a diagnostic strategy. Because numerous data suggested that more invasive diagnostic methods (e.g., quantitative cultures from bronchoalveolar lavage or BAL, mini-BAL specimens) allowed customization of antimicrobials compared with endotracheal aspirates, although still somewhat controversial, we chose the former method as our microbiologic approach to ascertain the etiology. In addition, we incorporated the clinical pulmonary infection score (CPIS) for purposes of establishing a clinical diagnosis for patients in whom a microbiologic diagnosis would not be possible. Based on these objective methods for diagnosing pneumonia, we created an algorithm that was clear to visualize thresholds for the BAL and the CPIS score. From there, the microbiology laboratory pulled isolates obtained from respiratory specimens collected in our ICUs and assembled an antibiogram from which empiric therapy was selected using a Chinese menu approach of one antimicrobial from column A (Gram-negative–directed), one from column B (Gram-negative–directed), and one from column C (MRSA-directed). Criteria for de-escalating the three drug empiric regimen (two drugs targeting Gram-negative pathogens, one drug targeting MRSA if risk factors exist) was outlined. If oral therapy is possible, criteria for transitioning parenteral-to-oral therapy was created. Finally, the duration of therapy was decided upon and measuring process and outcome measures were established. The *third step* involved the ASP taking responsibility to follow patients with pneumonia and to serve as human decision support for the treating teams, which include different surgery and pulmonary/ intensivist teams in the ICU and on the floors, hospitalist, medicine, or family practice services (each with rotating attendings and some with different residents). The ASP also served as a reminder that the microbiologic data have returned and offered recommendations, offered assistance with calculating the CPIS, and helped clinicians to feel more comfortable with de-escalating therapy or stopping it altogether. To this end, this represents an example of virtually all of the supplemental strategies that were rolled into one programmatic educational effort. Since our pathway's initial development, a collaborative effort with a medical education company designed to assist other healthcare facilities in developing their own locally customized pathway has taken place. Using a proprietary material called ClingZ® (Permacharge Corporation, Rio Rancho, New Mexico, U.S.) that uses static electricity so that it can be placed on any wall surface and is capable of being drawn upon and erased, individual parts of the algorithm (diagnosis, empiric therapy, de-escalation, duration of therapy) are able to be placed on display in a classroom to facilitate discussion and solidify multidisciplinary buy-in. The final product can then be transcribed onto a computer and then printed on pocket cards, placed on the intranet site, made into a poster campaign.

Thus, the role of an ASP can be to coordinate or facilitate the development of treatment guidelines by engaging a multidisciplinary group with an interest in the particular disease state (e.g., HAP/VAP/HCAP, sepsis, CDI). Because often times guidelines are not adhered to (96,110,112), the ASP may not only ensure that guidelines are created so that patients with HAP/VAP/HCAP or sepsis with risk factors for MDR pathogens receive combination antimicrobial therapy, but to identify these patients in the hospital prospectively and make sure that they are treated in accordance with guidelines (provide human decision support to prescribers serving as reminders) (21,32,99,114,115,121).

PROCESS AND OUTCOME MEASUREMENTS

The IDSA/SHEA guidelines for developing an institutional program to enhance antimicrobial stewardship recommend that outcomes be measured (54). This is the reason for having a data system and an information specialist to be able to assist the ASP members in quantifying their impact. Without this support, the ASP team members can spend more time justifying their positions and measuring outcomes than on the actual day-to-day functioning of the program and evaluating antimicrobial therapy, which is their primary purpose. Antimicrobial consumption can be measured for targeted (or all) antimicrobials. Using antimicrobial expenditure data has significant limitations, but is helpful to evaluate where the dollars are being spent. One measure of antimicrobial consumption has historically involved the use of DDD data, and standardized definitions are available at: http://www. whocc.no/atcddd. Converting grams of antibiotic used to DDD per 1000 patient days allows for a useful internal and external benchmark of antimicrobial consumption (see benchmarking Chapter 2). Other measures include antimicrobial days of therapy (122). Polk and colleagues demonstrated that days of therapy correlated best with antimicrobial use when compared with DDD data, primarily because it is not influenced by renal function and dosage adjustments (122). Currently, antimicrobial days are the most accurate means for measuring antimicrobial use. Regardless of mechanism chosen, establishing a baseline of antimicrobial use prior to program implementation allows one to track the progress of interventions on use over time. These measures can also be used to quantify the impact of interventions, including parenteral-to-oral conversions.

CONCLUSIONS

> ... On the whole, the position of antimicrobial agents in medical therapy is highly satisfactory. The majority of bacterial infections can be cured simply, effectively, and cheaply. The mortality and morbidity from bacterial diseases has fallen so low that they are no longer among the important unsolved problems of medicine. These accomplishments are widely known and appreciated.... (16)

This excerpt from a manuscript published in 1956 by Dr. Ernest Jawetz is ominous some 70 years into the "antibiotic era." A suitable conclusion for a similar paper today might read: *an increasing number of infections are no longer easily treated, morbidity and mortality are appreciable, and many ID have become unsolved problems of modern medicine.*

The problem of increasing antimicrobial resistance, due, in part, to suboptimal antimicrobial use, coupled with the fact that a growing number of pharmaceutical companies have abandoned anti-infective research and development, has resulted in a growing public health crisis. Because of the intensity of antimicrobial use in both institutional and community settings, they are target-rich environments for proactive interventions to improve antimicrobial stewardship. A variety of studies have concluded that programmatic means to steward the use of antimicrobials optimizes patient safety, addresses some of the contributing factors to escalating antimicrobial resistance such as reducing unnecessary antimicrobial use, and, as a side effect, minimizes direct and indirect costs to the healthcare system. The IDSA/SHEA guidelines for developing an institutional program to enhance antimicrobial stewardship serve as a starting place for institutions considering developing an ASP. This chapter complements the guidelines, hopefully giving the reader a practical viewpoint from the vantage point of someone who has developed, managed, and justified ASPs for more than 12 years. I often think of the words from Dr. Calvin Kunin, who once stated "... there are simply too many physicians prescribing antibiotics casually ... The issues need to be presented forcefully to the medical community and the public. Third-party payers must get the message that these programs (*referring to antimicrobial stewardship*) can save lives as well as money" (123). Regulatory agencies have selected measures to gauge the performance of healthcare facilities for specific infections. It is not too improbable to think that the same regulatory bodies will be considering in the near future whether or not an institution has an institutional program designed to oversee the appropriate use of these scarce resources as a core quality measure.

REFERENCES

1. Projan SJ. Why is big Pharma getting out of antibacterial drug discovery? Curr Opin Microbiol 2003; 6(5):427–30.
2. Levy SB. The 2000 Garrod lecture. Factors impacting on the problem of antibiotic resistance. J Antimicrob Chemother 2002; 49(1):25–30.
3. Gerding DN. The search for good antimicrobial stewardship. Jt Comm J Qual Improv 2001; 27(8):403–4.

4. Owens RC Jr. Risk assessment for antimicrobial agent-induced QTc interval prolongation and torsades de pointes. Pharmacotherapy 2001; 21(3):301–19.
5. Owens RC Jr. QT prolongation with antimicrobial agents: understanding the significance. Drugs 2004; 64(10):1091–124.
6. Owens RC Jr, Ambrose PG. Antimicrobial safety: focus on fluoroquinolones. Clin Infect Dis 2005; 41 (Suppl. 2):S144–57.
7. Owens RC Jr, Nolin TD. Antimicrobial-associated QT interval prolongation: pointes of interest. Clin Infect Dis 2006; 43(12):1603–11.
8. Owens RC. *Clostridium difficile*-associated disease: an emerging threat to patient safety. Insights from the Society of Infectious Diseases Pharmacists. Pharmacotherapy 2006; 26(3):299–311.
9. Owens RC. *Clostridium difficile*-associated disease: changing epidemiology and implications for management. Drugs 2007; 67(4):487–502.
10. Sarkar P, Gould IM. Antimicrobial agents are societal drugs: how should this influence prescribing? Drugs 2006; 66(7):893–901.
11. Fishman N. Antimicrobial stewardship. Am J Med 2006; 119(6 Suppl. 1):S53–61.
12. Gross R, Morgan AS, Kinky DE, Weiner M, Gibson GA, Fishman NO. Impact of a hospital-based antimicrobial management program on clinical and economic outcomes. Clin Infect Dis 2001; 33(3):289–95.
13. John JF Jr, Fishman NO. Programmatic role of the infectious diseases physician in controlling antimicrobial costs in the hospital. Clin Infect Dis 1997; 24(3):471–85.
14. Kollef MH. Inadequate antimicrobial treatment: an important determinant of outcome for hospitalized patients. Clin Infect Dis 2000; 31(Suppl. 4):S131–8.
15. Srinivasan A, Song X, Richards A, Sinkowitz-Cochran R, Cardo D, Rand C. A survey of knowledge, attitudes, and beliefs of house staff physicians from various specialties concerning antimicrobial use and resistance. Arch Intern Med 2004; 164(13):1451–6.
16. Jawetz E. Antimicrobial chemotherapy. Annu Rev Microbiol 1956; 10:85–114.
17. McGowan JE Jr, Finland M. Usage of antibiotics in a general hospital: effect of requiring justification. J Infect Dis 1974; 130(2):165–8.
18. Briceland LL, Nightingale CH, Quintiliani R, Cooper BW, Smith KS. Antibiotic streamlining from combination therapy to monotherapy utilizing an interdisciplinary approach. Arch Intern Med 1988; 148(9):2019–22.
19. Fraser GL, Stogsdill P, Dickens JD Jr, Wennberg DE, Smith RP Jr, Prato BS. Antibiotic optimization. An evaluation of patient safety and economic outcomes. Arch Intern Med 1997; 157(15):1689–94.
20. Fraser GL, Stogsdill P, Owens RC Jr. Antimicrobial stewardship initiatives: a programmatic approach to optimizing antimicrobial use. In: Owens RC Jr, Ambrose PG, Nightingale CH, eds. Antibiotic Optimization: Concepts and Strategies in Clinical Practice. 1st ed. New York: Marcel Dekker, 2005:261–326.
21. Owens RC Jr, Fraser GL, Stogsdill P. Antimicrobial stewardship programs as a means to optimize antimicrobial use. Insights from the Society of Infectious Diseases Pharmacists. Pharmacotherapy 2004; 24(7):896–908.
22. LaRocco A Jr. Concurrent antibiotic review programs—a role for infectious diseases specialists at small community hospitals. Clin Infect Dis 2003; 37(5):742–3.
23. Katz KC, McGeer AJ, Duncan CL, et al. Emergence of macrolide resistance in throat culture isolates of group a streptococci in Ontario, Canada, in 2001 1. Antimicrob Agents Chemother 2003; 47(7):2370–2.
24. Vanderkooi OG, Low DE, Green K, Powis JE, McGeer A. Predicting antimicrobial resistance in invasive pneumococcal infections. Clin Infect Dis 2005; 40(9):1288–97.
25. Anderson KB, Tan JS, File TM Jr, DiPersio JR, Willey BM, Low DE. Emergence of levofloxacin-resistant pneumococci in immunocompromised adults after therapy for community-acquired pneumonia. Clin Infect Dis 2003; 37(3):376–81.
26. Ambrose PG, Bast D, Doern GV, et al. Fluoroquinolone-resistant *Streptococcus pneumoniae*, an emerging but unrecognized public health concern: is it time to resight the goalposts? Clin Infect Dis 2004; 39(10):1554–6.
27. Fuller JD, Low DE. A review of *Streptococcus pneumoniae* infection treatment failures associated with fluoroquinolone resistance. Clin Infect Dis 2005; 41(1):118–21.

28. Marshall DA, McGeer A, Gough J, et al. Impact of antibiotic administrative restrictions on trends in antibiotic resistance. Can J Public Health 2006; 97(2):126–31.
29. Guidelines for the management of adults with hospital-acquired, ventilator-associated, and healthcare-associated pneumonia. Am J Respir Crit Care Med 2005; 171(4): 388–416.
30. Anon JB, Jacobs MR, Poole MD, et al. Antimicrobial treatment guidelines for acute bacterial rhinosinusitis. Otolaryngol Head Neck Surg 2004; 130(Suppl. 1):1–45.
31. Mandell LA, Wunderink RG, Anzueto A, et al. Infectious Diseases Society of America/American Thoracic Society consensus guidelines on the management of community-acquired pneumonia in adults. Clin Infect Dis 2007; 44 7(Suppl. 2):S27–S72.
32. Owens RC Jr, Rice L. Hospital-based strategies for combating resistance. Clin Infect Dis 2006; 42 (Suppl. 4):S173–81.
33. Fowler VG Jr, Boucher HW, Corey GR, et al. Daptomycin versus standard therapy for bacteremia and endocarditis caused by *Staphylococcus aureus*. N Engl J Med 2006; 355(7):653–65.
34. Draghi DC, Sheehan DJ, Hogan P, Sahm DF. In vitro activity of linezolid against key Gram-positive organisms isolated in the United States: results of the LEADER 2004 surveillance program. Antimicrob Agents Chemother 2005; 49(12):5024–32.
35. Jones RN, Ross JE, Fritsche TR, Sader HS. Oxazolidinone susceptibility patterns in 2004: report from the Zyvox Annual Appraisal of Potency and Spectrum (ZAAPS) Program assessing isolates from 16 nations. J Antimicrob Chemother 2006; 57(2): 279–87.
36. MacDougall C, Polk RE. Antimicrobial stewardship programs in health care systems. Clin Microbiol Rev 2005; 18(4):638–56.
37. Bell DM. Promoting appropriate antimicrobial drug use: perspective from the Centers for Disease Control and Prevention. Clin Infect Dis 2001; 33 (Suppl. 3):S245–50.
38. Levy SB, FitzGerald GB, Macone AB. Changes in intestinal flora of farm personnel after introduction of a tetracycline-supplemented feed on a farm. N Engl J Med 1976; 295(11):583–8.
39. Dinubile MJ, Friedland I, Chan CY, et al. Bowel colonization with resistant Gram-negative bacilli after antimicrobial therapy of intra-abdominal infections: observations from two randomized comparative clinical trials of ertapenem therapy. Eur J Clin Microbiol Infect Dis 2005; 24(7):443–9.
40. Dinubile MJ, Friedland I, Chan CY, et al. Bowel colonization with resistant Gram-negative bacilli after antimicrobial therapy of intra-abdominal infections: observations from two randomized comparative clinical trials of ertapenem therapy. Eur J Clin Microbiol Infect Dis 2005; 24(7):443–9.
41. Carling P, Fung T, Killion A, Terrin N, Barza M. Favorable impact of a multi-disciplinary antibiotic management program conducted during 7 years. Infect Control Hosp Epidemiol 2003; 24(9):699–706.
42. Pepin J, Valiquette L, Alary ME, et al. *Clostridium difficile*-associated diarrhea in a region of Quebec from 1991 to 2003: a changing pattern of disease severity. CMAJ 2004; 171(5):466–72.
43. Pepin J, Routhier S, Gagnon S, Brazeau I. Management and outcomes of a first recurrence of *Clostridium difficile*-associated disease in Quebec, Canada. Clin Infect Dis 2006; 42(6):758–64.
44. McDonald LC, Killgore GE, Thompson A, et al. An epidemic, toxin gene-variant strain of *Clostridium difficile*. N Engl J Med 2005; 353(23):2433–41.
45. Marra AR, Edmond MB, Wenzel RP, Bearman GM. Hospital-acquired *Clostridium difficile*-associated disease in the intensive care unit setting: epidemiology, clinical course and outcome 1. BMC Infect Dis 2007; 7:42.
46. Davey P, Brown E, Fenelon L, et al. Interventions to improve antibiotic prescribing practices for hospital inpatients. Cochrane Database Syst Rev 2005; (4):CD003543.
47. Gerding DN, Johnson S, Peterson LR, Mulligan ME, Silva J Jr. *Clostridium difficile*-associated diarrhea and colitis. Infect Control Hosp Epidemiol 1995; 16(8):459–77.
48. Wilcox MH, Fawley WN. Hospital disinfectants and spore formation by *Clostridium difficile*. Lancet 2000; 356(9238):1324.

49. Wilcox MH, Fawley WN, Wigglesworth N, Parnell P, Verity P, Freeman J. Detergent versus hypochlorite cleaning and *Clostridium difficile* infection. J Hosp Infect 2004; 56(4):331.
50. Hoffman JM, Shah ND, Vermeulen LC, et al. Projecting future drug expenditures— 2007. Am J Health Syst Pharm 2007; 64(3):298–314.
51. Glowacki RC, Schwartz DN, Itokazu GS, Wisniewski MF, Kieszkowski P, Weinstein RA. Antibiotic combinations with redundant antimicrobial spectra: clinical epidemiology and pilot intervention of computer-assisted surveillance. Clin Infect Dis 2003; 37(1): 59–64.
52. Cosgrove SE, Kaye KS, Eliopoulous GM, Carmeli Y. Health and economic outcomes of the emergence of third-generation cephalosporin resistance in *Enterobacter* species. Arch Intern Med 2002; 162(2):185–90.
53. Cosgrove SE. The relationship between antimicrobial resistance and patient outcomes: mortality, length of hospital stay, and health care costs. Clin Infect Dis 2006; 42(Suppl. 2):S82–9.
54. Dellit TH, Owens RC, McGowan JE Jr, et al. Infectious Diseases Society of America and the Society for Healthcare Epidemiology of America guidelines for developing an institutional program to enhance antimicrobial stewardship. Clin Infect Dis 2007; 44(2):159–77.
55. You JH, Lo LP, Chung IY, Marasinghe T, Lee N, Ip M. Effect of an antimicrobial stewardship programme on the use of carbapenems in a Hong Kong teaching hospital: a pilot study. J Hosp Infect 2007; 65(4):378–9.
56. von GV, Troillet N, Beney J, et al. Impact of an interdisciplinary strategy on antibiotic use: a prospective controlled study in three hospitals. J Antimicrob Chemother 2005; 55(3):362–6.
57. Zahar JR, Rioux C, Girou E, et al. Inappropriate prescribing of aminoglycosides: risk factors and impact of an antibiotic control team. J Antimicrob Chemother 2006; 58(3):651–6.
58. Wickens HJ, Jacklin A. Impact of the Hospital Pharmacy Initiative for promoting prudent use of antibiotics in hospitals in England. J Antimicrob Chemother 2006; 58(6):1230–7.
59. Struelens MJ. Multidisciplinary antimicrobial management teams: the way forward to control antimicrobial resistance in hospitals. Curr Opin Infect Dis 2003; 16(4):305–7.
60. Weller TM, Jamieson CE. The expanding role of the antibiotic pharmacist. J Antimicrob Chemother 2004; 54(2):295–8.
61. John JF Jr, Fishman NO. Programmatic role of the infectious diseases physician in controlling antimicrobial costs in the hospital. Clin Infect Dis 1997; 24(3):471–85.
62. Paterson DL. The role of antimicrobial management programs in optimizing antibiotic prescribing within hospitals. Clin Infect Dis 2006; 42(Suppl. 2):S90–5.
63. White AC Jr, Atmar RL, Wilson J, Cate TR, Stager CE, Greenberg SB. Effects of requiring prior authorization for selected antimicrobials: expenditures, susceptibilities, and clinical outcomes. Clin Infect Dis 1997; 25(2):230–9.
64. Calfee DP, Brooks J, Zirk NM, Giannetta ET, Scheld WM, Farr BM. A pseudo-outbreak of nosocomial infections associated with the introduction of an antibiotic management programme. J Hosp Infect 2003; 55(1):26–32.
65. Linkin DR, Paris S, Fishman NO, Metlay JP, Lautenbach E. Inaccurate communications in telephone calls to an antimicrobial stewardship program. Infect Control Hosp Epidemiol 2006; 27(7):688–94.
66. Carling PC, Fung T, Coldiron JS. Parenteral antibiotic use in acute-care hospitals: a standardized analysis of fourteen institutions. Clin Infect Dis 1999; 29(5):1189–96.
67. Ansari F, Gray K, Nathwani D, et al. Outcomes of an intervention to improve hospital antibiotic prescribing: interrupted time series with segmented regression analysis. J Antimicrob Chemother 2003; 52(5):842–8.
68. Ruttimann S, Keck B, Hartmeier C, Maetzel A, Bucher HC. Long-term antibiotic cost savings from a comprehensive intervention program in a medical department of a university-affiliated teaching hospital. Clin Infect Dis 2004; 38(3):348–56.

69. Lutters M, Harbarth S, Janssens JP, et al. Effect of a comprehensive, multidisciplinary, educational program on the use of antibiotics in a geriatric university hospital. J Am Geriatr Soc 2004; 52(1):112–6.

70. Bantar C, Sartori B, Vesco E, et al. A hospitalwide intervention program to optimize the quality of antibiotic use: impact on prescribing practice, antibiotic consumption, cost savings, and bacterial resistance. Clin Infect Dis 2003; 37(2):180–6.

71. Harris AD, Smith D, Johnson JA, Bradham DD, Roghmann MC. Risk factors for imipenem-resistant *Pseudomonas aeruginosa* among hospitalized patients. Clin Infect Dis 2002; 34(3):340–5.

72. Georges B, Conil JM, Dubouix A, et al. Risk of emergence of *Pseudomonas aeruginosa* resistance to beta-lactam antibiotics in intensive care units. Crit Care Med 2006; 34(6):1636–41.

73. Lesar TS, Briceland LL. Survey of antibiotic control policies in university-affiliated teaching institutions. Ann Pharmacother 1996; 30(1):31–4.

74. Scott RD, Solomon SL, Cordell R, Roberts RR, Howard D, McGowan JE Jr. Measuring the attributable costs of resistant infections in hospital settings. In: Owens RC Jr, Ambrose PG, Nightingale CH, eds. Antibiotic Optimization: Concepts and Strategies in Clinical Practice. 1st ed. New York: Marcel Dekker, 2005:141–79.

75. Parodi S, Rhew DC, Goetz MB. Early switch and early discharge opportunities in intravenous vancomycin treatment of suspected methicillin-resistant staphylococcal species infections. J Manag Care Pharm 2003; 9(4):317–26.

76. Itani KM, Weigelt J, Li JZ, Duttagupta S. Linezolid reduces length of stay and duration of intravenous treatment compared with vancomycin for complicated skin and soft tissue infections due to suspected or proven methicillin-resistant *Staphylococcus aureus* (MRSA). Int J Antimicrob Agents 2005; 26(6):442–8.

77. Li Z, Willke RJ, Pinto LA, et al. Comparison of length of hospital stay for patients with known or suspected methicillin-resistant *Staphylococcus* species infections treated with linezolid or vancomycin: a randomized, multicenter trial. Pharmacotherapy 2001; 21(3):263–74.

78. McKinnon PS, Sorensen SV, Liu LZ, Itani KM. Impact of linezolid on economic outcomes and determinants of cost in a clinical trial evaluating patients with MRSA complicated skin and soft-tissue infections. Ann Pharmacother 2006; 40(6):1017–23.

79. Owens RC Jr, Ambrose PG, Quintiliani R. Ceftazidime to cefepime formulary switch: pharmacodynamic and pharmacoeconomic rationale. Conn Med 1997; 61(4):225–7.

80. Lautenbach E, LaRosa LA, Marr AM, Nachamkin I, Bilker WB, Fishman NO. Changes in the prevalence of vancomycin-resistant enterococci in response to antimicrobial formulary interventions: impact of progressive restrictions on use of vancomycin and third-generation cephalosporins. Clin Infect Dis 2003; 36(4):440–6.

81. Lipworth AD, Hyle EP, Fishman NO, et al. Limiting the emergence of extended-spectrum beta-lactamase-producing enterobacteriaceae: influence of patient population characteristics on the response to antimicrobial formulary interventions. Infect Control Hosp Epidemiol 2006; 27(3):279–86.

82. Owens RC Jr, Ambrose PG, Jones RN. The antimicrobial formulary: reevaluating parenteral Cephalosporins in the context of emerging resistance. In: Owens RC Jr, Ambrose PG, Nightingale CH, eds. Antibiotic Optimization: Concepts and Strategies in Clinical Practice. 1st ed. New York: Marcel Dekker, 2005:383–430.

83. Valenti AJ. The role of infection control and hospital epidemiology in the optimization of antibiotic use. In: Owens RC Jr, Ambrose PG, Nightingale CH, eds. Antibiotic Optimization: Concepts and Strategies in Clinical Practice. 1st ed. New York: Marcel Dekker, 2005:209–59.

84. Nolin TD, Lambert DA, Owens RC Jr. Stability of cefepime and metronidazole prepared for simplified administration as a single product. Diagn Microbiol Infect Dis 2006; 56(2):179–84.

85. Harbarth S, Nobre V, Pittet D. Does antibiotic selection impact patient outcome?. Clin Infect Dis 2007; 44(1):87–93.

86. Moellering RC Jr, Wennersten C, Weinberg AN. Synergy of penicillin and gentamicin against *Enterococci*. J Infect Dis 1971; 124(Suppl):S207–9.

87. Zhou J, Chen Y, Tabibi S, Alba L, Garber E, Saiman L. Antimicrobial susceptibility and synergy studies of *Burkholderia cepacia* complex isolated from patients with cystic fibrosis 2. Antimicrob Agents Chemother 2007; 51(3):1085–8.

88. Yoon J, Urban C, Terzian C, Mariano N, Rahal JJ. In vitro double and triple synergistic activities of Polymyxin B, imipenem, and rifampin against multidrug-resistant *Acinetobacter baumannii*. Antimicrob Agents Chemother 2004; 48(3):753–7.

89. Tam VH, Louie A, Deziel MR, Liu W, Drusano GL. The relationship between quinolone exposures and resistance amplification is characterized by an inverted U: a new paradigm for optimizing pharmacodynamics to counterselect resistance. Antimicrob Agents Chemother 2007; 51(2):744–7.

90. Tam VH, Louie A, Fritsche TR, et al. Impact of drug exposure intensity and duration of therapy on the emergence of *Staphylococcus aureus* resistance to a quinolone antimicrobial. J Infect Dis 2007; 195(12):1818–27.

91. Drusano GL, Louie A, Deziel M, Gumbo T. The crisis of resistance: identifying drug exposures to suppress amplification of resistant mutant subpopulations. Clin Infect Dis 2006; 42(4):525–32.

92. Zimmerli W, Trampuz A, Ochsner PE. Prosthetic-joint infections. N Engl J Med 2004; 351(16):1645–54.

93. Zimmerli W, Widmer AF, Blatter M, Frei R, Ochsner PE. Role of rifampin for treatment of orthopedic implant-related staphylococcal infections: a randomized controlled trial. Foreign-Body Infection (FBI) Study Group. JAMA 1998; 279(19):1537–41.

94. Hyle EP, Lipworth AD, Zaoutis TE, Nachamkin I, Bilker WB, Lautenbach E. Impact of inadequate initial antimicrobial therapy on mortality in infections due to extended-spectrum beta-lactamase-producing enterobacteriaceae: variability by site of infection. Arch Intern Med 2005; 165(12):1375–80.

95. Coleman RW, Rodondi LC, Kaubisch S, Granzella NB, O'Hanley PD. Cost-effectiveness of prospective and continuous parenteral antibiotic control: experience at the Palo Alto Veterans Affairs Medical Center from 1987 to 1989. Am J Med 1991; 90(4):439–44.

96. Mol PG, Rutten WJ, Gans RO, Degener JE, Haaijer-Ruskamp FM. Adherence barriers to antimicrobial treatment guidelines in teaching hospital, the Netherlands. Emerg Infect Dis 2004; 10(3):522–5.

97. Paul M, uri-Silbiger I, Soares-Weiser K, Leibovici L. Beta-lactam monotherapy versus beta-lactam-aminoglycoside combination therapy for sepsis in immunocompetent patients: systematic review and meta-analysis of randomised trials. BMJ 2004; 328(7441):668.

98. Niederman MS. De-escalation therapy in ventilator-associated pneumonia. Curr Opin Crit Care 2006; 12(5):452–7.

99. Micek ST, Ward S, Fraser VJ, Kollef MH. A randomized controlled trial of an antibiotic discontinuation policy for clinically suspected ventilator-associated pneumonia. Chest 2004; 125(5):1791–9.

100. Ambrose PG, Bhavnani SM, Rubino CM, et al. Pharmacokinetics-pharmacodynamics of antimicrobial therapy: it's not just for mice anymore. Clin Infect Dis 2007; 44(1):79–86.

101. Lodise TP, Lomaestro BM, Drusano GL. Application of antimicrobial pharmacodynamic concepts into clinical practice: focus on beta-lactam antibiotics. Insights from the Society of Infectious Diseases Pharmacists. Pharmacotherapy 2006; 26(9):1320–32.

102. Lodise TP Jr, Lomaestro B, Drusano GL. Piperacillin-tazobactam for *Pseudomonas aeruginosa* infection: clinical implications of an extended-infusion dosing strategy. Clin Infect Dis 2007; 44(3):357–63.

103. Melmon KL, Blaschke TF. The undereducated physician's therapeutic decisions. N Engl J Med 1983; 308(24):1473–4.

104. Evans RS, Pestotnik SL, Classen DC, Burke JP. Evaluation of a computer-assisted antibiotic-dose monitor. Ann Pharmacother 1999; 33(10):1026–31.

105. Pestotnik SL, Classen DC, Evans RS, Burke JP. Implementing antibiotic practice guidelines through computer-assisted decision support: clinical and financial outcomes. Ann Intern Med 1996; 124(10):884–90.

106. Evans RS, Pestotnik SL, Classen DC, et al. A computer-assisted management program for antibiotics and other antiinfective agents. N Engl J Med 1998; 338(4):232–8.
107. Pestotnik SL. Expert clinical decision support systems to enhance antimicrobial stewardship programs. Insights from the society of infectious diseases pharmacists. Pharmacotherapy 2005; 25(8):1116–25.
108. Burke JP, Mehta RR. Role of computer-assisted programs in optimizing the use of antimicrobial agents. In: Owens RC Jr, Ambrose PG, Nightingale CH, eds. Antibiotic Optimization: Concepts and Strategies in Clinical Practice. 1st ed. New York: Marcel Dekker, 2005:327–52.
109. Samore MH, Bateman K, Alder SC, et al. Clinical decision support and appropriateness of antimicrobial prescribing: a randomized trial. JAMA 2005; 294(18):2305–14.
110. Stamm WE. Evaluating guidelines. Clin Infect Dis 2007; 44(6):775–6.
111. Taur Y, Smith MA. Adherence to the Infectious Diseases Society of America guidelines in the treatment of uncomplicated urinary tract infection. Clin Infect Dis 2007; 44(6):769–74.
112. Mol PG, Denig P, Gans RO, et al. Limited effect of patient and disease characteristics on compliance with hospital antimicrobial guidelines. Eur J Clin Pharmacol 2006; 62(4):297–305.
113. Warren JW, Abrutyn E, Hebel JR, Johnson JR, Schaeffer AJ, Stamm WE. Guidelines for antimicrobial treatment of uncomplicated acute bacterial cystitis and acute pyelonephritis in women. Infectious Diseases Society of America (IDSA). Clin Infect Dis 1999; 29(4):745–58.
114. Mol PG, Wieringa JE, Nannanpanday PV, et al. Improving compliance with hospital antibiotic guidelines: a time-series intervention analysis. J Antimicrob Chemother 2005; 55(4):550–7.
115. Owens RC Jr, Loew B, Soni S, Suissa S. Impact of interventions on non-evidence based treatment strategies during an outbreak of *Clostridium difficile*-associated disease due to BI/NAP1. In: Program and Abstracts of the 44th Annual Infectious Diseases Society of America, Toronto, Ontario, CA. 2006:60. [Abstract 687].
116. Stelfox HT, Bates DW, Redelmeier DA. Safety of patients isolated for infection control. JAMA 2003; 290(14):1899–905.
117. Saez-Llorens X, McCoig C, Feris JM, et al. Quinolone treatment for pediatric bacterial meningitis: a comparative study of trovafloxacin and ceftriaxone with or without vancomycin. Pediatr Infect Dis J 2002; 21(1):14–22.
118. Sunenshine RH, Wright MO, Maragakis LL, et al. Multidrug-resistant *Acinetobacter* infection mortality rate and length of hospitalization. Emerg Infect Dis 2007; 13(1): 97–103.
119. Nathwani D. Impact of methicillin-resistant *Staphylococcus aureus* infections on key health economic outcomes: does reducing the length of hospital stay matter? J Antimicrob Chemother 2003; 51(Suppl. 2):ii37–44.
120. McCollum M, Rhew DC, Parodi S. Cost analysis of switching from i.v. vancomycin to p.o. linezolid for the management of methicillin-resistant *Staphylococcus* species. Clin Ther 2003; 25(12):3173–89.
121. Solomon DH, Van HL, Glynn RJ, et al. Academic detailing to improve use of broad-spectrum antibiotics at an academic medical center. Arch Intern Med 2001; 161(15):1897–902.
122. Polk RE, Fox C, Mahoney A, Letcavage J, MacDougall C. Measurement of adult antibacterial drug use in 130 US hospitals: comparison of defined daily dose and days of therapy. Clin Infect Dis 2007; 44(5):664–70.
123. Kunin CM. Antibiotic armageddon. Clin Infect Dis 1997; 25(2):240–1.

16 Computer-Assisted Programs to Optimize Antimicrobial Use

Stanley L. Pestotnik and Jonathan B. Olson
TheraDoc, Incorporated, Salt Lake City, Utah, U.S.A.

At the dawn of the 21st century, the U.S. healthcare system is experiencing an information revolution. Scientific and clinical knowledge has expanded beyond the capacity of the average practitioner's ability to synthesize and apply knowledge at the bedside or in the clinic. The question that dominated healthcare at the dawn of the 20th century was how much of clinical practice was based on scientific evidence? The dominating question today is how much of the available evidence is applied at the front lines of patient care? The U.S. National Library of Medicine archives between 1500 and 3500 citations each day Tuesday through Saturday (1). One of the major obstacles facing clinicians is that much of the evidence base (knowledge) is unfiltered and in that state is often unreliable or irrelevant to daily practice (2). If evidence were properly filtered and combined with patient data at the time of clinical decision making, 30% to 60% of decisions would be different, resulting in improved care and reduced patient harm (2–6). Further complicating the situation is the observation that the unaided human mind can only process between four and seven simultaneous data constructs before sensory overload occurs (3,6).

Given this human limitation, the explosion of medical knowledge, and the complexities of illness, it is no wonder that the current state of affairs is wide variation in clinical practice, clinical error, and poor guideline compliance. It is simply unrealistic to believe that modern healthcare can continue to be delivered without the assistance of computers. The notion that a computer could serve as a consultant to help clinicians manage patients was put forth over three decades ago (7). Research in the field of clinical informatics (an application subfield of biomedical informatics) has led to the development of healthcare information technology (HIT) that enhances decision making by improving patient data management, knowledge integration, and real-time access by clinical care providers (8,9). This technology is known as clinical decision support systems (CDSS). Over the last two decades, the original intent of the investigator-pioneers in CDSS research and the fundamental definitions of CDSS have been diluted by "marketing messages" and other influences. A case in point is the observation that publishers now refer to their electronic referential textbooks and other materials as CDSS. This review of the technology and its application in infectious diseases adheres to the originally intended clinical informatics definitions and design requirements.

CDSS

Shortliffe (10), in a seminal paper in the field of clinical informatics, summarized the foundations, goals, and challenges of CDSS. In the broadest sense, these applications are tools that focus attention, manage information, and provide patient-specific consultation. A CDSS is software that uses individual patient data, population statistics, and computerized clinical knowledge to offer real-time, patient-specific information management, assessment, and recommendations. Six major levels of CDSS have been defined: (*i*) alerting, (*ii*) interpretating, (*iii*) assisting, (*iv*) critiquing, (*v*) diagnosing, and (*vi*) managing decision support (11). Complexity of the software and knowledge bases, as well as the data elements required, increases as the functionality moves from alerting to managing decision support.

Properly designed CDSS intelligently filter clinical knowledge and patient-related information, presenting alerts, interpretations, critiques, and recommendations at the appropriate time. CDSS operate on a continuum that includes access to intelligently filtered information, prompting when appropriate, offering guided choices to enhance care, and providing feedback of outcomes analysis. CDSS can either operate in an active or passive mode.

Active and Passive Modes

Active CDSS silently process data and information, automatically communicating with clinicians when current data indicates the need for intervention. Active CDSS provide guidance and decision support as a byproduct of monitoring or data-management activities. This mode of CDSS offers the greatest appeal to busy clinicians since little or no data entry is required of the clinician. Such capability requires that CDSS have embedded clinical knowledge and that the technology seamlessly interfaces or integrates with a comprehensive patient database [electronic medical record (EMR)] or all relevant ancillary clinical databases.

The power of active "knowledge-embedded" CDSS is that they operate in real-time and knowledge is brought to bear immediately without clinicians having to seek it. All six generic uses of CDSS can be accommodated in an active system. Active CDSS require careful design, and particular attention to detail is necessary so that the systems are not intrusive and noisy (e.g., generating false-positive alerts). Outputs should be actionable, pithy or concise, patient-specific, disease- or task-specific, and available at the time of care.

Passive CDSS require more clinician effort compared with active systems. First, clinicians need to recognize when consultation would be useful, and second, they must make a specific request of the system before receiving advice. Passive CDSS usually operate under three generic styles of use: critiquing, assisting, or diagnosing decision support. Most of the clinical use of passive CDSS occurs when clinicians want to use the technology as a sounding board for their own ideas or to rule out or limit competing alternatives. Poorly designed passive CDSS require significant data inputs by the user before generating advice; clinician acceptance is often suboptimal. Thus, like successful active CDSS, clinically accepted passive CDSS must interface or integrate with an EMR system or all applicable ancillary databases.

Design Features

Technology adoption follows a predictable course and the study of diffusion of innovation has a long history (12). Healthcare, as an industry, adopts technology in the same predictable fashion as other industries (13). Clinical decision support technology is no different in its path of adoption and diffusion throughout clinical practice. Clinical informatics research has identified eight design features that lead to successful adoption of CDSS in hospitals (Table 1) (14). First and foremost, the software must make clinicians' jobs easier; clinicians are always looking for easier

TABLE 1 Clinical Decision Support System Design Features

1. Makes the job easier
2. Educates
3. Patient-specific consultation with intelligent filtering of knowledge and data
4. Available in real-time, at the point-of-care
5. Allows on-line feedback and documentation
6. Allows for clinician choice and clinical judgment
7. Supports all six generic uses of CDSS
8. Adheres to standards for messaging and terminology

Source: Adapted from Ref. 14.

ways to perform daily tasks and will adopt technology that meets this objective. To accomplish this goal, CDSS must fit into clinical workflow and utilize intuitive, configurable user interfaces. Maximum time-saving benefits are realized when active clinical decision support is deployed. Second, an educational component within CDSS fosters user acceptance. Providing literature references as well as important caveats within the application increases adoption and acceptance of CDSS as convenient, credible, and trusted knowledge sources. Patient-specific consultation with intelligent filtering of knowledge and patient data is the third success criterion. A convenient scorecard for evaluating this criterion is the extent to which a CDSS addresses the five Ws (Table 2). Clinical decision support software that focuses attention and adds patient context to content (evidence-based) allows the clinician to focus on *who* they need to see, *what* data/information they need to look at, provides guidance as to *what* to do, supports the intervention with *why* it is necessary (literature), and finally allows for *what* should be documented to complete the intervention. Real-time operation at the point of care, at the moment and time of decision-making, is the fourth design criterion. On-line feedback and documentation within the application (fifth criterion) is equally important for both the user and the designer; this option allows for prompt identification and resolution of critical issues whether they are logical oversights in the knowledge base or software bugs. Presenting evidence-based clinical choices is the sixth design criterion that facilitates clinical adoption. Removing high-end knowledge workers such as physicians and pharmacists from the decision-making process is a mistake. They will resent or reject the system if it challenges their role or clinical autonomy. CDSS outputs should be recommendations rather than mandates. Recommendations should be pithy and supported with appropriately filtered referential material and patient data. Likewise, when an anticipated choice is contraindicated, presenting it in proper context, explicitly indicating that it is contraindicated secondary to patient-specific issues, fosters trust

TABLE 2 Five W Evaluation Targets for Clinical Decision Support Systems

Does the system identify:

1. Who (patient) the clinician needs to see?
2. What data elements to evaluate?
3. What course of action (recommendations) to take?
4. Why that action should be taken (evidence/literature)?
5. What should be documented?

and acceptance of the technology. Choice further enhances user acceptance because it recognizes the role of tacit knowledge in any decision-making process and guards against criticisms of cookbook medicine and loss of clinical judgment [(15), pp. 68–74]. Successfully implemented CDSS must provide for all six aforementioned generic uses (seventh criterion). CDSS that provide alerting, interpreting, assisting, critiquing, diagnosing, and managing decision support demonstrate maximum flexibility and have the broadest user appeal. Mandatory adherence to standards for messaging and clinical terminology (vocabulary) is the eighth criterion. Standards are the backbone of technology, assuring consistency between and interoperability of disparate information systems; standards are fundamental for accuracy and usability (16,17).

Messaging, Technical Standards, and Technical Architecture

Standards provide for two main levels of interoperability: functional and semantic. Functional or syntactic interoperability is accomplished through messaging standards, which provide a framework to allow two or more computer systems to exchange information so that it can be made human readable. Semantic interoperability relies on terminology standards and addresses the relationship between data and what that data means, similar to a dictionary. When information shared by different computer systems is understood at the level of formally defined domain concepts, semantic interoperability occurs between two or more computer systems. Within healthcare, the major communication standard for functional interoperability is the Health Level 7 (HL7) Messaging Standard (18). This data-interchange standard is built on protocols established in March 1987 and defines the message format of healthcare computing interfaces. Version 1.0 was published in September 1987 and on February 8, 1996 was approved by ANSI (American National Standards Institute) as the first healthcare data-interchange American National Standard. The current ANSI-approved version of the HL7 Messaging Standard is 2.5, with Version 3 under development (19).

A variety of clinical terminology standards exist in healthcare, giving meaning to raw data and allowing for semantic interoperability. Systematized Nomenclature of Medicine (SNOMED) (20) clinical terms are one example of a clinical reference terminology that provides for semantic interoperability. SNOMED is the most comprehensive international and multilingual clinical reference terminology available in the world. SNOMED serves as a taxonomy for a specific set of concepts (e.g., organisms, allergies, device procedures, symptoms, and so on) with unique meaning; the current core terminology contains over 357,000 healthcare concepts. Other examples of terminology standards include LOINC (Logical Observation Identifiers Names and Codes) (21) and RxNorm (22). Table 3 is a summary of key standards and the organizations responsible for developing and maintaining them (23). Without strict adherence to standards it is unlikely that CDSS will function properly and satisfy the first design feature, let alone the other six.

The minimum required technical architecture for these systems includes a communication engine to access disparate data for functional interoperability, a vocabulary engine to accomplish semantic interoperability, a decision support-optimized patient database, a modular knowledge base, and inference engines that interpret and filter patient data and knowledge (Fig. 1). Clinicians access and receive alerts, reminders, and guidance from CDSS through a variety of mechanisms such as email, secure paging, handheld personal data assistants, and web browsers.

TABLE 3 Summary of Key Standards and Developer Organizations

Standard	Acronym	Description	Developer
Data exchange/messaging			
Health Level Seven Messaging Standards Version 2 and 3	HL7 V2.x and V3	Electronic message formats for clinical, financial, and administrative data; V2 is common in commercially available software; V3 was launched in January 2005	Health Level Seven, www.hl7.org
Digital Imaging and Communications in Medicine Committee	DICOM	Format for communicating radiology images and data	National Electronics Manufacturers Association, www.nema.org
Clinical Data Interchange Standards Consortium	CDISC	Format for reporting data collected in clinical trials	Clinical Data Interchange Standards Consortium, www.cdisc.org
National Council for Prescription Drug Programs	NCPDP	Structure for transmitting prescription requests and fulfillment	The National Council for Prescription Drug Programs, www.ncpdp.org
Accredited Standards Committee X12	ASC X12	Electronic messages for claims, eligibility, and payments	American National Standards Institute, Accredited Standards Committee, www.x12.org/x12org/index.cfm
Institute of Electrical and Electronics Engineers Standard 1073	IEEE 1073	Messages for medical device communications	Institute of Electrical and Electronics Engineers Standards Association, standards.ieee.org/sa/sa-view.html
Terminology			
International Classification of Diseases-9 and 10	ICD-9, ICD-10	Diagnosis and disease codes commonly used in billing and claims; version 9 is often used in the U.S. for billing and reimbursement.	World Health Organization, www.who.int/en
Current Procedural Terminology	CPT	Procedure codes commonly used in billing and claims	American Medical Association, www.amaassn.org/ama/pub/category/3113.html
Logical Observation Identifiers Names and Codes	LOINC	Concept-based terminology for lab orders and results	Regenstrief Institute for HealthCare, www.loinc.org
Systematized Nomenclature of Medicine	SNOMED	Mapping of clinical concepts with standard descriptive terms	College of American Pathologists, www.cap.org
Unified Medical Language System®	UMLS®	Database of over 100 medical terminologies with concept mapping tools	National Library of Medicine, www.nlm.gov
RxNorm	RxNorm	Provides standard names for clinical drugs and for dose forms as administered to a patient	National Library of Medicine, www.nlm.gov

Source: Adapted from Ref. 23.

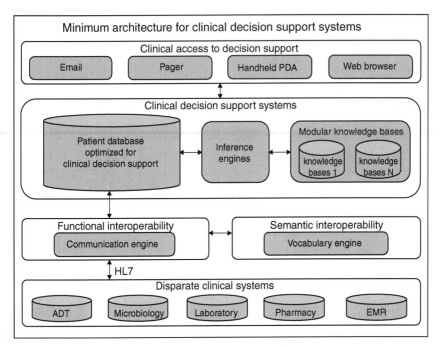

FIGURE 1 Minimum architecture for clinical decision support systems. *Abbreviations*: ADT, admission, discharge, transfer; EMR, electronic medical records; HL7, Health Level 7, Messaging Standard; PDA, personal digital assistant.

Historical Barriers to System Adoption

The historical barriers for widespread adoption of CDSS are well known (Table 4) (24–26). Seven primary historical barriers have been identified: (*i*) lack of a HIT infrastructure uniformly using HL7 as the communication standard for functional interoperability; (*ii*) slow adoption of clinical terminology standards for semantic interoperability; (*iii*) cost of implementation; (*iv*) HIT infrastructure that is optimized for transaction processing; (*v*) perceived increased liability risks; (*vi*) suboptimal models for embedding, sharing, and maintaining knowledge; and (*vii*) fundamental development/design knowledge has been the purview of a few academic groups. Significant reductions in implementation costs can be realized if

TABLE 4 Historical Barriers for Adoption of Clinical Decision Support Systems

i.	Lack of adoption of communication standards (HL7)
ii.	Lack of adoption of terminology standards
iii.	Cost of implementations
iv.	HIT infrastructure that is optimized for transaction processing
v.	Perceived increase liability risks
vi.	Suboptimal models for embedding, sharing and maintaining knowledge
vii.	Fundamental design knowledge an academic pursuit

Abbreviations: HIT, healthcare information technology; HL7, health level 7 messaging standard.

standards for functional and semantic interoperability are widely adopted. This is particularly true for electronic microbiology data, which tends to vary widely in quality and integrity from institution to institution. Most laboratory information systems do not require discrete microbiology data and as such this creates a significant cost issue when implementing CDSS in the domain of infectious diseases. The U.S. federal government is taking a large role in promulgating interoperability standards and has issued a call for most Americans to have electronic health records by the year 2014, and the Department of Health and Human Services (HHS) is responding by setting standards to make health records interoperable and certifying HIT vendors to ensure quality (27). HHS is encouraging healthcare institutions to adopt clinical vocabulary standards by agreeing with the College of American Pathologists (CAP) in 2003 to provide SNOMED to U.S. users at no cost through the National Library of Medicine's Unified Medical Language System (UMLS). The existing agreement lasts until 2008 (28). Despite government assistance, adoption of these vocabulary systems is slow due to the resource investments required by healthcare institutions and vendors alike. There are a few standard approaches to representing and sharing knowledge, but these are rarely being adopted in practice outside of academic endeavors. Arden syntax (29) is an HL7-supported standard for sharing knowledge that has technical limitations and limited adoption. Guideline Interchange Format (GLIF) (30–32) also aims to enable knowledge sharing, but focuses on the temporal aspects intrinsic to healthcare (33). Ancillary information systems (such as laboratory and pharmacy information systems) as well as EMR systems are optimized to process large volumes of transactions on a day-to-day basis, often called online transaction processing (OLTP). The business operations of individual departments and the institution at large are heavily reliant on the capability of these systems to process transactions. Technically and operationally, it is difficult for OLTP systems to deliver the six generic uses of CDSS. Successful CDSS are optimized to automatically analyze all relevant data (regardless of the source) and process knowledge rather than transactions.

Skeptics have traditionally resisted adopting CDSS because of the perception of increased risks of liability if the system is not accessed or the advice is not followed. With respect to the former there is a growing body of scientific evidence supporting the use of technology, particularly CDSS to improve patient safety and quality of care (34). Computerized provider order entry (CPOE) is becoming the touchstone of patient safety initiatives (35). The U.S. federal government has demonstrated a growing interest in fostering the development and diffusion of information technology to improve the delivery of healthcare (36). In aggregate these forces and the maturation of HIT are driving the standard of care. As HIT and CDSS become more pervasive, negligence may arise from a failure to use these technologies to prevent patient harm: the *Hooper* principle applied to HIT (37). The perception of increased liability risks when advice is not followed can be mitigated by documenting within the CDSS the reasons for dismissing the alert and/or advice, assuming that those reasons are clinically justifiable. Furthermore, most CDSS on the market are "open-looped" systems, which means that there is clinician intermediation before a recommendation is followed, for example, prescribing a drug.

Improved knowledge engineering techniques as well as modern software development tools and architectures have facilitated the development and maintenance of today's CDSS. Regardless of the individual barriers, the diffusion of innovations is a major challenge in all industries. Reassuringly, CDSS, like all technologies follow a predictable rate of spread called the technology adoption life cycle, based statistically on the number of standard deviations from the mean adoption time [(12), p. 262]. Sufficient evidence exists to support the use of CDSS as tools for focusing attention, managing information, and augmenting clinical decision making to improve patient outcomes (38–41). Furthermore, recent investigations have observed increased errors and adverse drug events with CPOE implementations that lack CDSS (42,43). This growing body of evidence is systematically dismantling the historical barriers to adoption and redefining the base level of care.

INFECTIOUS-DISEASE–SPECIFIC CLINICAL DECISION SUPPORT SYSTEMS

The management of infectious diseases crosses all specialty boundaries, involves a multitude of causative pathogens and hundreds of generic anti-infective compounds, and usually requires management by clinicians without special training in infectious diseases. Anti-infective agents are usually chosen in a setting of incomplete knowledge of the causative pathogen and a lack of appreciation for the unique pharmacokinetic and pharmacodynamic properties of the drugs. Antimicrobial drugs are a leading cause of adverse drug events and thus are a target of patient safety efforts in improving medication use (14,44,45).

Equally troubling is the observation that as much as 50% of antimicrobial drug use is inappropriate (46–48). Suboptimal use and misuse of antimicrobial drugs as well as other factors have resulted in an alarming rise in resistant healthcare-associated infections (HAIs) (49–52). According to the Centers for Disease Control and Prevention more than 70% of bacteria that cause HAIs are resistant to at least one of the drugs most commonly used to treat the infection (51). Inadequate or inappropriate treatment of HAIs, particularly in the intensive care setting, is an important determinant of death in the hospital (53,54). Patients isolated for certain infectious processes are twice as likely to experience a non-infectious adverse event, of which 73% are preventable, compared to cohorts who are not in isolation (55).

The financial burdens placed on the healthcare delivery system as a result of HAIs and antimicrobial misuse is of great concern. Prevention and management of HAIs is one of the largest cost drivers in U.S. hospitals, with annual economic costs of $6.7 billion in 2002 dollars (56). In addition to the extra costs attributed to the management of HAIs there are additional extra costs associated with adverse drug events that result from antimicrobials. Studies have demonstrated that the attributable excess cost of hospital-associated adverse drug events range from $2013 for actual events (57) to $4685 for preventable adverse drug events (58). Likewise, there are costs associated with treating antimicrobial-resistant nosocomial infections. Recent estimates place annual U.S. costs at $4 billion (59). Because of the potentially destabilizing economic consequences of antimicrobial resistance, both the CIA and the World Bank have declared antimicrobial resistance as a national security risk for the United States (59). In addition, systemic anti-infectives are the largest therapeutic drug class expenditure in non-federal U.S. hospitals (60).

Patient safety, economic and environmental burdens placed on the healthcare system by HAIs, and antimicrobial misuse have led many to outline strategies to improve antimicrobial use, stem the tide of antimicrobial resistance, and prevent infections (51,61–70). These strategies have included: formulary manipulations, antibiotic order forms, selective susceptibility reporting, academic counter detailing (education), restriction of pharmaceutical representatives, prior approval, concurrent review with feedback, antibiotic streamlining programs, and antibiotic cycling, to name the most popular. Most if not all of these strategies have demonstrated initial impacts; however, holding and sustaining the gains have been difficult, to say the least. The future of sustainable antimicrobial stewardship programs appears, like all of healthcare, to rely heavily on information technology. CDSS offer the greatest potential to improve clinical knowledge management and identify situations of antimicrobial misuse. CDSS have been shown to improve the empiric, therapeutic, and surgical prophylactic use of antimicrobials (14,71–93).

The hallmark of these systems is the capability to address patient-specific problems while accounting for institutional and individual variances. CDSS that target infectious diseases and antimicrobial drug use must adhere to the eight aforementioned design features as well as domain-specific specifications. The infectious diseases domain-specific components include: organism and drug name hierarchy lexicons, intrinsic and cross-resistance rules, automated antibiograms, antibiotic selection rules, mitigating factor rules, equivalent and alternative agent rules, contraindication rules, drug interaction rules, formulary matching rules, dosing rules, duration of use rules, explicit logic and caveat statements, literature references and structured feedback tailored at the syndrome, and disease and recommendation levels. Some of these components are technically trivial, whereas others require sophisticated architectures and design.

The mandatory adherence to organism and drug name hierarchy lexicons (clinical terminology standards) is critical for semantic interoperability. Sophisticated inference engines are required to automatically handle redundant antimicrobial spectra drug combinations and to automatically recognize resistance patterns based on microbial phenotypes. Early systems were designed to examine the susceptibility results of individual antibiotics; more advanced modern expert systems reason across susceptibility results, analyze the data, and infer resistance patterns by predicting the underlying mechanism(s) of resistance. The advantage of the latter approach is that anomalous combinations of phenotypes and organisms can be considered, which allows for more precise predictions of antimicrobial drug choice.

The target functional specifications for a comprehensive CDSS in infectious diseases should be the CDC's 12-step program to prevent antimicrobial resistance among hospital patients (Table 5) (51). CDSS that meet these functional specifications should generate vaccination reminders (Step 1) and catheter extended-use alerts (Step 2). The computer algorithms of CDSS should be able to automatically screen for and alert on inconsistencies between patients' antimicrobial drug therapies and their microbiology susceptibility test results, in addition to generating alerts that narrow the drug spectrum when appropriate (Step 3). To further meet the spirit of Step 3, these technologies should contain sophisticated inference engines that can analyze data to infer infectious processes, prompting for proper selection, dosage, and administration of drugs.

CDSS should recognize the limitations of their knowledge bases and the complexities of patient factors, recommending human expert consultation in these scenarios (Step 4). Parenteral-to-oral antimicrobial switch alerts, automated formulary checking, and evidence-based recommendations for prophylaxis and treatment of defined infections should be standard functions (Step 5).

Infectious disease-specific CDSS should also automatically produce institution-wide and location-specific antibiograms that conform to the latest performance standards of the Clinical and Laboratory Standards Institute (formerly NCCLS), currently the M39-A2 guidelines (94). The technology should use local antimicrobial resistance data derived from CDSS-generated antibiograms to guide empiric drug selection and track emerging resistance (Step 6). Well-designed inference engines (75,76) can discriminate between contaminated and colonized microbiology test results, suggesting interventions other than drugs when contamination or colonization occurs (Steps 7 and 8). Target drug alerts for vancomycin (Step 9) as well as alerts for duration of therapy or prophylaxis (Step 10) are well within the functional capabilities of CDSS. Finally, comprehensive CDSS in the domain of infectious diseases management should include components that alert and recommend for infection control activities (Steps 11 and 12).

The major technical limitation to accomplishing these target functional specifications is the availability of electronic data from an EMR or ancillary information systems. The minimum data for technical feasibility is admission, discharge, and transfer (ADT) data, pharmacy data, and laboratory data, including microbiology. The availability of electronic surgery and radiology data enhances the clinical utility of an infectious diseases-specific CDSS.

CLINICAL EXPERIENCE

Published clinical experience with CDSS in infectious diseases has primarily come from one group (14,48,72–79,81–83); however, other investigators (71,80,84–93) have reported on their use of this technology to enhance antimicrobial stewardship programs and HAIs surveillance. A wide variety of interventions are facilitated by applying the six generic uses of CDSS. Alerting decision support has demonstrated benefit in increasing influenza vaccination rates (85), improving the delivery time of preoperative antibiotics (72), as well as improving intraoperative dosing (87,88) and reducing the duration of postoperative antibiotic use (74). Alerts for parenteral to oral switching, discontinuation of therapy, and the need to change from broad-spectrum to specific therapy have enhanced the effectiveness of antimicrobial stewardship programs (80). Alerting decision support has been shown to improve the capacity of clinicians to monitor for renal function changes that dictate dosage adjustments and pharmacokinetic monitoring (77,80,83,90). CDSS have aided clinicians in monitoring microbiology data and managing inappropriate treatment approaches (73,84,90,93). Comprehensive CDSS that encompass all six levels of clinical decision support have demonstrated statistically significant improvements in the quality and safety of inpatient care, as well as reducing the cost to deliver care (14,81). Two recent investigations have demonstrated the utility of antimicrobial decision support systems in the rural, ambulatory setting (91,92). Samore et al. (91), in a randomized trial of a CDSS for antimicrobial prescribing for the treatment of acute respiratory tract infections, found statistically significant improvements in the appropriateness of antimicrobial selection in the CDSS-intervention arm as compared to controls.

CDSS are quickly becoming an essential element in the enlarging role of infectious diseases specialized clinicians, whether they are physicians or pharmacists. These tools and the documentation of the interventions that result from their use will enhance and support the role of clinicians in consultation and patient care.

TABLE 5 Functional Specifications of Infectious Diseases CDSS in relation to CDC[a] 12-Step Program

CDC 12-steps	CDSS functional requirement (CDC equivalent)
Prevent infections	
1. Vaccinate	Vaccinate reminders (Step 1)
2. Get the catheters out	Catheter extended-use alerts (Step 2)
Diagnose and treat infections effectively	
3. Target the pathogen	Drug-bug mismatch alerts (Step 3)
	Drug-spectrum alerts (Step 3)
	Infer infections (Step 3)
	Timing of therapy alerts (Step 3)
	Timing of prophylaxis alerts (Step 3)
	Drug dosage alerts (Step 3)
4. Access the experts	Recommend ID consultation when appropriate (Step 4)
Use antimicrobials wisely	
5. Practice antimicrobial control	Parenteral to oral switch alerts (Step 5)
	Automated formulary checking (Step 5)
	Automated recommendations for defined infections (Step 5)
	Automated recommendation for prophylaxis (Step 5)
	Evidence-based knowledge bases (Step 5)
6. Use local data	Automated antibiograms (Step 6)
	Automated empiric recommendations (Step 6)
	Track and alert on emerging resistance (Step 6)
7. Treat infection, not contamination	Infer contamination of specimens (Step 7)
8. Treat infection, not colonization	Infer colonization (Step 8)
9. Know when to say "no" to vancomycin	Target drug alerts (Step 9)
10. Stop treatment when infection is cured or unlikely	Duration of therapy alerts (Step 10)
	Duration of prophylaxis alerts (Step 10)
Prevent transmission	
11. Isolate the pathogen	Patient isolation alerts (Step 11)
	Infection control precaution reminders (Step 11)
	HAIs case-finding alerts (Step 11)
	Patient-based location tracking (Step 11)
	Population-based location tracking (Step 11)
	Clonal detection and alerting (Step 11)
	Target organism alerts (Step 11)
12. Break the chain of contagion	Hand washing reminders (Step 12)
	Online infection control information (Step 12)

[a]CDC 12-step program to prevent antimicrobial resistance among hospitalized adults.
Abbreviations: CDC, Centers for Disease Control and Prevention; CDSS, clinical decision support systems; HAI, hospital-acquired infection; ID, infections disease.
Source: Adapted from Ref. 51.

The technology will also allow clinical providers to demonstrate the value of their contributions in anti-infective management, patient safety, and the detection and control of HAIs. The critical role of CDSS in successful antimicrobial stewardship programs is self-evident; rather than replacing clinicians they will greatly assist both the generalist and specialist increasing their capacities and the reach of their influences.

CONCLUSION

The emergence of CDSS as paradigm-shifting technologies that play a deterministic role in the selection of best practices is an encouraging development (14,34,81). CDSS have been shown to change behavior in a non-threatening, defensible manner. These systems facilitate adherence to best practices and increase compliance with guidelines. Although they offer no panacea, such technologies offer the greatest potential to make care safer (34). Providing reliable, efficient, and individualized infection management and antimicrobial stewardship requires a mastery of data, information, and knowledge that is achievable with the increased use of CDSS. The design and functional requirements described above can be used to assess CDSS for overall clinical use as well as antimicrobial stewardship.

REFERENCES

1. Fact Sheet Medline®. (Accessed September 29, 2006 at http://www.nlm.nih.gov/pubs/factsheets/medline.html).
2. Djulbegovic B. Lifting the fog of uncertainty from the practice of medicine: strategy revolves around evidence, decision making, and leadership [editorial]. Br Med J 2004; 329:1419–20.
3. Morris AH. Developing and implementing computerized protocols for standardization of clinical decisions. Ann Intern Med 2000; 132:373–83.
4. Covell DG, Uman GC, Manning PR. Information needs in office practice: are they being met? Ann Intern Med 1985; 103:596–9.
5. Redelmeier DA, Shafir E. Medical decision making in situations that offer multiple alternatives. JAMA 1995; 273:302–5.
6. McDonald CJ. Protocol-based computer reminders, the quality of care and the non-perfectibility of man. N Engl J Med 1976; 295:1351–5.
7. Bleich HL. The computer as a consultant. N Engl J Med 1971; 284:141–7.
8. Hersh WR. Medical informatics: improving health care through information. JAMA 2002; 288:1955–8.
9. Pestotnik SL. Medical informatics: meeting the information challenge of a changing health care system [editorial]. J Inform Pharmacother 2000; 2:1.
10. Shortliffe EH. Computer programs to support clinical decision making. JAMA 1987; 258:61–6.
11. Pryor TA. Development of decision support systems. Int J Clin Monit Comput 1990; 7:137–46.
12. Rogers EM. Diffusion of Innovations. 4th ed. New York, NY: Free Press, 1995.
13. Berwick DM. Disseminating innovations in health care. JAMA 2003; 289:1969–75.
14. Pestotnik SL, Classen DC, Evans RS, Burke JP. Implementing antibiotic practice guidelines through computer-assisted decision support: clinical and financial outcomes. Ann Intern Med 1996; 124:884–90.
15. Stewart TA. Intellectual Capital: The New Wealth of Organizations. New York, NY: Currency-Doubleday, 1997.
16. Gardner M. Why clinical information standards matter: because they constrain what can be described [editorial]. Br Med J 2003; 326:1101–2.
17. Hammond WE. The making and adoption of health data standards. Health Affairs 2005; 24:1205–13.
18. Dolin RH, Alschuler L, Beebe C, et al. The HL7 clinical document architecture. J Am Med Inform Assoc 2001; 8:552–69.
19. HL7. About Page. (Accessed October 14, 2006 at http://www.hl7.org/about/hl7about.html).
20. SNOMED about page and frequently asked questions. (Accessed October 12, 2006 at http://www.snomed.org/about/index.html).
21. LOINC. Home page. (Accessed July 29, 2006 at http://www.loinc.org/).

22. UMLS. RxNorm page. (Accessed July 29, 2006 at http://www.nlm.nih.gov/research/umls/rxnorm/).
23. California Health Care Foundation. Clinical Data Standards in Health Care: Five Case Studies. (Accessed October 14, 2006 at http://www.chcf.org/topics/view.cfm?item-ID=112795).
24. Osheroff JA, Pifer EA, Sittig DF, Jenders RA, Teich JM. Clinical decision support implementer's workbook. (Accessed September 29, 2006 at http://www.himss.org/ASP/topics_cds_workbook.asp?faid=108&tid=14).
25. Sim I, Gorman P, Greenes RA, et al. Clinical decision support systems for the practice of evidence-based medicine. J Am Med Inform Assoc 2001; 8:527–34.
26. Bates DW, Kuperman GJ, Wang S, et al. Ten commandments for effective clinical decision support: making the practice of evidence-based medicine a reality. J Am Med Inform Assoc 2003; 10:523–30.
27. Office of the National Coordinator for Health Information Technology. Home Page. (Accessed July 29, 2006 at http://www.hhs.gov/healthit/).
28. UMLS. SNOMED announcement page. (Accessed July 29, 2006 at http://www.nlm.nih.gov/research/umls/Snomed/snomed_announcement.html).
29. Open Clinical. Arden Syntax page. (Accessed July 29, 2006 at http://www.openclinical.org/gmm_ardensyntax.html).
30. Open Clinical. GLIF page. (Accessed July 29, 2006 at http://www.openclinical.org/gmm_glif.html).
31. GLIF. Home page. (Accessed July 29, 2006 at http://www.glif.org/glif_main.html).
32. Stanford University. Protégé home page. (Accessed July 29, 2006 at http://protege.stanford.edu/).
33. Peleg M, Boxwalla AA, Bernstam E, Tu S, Greenes RA, Shortliffe EH. Representation of clinical guidelines in GLIF: relationship to the Arden Syntax. J Biomed Inform 2001; 34(3):170–81.
34. Bates DW, Gawande AA. Improving safety with information technology. N Engl J Med 2003; 348:2526–34.
35. Leapfrog Group for Patient Safety. Home page. Available from http://www.leapfroggroup.org. Accessed October 10, 2006.
36. Department of Health and Human Services Web site. The decade of health information technology: delivering consumer-centric and information-rich health care. (Accessed September 29, 2006 at http://www.hhs.gov/onchit/framework/hitframework.pdf).
37. Osler, Hoskin & Harcourt. Ten commandments of computerization. (Accessed August 15, 2006 at http://www.e-privacy.ca/TenComma.htm).
38. Rind DM, Safran C, Phillips RS, et al. Effect of computer-based alerts on the treatment and outcomes of hospitalized patients. Arch Intern Med 1994; 154:1511–17.
39. Overhage JM, Tierney WM, McDonald CJ. Computer reminders to implement preventive care guidelines for hospitalized patients. Arch Intern Med 1996; 156:1551–6.
40. Hunt DL, Haynes RB, Hanna SE, Smith K. Effects of computer-based clinical decision support systems on physician performance and patient outcomes. A systematic review. JAMA 1998; 280:1339–46.
41. Garg AX, Adhikari NK, McDonald H, et al. Effects of computerized clinical decision support systems on practitioner performance and patient outcomes. A systematic review. JAMA 2005; 293:1223–38.
42. Bobb A, Gleason K, Husch M, et al. The epidemiology of prescribing errors. The potential impact of computerized prescriber order entry. Arch Intern Med 2004; 164:785–92.
43. Nebeker JR, Hoffman JM, Weir CR, Bennett CL, Hurdle JF. High rates of adverse drugs events in a highly computerized hospital. Arch Intern Med 2005; 165:1111–6.
44. Classen DC, Pestotnik SL, Evans RS, Burke JP. Computerized surveillance of adverse drug events in hospital patients. JAMA 1991; 266:2847–51.
45. Lesar TS, Briceland L, Stein DS. Factors related to errors in medication prescribing. JAMA 1997; 277:312–7.
46. Gerding DN. The search for good antimicrobial stewardship. Joint Commission J Qual Improv 2001; 27:403–4.

47. Avorn J, Solomon DH. Cultural and economic factors that (mis)shape antibiotic use: the nonpharmacologic basis of therapeutics. Ann Intern Med 2000; 133:128–35.

48. Classen DC, Evans RS, Pestotnik SL, Horn SD, Menlove RL, Burke JP. The timing of prophylactic administration of antibiotics and the risk of surgical-wound infections. N Engl J Med 1992; 326:281–6.

49. Weinstein RA. Nosocomial infection update. Emerg Infect Dis 1998; 4:416–20.

50. Weinstein RA. Controlling antimicrobial resistance in hospitals: infection control and use of antibiotics. Emerg Infect Dis 2001; 7:188–92.

51. Centers for Disease Control and Prevention. Slide presentation: 12-steps to prevent antimicrobial resistance among hospitalized adults. (Accessed September 29, 2006 at http://www.cdc.gov/drugresistance/healthcare/).

52. Muto CA, Pokrywka M, Shutt K, et al. A large outbreak of *Clostridium difficile*-associated disease with an unexpected proportion of deaths and colectomies at a teaching hospital following increased fluoroquinolone use. Infect Control Hosp Epidemiol 2005; 26:273–80.

53. Kollef MH, Sherman G, Ward S, Fraser VJ. Inadequate antimicrobial treatment of infections: a risk factor for hospital mortality among critically ill patients. Chest 1999; 115:462–74.

54. Ibrahim EH, Sherman G, Ward S, Fraser VJ, Kollef MH. The influence of inadequate antimicrobial treatment of bloodstream infections on patient outcomes in the ICU setting. Chest 2000; 118:146–55.

55. Stelfox HT, Bates DW, Redelmeier DA. Safety of patients isolated for infection control. JAMA 2003; 290:1899–905.

56. Graves N. Economics and preventing hospital-acquired infection. Emerg Infect Dis 2004; 10:561–6.

57. Classen DC, Pestotnik SL, Evans RS, Lloyd JF, Burke JP. Adverse drug events in hospitalized patients: excess length of stay, extra costs, and attributable mortality. JAMA 1997; 277:301–6.

58. Bates DW, Spell N, Cullen DJ, et al. The costs of adverse drug events in hospitalized patients. Adverse drug events prevention study group. JAMA 1997; 277:307–11.

59. Smith RD. What does economics have to offer in the war against antimicrobial resistance? In: Knobler SL, Lemon SM, Najafi M, Burroughs T, (Eds.) The Resistance Phenomenon in Microbes and Infectious Disease Vectors: Implications for Human Health and Strategies for Containment. Washington, DC: National Academy Press, 2003:108–18.

60. Hoffman JM, Shah ND, Vermeulen LC, et al. Projecting future drug expenditures – 2006. Am J Health-Syst Pharm 2006; 63:123–38.

61. Shales DM, Gerding DN, John JF, et al. Society for Healthcare Epidemiology of American and Infectious Diseases Society of America Joint Committee on the Prevention of Antimicrobial Resistance: guidelines for the prevention of antimicrobial resistance in hospitals. Clin Infect Dis 1997; 25:584–99.

62. Goldmann DA, Weinstein RA, Wenzel RP, et al. Strategies to prevent and control the emergence and spread of antimicrobial-resistant microorganisms in hospitals: a challenge to hospital leadership. JAMA 1996; 275:234–40.

63. John JF, Fishman NO. Programmatic role of the infectious diseases physician in controlling antimicrobial costs in the hospital. Clin Infect Dis 1997; 24:471–85.

64. Gums JG, Yancey RW, Hamilton CA, Kubilis PS. A randomized, prospective study measuring outcomes after antibiotic therapy intervention by multidisciplinary consult team. Pharmacotherapy 1999; 19:1369–77.

65. Fishman NO. Methods and strategies for effective treatment of community-acquired mixed infections. Adv Stud Med 2002; 2:117–25.

66. Safdar N, Maki DG. The commonality of risk factors for nosocomial colonization and infection with antimicrobial-resistant *Staphylococcus aureus*, Enterococcus, Gram-negative bacilli, *Clostridium difficile*, and *Candida*. Ann Intern Med 2002; 136:834–44.

67. Owens RC, Fraser GL, Stogsdill P. Antimicrobial stewardship programs as a means to optimize antimicrobial use: insights from the Society of Infectious Diseases Pharmacists. Pharmacotherapy 2004; 24:896–908.

68. Gaynes R, Richards C, Edwards J, et al. Feeding back surveillance data to prevent hospital-acquired infections. Emerg Infect Dis 2001; 7:295–8.
69. Bratzler DW, Hunt DR. The surgical infection prevention and surgical care improvement projects: national initiatives to improve outcomes for patients having surgery. Clin Infect Dis 2006; 43:322–30.
70. Owens RC. *Clostridium difficile*-associated disease: an emerging threat to patient safety. Pharmacotherapy 2006; 26(3):299–311.
71. Yu VL, Fagan LM, Wraith SM, et al. Antimicrobial selection by a computer. A blinded evaluation by infections diseases experts. JAMA 1979; 242:1279–82.
72. Larsen RA, Evans RS, Burke JP, Pestotnik SL, Gardner RM, Classen DC. Improved perioperative antibiotic use and reduced surgical wound infections through use of computer decision analysis. Infect Control Hosp Epidemiol 1989; 10:316–20.
73. Pestotnik SL, Evans RS, Burke JP, Gardner RM, Classen DC. Therapeutic antibiotic monitoring: surveillance using a computerized expert system. Am J Med 1990; 88:43–8.
74. Evans RS, Pestotnik SL, Burke JP, Gardner RM, Larsen RA, Classen DC. Reducing the duration of prophylactic antibiotic use through computer monitoring of surgical patients. DICP 1990; 24:351–4.
75. Evans RS, Burke JP, Classen DC, et al. Computerized identification of patients at high risk for hospital-acquired infection. Am J Infect Control 1992; 20:4–10.
76. Evans RS, Pestotnik SL, Classen DC, Burke JP. Development of an automated antibiotic consultant. MD Comput 1993; 10:17–22.
77. Pestotnik SL, Classen DC, Evans RS, Stevens LE, Burke JP. Prospective surveillance of imipenem-cilastatin use and associated seizures using a hospital information system. Ann Pharmacother 1993; 27:497–501.
78. Evans RS, Classen DC, Pestotnik SL, Lundsgaarde HP, Burke JP. Improving empiric antibiotic selection using computer decision support. Arch Intern Med 1994; 154:878–84.
79. Evans RS, Pestotnik SL, Classen DC, Horn SD, Bass SB, Burke JP. Preventing adverse drug events in hospitalized patients. Ann Pharmacother 1994; 28:523–7.
80. Jozefiak ET, Lewicki JE, Kozinn WP. Computer-assisted antimicrobial surveillance in a community teaching hospital. Am J Health-Syst Pharm 1995; 52:1536–40.
81. Evans RS, Pestotnik SL, Classen DC, et al. A computer-assisted management program for antibiotics and other antiinfective agents. N Engl J Med 1998; 338:232–8.
82. Burke JP, Pestotnik SL. Antibiotic use and microbial resistance in intensive care units: impact of computer-assisted decision support. J Chemother 1999; 11:530–5.
83. Evans RS, Pestotnik SL, Classen DC, Burke JP. Evaluation of a computer-assisted antibiotic dose monitor. Ann Pharmacother 1999; 33:1026–31.
84. Bailey TC, McMullin ST. Using information systems technology to improve antibiotic prescribing. Crit Care Med 2001; 29:4(Suppl.):N87–91.
85. Dexter PR, Perkins S, Overhage JM, Maharry K, Kohler RB, McDonald CJ. A computerized reminder system to increase the use of preventative care for hospitalized patients. N Engl J Med 2001; 345:965–70.
86. Barenfanger J, Short MA, Groesch AA. Improved antimicrobial interventions have benefits. J Clin Microbiol 2001; 39:2823–8.
87. Platt R, Yokoe DS, Sands KE, et al. Automated methods for surveillance of surgical site infections. Emerg Infect Dis 2001; 7:211–6.
88. Zanetti G, Flanagan HL, Cohn LH, Giardina R, Platt R. Improvement of intraoperative antibiotic prophylaxis in prolonged cardiac surgery by automated alerts in the operating room. Infect Control Hosp Epidemiol 2003; 24:13–6.
89. Trick WE, Zagorski BM, Tokars JI, et al. Computer algorithms to detect bloodstream infections. Emerg Infect Dis 2004; 10:1612–20.
90. Wilson JW, Oyen LJ, Ou NN, et al. Hospital rules-based system: the next generation of medical informatics for patient safety. Am J Health-Syst Pharm 2005; 62:499–505.
91. Samore MH, Bateman K, Alder SC, et al. Clinical decision support and appropriateness of antimicrobial prescribing: a randomized trial. JAMA 2005; 294:2305–14.
92. Stevenson KB, Barbera J, Moore JW, Samore MH, Houck P. Understanding keys to successful implementation of electronic decision support in rural hospitals: analysis of a pilot study for antimicrobial prescribing. Am J Med Qual 2005; 20:313–8.

93. McGregor JC, Weekes E, Forrest GN, et al. Impact of computerized clinical decision support system on reducing inappropriate antimicrobial use: a randomized controlled trial. J Am Med Inform Assoc 2006; 13:378–84.
94. Clinical and Laboratory Standards Institute. Analysis and Presentation of Cumulative Antimicrobial Susceptibility Test Data; Approved Guideline, 2nd ed. Wayne, Pennsylvania: NCCLS document M39-A2; 2005.

17 Practical Application of Pharmacodynamic Principles to Optimize Therapy and Treat Resistant Organisms: A Focus on Beta-Lactam Antibiotics

Thomas P. Lodise
Albany College of Pharmacy, Albany, New York, U.S.A.

Ben M. Lomaestro
Albany Medical Center Hospital, Albany, New York, U.S.A.

George L. Drusano
Ordway Research Institute and New York State Department of Health, Albany, New York, U.S.A.

INTRODUCTION

Recent research has greatly enhanced our understanding of the relationship between beta-lactam pharmacodynamics and the microbiologic response. For beta-lactams, in vitro and animal studies have demonstrated that the time at which the "free" or non-protein-bound concentration exceeds the organism's minimum inhibitory concentration (fT > MIC) is the best predictor of bacterial killing and microbiologic response. Using population pharmacokinetic modeling and Monte Carlo simulation, it is now possible to integrate pharmacokinetics, the pharmacodynamic target, and microbiologic surveillance data to generate empiric beta-lactam dosing strategies to determine the fT > MIC associated with near-maximal bactericidal effect against the range of pathogens encountered in clinical practice.

Such mathematical modeling techniques were used at Albany Medical Center Hospital (AMCH) to devise alternative dosing schemes for piperacillin/tazobactam, meropenem, and cefepime. These new dosing schemes optimized fT > MIC at a total daily dose less than traditional dosing methods and achieved the targeted fT > MIC with less administration time per day than continuous infusion. This chapter provides an overview of the latest advances in beta-lactam pharmacodynamics and highlights AMCH's experience implementing these new dosing schemes into clinical practice.

Antimicrobial pharmacodynamics (PD) is a term used to describe the relationship between drug exposure and antimicrobial activity, and the past two decades have seen tremendous progress in understanding this complex relationship. The PD target associated with maximal effect has been identified for most antimicrobials, including the beta-lactams. With advances in computer technology and mathematical modeling (population pharmacokinetics and Monte Carlo simulation), it is now possible to apply PD principles to clinical practice. Specifically, mathematical modeling can allow one to design antimicrobial regimens that optimize the probability of achieving the PD target associated with maximal effect. These mathematical modeling techniques have an array of other utilities and have become the standard methodology for assessing the clinical viability of both experimental and approved antimicrobials.

Unfortunately, the most prevalent beta-lactam antibiotics were developed prior to this contemporary understanding of beta-lactam pharmacodynamics. Thus, many of the conventional beta-lactam dosing schemes too often yield a concentration–time profile with a low probability of achieving the PD endpoint linked with a favorable outcome in the targeted patient population. In an effort to maximize the PD profile of beta-lactam antibiotics and ensure the highest probability of the desired patient response, alternative dosing schemes for piperacillin/tazobactam, meropenem, and cefepime were devised using population pharmacokinetic modeling and Monte Carlo simulation, then were adopted into clinical practice at Albany Medical Center Hospital (AMCH).

The reader will find this chapter is structured to meet the following goals:

- Discuss advances in our current knowledge of beta-lactam pharmacodynamics
- Provide an overview of the mathematical modeling techniques used to develop alternative dosing schemes for piperacillin/tazobactam, meropenem, and cefepime
- Discuss how these novel dosing schemes were adopted and implemented into clinical practice at AMCH
- Discuss the rationale for the beta-lactam dosing regimens selected
- Present the supporting outcomes data

BACKGROUND

Historically, the measure most often used to characterize antimicrobial activity is the minimal inhibitory concentration, or MIC. This is the antimicrobial concentration that inhibits visible microbial growth in an artificial media following a fixed time of incubation. Although the MIC is a useful parameter, it is often viewed as an "all-or-none" (growth vs. no growth) phenomena and has several key limitations. First, the MIC does not provide information on the time course of antimicrobial activity and does not account for the changing concentrations throughout the dosing interval (1). Second, the fixed MIC concentration does not capture inherent inter-patient pharmacokinetic (PK) variability. Third, the MIC does not provide information on the potential for persistent anti-infective activity after the concentration at the site has dropped below the MIC or on the additive effects of the immune system. Fourth, the MIC does not reflect the rate that bacteria are killed nor does it offer insights as to whether bactericidal activity is further enhanced at higher concentrations; the MIC only quantifies net growth over an 18- to 24-hr observation period, so killing and regrowth may well occur during this period, as long as the net growth is zero (1).

For antimicrobials, integration of PK parameters with MIC overcomes many of the MIC limitations and has been shown to be a more reliable predictor of outcomes. Recent research has focused on the relationship between the PD of beta-lactams and microbiologic response (2,3). The beta-lactams, in contrast to the aminoglycosides and fluoroquinolones, exhibit little concentration-dependent bacterial killing (2–11). This phenomenon was observed in the earliest *S. aureus* time kill-curve studies, which demonstrated that the rate of bacterial kill was not improved by increasing the concentration of penicillin (12).

For beta-lactams, in vitro and animal studies have demonstrated that the time at which the "free" or non-protein-bound concentration exceeds the organism's minimum inhibitory concentration ($fT > MIC$) is the best predictor of bacterial killing and microbiologic response (2,3,5–8). These studies have consistently shown that free beta-lactam concentrations do not have to remain above the MIC for the entire dosing interval and the fraction of the dosing interval required for maximal bacterial effect varies according to beta-lactam type. Although the precise $fT > MIC$ varies for different drug-bacteria combinations, bacteriostatic effects are typically observed when the free drug concentration exceeds the MIC for 35% to 40%, 30%, and 20% of the dosing interval for the cephalosporins, penicillins, and carbapenems, respectively. Near-maximal bactericidal effects require 60% to 70%, 50%, and 40% $fT > MIC$, respectively, for these beta-lactam classes (2,3,5–8).

POPULATION PHARMACOKINETIC MODELING AND MONTE CARLO SIMULATION: INTEGRATION OF PK, PD, AND MICROBIOLOGIC DATA

With advances in computer technology and software, it is now possible to integrate PK, a PD target, and microbiologic surveillance data to determine the probability of PD target attainment for different antibiotic regimens (2,13–22). More importantly, it is now possible to generate empiric antibiotic dosing strategies that maximize the likelihood that an antibiotic regimen achieves the desired PD target (e.g., 50% $fT > MIC$, AUC/MIC >125, etc.) against the range of pathogens encountered in the patient population of interest (14,17,18,23,24).

The first step of this integration process is obtaining estimates and associated dispersions of the PK parameters for the patient group. The two methods primarily used to obtain estimates of PK parameters are the standard two-stage pharmacokinetic modeling approach and population pharmacokinetic modeling. While the two-stage approach of PK modeling has been the traditional method of generating PK values and is much less computationally intensive, population pharmacokinetic modeling provides several distinct advantages over the standard two-stage modeling approach. The major advantage is that population modeling explicitly deals with populations of patients rather than with individual patients and aims to estimate the distribution of the parameters. In other words, population pharmacokinetics explicitly estimates between-patient variability in PK parameters for the population pharmacokinetic model. Population modeling also seeks to estimate covariance among the PK parameters. The standard two-stage approach determines the PK estimates for each patient first and then uses descriptive statistics on the results to generate the dispersion surrounding PK estimates. While fitting an individual subject, the standard two-stage approach ignores the existence of all other individuals within the population. Mean estimates of parameters are usually unbiased, but the random effects (variance and covariance) are likely to be overestimated in realistic situations. As a result, the estimates of model parameter dispersion and simulated drug exposures are more precise by the population-modeling technique (25).

Another advantage of population pharmacokinetic modeling over the standard two-stage approach is its improved ability to estimate population pharmacokinetic parameters for subjects with limited sampling times by using data from other subjects when estimating the mean parameter vector and its associated dispersions. In essence, population modeling "borrows" PK information from other subjects within the dataset to estimate the most likely population parameters. Because of these methodological differences, population pharmacokinetic modeling has become the standard methodology for estimating population pharmacokinetic parameters and associated dispersions (25,26).

Once the values for PK parameters and their dispersion are estimated, Monte Carlo simulation is used to characterize the PD profile of the antibiotic. Specifically, Monte Carlo simulation is a technique that incorporates the PK variability among potential patients (between-patient variability) when predicting antibiotic exposures and allows calculation of the probability for obtaining a critical target exposure for the range of possible MIC values. If a number of volunteers or patients are given an antibiotic, there will be true variability in the observed concentration time profiles between people. For example, the peak serum concentrations and drug clearance will vary between individuals. In essence, Monte Carlo simulation is a mathematical modeling technique that is used to simulate the dispersion or full spread of values [e.g., peak concentration, area under the curve (AUC)] that would be seen in a large population after the administration of a specific drug dose and allows one to estimate the ability that a dosing regimen achieves the critical PD target (2,11).

There are several steps involved in the Monte Carlo simulation process. First, the mean PK parameters and their associated variability (variance and covariance) are used to create a multivariate distribution of PK parameters. From this multivariate distribution, Monte Carlo simulation randomly draws a set of PK parameters for a single subject (this is why it is extremely important to have reasonable estimates of the dispersion surrounding PK parameters). Second, these randomly selected parameters are used to simulate a concentration time profile for that subject based on the desired antibiotic dosing regimen. Based on this simulated concentration time profile, it is determined whether the target was reached or not in this virtual patient (e.g., 50% $fT > \text{MIC}$ for different MICs). This process is repeated a specified number of times (e.g., 10,000 times) to simulate concentration time profiles for a virtual patient population. Once the simulations are complete, the model calculates the proportion of virtual patients who reached the target, generating the frequency of target attainment at each MIC value over the specified MIC range. The frequency of target attainment is used to estimate the probability of PD target attainment (e.g., 50% $fT > \text{MIC}$) at each MIC for a given MIC range.

In clinical practice, a distribution of MICs is encountered for a given organism and/or infection. The final step, therefore, is determining the overall probability of target attainment for a distribution of organisms encountered clinically. As previously mentioned, the probability of target attainment at each MIC value found in the distribution of the target pathogen(s) is computed in the previous step. Because the fraction of organisms collected at each MIC is known, a weighted average (expectation) of the target attainment rates can be calculated by multiplying the probability of target attainment for a specific MIC and the frequency of occurrence for this MIC. This product is calculated for each MIC of interest. The overall probability of target attainment for the MIC distribution is then calculated by summing the product of probability of target attainment and probability of MIC occurrence for each respective MIC.

As previously mentioned, a key element for these simulations is the estimation of the PK parameters and their associated dispersion (variance and covariance). Pharmacokinetic data, especially for new compounds, is usually limited to data from healthy volunteer studies. Caution should be exercised when generalizing the results of volunteer studies to the population of interest. Volunteer studies are often considered as the most conservative evaluation that can be considered for a new drug, in that volunteers are young and healthy, likely to have the highest drug clearances and shortest half lives. However, when one performs Monte Carlo simulation, the measure of central tendency (high drug clearance, short half-lives) is only part of the story. Because Monte Carlo simulations are explicitly creating a distribution, it is important to understand the measure of dispersion. Secondary to the limited variation surrounding PK parameters from healthy volunteer studies, it is possible that they overestimate the probability of target attainment. Applicability to the target population must always be considered.

Monte Carlo simulation has been applied to a variety of situations, such as determining the PD profile of both approved and study antimicrobials, optimizing antimicrobial dosing against a known or suspected MIC distribution of organism(s), establishing the optimal dose for a new compound, and estimating the ability of antimicrobials to penetrate the site of infection (2,16–21,23,24,26,27). Monte Carlo simulation is also used by the Clinical Laboratory Standards Institute (CLSI, formerly known as NCCLS), to establish antibiotic susceptibility breakpoints for new antibiotics and to assess the validity of existing breakpoints for U.S. Food and Drug Administration-approved antibiotics (20,28,29).

TRANSLATION OF PRINCIPLES INTO PRACTICE

The AMCH antibiotic subcommittee catalyzed development of the new beta-lactam dosing schemes for clinical practice. At the time, the antibiotic subcommittee consisted of physicians, pharmacists, and epidemiologists with considerable expertise in antimicrobial PK/PD principles and modeling, and these techniques were used to devise alternative dosing schemes for piperacillin/tazobactam, meropenem, and cefepime (16,17,23). To reduce potentially harmful variation in dosing practice, the antibiotic subcommittee implemented an automatic substitution program using a preprinted antibiotic order sheet (Fig. 1); this system ensured standardization to the newly approved dosing schemes. Preprinted antibiotic order sheets for therapeutic substitutions had been well accepted by the both the AMCH medical attending and house staff in the past. When the prescriber did not adhere to the specified dose and frequency, the preprinted antibiotic order sheets allowed the pharmacist to automatically convert the written order to the newly adapted protocols. This feature was critical to patient safety because it eliminated dosing discrepancies or potential delays in therapy.

Once a consensus was reached on the novel beta-lactam dosing protocol, the proposed policy was presented to both the Pharmacy and Therapeutics and Medical Executive Committees for approval. The support of hospital administration and medical attending staff was crucial to minimize the likelihood of liability concerns being raised by practitioners. The final implementation process component was pharmacy and medical staff education, and the new process was seamlessly integrated into ongoing house staff education.

The three-step implementation process of mathematical modeling, committee approval, and staff education resulted in a smooth migration of the new beta-lactam dosing principles into clinical practice. It is noteworthy that the novel beta-lactam dosing schemes were adopted into practice solely based on the strength of the Monte

Carlo simulation studies and expected patient benefit; no pilot data were collected prior to implementation. Because of the collective expertise in PK and PD on the antibiotic subcommittee, the Pharmacy and Therapeutics and Medical Executive Committees were highly supportive of the new beta-lactam dosing protocols.

Detailed reviews of the Monte Carlo simulation and supporting outcomes data are provided under each of the respective antibiotic sections, with emphasis on the piperacillin/tazobactam experience. Since the processes were similar for meropenem and cefepime, the discussions for these protocols are abbreviated. Other institutions have utilized similar methodology to develop unique protocols

---

Albany Medical Center

PHARMACY THERAPEUTIC SUBSTITUTION ORDER SHEET

Name:_____

Location:_____

Serial #:_____

MR #:_____

Date of Birth: ____/____/____

Instructions:
1. Imprint patient's plate before placing in chart
2. Sign bottom of form.
3. Kardex order as substitution.

ALLERGIES: WEIGHT   lb.   kg. HEIGHT: cm BSA: m^2

ANTIBIOTIC Therapeutic Substitution
Piperacillin/Tazobactam (Zosyn®) (Adult)
BY DIRECTION OF THE ALBANY MEDICAL CENTER FORMULARY COMMITTEE, THESE AGENTS ARE DESIGNATED THERAPEUTIC EQUIVALENTS FOR AUTOMATIC SUBSTITUTION.

Nursing – Please discontinue:

Piperacillin/Tazobactam _____ g IV q _____ h
                                      (dose)   (frequency)
Nursing – Please start:

Piperacillin/Tazobactam 3.375g IV   ☐ **q8h** *over 4h*   ☐ **q12h** *over 30min*   **for** _____ **days.**

Pharmacist Signature: _____   Date:_____ Time:_____

Print Name: _____

RN Signature:_____   Date:_____ Time:_____

Print Name:_____

FOR REFERENCE ONLY

Dose in Renal Impairment

(A)

CrCl (ml/min)	Over 20	Under 20, peritoneal, hemodialysis	CRRT
Dose:	3.375g over 4 hours q8h	3.375g over 30min q12h	3.375g over 4 hours q8h

FIGURE 1 A–C   Albany Medical Center Hospital dosing protocol for **(A)** piperacillin/tazobactam. (*Continued*)

Albany Medical Center

PHARMACY THERAPEUTIC SUBSTITUTION ORDER SHEET

Instructions:
4. Imprint patient's plate before placing in chart.
5. Sign bottom of form.
6. Kardex order as substitution.

ALLERGIES: WEIGHT   lb.   kg. HEIGHT: cm BSA: m^2

ANTIBIOTIC THERAPEUTIC SUBSTITUTION

MEROPENEM - IMIPENEM/CILASTATIN (ADULT & PEDIATRIC)

BY DIRECTION OF THE ALBANY MEDICAL CENTER FORMULARY COMMITTEE, THESE AGENTS ARE DESIGNATED THERAPEUTIC EQUIVALENTS FOR AUTOMATIC SUBSTITUTION.

Nursing – Please discontinue:

☐ Imipenem/cilastatin (Primaxin®) _____ IV _____
                                        (dose)   (frequency)

☐ Meropenem (Merrem®) 1g IV q8h*

Nursing – Please start:

☐ **Meropenem (Merrem®)**   ☐ **500mg IV over 30 min**   ☐ **1g over 3h**   ☐ **2g over 3 h**

                    ☐ **q6h**   ☐ **q8h**   ☐ **q12h** ☐ **q24h**   for ___ days

☐ **Meropenem** ____mg (___mg/kg) **IV over 30 min** ☐ **q6h** ☐ **q8h** ☐ **q12h** ☐ **q24h for** ___days

Pharmacist Signature: _____ Date:_____ Time:_____

Print Name: _____

For reference only

Renal impairment dose adjustment for adults and children (not neonates):

CrCl (ml/min)	26–50	10–25	Under 10, peritoneal, hemodialysis	CRRT
Dose:	Normal dose q8h	Normal dose q12h	Normal dose q24h	Normal dose q8h

Normal dose (Adult): 500mg IV q6h

*NOTE: Adult patients ordered on meropenem 1g IV q8h should be substituted to 500mg q6h except in CF and meningitis for cystic fibrosis patients: 1g over 3h IV q8h max (normal renal function)

For meningitis: 2g over 3 h IV q8h max (normal renal function)

Normal dose: Pediatrics:	Sepsis and other indications	Meningitis
Neonates under 7 days	20mg/kg/dose q12h	40mg/kg/dose IV q12h
Neonates 7 days and over	20mg/kg/dose q8h	40mg/kg/dose (max 2g) IV q8h
Children	15mg/kg/dose (max 500mg) q6h	

(B)

FIGURE 1 A–C   **(B)** Dosing protocol for meropenem. (*Continued*)

Name:_____

Location:_____

Serial #:_____

MR #:_____

Date of Birth: ____/__/____

Albany Medical Center

PHARMACY THERAPEUTIC SUBSTITUTION ORDER SHEET

Instructions:
7. Imprint patient's plate before placing in chart.
8. Sign bottom of form.
9. Kardex order as substitution.

ALLERGIES: WEIGHT   lb.   kg. HEIGHT: cm BSA: m²

ANTIBIOTIC THERAPEUTIC SUBSTITUTION

Cefepime (Maxipime®)

BY DIRECTION OF THE ALBANY MEDICAL CENTER FORMULARY COMMITTEE, THESE AGENTS ARE DESIGNATED THERAPEUTIC EQUIVALENTS FOR AUTOMATIC SUBSTITUTION.

Discontinue:
•Ceftazidime •500mg •1g •2g •_____mg (_____mg/kg/dose) IV q _____h

•Cefepime 2g IV q8h

Start:
•Cefepime 1g IV q _____ h for _____ days
                                       (frequency)

•Cefepime _____mg (25mg/kg/dose, max 1000mg) IV q _____ h for _____ days
                                                                          (frequency)

•Febrile, Neutropenic Patient in the Children's Hospital

Cefepime _____mg (50mg/kg/dose, max 2000mg) IV q _____ h for _____ days
                                                                       (frequency)

Pharmacist Signature: _____ Date:_____Time:_____

Print Name: _____

For reference only

Cefepime (Maxipime®) Therapeutic Substitution Table					
Cr Cl (ml/min)	Over 50	30–50	15–29	Under 15, peritoneal, hemodialysis	CRRT
Cefepime Dose* ADULT	1g q6h	1g q8h	1g q12h	1g q24h	1g q8h
Cefepime Dose* PEDIATRIC	25mg/kg/ dose q6h	25mg/kg/ dose q8h	25mg/kg/ dose q12h	25mg/kg/ dose q24h	25mg/kg/ dose q8h
Cefepime Dose PEDIATRIC Febrile Neutropenic in Children's Hospital	50mg/kg/ dose q8h	50mg/kg/ dose q8h	50mg/kg/ dose q12h	50mg/kg/ dose q24h	50mg/kg/ dose q8h
Substituted for: Ceftazidime	Ordered doses				

(C)   * Do NOT substitute for Ceftazidime for Cystic Fibrosis Patients.

FIGURE 1 A–C   (C) Dosing protocol for cefepime.

for their institutions, but this discussion is limited to our experience at AMCH (30,31).

Piperacillin/Tazobactam

One of the major goals for AMCH was to maximize $fT > MIC$ for piperacillin/ tazobactam by altering the mode of administration. Similar to other institutions, piperacillin/tazobactam is frequently used as first-line empiric therapy for patients with documented or suspected *Pseudomonas aeruginosa* infections. While the AMCH antibiogram suggested that piperacillin/tazobactam was a suitable agent for *P. aeruginosa*, there were concerns that the traditional dosing strategies (3.375 g IV every 4 or 6 hr as a 0.5-hr infusion) may not attain the target of 50% $fT > MIC$ for the full range of MICs deemed susceptible by the CLSI. The concerns were precipitated by the current CLSI susceptibility breakpoints for *P. aeruginosa* (susceptible: ≤ 64 mg/L; intermediate: 128 mg/L; and resistant ≥ 256 mg/L) and validated by the Monte Carlo simulation results (23).

Since the breakpoints were set by CLSI, a global, guideline development organization, the antibiotic subcommittee chose not to adjust the CLSI suscept- ibility breakpoint for piperacillin/tazobactam and rather decided to optimize the PD profile against the range of MICs considered susceptible by CLSI. It was recognized that optimal target attainment against non-lactose fermentors (for which the susceptibility breakpoint is 64 mg/L) would be difficult with the proposed regimen, but hopefully at least superior to conventional dosing.

To maximize the PD profile of piperacillin/tazobactam, the beta-lactam dose optimization strategies considered were doubling the dose, more frequent dosing, and prolonging the infusion time (continuous and extended infusion) (22,32,33). As shown in Figure 2, increasing the dose proved to be ineffective because it only increases the $fT > MIC$ one half-life, which is typically 1 or 2 hr for most beta-lactams, including piperacillin (32). The antibiotic subcommittee also knew that more frequent dosing of piperacillin/tazobactam was not a viable

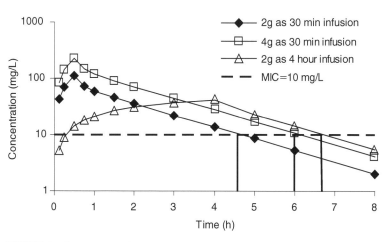

FIGURE 2   Comparison of time above the MIC (10 mg/L) between piperacillin 2 g as a 30-minute infusion, piperacillin 4 g as a 30-minute infusion, and piperacillin 2 g as a 4-hr infusion. *Abbreviation*: MIC, minimum inhibitory concentration.

option from a nursing and pharmacy perspective due to increased administration and preparation time given that piperacillin/tazobactam was already dosed four to six times per day.

The antibiotic subcommittee finally arrived at extended infusion as the most viable option to maximize $fT > MIC$ for piperacillin/tazobactam (22). Consistent with most healthcare institutions, piperacillin/tazobactam was being infused over 0.5 hr at AMCH. Administering a dose of a beta-lactam agent as an infusion longer than the conventional 0.5 to 1.0 hr infusion duration has two main effects (Fig. 2). First, it produces lower peak concentration of the drug. Because the bacterial kill rate for these agents is not concentration dependent, this does not present a major disadvantage (2,3,5,6,34). Second, the drug concentrations remain in excess of the MIC for a longer period of time. Because this is what drives antibacterial effect for beta-lactams, this should yield a higher probability of attaining a good clinical outcome. It should also be noted that this can be done with less frequent drug dosing.

Continuous infusion was also considered but prolonged infusion was selected secondary to the several advantages it offers over continuous infusion. Although continuous infusion is a rational method to optimize $fT > MIC$, it is not always realistic for multiple reasons. For example, an intravenous line or lumen of an intravenous catheter must be dedicated to infuse the antibiotic and this is not always practical, especially for patients with limited intravenous access or patients requiring multiple daily infusions (with other concerns such as compatibility and access site issues). Administration of the infusion for a prolonged time, but not continuously, obviates the need to have a dedicated intravenous line for the patient just for beta-lactam continuous infusion. In addition, the extended infusion beta-lactam administration allows time within each dosing interval when other agents could be administered through the same intravenous line, circumventing many of the aforementioned issues of the continuous infusion approach while achieving the targeted $fT > MIC$ at a total daily dose less than standard beta-lactam dosing methods.

Based on a Monte Carlo simulation that used PK data for healthy male volunteers, piperacillin/tazobactam 3.375 g administered over a 4-hr period every 8 hr (extended infusion piperacillin/tazobactam) was identified as an alternative means to the traditional dosing of piperacillin/tazobactam 3.375 g administered over 30 minutes every 4 or 6 hr (traditional piperacillin/tazobactam, Fig. 3A) (16,23). The PD endpoint selected for this simulation was 50% $fT > MIC$ target correlated with maximal bactericidal activity for penicillins. The Monte Carlo simulation revealed that the probability of target attainment for extended infusion piperacillin/tazobactam was 92% at 16 mg/L and was 100% for lower MICs. For traditional piperacillin/tazobactam every 4 hr, the probability of target attainment was >90% only for ≤8 mg/L and was substantially less for higher MICs. For traditional piperacillin/tazobactam every 6 hr, the probability of target attainment was >90% only for 1 mg/L. All regimens were suboptimal for MICs ≥ 32 mg/L.

Given the low probabilities of target attainment for MICs ≥ 32 mg/L, several other extended infusion piperacillin/tazobactam regimens were evaluated (piperacillin/tazobactam 3.375 g IV q6h as a 2- to 4-hr infusion). For all additional regimens examined, the probability of target attainment was <50% for MICs ≥ 32 mg/L (data not shown). Given the minimal gain in probability of target attainment and higher drug acquisition costs and workload associated with more frequent dosing, the committee decided to endorse piperacillin/tazobactam 3.375 g q8h as a 4-hr infusion as the preferred dosing strategy. It is important to note that

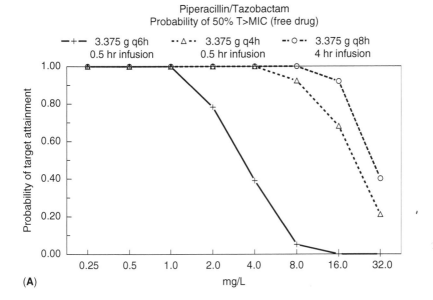

(A)

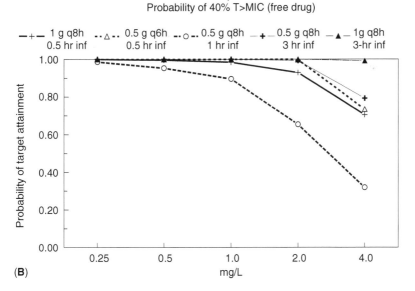

(B)

FIGURE 3 A–C Results of probabilities of target attainment analyses for (**A**) piperacillin/tazobactam and (**B**) meropenem. *Source*: (**A**) Adapted from Ref. 23. (*Continued*)

only the piperacillin component of piperacillin/tazobactam was simulated. The PD profile of tazobactam was not examined because current doses of tazobactam in the piperacillin/tazobactam formulation have been shown to be sufficient for an antibacterial effect when the target is fT > MIC (35).

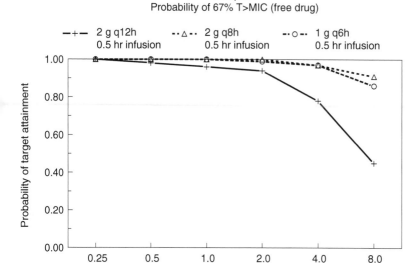

FIGURE 3 A–C (**C**) Results of probabilities of target attainment analyses for cefepime.

In addition to the superior PD profile, the extended infusion piperacillin/tazobactam administration allowed 4 hr within each 8 hr dosing interval when other agents could be administered through the same intravenous line. The extended infusion strategy also economized drug costs by eliminating the need for one to three doses per day. During 2001 (year before conversion), piperacillin/tazobactam purchases totaled approximately $275,000; reducing the total daily dose by 25% to 50% (one to three doses per day) represents a potential savings of approximately $68,750 to $135,750 in annual direct drug acquisition costs. In February 2002, a hospital-wide, automatic substitution program was implemented to allow automatic conversion of written orders for intermittent infusion of piperacillin/tazobactam to be dosed as extended-infusion piperacillin/tazobactam.

An assessment of the automatic substitution program was conducted to evaluate the impact among critically ill adult patients who received piperacillin/tazobactam for a *Pseudomonas aeruginosa* infection between January 2000 and June 2004 at AMCH (36). Prior to February 2002, all patients received traditional-infusion piperacillin/tazobactam; after this time, all patients received extended-infusion piperacillin/tazobactam. The study only included patients with a positive *P. aeruginosa* culture and who (*i*) were ≥ 18 years old, (*ii*) had an absolute neutrophil count ≥ 1000 cells/mm), (*iii*) had a positive culture for *P. aeruginosa*, (*iv*) met the CDC criteria for infection (37), (*v*) were administered piperacillin/tazobactam within the first 72 hr of the onset of *P. aeruginosa* infection, and (*vi*) were administered piperacillin/tazobactam ≥ 48 hr. Patients were excluded if (*i*) they received more than 1 day of intermittent infusion of piperacillin/tazobactam before conversion to the extended infusion protocol, (*ii*) they received a concurrent beta-lactam antibiotic with *P. aeruginosa* activity within five days of initiation of piperacillin/tazobactam (fluoroquinolones and aminoglycosides were acceptable), (*iii*) the

P. aeruginosa isolate was resistant to piperacillin/tazobactam, (*iv*) there was a necessity for dialysis, (*v*) they received a solid organ or bone marrow transplant, or (*vi*) they were diagnosed with cystic fibrosis. For patients with multiple *P. aeruginosa* clinical cultures, only the first set of cultures were considered for the study.

Since piperacillin/tazobactam is often used empiric in critically ill patients, we felt it was important to examine the impact of extended-infusion piperacillin/tazobactam among the most vulnerable patients. Patients at greatest risk for deleterious outcomes were identified by classification and regression tree (CART) analysis (Fig. 3). With CART, the best predictors of outcome are identified, and the entire population was divided into two groups: those who have a high likelihood of the outcome of interest and those who do not. Once the populations are identified, the influence of piperacillin/tazobactam was examined within the resultant risk-stratified populations. To further ensure that the study hypothesis was clearly addressed, we limited the study to patients with documented *P. aeruginosa* infections. The study was restricted to *P. aeruginosa* infections for several reasons. First, patients with *P. aeruginosa* who met the inclusion/exclusion criteria represented a relatively homogenous patient population; this attribute minimized confounding and increased the ability to detect differences between treatment groups according to intervention. Second, patients with *P. aeruginosa* infections are more dependent on antimicrobial therapy than other populations because *P. aeruginosa*-infected patients are frequently critically ill and often have an impaired innate immune system (38,39). Third, *P. aeruginosa* isolates typically have a higher range of MICs to piperacillin/tazobactam than other organisms and the benefits of optimizing $fT >$ MIC were better elucidated in this patient population (40,41).

During the specified enrollment period, 194 patients satisfied the study criteria (102 extended and 92 intermittent). No differences in clinical characteristics were noted between groups. The results of the CART analysis are displayed in

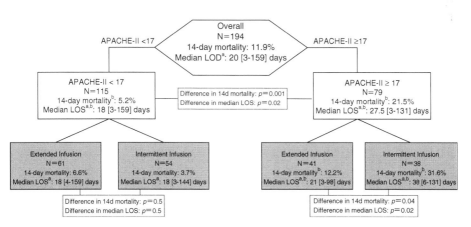

FIGURE 4 Comparison of outcomes between patients that received extended infusion piperacillin/tazobactam and intermittent infusion piperacillin/tazobactam among patients with APACHE-II score $\geq$ 17 and patients with APACHE-II score < 17 (CART-derived breakpoint). *Notes*: [a]Excludes patients that died within 14 days of collection of *P. aeruginosa* culture. [b]Comparison between APACHE-II $\leq$17 versus APACHE-II $\geq$ 17 was $p \leq 0.05$. [c]Comparison between extended versus intermittent infusion was $p \leq 0.05$. *Abbreviations*: APACHE-II, Acute Physiology and Chronic Health Evaluation II; CART, classification and regression tree; LOD, limit of direction; LOS, limit of sensitivity.

Figure 4. An Acute Physiology and Chronic Health Evaluation II (APACHE-II) score ≥ 17 was the most important predictor of 14-day mortality: the 14-day mortality among patients with an APACHE-II score ≥ 17 versus patients with an APACHE-II score < 17 was 21.5% versus 5.2%, respectively, $p < 0.01$. Comparison of 14-day mortality and hospital length of stay post–culture-collection are also shown in Figure 4. In patients with APACHE-II scores ≥ 17, 14-day mortality was significantly lower in extended versus intermittent infusion patients (12.2% vs. 31.6%, respectively; $p = 0.04$) and median hospital length of stay post–culture-collection was significantly shorter among extended infusion versus intermittent infusion patients (21 days versus 38 days, $p = 0.02$). No differences in outcomes were noted for patients with APACHE-II score < 17.

Based on these findings, and that of others who performed similar evaluations (30), extended infusion piperacillin/tazobactam was deemed a safe and effective alternative dosing strategy to traditional piperacillin/tazobactam intermittent dosing, and the program continued based on the improved outcomes and substantial cost savings associated with the extended infusion method.

Meropenem

In 2001, conventional imipenem/cilastatin dosing was switched to meropenem 500 mg q8h as a 30-minute infusion or 1000 mg IV q8h as a 3-hr infusion (extended infusion meropenem) (17). Based on a Monte Carlo simulation that used healthy volunteer pharmacokinetic data, Lomaestro and Drusano showed that extended-infusion meropenem provided more robust target attainment probabilities than conventional meropenem dosing regimens and imipenem 500 mg IV q6h (1-hr infusion) (17). Using the global Meropenem Yearly Susceptibility Testing Information Collection (MYSTIC) surveillance data as the measure of MIC distribution and frequency, the overall probability of target attainment was calculated for various nosocomial pathogens (Table 1). Meropenem 500 mg IV q8h (1- and 3-hr infusions) had excellent coverage against all nosocomial pathogens examined, except *P. aeruginosa* and *Acinetobacter* spp. For these pathogens, meropenem 1000 mg IV q8h (3-hr infusion) provided higher probabilities of target attainment. The PD profile of imipenem/cilastatin 500 mg IV q6h (1-hr infusion) was similar to meropenem 500 mg IV q8h (1- and 3-hr infusions). Prolonged infusion

TABLE 1 Probability of Target Attainment (40% f T>MIC) of Extended Infusion Meropenem (500–1000 mg q8h as a 3-Hour Infusion) and Imipenem 500 mg IV q6h (1-hr Infusion) Against Target Organisms Isolated from the MYSTIC Surveillance Program

Organisms	Imipenem 500 mg q6h (1-hr infusion)	Meropenem 500 mg q8h (1-hr infusion)	Meropenem 500 mg q8h (3-hr infusion)	Meropenem 1,000 mg q8h (3-hr infusion)
Staphylococcus aureus	98.5%	95.0%	98.4%	98.8%
Klebsiella spp.	99.0%	97.5%	99.5%	99.6%
Enterobacter spp.	98.0%	97.3%	99.5%	99.8%
Serratia spp.	97.5%	96.2%	99.4%	99.6%
Acinetobacter spp.	76.0%	76.4%	77.1%	83.0%
Pseudomonas aeruginosa	73.0%	76.0%	79.3%	86.4%

Abbreviations: MIC, minimum inhibitory concentration; MYSTIC, Meropenem Yearly Susceptibility Test Information Collection.
Source: Adapted from Ref. 17.

simulation for imipenem/cilastatin was not performed because of stability issues cited in the package insert (17).

Based on the above information, conventional meropenem dosing was changed to meropenem 500 mg IV q8h (1-hr infusion), with meropenem 1 g q8h (3-hr infusion) reserved for documented or suspected infections when either *P. aeruginosa* or *Acinetobacter* spp. For situations when meropenem 1 g q8h (3-hr infusion) was not warranted, the antibiotic subcommittee opted to infuse meropenem 500 mg IV q8h over 1 hr rather than 3 hr due to the similar probability of target attainment and reduced administration time.

After gaining approval by both the Pharmacy and Therapeutics and Medical Committees in April 2001, a hospital-wide automatic substitution program was implemented to allow automatic conversion of written orders for conventional infusion meropenem and imipenem/cilastatin to be dosed as extended infusion meropenem. The meropenem extended-infusion program continued until the national meropenem shortage in February 2004. During the shortage, meropenem orders were changed to imipenem/cilastatin 500 mg IV q6h. Once the meropenem supply resumed, the imipenem/cilastatin orders were converted to meropenem 500 mg IV q6h (0.5 hr infusion). The current AMCH dosing protocol for meropenem can be found in Figure 1B.

There were several reasons for the conversion from extended-infusion meropenem to meropenem 500 mg IV q6h after the meropenem shortage lifted. First, meropenem 500 mg IV q6h (0.5 hr infusion) had a high likelihood of achieving 40% $fT > MIC$ for the full range of MICs deemed susceptible by CLSI (Fig. 3C). Second, a growing amount of literature supported the AMCH Monte Carlo simulation results for meropenem 500 mg IV q6h. A Monte Carlo simulation by Kuti et al. noted that meropenem 500 mg q6h and meropenem 1g q8h achieved a similar percentage of $fT>MIC$ (13). The Monte Carlo simulation by Kays et al. also found similar probabilities of target attainment ($fT > MIC$ 50% or 70%) for meropenem 500 mg q6h and meropenem 1g q8h against clinical isolates of *P. aeruginosa* (42). Using data obtained from neutropenic patients, Ariano et al. also observed similar $fT > MIC$ between meropenem 500 mg q6h and meropenem 1000 mg q8h (43).

The third reason for the conversion to meropenem 500 mg IV q6h was the shorter infusion time (0.5 hr). Although the extended infusion method circumvented many of the practical limitations of the continuous-infusion methodology, it still required a dedicated line for a majority of the day. As previously discussed, the need for an intravenous line for the sole purpose of delivering antibiotics is associated with infection risk, and limits both patient mobility and nursing staff availability. Upon reviewing the Monte Carlo simulation data, the AMCH antibiotic subcommittee decided that the slightly higher probability of target attainment observed with extended-infusion meropenem did not merit these additional risks and logistical issues (Fig. 3C).

The fourth and final reason that factored into the decision-making process was the projected daily drug cost savings when compared to meropenem 1000 mg IV q8h (one less gram dose per day). When the drug acquisition costs were projected, the committees realized that reducing just 1g per day could save at least $40,000 per year. More importantly, there were clinical data available that suggested that meropenem 500 mg IV q6h was a suitable alternative to meropenem 1000 mg IV q8h. In an outcomes study by Kotapati et al., clinical and microbiologic successes were similar between patients who received meropenem

500 mg IV q6h group and meropenem 1000 mg IV q8h, while level one costs (drug-related costs) were reduced by $406 per patient in the meropenem 500 mg IV q6h arm (31). The outcomes of this revised meropenem dosing program are currently being assessed by AMCH researchers.

Cefepime

Using 67% $fT>MIC$ as the PD target (9,24), cefepime 1000 mg IV q6h as a 0.5-hr infusion was identified as an alternative to conventional cefepime dosing (Fig. 3C). Multiple extended infusion regimens were evaluated and all cefepime dosing schemes provided high probability of target attainment against the range of MICs deemed susceptible by CLSI. Cefepime 1000 mg IV q6h as a 0.5-hr infusion was adopted as the new dosing strategy for several reasons. First, it provided more robust probabilities of target attainment than conventional cefepime dosing (1000 mg IV q12h as a 0.5-hr infusion). Second, cefepime 1000 mg IV q6h had a similar probability of target attainment profile as maximal cefepime dosing (2000 mg IV q8h as a 0.5-hr infusion) but optimized $fT>MIC$ at two fewer grams per day. Given that drug acquisition cost of cefepime is approximately $12.50 per gram, the projected drug acquisition cost savings were considerable. Finally, cefepime 1000 mg IV q6h achieved the targeted $fT>MIC$ with less administration time per day than prolonged infusion and continuous infusion. Again, the use of prolonged infusion is only justifiable when the benefits outweigh the risks, and the antibiotic subcommittee decided that the slightly higher probability of target attainment observed with extended infusion cefepime did not merit the additional risks. The conversion from conventional cefepime dosing to cefepime 1000 mg IV q6h as a 0.5-hr infusion occurred in 2004, and research is underway to evaluate the outcomes of this program. We are unaware of any supporting clinical data from other institutions.

SUMMARY

These case studies demonstrate the power of mathematical modeling to develop new beta-lactam dosing strategies that optimize drug delivery, minimize costs, and maximize patient outcomes. At AMCH, these modeling techniques were used to devise new dosing schemes for piperacillin/tazobactam, meropenem, and cefepime. Even though PD simulations cannot replace well-controlled clinical studies, they can be used to assess the viability of a new agent or dosing method. They can also be used to compare antimicrobials to each other or to other published data. Clinical outcomes should be conducted to validate the model predictions.

REFERENCES

1. Ebert SC, Craig WA. Pharmacodynamic properties of antibiotics: application to drug monitoring and dosage regimen design. Infect Control Hosp Epidemiol 1990; 11:319–26.
2. Drusano GL. Antimicrobial pharmacodynamics: critical interactions of "bug and drug." Nat Rev Microbiol 2004; 2:289–300.
3. Craig WA. Pharmacokinetic/pharmacodynamic parameters: rationale for antibacterial dosing of mice and men. Clin Infect Dis 1998; 26:1–10; quiz 11–2.
4. Drusano GL, Preston SL, Fowler C, Corrado M, Weisinger B, Kahn J. Relationship between fluoroquinolone area under the curve: minimum inhibitory concentration ratio

and the probability of eradication of the infecting pathogen, in patients with nosocomial pneumonia. J Infect Dis 2004; 189:1590–7.

5. Craig WA, Andes D. Pharmacokinetics and pharmacodynamics of antibiotics in otitis media. Pediatr Infect Dis J 1996; 15:255–9.

6. Craig WA. Interrelationship between pharmacokinetics and pharmacodynamics in determining dosage regimens for broad-spectrum cephalosporins. Diagn Microbiol Infect Dis 1995; 22:89–96.

7. Leggett JE, Fantin B, Ebert S, et al. Comparative antibiotic dose–effect relations at several dosing intervals in murine pneumonitis and thigh-infection models. J Infect Dis 1989; 159:281–92.

8. Leggett JE, Ebert S, Fantin B, Craig WA. Comparative dose–effect relations at several dosing intervals for beta-lactam, aminoglycoside and quinolone antibiotics against Gram-negative bacilli in murine thigh-infection and pneumonitis models. Scand J Infect Dis Suppl 1990; 74:179–84.

9. Tam VH, McKinnon PS, Akins RL, Rybak MJ, Drusano GL. Pharmacodynamics of cefepime in patients with Gram-negative infections. J Antimicrob Chemother 2002; 50:425–8.

10. Kashuba AD, Nafziger AN, Drusano GL, Bertino Jr JS. Optimizing aminoglycoside therapy for nosocomial pneumonia caused by Gram-negative bacteria. Antimicrob Agent Chemother 1999; 43:623–9.

11. Preston SL, Drusano GL, Berman AL, et al. Pharmacodynamics of levofloxacin: a new paradigm for early clinical trials. JAMA 1998; 279:125–9.

12. Kirby WN. Bacteriostatic and lytic actions of penicillins on sensitive and resistant staphylococci. J Clin Invest 1945; 24:165–9.

13. Kuti JL, Dandekar PK, Nightingale CH, Nicolau DP. Use of Monte Carlo simulation to design an optimized pharmacodynamic dosing strategy for meropenem. J Clin Pharmacol 2003; 43:1116–23.

14. Kuti JL, Nightingale CH, Nicolau DP. Optimizing pharmacodynamic target attainment using the MYSTIC antibiogram: data collected in North America in 2002. Antimicrob Agents Chemother 2004; 48:2464–70.

15. Kuti JL, Florea NR, Nightingale CH, Nicolau DP. Pharmacodynamics of meropenem and imipenem against Enterobacteriaceae, *Acinetobacter baumannii*, and *Pseudomonas aeruginosa*. Pharmacotherapy 2004; 24:8–15.

16. Lodise Jr TP, Lomaestro B, Rodvold KA, Danziger LH, Drusano GL. Pharmacodynamic profiling of piperacillin in the presence of tazobactam in patients through the use of population pharmacokinetic models and Monte Carlo simulation. Antimicrob Agent Chemother 2004; 48:4718–24.

17. Lomaestro BM, Drusano GL. Pharmacodynamic evaluation of extending the administration time of meropenem using a Monte Carlo simulation. Antimicrob Agent Chemother 2005; 49:461–3.

18. Tam VH, Louie A, Lomaestro BM, Drusano GL. Integration of population pharmacokinetics, a pharmacodynamic target, and microbiologic surveillance data to generate a rational empiric dosing strategy for cefepime against *Pseudomonas aeruginosa*. Pharmacotherapy 2003; 23:291–5.

19. Drusano GL, D'Argenio DZ, Preston SL, et al. Use of drug effect interaction modeling with Monte Carlo simulation to examine the impact of dosing interval on the projected antiviral activity of the combination of abacavir and amprenavir. Antimicrob Agents Chemother 2000; 44:1655–9.

20. Drusano GL, Preston SL, Hardalo C, et al. Use of preclinical data for selection of a phase II/III dose for evernimicin and identification of a preclinical MIC breakpoint. Antimicrob Agent Chemother 2001; 45:13–22.

21. Drusano GL, Moore KH, Kleim JP, Prince W, Bye A. Rational dose selection for a nonnucleoside reverse transcriptase inhibitor through use of population pharmacokinetic modeling and Monte Carlo simulation. Antimicrob Agent Chemother 2002; 46:913–6.

22. Drusano GL. Prevention of resistance: a goal for dose selection for antimicrobial agents. Clin Infect Dis 2003; 36:S42–50.

23. Lomaestro BM, Drusano GL. Pharmacodynamic evaluation of extending the infusion time of piperacillin/tazobactam doses using Monte Carlo Analysis. 41st Annual Interscience Conference on Antimicrobial Agents and Chemotherapy 2002; Abstract A-2190.

24. Tam VH, McKinnon PS, Akins RL, Drusano GL, Rybak MJ. Pharmacokinetics and pharmacodynamics of cefepime in patients with various degrees of renal function. Antimicrob Agent Chemother 2003; 47:1853–61.

25. Tam VH, Preston SL, Drusano GL. Comparative pharmacokinetic analysis by standard two-stage method versus nonparametric population modeling. Pharmacotherapy 2003; 23:1545–9.

26. Drusano GL, Preston SL, Gotfried MH, Danziger LH, Rodvold KA. Levofloxacin penetration into epithelial lining fluid as determined by population pharmacokinetic modeling and Monte Carlo simulation. Antimicrob Agents Chemother 2002; 46:586–9.

27. Krueger WA, Bulitta J, Kinzig-Schippers M, et al. Evaluation by Monte Carlo simulation of the pharmacokinetics of two doses of meropenem administered intermittently or as a continuous infusion in healthy volunteers. Antimicrob Agent Chemother 2005; 49:1881–9.

28. Dudley MN, Ambrose PG. Monte Carlo PK-PK simulation and new cefotaxime, ceftriaxone, and cefipime susceptibility breakpoints for S. pneumoniae, including strains with reduced susceptibility to penicillin. 42nd Annual Interscience Conference on Antimicrobial Agents and Chemotherapy, San Diego, California 2002; Abstract A-1263.

29. Owens Jr RC, Bhavnani SM, Ambrose PG. Assessment of pharmacokinetic-pharmacodynamic target attainment of gemifloxacin against Streptococcus pneumoniae. Diagn Microbiol Infect Dis 2005; 51:45–9.

30. Grant EM, Kuti JL, Nicolau DP, Nightingale C, Quintiliani R. Clinical efficacy and pharmacoeconomics of a continuous-infusion piperacillin-tazobactam program in a large community teaching hospital. Pharmacotherapy 2002; 22:471–83.

31. Kotapati S, Nicolau DP, Nightingale CH, Kuti JL. Clinical and economic benefits of a meropenem dosage strategy based on pharmacodynamic concepts. Am J Health Syst Pharm 2004; 61:1264–70.

32. Visser LG, Arnouts P, van Furth R, Mattie H, van den Broek PJ. Clinical pharmacokinetics of continuous intravenous administration of penicillins. Clin Infect Dis 1993; 17:491–5.

33. Craig WA, Ebert SC. Continuous infusion of beta-lactam antibiotics. Antimicrob Agent Chemother 1992; 36:2577–83.

34. Drusano GL. How does a patient maximally benefit from anti-infective chemotherapy? Clin Infect Dis 2004; 39:1245–6.

35. Strayer AH, Gilbert DH, Pivarnik P, Medeiros AA, Zinner SH, Dudley MN. Pharmacodynamics of piperacillin alone and in combination with tazobactam against piperacillin-resistant and -susceptible organisms in an in vitro model of infection. Antimicrob Agent Chemother 1994; 38:2351–6.

36. Lodise TP, Lomaestro BM, Drusano GL. Piperacillin/Tazobactam for Pseudomonas aeruginosa infections: clinical implications of an extended infusion dosing strategy. Clin Infect Dis, in press.

37. Garner JS, Jarvis WR, Emori TG, Horan TC, Hughes JM. CDC definitions for nosocomial infections, 1988. Am J Infect Control 1988; 16:128–40.

38. Mohr JF, Wanger A, Rex JH. Pharmacokinetic/pharmacodynamic modeling can help guide targeted antimicrobial therapy for nosocomial Gram-negative infections in critically ill patients. Diagn Microbiol Infect Dis 2004; 48:125–30.

39. Micek ST, Lloyd AE, Ritchie DJ, Reichley RM, Fraser VJ, Kollef MH. Pseudomonas aeruginosa bloodstream infection: importance of appropriate initial antimicrobial treatment. Antimicrob Agent Chemother 2005; 49:1306–11.

40. Streit JM, Jones RN, Sader HS, Fritsche TR. Assessment of pathogen occurrences and resistance profiles among infected patients in the intensive care unit: report from the SENTRY Antimicrobial Surveillance Program (North America, 2001). Int J Antimicrob Agents 2004; 24:111–8.

41. Rhomberg PR, Jones RN, Sader HS. Results from the Meropenem Yearly Susceptibility Test Information Collection (MYSTIC) Programme: report of the 2001 data from 15 United States medical centres. Int J Antimicrob Agents 2004; 23:52–9.
42. Kays MB, Burgess DS, Denys GA. Pharmacodynamic evaluation of six beta-lactams against recent clinical isolates of *Pseudomonas aeruginosa* using Monte Carlo analysis. 42nd Annual Interscience Conference on Antimicrobial Agents and Chemotherapy, San Diego, CA, 2002; Abstract A-642.
43. Ariano RE, Nyhlen A, Donnelly JP, Sitar DS, Harding GK, Zelenitsky SA. Pharmacokinetics and pharmacodynamics of meropenem in febrile neutropenic patients with bacteremia. Ann Pharmacother 2005; 39:32–8.

18 Shorter Course Antibiotic Therapy (SCAT): Principles, Current Data, and Caveats

Donald E. Craven, Daniel P. McQuillen, and Winnie W. Ooi
Department of Infectious Diseases, Lahey Clinic Medical Center, Burlington, Massachusetts and Tufts University School of Medicine, Boston, Massachusetts, U.S.A.

George A. Jacoby
Department of Infectious Diseases, Lahey Clinic Medical Center, Burlington, Massachusetts and Harvard Medical School, Boston, Massachusetts, U.S.A.

Efren L. Rael
Department of Medicine, Lahey Clinic Medical Center, Burlington, Massachusetts, U.S.A.

Kathleen Steger Craven
Consultant in Infectious Diseases and Public Health, Wellesley, Massachusetts, U.S.A.

> *Clinical medicine seems to consist of a few things we think we know and lots of things we don't know.*
>
> C. D. Naylor (1)

INTRODUCTION

The population in the United States in the 21st century is at greater risk for infections due to increased longevity coupled with more chronic underlying diseases, aggressive medical and surgical procedures, solid organ transplantation, immunosuppressive therapy, and a highly mobile modern society. The current population is also at greater risk of infection from obesity, diabetes mellitus, and cardiovascular diseases. Therapies for various diseases may include antibiotics, steroids, chemotherapy, and a spectrum of monoclonal immune modulators that may increase colonization with antibiotic-resistant bacteria or alter the host immune system. As the result of these pressures, there have been well-documented increases in infections caused by multidrug-resistant (MDR) pathogens both in the community and healthcare settings (2). Some of the more common MDR pathogens include methicillin-resistant *Staphylococcus aureus* (MRSA), *Streptococcus pneumoniae*, extended-spectrum beta-lactamase-positive (ESBL+) *Klebsiella pneumoniae*, *Pseudomonas aeruginosa*, and vancomycin-resistant *Enterococcus faecalis* (VRE). The widespread use and frequent misuse of antibiotics provide persistent selection pressure for expansion and transmission of MDR pathogens both within and outside of healthcare settings (3–5).

Prevention strategies for reducing antibiotic resistance and improving patient outcomes should focus on reducing inappropriate initiation of antibiotics as well as on using shorter course antibiotic therapy (SCAT) (6). Significant progress has been made in our understanding of SCAT for treating outpatient infections such as sexually transmitted diseases (STDs), urinary tract infections (UTIs), surgical prophylaxis, and selected gastrointestinal and respiratory tract infections (6). Perhaps the best example of the success of SCAT has been the use of combination therapy regimens containing rifampin for the treatment of *Mycobacterium tuberculosis* (TB). The length of treatment for TB in immunocompetent individuals has decreased from 18 to 24 months to 4 to 6 months and also has included the use of directly observed therapy (DOT) administered three times per week. These changes underscore the importance and impact of SCAT for improving quality of life, adherence, and reducing the plague of MDR disease pathogens, toxicity, and cost (Fig. 1) (7,8). Although sufficient data supporting the use of SCAT for many other infectious diseases or for defining populations that would be most likely to benefit from SCAT is lacking, there is potential to save enormous resources, reduce healthcare costs, and improve clinical outcomes. The lack of compelling data to support SCAT is related, in part, to a lack of funds to support randomized clinical trials. Unfortunately, pharmaceutical companies may lack the incentives to support the conduct of such trials, but perhaps a federal-government administered and pharmaceutical-supported collaborative group, similar to the AIDS clinical trials group (ACTG) model should be established to evaluate a broader spectrum of optimal infectious disease management. Important considerations regarding the use of SCAT include host variables, the specific pathogen(s), site and type of infection, antibiotic pharmacokinetics, and antibiotic sensitivity of the infecting organism(s) (Fig. 2). Effective use of SCAT should decrease the number and amount of antibiotics prescribed, improve outcomes, particularly in terms of better adherence, and reduce adverse effects, complications, and selection of antibiotic-resistant pathogens (Table 1). SCAT also provides enormous economic benefits related to reduced costs for drug acquisition and administration and fewer office visits for laboratory tests and treatments for adverse events, and reduced complications secondary to more prolonged antibiotic use. Potential disadvantages of SCAT may include reduced treatment efficacy related to incomplete therapy that could result in complications and prolonged carriage or potential transmission of the pathogen (9).

This chapter provides an overview of the background and available evidence for the use of SCAT for selected infectious diseases. Our primary focus is the use of SCAT in adults with bacteremia, genitourinary, gastrointestinal, and respiratory tract infections acquired in both the community and healthcare settings. A summary of key points with references is included at the end of each section.

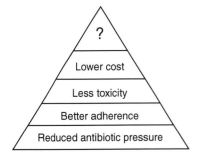

FIGURE 1 Advantages of shorter course antimicrobial therapy (SCAT) are numerous. These advantages must be balanced by the potential disadvantages of complications related to untreated infection, the possibility of prolonged carriage, or colonization with the potential spread to others.

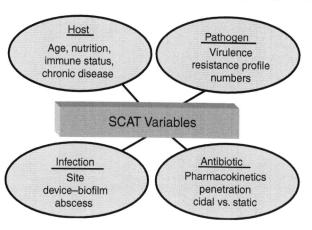

FIGURE 2 Considerations for the use of shorter course antimicrobial therapy (SCAT) involve host factors, specific type and extent of the infection, the infecting pathogen, and the characteristics and efficacy of the antimicrobial agent prescribed.

BACKGROUND ISSUES

Since antibiotics were first introduced nearly 70 years ago, there have been a number of antimicrobial agents developed to inhibit or kill bacteria causing human infections. Sulfonamides were the first modern antimicrobials used, but it was Fleming's observation that a mold (penicillin) could inhibit bacterial growth, that ushered in the antibiotic era that is such an integral part of modern medicine. The use of penicillin and other antibiotics has had an enormous effect on reducing patient morbidity and mortality, but these successes have been countered, in part, by the widespread misuse of antimicrobial agents, resulting in the sustained emergence of MDR bacteria. It is estimated that 40% to 50% of antibiotic use in hospitals is inappropriate in terms of timing, indications, and proper dosing (10,11). Solutions to this problem include wiser and more effective use and monitoring of antibiotics, coupled with better primary and secondary prevention strategies (12,13).

Strategies to Reduce Antibiotic Use

Appropriate antibiotic therapy should target bacterial pathogens rather than viruses, treating individuals who are symptomatic or have evidence of infection rather than those with colonization, streamlining, or de-escalating antibiotic therapy when possible, and discontinuing antibiotics in patients with undocumented infection (14,15). Implementing such strategies will require better education of healthcare providers and consumers about the risks of antibiotic misuse, along

TABLE 1   General Principles of Antibiotic Therapy and for the Use of Shorter-Course Antibiotic Therapy (SCAT)

Identify the site of infection, pathogen, and the antibiotic sensitivity pattern
Evaluate host factors: age, pregnancy, drug allergies, renal, hepatic, and immune status
Assess antibiotic dose, route, synergy, antagonism, pharmacokinetics, drug interactions, and adverse events
Assess the patient's response to therapy and need to alter, streamline, or stop antibiotic therapy
Assess for SCAT as recommended in guidelines and follow patient for relapse, reinfection, or complications

with more effective systems to monitor and control antibiotic use. Use of a computerized pharmacy surveillance system or the use of targeted surveillance by pharmacists have also been cost-effective intervention strategies (16).

Antibiotic Pharmacokinetics and Pharmacodynamics
An understanding of antibiotic pharmacokinetics and pharmacodynamics is critical, but these processes are complicated and may vary among classes of antibiotics and individual agents within the class. Pharmacokinetics refer to the serum and tissue levels of antibiotics, whereas pharmacodynamics refer to the antibiotics' abilities to inhibit and or kill bacterial pathogens (17,18). Pharmacodynamic properties of specific antibiotics should be considered in selecting an optimal dosing regimen. For example, while some antibiotics penetrate well and achieve high local concentrations at specific sites, others do not. Many antibiotics do not achieve therapeutic levels in specific tissues, like the prostate (ampicillin and cephalosporins), the lung (daptomycin), or the central nervous system (first- and second-generation cephalosporins), despite being reported as "sensitive" by in vitro laboratory testing. Also, most beta-lactam antibiotics achieve less than 50% of their serum concentration in the lung, but fluoroquinolones, macrolides, and oxazolazidones, such as linezolid, equal or exceed their serum concentration in bronchial secretions. Penicillins, sulfonamides, and most cephalosporins achieve high concentrations in the urine while other antibiotics, such as ceftriaxone, or the macrolides and linezolid, which are detoxified in the liver, may be excreted into the bile and gastrointestinal tract.

Antimicrobials may be bactericidal (kill bacteria) or bacteriostatic (inhibit growth, but do not kill) microorganisms (17,18). These differences may be important for treating selected infections, such as endocarditis, which requires bactericidal antibiotics, but are less important for urinary or respiratory tract infections for which host defenses play a greater role. Even among bactericidal agents, several mechanisms of killing can be present. For example, agents such as the aminoglycosides and quinolones are bactericidal in a concentration-dependent fashion, defined as killing more rapidly at higher concentrations. By comparison, vancomycin and the beta-lactams kill in a time-dependent fashion, defined as the time above the organism's minimal inhibitory concentration (MIC). Other antibiotics also have a postantibiotic effect (PAE), in which they are able to suppress bacterial growth even after the antibiotic level falls below the MIC of the organism. With Gram-negative bacilli, a prolonged PAE occurs with the use of aminoglycosides and quinolones, and a limited effect is seen with beta-lactam antibiotics, excluding the carbapenems (imipenem or meropenem). Therefore, beta-lactam antibiotics (penicillins, cephalosporins) are most effective when levels remain above the MIC of the infecting organism for as long as possible, while quinolones and aminoglycosides can be dosed less frequently due to a prolonged PAE (17,18).

Emergence of MDR Pathogens
In the past decade, there has been a notable escalation of infections due to MDR strains in the community and healthcare institutions (2,19). Examples of MDR Gram-negative bacilli include *K. pneumoniae* and *Escherichia coli* with ESBL+, *P. aeruginosa* and *Acinetobacter baumannii* (4,20). There has also been a rapid increase in infections due to MDR Gram-positive cocci, such as *S. pneumoniae*,

community-acquired (CA) and healthcare-associated (HA) MRSA, and vancomycin-resistant strains, such as VRE and *S. aureus* with intermediate resistance (VISA) or a smaller number of isolates that have high resistance (VRSA) (2).

Infections due to MDR pathogens may delay early initiation of appropriate antibiotic therapy, often increasing patient morbidity and mortality, and result in higher healthcare costs related to complications and increased length of hospital stay (4). MDR pathogens are more commonly isolated from patients with: chronic diseases, immunosuppression, prior antibiotic therapy, prior hospitalization, intensive care stay, or long-term healthcare facility admissions (4). Many of these patients are merely colonized with MDR bacteria and thus may be a reservoir for transmission to others, but have no evidence of infection. Antibiotic use increases the selection pressure for growth and spread of MDR pathogens by increasing the numbers of organisms, colonization, and environmental contamination (3). More recently, these concerns have been compounded by rapid emergence and spread of community-acquired MDR infections caused by *S. pneumoniae* and MRSA (21,22).

In Vitro Vs. In Vivo or Clinical Resistance

There has been a continued emergence of antibiotic resistance among numerous bacteria, mycobacteria, viruses, fungi, and parasites. Many bacterial resistance studies have focused primarily on trends toward greater in vitro resistance among different species of bacteria. In vitro or laboratory-related antibiotic sensitivities, as measured by MIC, represents the concentration of antibiotic required to prevent the growth of a selected inoculum of bacteria in a test tube or on an agar plate. The MIC thus represents the concentration of antibiotic that should be present for treating bacteremia, and does not account for penetration of the antibiotic into tissues, such as the central nervous system, lung, prostate, or bone (23). It is important to emphasize that such in vitro data may not be applicable to infections involving invasive devices, such as central venous or urinary catheters or endotracheal tubes that may have bacteria embedded in biofilm, impairing antibiotic penetration or reducing bacterial killing by phagocytic cells, antibodies, and complement (24).

UPPER RESPIRATORY TRACT INFECTIONS
Tonsillopharyngitis

Group A streptococcus (GAS) is the most common cause of tonsillopharyngitis requiring antibiotic therapy (25). GAS is associated with both suppurative and nonsuppurative complications (26). Suppurative complications include local cellulitis, abscess formation, myositis, fasciitis, otitis media, and sinusitis. Nonsuppurative complications include rheumatic fever, streptococcal toxic shock syndrome, and glomerulonephritis. Prevention of acute rheumatic fever is the principle goal of treatment, but antibiotic therapy also reduces severity and duration of symptoms, shortens the infective period, and reduces suppurative complications.

The literature on SCAT for tonsillopharyngitis is difficult to interpret, due to differences in study design, adherence issues, and inconsistent endpoints. Poor adherence to a 10-day regimen is probably the most common cause for treatment failure (27). In addition, the long-term sequelae of GAS infections remain of great concern.

Penicillin

The American Heart Association (AHA) and the Infectious Diseases Society of America (IDSA) recommend treatment with penicillin for 10 days, which has been the "gold standard" since 1951 (28). However, failure rates of 10% to 25% have been reported, due in part to poor adherence (27). Symptomatic improvement is often achieved within 24 to 48 hr after initiating therapy, which often results in the patient not completing the course of therapy or perhaps saving the medication for a future infection.

Early studies by Wannamaker in military recruits suggested that treatment of GAS tonsillopharyngitis with intramuscular benzathine penicillin had a higher eradication rate than patients who were treated with oral penicillin for longer periods (29,30). Schwartz and coworkers compared patients treated with 7 versus 10 days of oral penicillin V every 8 hr and concluded that 10 days was preferable because of higher bacterial eradication rates (31). Gerber and coworkers compared patients treated with penicillin V for 5 versus 10 days in a randomized, controlled trial. Patients in the two treatment groups were comparable with respect to clinical findings, compliance, and serologic response to GAS, but the same serotype of GAS was later identified in 18% of the 73 patients treated for 5 days versus 6% of the 99 patients treated for 10 days, suggesting persistent carriage of GAS (32). In general, results of SCAT therapy for GAS tonsillopharyngitis with oral penicillins other than amoxicillin have been disappointing. The use of a single injection of intramuscular benzathine penicillin G is recommended for patients who are unlikely to complete a 10-day course of therapy.

Cephalosporins

In contrast to the experience with penicillin, several studies of tonsillopharyngitis with cephalosporins given orally for 4 to 7 days had similar outcomes and were more effective eradicating GAS than 10 days of therapy with oral penicillins, but none of these studies examined the impact on preventing rheumatic fever (28,33).

Two recent large-scale European trials of 4782 culture-proven cases of GAS pharyngitis compared 10-days of penicillin versus SCAT with 5 days of treatment with one of six different antibiotic regimens (amoxicillin/clavulanate, ceftibuten, cefuroxime axetil, loracarbef, clarithromycin, or erythromycin estolate) (34). Bacteriologic eradication and clinical success rates were equivalent, but there were three cases of rheumatic fever and one of acute glomerulonephritis in the SCAT group versus one patient with acute glomerulonephritis in the 10-day group.

A meta-analysis of 19 studies concluded that although oral cephalosporins were at least as effective as penicillin for eradicating GAS, because of cost and the potential risk of poststreptococcal sequelae, 10-days of oral penicillin V should remain the treatment of choice (26).

Macrolides

Macrolide therapy has been recommended for patients who are allergic to penicillin. Macrolides, such as clarithromycin and azithromycin, appear to be more effective in eradicating GAS than penicillin, but have been associated with higher rates of antibiotic resistance, resulting in higher failure rates (22% for macrolides vs. 6% for penicillin) (35). SCAT with azithromycin administered for 3 days at a dose of 10 mg/kg has produced unacceptably low clinical responses (<80% in 2 of 5 studies) and bacteriologic cures (80% in 4/5 studies) (28). However, Casey and

Pichichero reported a recent meta-analysis of SCAT in patients treated with 3 or 5 days of azithromycin versus 10 days for a comparator antibiotic. Children treated with azithromycin had statistically significant better outcomes (clinical cure and bacterial eradication rates) than a comparator drug administered for 10 days. Bacteriologic failures were reduced fivefold in the high-dose SCAT group. Three-day regimens of azithromycin (500 mg/day) demonstrated a trend over the 10-day comparator group, but the use of 5 days of azithromycin demonstrated the best result. In adults, azithromycin dosed at 10 mg/kg/day for 3 days was equivalent to the 10-day comparator in terms of bacteriologic cure rate while the 5-day "Z-pak" (500 mg orally followed by 250 mg/day for 4 days) was significantly inferior to the 10-day comparator. These data underscore the importance of weight-based dosing of azithromycin for the treatment of GAS tonsillopharyngitis in children, but these data cannot be extrapolated to adults, especially in the presence of increasing rates of macrolide resistance in the United States and Europe (25).

Key Points:

- AHA, IDSA, and other organizations recommend 10 days of penicillin V for tonsillopharyngitis. The increased cost of other regimens (cephalosporins and macrolides) also favors the use of penicillin. Single-dose intramuscular therapy with benzathine penicillin is also highly effective (26).
- Poor adherence with 10 days of antibiotic therapy is one of the major causes of treatment failure of GAS tonsillopharyngitis. SCAT with cephalosporins may be an alternative for patients with a penicillin allergy. Higher doses of azithromycin (60 mg/kg) given for 5 days in children appear superior to a comparator regimen given for 10 days. Such a program would be an acceptable alternative for individuals allergic to penicillin (25). Unfortunately, the increased rates of macrolide resistance may limit such use.
- Two recent large-scale European trials of 4782 culture-proven cases of GAS pharyngitis compared 10 days of penicillin versus SCAT with 5 days of six different antibiotic regimens (amoxicillin/clavulanate, ceftibuten, cefuroxime axetil, loracarbef, clarithromycin, and erythromycin estolate). Bacteriologic eradication and clinical success rates were equivalent, but there were three cases of rheumatic fever and one patient with acute glomerulonephritis in the SCAT group versus one patient with glomerulonephritis in the 10-day group, raising concern (34).

Acute Sinusitis

Acute bacterial rhinosinusitis is a common upper respiratory tract infection, with more than 20 million cases reported annually in the United States (6). Many of these infections are associated with viral illnesses that are occasionally complicated by bacterial superinfection. Data suggest that only about 2% of patients with viral sinusitis develop clinically significant bacterial superinfection.

Common presenting signs and symptoms include facial pain, headache, nasal discharge, and fever. It is generally believed that patients with acute symptoms (<7 days) are unlikely to have bacterial infection. Distinguishing between viral and bacterial etiologies and the ability to isolate a specific pathogen are difficult.

Acute bacterial sinusitis is often caused by pneumococci, *Haemophilus* spp., or *S. aureus*, and many infections are mixed. Chronic infections also may be caused by *S. aureus*, anaerobic bacteria, or aerobic Gram-negative bacilli. Frequent antibiotic exposure increases the risk of MDR pathogens, anaerobic bacteria, and opportunistic pathogens. The specific antibiotics prescribed should be based on the prevalence of antibiotic resistant organisms and prior antibiotic use within the past 3 to 6 months.

Optimal duration of therapy for acute bacterial sinusitis has not been well-defined, but most textbooks recommend a 7- to 14-day course (6,28). Problems include the uncertainty of diagnosis using clinical assessment, radiography, ultrasound or computerized tomography, and difficulty differentiating bacterial sinusitis from viral or allergic rhinitis. In addition, most studies have involved acute maxillary sinusitis and it is not clear that these data can be applied to frontal, ethmoid, and sphenoid sinusitis.

Studies of Acute Maxillary Sinusitis in Adults

At least four studies have examined SCAT for the treatment of acute maxillary sinusitis in adults (36). Williams and coworkers carried out a randomized trial of 80 adults with acute maxillary sinusitis treated with 3 versus 10 days of trimethoprim-sulfamethoxazole (TMP-SMX) and reported 76% cure rates and bacteriologic eradication in both groups. The authors concluded that afebrile, immunocompetent adults could receive a 3-day course of TMP-SMX. Nonresponders should be re-evaluated and treated for 10 days (36). Casiano and coworkers performed a study of acute maxillary sinusitis in 78 adults treated with azithromycin 500 mg on day 1 followed by 4 days of 250 mg compared to those with amoxicillin 500 mg three times daily for 10 days (37). Clinical diagnosis was confirmed by transantral maxillary sinus aspiration. Bacteriologic cure was reported as 100% in each group and clinical cure was 74% and 73%, respectively. Khong and coworkers evaluated 386 patients randomized to cefpodoxime proxetil for 5 days versus amoxicillin/clavulanic acid for 8 days (38). Clinical cure rates were 83% and 86%, respectively.

Guidelines from the Sinus and Allergy Health Partnership suggest stratifying patients by severity of disease, rate of progression, and prior treatment with antibiotics (39). Traditionally, the duration of therapy for acute bacterial rhinosinusitis has been 7 to 14 days. In the controlled studies discussed, SCAT for fewer than 7 days was equivalent to longer courses. Risk factors for failure in the SCAT group included a history of more than 4 episodes of sinusitis over a 2-year period and a history of surgical drainage. Longer treatment courses may be beneficial for these groups and non-responders to initial therapy.

Key Points:

■ Data suggest that optimal therapy for acute sinusitis has not been well defined, but most textbooks recommend 7 to 14 days. The Guidelines from the Sinus and Allergy Health Partnership suggest stratifying patients by severity of disease, rate of progression, and recent antibiotic and local resistance data (6).

■ Four studies have examined SCAT for 3 versus 10 days for acute maxillary sinusitis in adults (42–45). The data suggest that afebrile, immunocompetent adults could receive a 3-day course of TMX-SMX but that nonresponders should be re-evaluated and treated for 10 days (6).

- Longer courses of antibiotic therapy may be needed in nonresponders and those with multiple recurrences (6).

LOWER RESPIRATORY TRACT INFECTIONS
Exacerbation of COPD and Bronchitis
Most of the bacterial species isolated from sputum during acute exacerbations of chronic obstructive pulmonary disease (AE-COPD) colonize the oral cavity or nasopharynx, and approximately 25% of patients with stable COPD have lower airway bacterial colonization, which may increase to 50% during an exacerbation (40,41). AE-COPD is common in these patients and appears to result in greater morbidity and mortality (28,42). Benefits of antibiotic therapy have been shown in several randomized trials as well as by meta-analysis. The etiologic agents are often *Haemophilus influenzae, S. pneumoniae*, and *Moraxella catarrhalis*, but atypical pathogens and viruses also play a role. About half of the exacerbations yield positive sputum cultures with higher bacterial counts, and rates of infection are increased when the sputum is purulent. Bacteria are associated with airway inflammation in both the stable state and with AE-COPD, but it is not clear if there is a cause and effect relationship or if the bacteria are "along for the ride" and taking advantage of mucosal damage (41). Recent observations in a longitudinal study by Murphy and coworkers suggest that AE-COPD by *M. catarrhalis* appears to be related to the acquisition of a new strain that was not recognized by the immune system, resulting in greater inflammation. In addition, the exacerbation-associated strain of *M. catarrhalis* generated a systemic antibody response, suggesting a causative role in the exacerbation (43). Of course, AE-COPD is very complex and may also be due to differences in airway colonization factors, host immune responses to different bacterial species, or coinfection with viruses and/or atypical pathogens.

There are a number of problems with the clinical trials of AE-COPD, including lack of comparisons to placebo, the concurrent use of different corticosteroid regimens, lack of clear documentation of the etiologic agent, the emergence of antibiotic-resistant or MDR pathogens, variable time to recurrence, and lack of data on long-term outcomes. The duration of therapy for AE-COPD has varied from 10 to 14 days to the more recent use of 7 days or less. Most studies have compared different antibiotics in patients treated more or less than 7 days.

In a series of studies conducted from 1988 to 2001, the clinical and bacteriologic efficacy for antibiotics given for 3 to 5 days compared to 8 to 14 days was essentially equivalent (Table 2) (28). Quinolones and macrolides are frequently prescribed because of their spectrum of activity against pneumococci, *H. influenzae*, and atypical pathogens. These agents also have favorable pharmacokinetics and achieve high concentrations in lung tissue. The anti-inflammatory effect of macrolides may also be beneficial, and azithromycin, in particular, has a long half-life that is ideal for SCAT. Thus, shorter courses of quinolones (5 days) and perhaps azithromycin for 3 days appear to have equivalent efficacy and benefits when compared to 10- to 14-day courses for treatment of AE-COPD with other comparators (28,44–46).

Key Points:

- AE-COPD is a complex disease process involving several different pathogens. There are a number of problems with the clinical trials for AE-COPD,

TABLE 2 Selected Studies of SCAT for Acute Bacterial Exacerbations of Chronic Bronchitis

Guay study number	Drug regimens	No. of patients	Clinical response (% cure/improvement)
1	Amoxicillin 3d	41	85
	Amoxicillin 7d		86
2	Cefdinir 5d	281	80
	Cefprozil 10d		72
3	Cefixime 5d	160	91
	Cefixime 10d		89
4	Levofloxacin 5d	482	91
	Levofloxacin 7d		88
5	Moxifloxacin 5d	512	96
	Amox/Clav 7d		92
6	Moxifloxacin 5d	855	95
	Moxifloxacin 10d		95
	Clarithromycin 10d		94
7	Gemifloxacin 5d	709	80
	Clarithromycin 7d		78
8	Dirithromycin 5d	321	95
	Amox/Clav 7–10d		93
9	Dirithromycin 5d	191	90
	Clarithromycin 7d		95
10	Dirithromycin 5d	80	90
	Azithromycin 3d		93
11	Azithromycin 3d	120	98
	Amox/Clav 10d		89
12	Azithromycin 3d	137	96
	Amox/Clav 5–10d		80
13	Azithromycin 3d	138	95
	Clarithromycin 10d		97

Note: There are little differences in clinical response rates reported for the different antibiotic regimens studied.
Abbreviations: Amox, amoxicillin; Clav, clavulanic acid; SCAT, shorter-course antibiotic therapy.
Source: From Ref. 28.

including lack of comparisons to placebo, the concurrent use of different corticosteroid regimens and lack of clear documentation of the etiologic agent, the increase in antibiotic-resistant or MDR pathogens, high rates of recurrent infection, and the need for better data on long-term outcomes.

- Accumulating evidence supports the use of Food and Drug Administration (FDA)-approved SCAT for adults with AE-CB, (≤5 days for most agents and ≤3 days for azithromycin) as an alternative to 7 to 14 days of therapy with amoxicillin, TMP-SMX, cephalosporins, fluoroquinolones, ketolides, and macrolides. Clearly, better placebo-controlled, double-blind trials using standardized doses of corticosteroids are needed.

Community-Acquired Pneumonia (CAP)

CAP results in more than 10 million visits to physicians, 64 million days of limited activity, and more than 600,000 hospitalizations annually in the United States (47,48). Most patients with CAP are treated as outpatients with oral antibiotics. This group has a mortality of about 1%, which is a considerably better prognosis than for the elderly or for those who are admitted to the hospital or the intensive care unit for whom mortality rates may range from 12% to 29%. CAP is a major cause of morbidity and mortality (47,48). Mild infections can be managed in the community with oral antibiotics. Patients with more serious infections, as manifest by the pulmonary severity index, may require hospitalization and treatment with intravenous antibiotics or admission to a critical care unit with assisted ventilation.

There is a wide spectrum of individuals with special risk factors and exposure to a variety of pathogens. *S. pneumoniae* is the most common bacterial pathogen isolated and other common bacterial pathogens include *H. influenzae*, *M. catarrhalis*, and *S. aureus*. There are also atypical pathogens that include *Legionella pneumophila*, *Chlamydia pneumoniae*, and *Mycoplasma pneumoniae*, which may occur alone or in combination with the more "typical" bacterial pathogens, listed above. Antibiotic and MDR pathogens of note include *S. pneumoniae* and more recently community-acquired MRSA (21,49). Unfortunately, no bacterial pathogen can be identified in 30% to 40% of CAP patients, impeding evaluation of clinical eradication and clinical efficacy difficult.

Guidelines for the Management of CAP were published by IDSA and the American Thoracic Society (ATS) in 2007 (48). Outpatient therapy for reasonably healthy adults includes doxycycline, an oral macrolide (azithromycin or clarithromycin), or a ketolide or a fluoroquinolone, such as levofloxacin, moxifloxacin, or gemifloxacin. By comparison, patients admitted to the hospital with CAP may be treated with either levofloxacin or ceftriaxone and azithromycin. Those patients admitted to the ICU should have their antibiotics expanded to include an antipseudomonal cephalosporin, carbapenem or beta-lactam–beta-lactamase inhibitor combination, plus vancomycin or linezolid, if MRSA is suspected.

Evidence for SCAT Therapy

In the era of evidence-based medicine, there are few studies that have examined the duration of therapy for CAP, and generally physicians have treated patients with CAP from 7 to 14 days for common bacterial pathogens and perhaps a bit longer for patients with atypical pathogens, such as *L. pneumophila*. SCAT may be possible and should be studied in patients with no underlying diseases who are currently treated as outpatients and those who are younger or have a prompt response to initial therapy.

A recent meta-analysis of CAP therapies for >7 versus ≤7 days reported no differences in mortality or bacteriological eradication and suggested that SCAT may reduce resistance costs and also increase adherence and tolerability (122).

Recently, Dunbar examined 528 patients with CAP who were randomized to therapy with levofloxacin 750 mg/day IV or PO for 5 days versus levofloxacin 500 mg/day IV or PO for 10 days (49,50). Patients with previous quinolone therapy, pneumonia acquired in the hospital, aspiration, pregnancy, HIV infection with a CD4 count <200/mL empyema, or need for a chest tube were excluded (50). Clinical efficacy was evaluated in 77% of the high-dose SCAT group versus 71% in the longer therapy group and microbiologic data were evaluated in 40% and 34% of each group, respectively. Clinical success rates were similar in each group (92% vs. 91%), but the higher-dose 5-day SCAT group had a significantly higher rate of defervescence by day 3 of therapy than the 10-day group treated with a 500 mg dose. Microbiologic eradication, relapse, and adverse events were similar in both groups for all pathogens.

Because levofloxacin is a concentration-dependent antibiotic in which therapeutic success is associated with the AUC/MIC and C_{max}/MIC, higher doses may be more effective in helping prevent resistance (49,50). Also, the mean epithelial lining fluid concentration was 9.9 µg/mL with the 500 mg low dose levofloxacin versus 22.1 µg/mL for the 750 mg group. Higher dose and SCAT for 5 days may also increase compliance and prevent the emergence of resistance. Higher doses of levofloxacin in this study were not associated with greater adverse effects than in the lower dose control group. Notably, the overall mortality rate was increased twofold in the longer course 500 mg group (3.4% vs. 1.9%), but the difference was not statistically significant.

Although the data presented by Dunbar and coworkers suggest that SCAT is effective, it is not clear if the results reflect the higher dose of levofloxacin or the shorter course of therapy. This could have been gleaned if a third group had been randomized to 500 mg daily for 5 days. Also, it would be interesting to determine if SCAT decreases the risk of colonization with MDR pathogens or lowers the risk of other complications, such as *Clostridium difficile* colitis. Clearly, all patients with CAP who are treated with SCAT should be carefully monitored for recurrence of infection or longer term complications.

A recently published study reported that gemifloxacin (320 mg, orally daily) for 5 days had similar outcomes to patients treated for 7 days with respect to clinical, bacteriological, and radiological efficacy (123).

Recently, Tellier et al. found that the clinical and bacteriological efficacy of telithromycin, 800 mg once daily for 5 (n=193) or 7 days (n=196) was as effective as a 10-day course of oral dosage clarithromycin 500 mg bid (n=187) (51). Data to be presented at the infectious disease meetings by File and coworkers indicated that a 5-day course of gemifloxacin (320 mg daily) gave comparable results to a 7-day course of gemifloxacin in 468 patients who participated in a randomized, double-blind multicenter trial of mild to moderate CAP. Furthermore, the incidence of drug rash was lower in the 5-day group (0.4% vs. 2.8%), supporting the use of a 5-day regimen in terms of efficacy, side effects, and cost (52). In addition, O'Doherty and coworkers compared SCAT therapy with azithromycin (n=101) 500 mg daily for 3 days with clarithromycin 250 mg bid for 10 days (53). Satisfactory clinical response was 94% and 95% in each group, with bacterial eradication rates of 97% and 91%, respectively. Furthermore, preliminary data using a single 2 g dose of an extended release formulation of azithromycin indicated efficacy equivalent to 7 days of clarithromycin XL for mild to moderate CAP (54).

Additional studies of SCAT therapy for CAP are planned or underway. Note also that data discussed below for hospital-acquired pneumonia (HAP) and VAP also suggest that SCAT is an effective strategy for the management of CAP or tracheobronchitis. Outpatients with lower disease severity, such as Pulmonary Severity Score (PSI) (classes I–III) may be a good target group to study (48,55). It should also be emphasized that intravenous antibiotics can often be streamlined and switched to oral therapy within 48 hr for responders, and that the use of pneumococcal and influenza vaccines should be strongly encouraged (47,55).

Key Points:

■ Data are available to support the use of SCAT for outpatient therapy of mild to moderate CAP. Dunbar concluded that treatment with levofloxacin 750 mg daily for 5 days was comparable to a dose of 500 mg daily for 10 days (50), and Tellier found that treatment with 800 mg of telithromycin for 5 days was similar to clarithromycin 500 mg bid for 10 days (56).

■ O'Doherty and coworkers reported that patients with mild to moderate CAP who were randomized to therapy with oral azithromycin 500 mg daily for 3 days had similar outcomes when compared to those treated with 10 days of oral clarithromycin 250 mg bid (53).

■ Data appear to support the use of SCAT with selected antibiotics, such as azithromycin, and fluoroquinolones, such as levofloxacin and gemifloxacin.

Hospital-Acquired, Ventilator-Associated, and Healthcare-Associated Pneumonia

HAP is the second most common nosocomial infection, accounting for about 27% of cases in the series by Richards, but resulting in the highest mortality and morbidity (19). Treatment of HAP and ventilator-associated pneumonia (VAP) account for the majority of the antibiotics used in the ICU. Patients who are intubated have a 6- to 21-fold increased risk of pneumonia and increased mortality rates that range from 20% to 50% (4,57). In contrast to CAP, HAP and VAP are more likely to be caused by MDR pathogens, especially if the patient has risk factors, such as prior antibiotic therapy, prior hospitalization or residence in a nursing home or chronic care facility, the presence of an immunosuppressive disease or immunosuppressive therapy, or late-onset disease (≥ 5 after admission or intubation). Common MDR pathogens causing HAP and VAP include Gram-negative bacteria, such as *P. aeruginosa, Acinetobacter* spp., or ESBL + *K. pneumoniae*, or Gram-positive bacteria, such as MRSA (4). Guidelines for the management of HAP, VAP, and healthcare-associated pneumonia (HCAP) have emphasized initial early and appropriate therapy with adequate doses of each antibiotic coupled with streamlining therapy, based on the clinical response of the patient and microbiologic data (4).

Evidence for SCAT

In the past, many patients with HAP and VAP were treated with 14 to 21 days of therapy. The recent ATS/IDSA Guideline has recommended 7 to 8 days of therapy in patients who are responding clinically (4). Efforts to reduce the duration of therapy for VAP are justified by studies of the natural history of the response to therapy. Dennesen and colleagues demonstrated that when VAP was caused by *H. influenza* and *S. pneumoniae*, the organisms could be rapidly eradicated from tracheal aspirates, whereas Enterobacteriaceae, *S. aureus*, and *P. aeruginosa* persisted longer despite in vitro susceptibility to the antibiotics administered (58). Significant improvements were observed for all clinical parameters, generally within the first 6 days after initiation of antibiotics. The consequence of prolonged therapy to 14 days or more was newly acquired colonization, especially with *P. aeruginosa* and Enterobacteriaceae, generally during the second week of therapy.

Luna et al., using serial clinical pulmonary infection score (CPIS) measurements, found that patients who survived VAP after receiving adequate therapy tended to have a clinical improvement by 3 to 5 days, especially reflected by improved PaO_2/FiO_2 ratio, while nonresponders did not have such a response during the same time period (59). These data support the premise that most patients with VAP who receive appropriate antimicrobial therapy have a good clinical response within the first 6 days and prolonged therapy simply leads to colonization with antibiotic-resistant bacteria, which may precede a recurrent episode of VAP.

Micek and coworkers performed a randomized, controlled trial of an antibiotic discontinuation policy for clinically suspected VAP in 290 patients (60). Patients were randomized to have their duration of therapy determined by an antibiotic discontinuation policy (discontinuation group) or by their treating physician (conventional group). The randomized groups were similar, but the duration of therapy of VAP was statistically shorter among patients in the discontinuation group (6.0 vs. 8.0 days, $p < 0.001$) and the incidence of recurrent episodes was not statistically different between the discontinuation and conventional groups (17.3% vs. 19.3%). Also, there were no significant differences by specific pathogen isolated. Other similar outcomes were found in terms of hospital mortality (32.0% vs. 37.1%) and ICU length of stay (6.8 vs. 7.9 days).

Reducing duration of therapy in patients with VAP has led to good outcomes with less antibiotic use with a variety of strategies. Singh et al. used a modification of the CPIS scoring system to identify low-risk patients (CPIS ≤ 6) with suspected VAP who could be treated with 3 days of antibiotics as opposed to the conventional practice of 10 to 21 days of antibiotic therapy (61). Patients receiving the SCAT had better clinical outcomes than patients receiving longer therapy, with fewer subsequent superinfections attributed to antibiotic-resistant pathogens (Fig. 3). This study needs further validation, and it has been suggested that some of the patients having a CPIS score < 6 may not have had pneumonia.

Perhaps the most compelling data are from a recent multicenter, randomized, controlled trial showing that patients who received appropriate, initial empiric therapy of VAP for 8 days ($n=197$) had similar outcomes in terms of survival and several other parameters when compared to patients who received therapy for 15 days ($n=203$) (Fig. 4) (62). In addition, the patients treated with the shorter course of therapy had significantly fewer resistant organisms and recurrence (42% vs. 62%, $p < 0.04$) than the 15-day group. For patients infected with *P. aeruginosa*, however, there was a trend toward greater rates of relapse in the shorter course group (41% vs. 25%) compared with the 15-day group. Clearly, all patients need careful follow-up after antibiotics are discontinued, and those who do not receive appropriate initial therapy or those who do not have a clinical response may need longer courses of the antibiotic therapy. There are opportunities for further studies on the optimal duration of antibiotic therapy of different patient populations.

One of the difficult decisions is trying to determine which patients may benefit from longer therapy. Singh and coworkers used the repeat CPIS score at day 3 to determine the need for further therapy, and Luna and colleagues demonstrated that the modified CPIS could differentiate at day 3 between patients with poor versus good clinical outcomes. Notable improvement was strongly associated with PaO_2/FiO_2; other clinical markers such as the temperature, radiologic results, and WBC counts did not correlate well with outcome. In a more recent study, Harbarth and coworkers suggested that elevated procalcitonin (PCT) concentration in serum was an effective indicator of sepsis and was superior to levels of interleukin-6 (IL-6) or IL-8 (63). Duflo and coworkers evaluated markers of oxidative stress in the plasma and bronchoalveolar samples from 36 patients with VAP and 42 patients without VAP and reported that thiobarbituric acid-reactive substances and glutathione peroxidase were higher in patients with VAP than those without, but there was no evaluation of survivors versus nonsurvivors (64). More recently, Luyt and coworkers, reported data from a prospective, observational study that evaluated PCT as a prognostic marker of outcomes during VAP (65). The data suggested that levels of PCT generally decreased during the clinical course of VAP from days 1 to 7, except in patients with an unfavorable outcome. In this study, 690 patients were admitted to the ICU, 290 (42%) were ventilated for 48 hr or more, 172 were suspected of VAP, but only 69 (40%) had microbiological confirmation, and 6 patients who died before day 3 were not included in the analysis. Of the 63 patients, 38 (60%) had unfavorable outcome (14 deaths, 21 recurrences, and 3 documented extrapulmonary infections). Early identification of patients with a high risk of an unfavorable outcome using PCT levels at days 1, 3, and 7 was an independent predictor of outcome that could provide an opportunity to change or alter treatment strategies to improve outcomes or conversely could be taken as an indicator to shorten therapy.

Key Points:

■ There are several observational studies and one randomized-controlled study supporting treatment of most patients with HAP, VAP, and HCAP for 7 to 8 days. The 2005 ATS/IDSA guidelines support the use of SCAT (4,62).

■ One randomized study suggested that patients with suspected HAP or VAP who have a sustained CPIS score of <6 may be treated with SCAT therapy for 3 days (61).

■ Further research is needed to identify the best candidates for SCAT and perhaps even shorter courses of antibiotic therapy. All patients require close follow-up and an emphasis for prevention is of paramount importance.

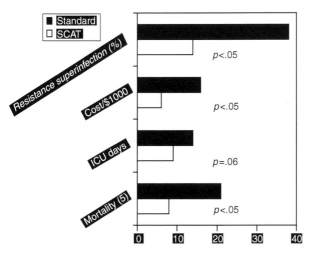

FIGURE 3 Shorter course antimicrobial therapy (SCAT) outcomes for patients with a clinical pulmonary infection score <6 who were randomly assigned to SCAT with intravenous ciprofloxacin for hospital-acquired pneumonia (HAP) versus standard therapy ordered by the intensive care unit (ICU) team. *Source*: From Ref. 61.

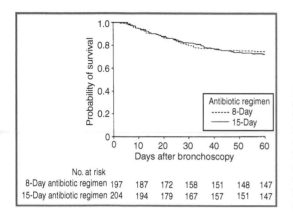

FIGURE 4 Data taken from a multicenter, randomized study of antibiotic therapy for ventilator-associated pneumonia (VAP) where patients were randomized to 8 versus 15 days of therapy. Notice that the Kaplan–Meier survival curves for the two groups are virtually superimposed. Data collected for other outcomes variable were also similar. *Source*: From Ref. 62.

URINARY TRACT INFECTIONS

Symptomatic UTIs are among the most common bacterial infections requiring antimicrobial treatment. Optimal duration of treatment for acute uncomplicated bacterial cystitis and acute pyelonephritis in women has been thoroughly studied. Less comprehensive information is available concerning treatment of pregnant women, older women, diabetics, patients with spinal cord injuries, and men.

In 1999, the IDSA published guidelines for antimicrobial treatment of uncomplicated acute bacterial cystitis and acute pyelonephritis in otherwise healthy adult women. The authors reviewed 76 studies of acute cystitis and 9 studies of acute pyelonephritis that met their strict screening criteria. Treatment with TMP-SMX (or TMP alone for the sulfonamide-intolerant patient) for 3 days was recommended as standard therapy (Table 3) (64). Since 1999, increasing resistance to TMP-SMX has forced consideration of other treatment options (67). A 3-day course of a fluoroquinolone (in the United States, commonly ciprofloxacin, levofloxacin, or, to a lesser extent-gatifloxacin) is as effective as a similar course of TMP-SMX, but it is more expensive and increasing resistance is also a concern. A single 3 g dose of fosfomycin or a 5- to 7-day course of nitrofurantoin are additional recommended options. Beta-lactam agents may also be useful, but in a recent trial a 3-day regimen of amoxicillin-clavulanate was not as effective as a 3-day regimen of ciprofloxacin for either clinical or microbiological cure of women with uncomplicated cystitis (68). Treatment with a single dose of an antibacterial agent for acute cystitis has also been studied but has a lower rate of eradication and a higher rate of recurrence than treatment using the same agent for a longer period of time, but also had a lower rate of adverse effects. For most agents, therapy for longer than 3 days provided no added benefits.

The IDSA guidelines recommended a 14-day course of therapy for young nonpregnant women with normal urinary tracts who presented with acute pyelonephritis. Mild cases could be managed with SCAT oral therapy. A fluoroquinolone or, if the causative bacteria were known to be susceptible, TMP-SMX was recommended for Gram-negative infections, while amoxicillin or amoxicillin/clavulanic acid were recommended for Gram-positive infections (66). Courses shorter than 14-days had a higher rate of recurrence while treatment >14 days provided no added benefit.

UTIs are common in pregnancy, but treatment options need to be modified because of exposure to the developing fetus. Quinolones, tetracycline, trimethoprim (in the first trimester), and sulfonamides (in the last trimester) should not be used (69). Consequently amoxicillin, cephalosporins, fosfomycin, or nitrofurantoin have been recommended, but there are no data on appropriate duration of therapy.

Optimal antibiotic duration to treat uncomplicated, symptomatic lower UTIs in elderly women has recently been reviewed (70). No difference in clinical cure rate or persistence of bacteriuria at long term was found between short (3 to 6 days) and long course (7 to 14 days) although the rate of persistent bacteriuria was lower 2 weeks post-treatment with long course treatment. Single dose therapy was less effective than treatment for 3 to 6 days in terms of the rate of persistent bacteria at 2 weeks post-treatment, but the rate of persistent bacteriuria at long term was similar in the two groups and a statistically significant difference in clinical cure rate was not evident. In a recent double-blind, randomized-controlled trial of 183 women aged 65 or over with an acute uncomplicated UTI, bacterial eradication was the same whether treatment with ciprofloxacin was of 3 or 7 days duration (71).

Patients with diabetes mellitus are more likely to have UTIs caused by atypical or resistant organisms and to have anatomic or functional abnormalities of the urinary tract. Hence, initial therapy should be based on urine Gram stain

TABLE 3 Recommended Agents and Duration of Treatment for Urinary Tract Infections (UTIs)

Condition	Population	Agents	Duration
Acute cystitis	Young, healthy, nonpregnant women	Trimethoprim-sulfamethoxazole or trimethoprim alone[a]	3 days
		Fluoroquinolone[b]	3 days
		Fosfomycin[c]	Single dose
		Nitrofurantoin[c]	5–7 days
	Healthy, postmenopausal women	Same agents as for young women	3 days
	Diabetic women	Choice based on urine Gram stain and culture Empiric fluoroquinolone	7 days
	Men	Same agents as for young women	7 days[d]
	Men or women with spinal cord injury	Same agents as for diabetic women	14 days
	Pregnant women	Amoxicillin[e] Cephalosporins Fosfomycin Nitrofurantoin	
Acute pyelonephritis	Young, healthy, nonpregnant women	Same agents as for cystitis[f] and amoxicillin or amoxicillin/clavulanic acid for Gram-positive infections	14 days

[a]In communities where the frequency of resistance to these agents is < 20%.
[b]Ciprofloxacin, levofloxacin, others.
[c]Limited studies.
[d]Increased duration to treat possible prostatitis.
[e]Quinolones, tetracycline, trimethoprim (in the first trimester), and sulfonamides (in the last trimester) should not be used during pregnancy (69).
[f]Nitrofurantoin excepted.
Source: Adapted from Ref. 66.

and culture. Empiric therapy with a fluoroquinolone is reasonable for patients likely to have a susceptible organism and 7 days of therapy is recommended (72). Complications are more likely in this group than in the nondiabetic patient, so close follow-up is recommended.

Because of the rarity of UTIs in men, data from controlled treatment trials are lacking, but since the etiologic agents and their susceptibility are similar to what is found in women, the same agents for empiric treatment apply, and a 7-day regimen has been recommended to manage possible prostatic involvement (73).

In men and women with spinal cord injury, asymptomatic bacteriuria is common, but usually does not require treatment. Treatment of symptomatic bacteriuria in such patients is complicated by the increased likelihood of antibiotic-resistant organisms, recurrence of past infections, catheter drainage, and functional abnormalities. Antibiotic choice should be based on Gram stain and culture of the urine and knowledge of local infecting organisms and their resistance (74). Prolonged duration of treatment is advisable. In a study of acute symptomatic UTI in spinal cord patients, treatment with ciprofloxacin for 14 rather than 3 days produced better microbiological cure rates and a lower rate of relapse at long-term follow-up (75).

Adherence to recommendations is surprisingly low. In a study in Israel involving more than 7000 physician–patient encounters, TMP-SMX was the most frequently prescribed agent to treat acute UTIs in women, followed by fluoroquinolones, but cephalosporins, which were not specifically recommended, were used almost as often (76). Treatment with TMP-SMX was most often prescribed for 5 days, next for 10 days, and in less than 4% of the cases for the recommended 3 days. Similarly fluoroquinolone was most often given for 5 or 10 days and in only 4% of cases for the recommended 3 days. Overall, in only 8.7% of cases were treatment guidelines accurately followed. In a survey of almost 9000 physicians in the United States reported in 1999, duration of treatment for newly diagnosed cystitis was 2 to 5 days for 52% of the cases but 41% were treated for 6 to 10 days, and 2% for >10 days (77).

Key Points:

- Recommended therapy for women with uncomplicated acute, bacterial cystitis is 3 days of TMP-SMX, or if that agent cannot be used because of intolerance or resistance in the community, 3 days of a fluoroquinolone or 7 days of nitrofurantoin (66,68,73).
- For nonpregnant women with acute pyelonephritis and normal urinary tracts, 14 days of treatment with TMP-SMX or a fluoroquinolone is recommended (66). UTIs in pregnancy, diabetes, the elderly, and those with spinal cord injury are special situations generally requiring 7 to 14 days of therapy.
- Despite published standards, the recommended duration of therapy is often exceeded (76,77).

GASTROINTESTINAL INFECTIONS
Helicobacter pylori
H. pylori is the causative agent of chronic active gastritis and peptic ulcer disease (78,79). *H. pylori* are also implicated in about 70% of gastric ulcers and there is increasing evidence to indicate its association with the development of gastric

adenocarcinoma, and gastric mucosa-associated lymphoid tissue (MALT) lymphoma. This infection is common in the general population, with most infected individuals being asymptomatic. Currently, combination therapy aimed at *H. pylori* is known to cure and to prevent recurrence of peptic ulcer disease and gastritis. Therapy has also been associated with regression of gastric MALT lymphoma.

The goal of treatment is the complete elimination of *H. pylori*. Once this is achieved, the reinfection rates in industrialized countries are low. Combination drug regimens were found to be important to increase eradication rates and to minimize the risk of inducing drug resistance. Triple therapies (a proton pump inhibitor with two out of three antibiotics, metronidazole, clarithromycin, or amoxicillin) are regarded as standard therapy in industrialized countries, achieving eradication rates of >80% (based on intent-to-treat analysis) to >90% (per protocol basis) (78,80). The duration of therapy, however, remains controversial. Multiple eradication trials utilizing different regimens at varying doses for different durations in populations that have varying underlying diseases attributable to *H. pylori* have made the analysis of the available data difficult to interpret. This is compounded by small numbers of patients in each study with different study designs and different percentages of patients with resistant organisms to metronidazole and clarithromycin in each trial.

Currently, the typical three-drug regimens consisting of a proton pump inhibitor (e.g., lansoprazole 30 mg twice daily, omeprazole 20 mg twice daily, or esomeprazole 40 mg once daily), amoxicillin (1 g twice daily), and clarithromycin 500 mg twice daily are recommended for 7 days in Europe versus 10 to 14 days in the United States (76–80). Shorter therapy is beneficial in increasing compliance, decreasing cost, and causing fewer side effects (especially when multiple drugs are necessary), and may reduce secondary antibiotic resistance. Failed eradication therapy from either drug resistance or insufficient duration of therapy have been shown to induce secondary antibiotic resistance with metronidazole and clarithromycin (81,82). Eradication rates are significantly reduced when *H. pylori* isolates are resistant to metronidazole or clarithromycin alone. Primary resistances to clarithromycin and metronidazole have decreased rates of cure by 37% and 50%, respectively, in regimens using these agents. Increasing drug resistance, primarily to metronidazole (36% to 45%) and clarithromycin (11% to 12%), has been reported in the United States (83,84). By comparison, resistance to amoxicillin or tetracycline appears to be rare. Since sensitivity testing for *H. pylori* is not routinely done or available clinically, metronidazole (500 mg twice daily) is therefore recommended only in penicillin allergic patients. High rates of metronidazole resistance in Europe have also led to 7-day triple therapy with omeprazole, clarithromycin, and amoxicillin. This triple combination regimen has also been found to have equivalent eradication rates when compared to classic quadruple bismuth-based regimens (85). The >50% rate of resistance of *H. pylori* isolates to metronidazole has also rendered this antibiotic of limited utility for treatment in the developing world, where reinfection rates are also higher (86). It has been suggested that *H. pylori* should be cultured and tested for clarithromycin susceptibility in patients who have failed therapy containing clarithromycin (87). Any previous use of macrolides should also be taken into account when clarithromycin is chosen for eradication of *H. pylori* since this may increase the possibility of primary drug resistance for this organism (88).

The success of 7-day triple therapy regimens has been well documented in European populations but U.S. guidelines for initial treatment of *H. pylori* infection recommend treatment for 10 to 14 days because of inconsistent results in trials in the United States with 7-day therapy. Some U.S.-based randomized trials have demonstrated that there was no statistical difference between eradication rates in 7-day regimens versus 14-day regimens (89). But the 7-day regimen had a numerically lower eradication rate and it was believed this trial may have lacked the power to demonstrate a difference even if one was present. Based on trials using the four-drug regimens reported by de Boer et al. (90), 1-week quadruple therapy using the traditional bismuth therapy with the addition of a proton pump inhibitor has also been accepted in the U.S. guidelines. More recent U.S. studies to assess the relative efficacy of shorter course 7-day triple therapy in comparison to standard 10 day therapy with omeprazole, amoxillin, and clarithromycin have shown similar efficacy (91). This is supported by a recent Cochrane review where 53 randomized, controlled trials of eradication therapy for *H. pylori* versus long-term treatment of peptic ulcer disease in *H. pylori*-infected adults were analyzed (92). Trials involving at least 1-week eradication treatments of at least 1 week's duration were included to evaluate whether eradication therapy was effective for patients with *H. pylori* peptic ulcer disease compared with an ulcer-healing drug, placebo, or no treatment. The data suggested that a 1- to 2-week course of *H. pylori* eradication therapy was effective. While this review did not specifically address the issue of 1- versus 2-week treatment for eradication of *H. pylori* infection, it showed that 1 week appeared to be as effective as maintenance therapy with ulcer-healing drugs in preventing recurrent duodenal ulcer disease.

Shorter triple drug regimens using 5-day treatment durations have been studied showing greater than 80% success on an intention-to-treat basis in small numbers of patients (93). A 4-day quadruple therapy consisting of a proton pump inhibitor, a bismuth salt, tetracycline, and metronidazole achieves >95% cure rate in metronidazole-sensitive strains but may be a problem in areas with a high prevalence of metronidazole resistance (93,94). Due to increasing concerns about drug resistance and limited numbers of randomized trials and small sample sizes, triple drug regimens of fewer than 7 days duration cannot be recommended at this time.

Key Points:

- Current evidence for SCAT supports the use of 1-week treatment regimens for initial eradication treatment of *H. pylori* infections using a proton pump inhibitor and clarithromycin, in combination with amoxillin, metronidazole, or tetracycline (depending on regional resistance patterns). The addition of a proton pump inhibitor to the traditional bismuth-based regimen of bismuth, tetracycline, and metronidazole for 1-week is also recommended (78,79).
- SCAT regimens for less than 5 to 7 days need further study with larger controlled clinical trials (96).

Typhoid Fever

Typhoid fever is a systemic infection with the bacterium *Salmonella enterica*, serotype typhi commonly known as *S. typhi*. It is a significant cause of morbidity and mortality worldwide, causing an estimated 16 million cases and 600,000 deaths annually. The number of travel-related cases has increased in the United States, but the total number of cases has dropped (97). MDR isolates (i.e., resistant to chloramphenicol, ampicillin, and cotrimoxazole) of *S. enterica*, serotype typhi is an increasing problem and has emerged as a predominant clone in Southeast Asia and the Indian subcontinent, leading to the use of quinolones as the first line of drug treatment (98).

Fluoroquinolones, which achieve high concentrations in macrophages and in bile, have been shown in randomized clinical trials to be rapidly effective for treatment of quinolone-sensitive infections of *S. typhi* using SCAT ranging from 3 to 7 days (6,99) achieving cure rates of greater than 90%. SCAT with fluoroquinolones appears to be rapidly effective and was associated with lower rates of stool carriage than the use of other first-line drugs. Unfortunately, strains of *S. enterica*, serotype typhi with reduced susceptibility to fluoroquinolones (as indicated by resistance to nalidixic acid), have become endemic in many Asian countries. Among patients with quinolone-resistant *S. enterica* serotype typhi infection, the rate of treatment failure is higher for patients treated with fluoroquinolones for <7 days (100). The median time to fever clearance is longer and relapse rates are higher when quinolones are used to treat these infections. This has led to clinical trials using azithromycin, which is active in vitro against many enteric bacterial pathogens and is also concentrated inside neutrophils and other phagocytic cells. In one open label, randomized study of SCAT with azithromycin (1 g daily for 5 days at 20 mg/kg/day), this drug was 95% effective for the treatment of uncomplicated enteric fever due to MDR and nalidixic acid-resistant, *S. enterica*, serotype typhi in adults (101). In severe or complicated typhoid fever, ceftriaxone, given intravenously once daily in 4 g doses for 5 days, achieved cure rates of only 79% in a randomized clinical trial compared to the traditional therapy of chloramphenicol given for 14 days (102). No data are available to support SCAT in HIV-infected patients who are at increased risk for this infection.

Key Points:

- Despite small numbers of patients in each study, multiple publications suggest that SCAT for uncomplicated typhoid fever with a quinolone for 5 days can be recommended for *S. enterica*, serotype typhi that are sensitive to nalidixic acid. For nalidixic acid-resistant strains, SCAT with azithromycin for 5 days has also been demonstrated to be effective (101).
- SCAT for complicated typhoid fever in the normal host or uncomplicated infections in the HIV-infected patient cannot be recommended based on currently available evidence (102).

SEXUALLY TRANSMITTED DISEASES

SCAT has been extensively studied for the treatment STDs, where ease of administration, tolerability, and cost has had a great influence. The literature is most robust for *Neisseria gonorrhoeae* and *Chlamydia trachomatis* infections. A recent review found clinical trial evidence for 30 regimens that were >95% effective in eradicating gonococcal infection (103). Despite a rising incidence of antibiotic resistance among strains of *N. gonorrhoeae*, highly active and effective single-dose regimens are available for both of these pathogens, which support the effective use of DOT. DOT greatly increases compliance and decreases secondary transmission when compared with longer courses of antibiotic therapy.

Uncomplicated Gonococcal Infections

Ceftriaxone in a single intramuscular injection of 125 mg provides sustained high bactericidal levels in the blood. Extensive clinical experience indicates that ceftriaxone is safe and effective for the treatment of uncomplicated gonorrhea at all anatomic sites, curing 99.1% of uncomplicated urogenital and anorectal infections in published clinical trials (101). Until 2006, ciprofloxacin was also effective against most strains of *N. gonorrhoeae* in the United States (excluding Hawaii). A ciprofloxacin dose of 500 mg provides sustained bactericidal levels in the blood and has cured 99.8% of uncomplicated urogenital and anorectal infections in published clinical trials.

Ciprofloxacin is safe, inexpensive, and can be administered orally. The CDC has recommended single-dose fluoroquinolone regimens for the treatment of gonococcal infections since 1993. Although quinolone-resistant *N. gonorrhoeae* (QRNG) was identified as a problem in Asia in 1991, and was first identified in Hawaii in the same year, only sporadic occurrences were noted in the continental United States during the 1990s (102,103). However, since 1999, increasing resistance of *N. gonorrhoeae* to fluoroquinolones has been observed, first in Hawaii, then in California and other Western states, then among MSM, and now in other populations and regions. During the first six months of 2006, QRNG was identified in 25 out of 26 Gonococcal Isolate Surveillance Project (GISP) sites, and increases in the prevalence of QRNG were observed among isolates from heterosexual males and MSM in most regions of the country. As a result, the CDC no longer recommends fluoroquinolones for treatment of gonorrhea in the United States. The CDC has changed treatment recommendations when QRNG prevalence has reached >5% in defined groups and locations, a threshold used so that all recommended treatments for gonorrhea can be expected to cure >95% of infections (104).

Because fluoroquinolones are no longer recommended, the options for treating gonococcal infections in the United States are limited (104). For the treatment of uncomplicated urogenital and anorectal gonorrhea, the CDC now recommends a single intramuscular dose of ceftriaxone 125 mg or a single oral dose of cefixime 400 mg. However, 400 mg tablets of cefixime are not available; cefixime is only available in a suspension formulation. Some evidence suggests that a single oral dose of cefpodoxime 400 mg or cefuroxime axetil 1 g might be additional oral alternatives for the treatment of urogenital and anorectal gonorrhea (104).

Spectinomycin, 2 g injected in a single intramuscular dose, is expensive and cures 98.2% of uncomplicated urogenital and anorectal gonococcal infections. Spectinomycin is clinically useful for treatment of patients who cannot tolerate cephalosporins, but it is not currently available in the United States.

Azithromycin 2 g as a single oral dose has demonstrated an efficacy of 99.2% (95% CI; 97.2–99.9%) for urogenital and rectal infections, and treatment efficacy of 100% for pharyngeal infection (95% CI; 82.3–100%) but is not recommended because of expense, frequency of gastrointestinal intolerance, and concerns regarding rapid emergence of resistance, as evidenced by the increase in azithromycin MICs documented since 1999 in the United States and internationally (103,104). Treatment with 1 g of azithromycin is insufficiently effective and is not recommended. Azithromycin remains a treatment option in patients with documented severe allergic reactions to beta-lactams.

Alternative single-dose cephalosporin regimens (other than ceftriaxone 12 mg IM) that are safe and highly effective against uncomplicated urogenital and anorectal gonococcal infections include ceftizoxime (500 mg, administered IM), cefoxitin (2 g, administered IM with probenecid 1 g orally), and cefotaxime (500 mg, administered IM) (104). None of the injectable cephalosporins offer any advantage over cefiriaxone.

Uncomplicated Chlamydial Infections
Chlamydial urethritis is characterized by urethral discharge of mucopurulent or purulent material and sometimes by dysuria or urethral pruritis. Asymptomatic infections are common. All patients who have urethritis should be evaluated for the presence of gonococcal and chlamydial infection. Treatment should be initiated as soon as possible after diagnosis. Single-dose regimens have the advantage of improved compliance and permit DOT. The medication should be provided in the clinic or healthcare provider's office. Recommended regimens include azithromycin 1 g orally in a single dose or doxycycline 100 mg orally twice a day for 7 days. Again, the 2 g single oral dose of azithromycin has not been recommended, due to its increased expense and frequency of gastrointestinal intolerance. Alternative regimens include erythromycin base 500 mg orally four times a day for 7 days, erythromycin ethylsuccinate 800 mg orally four times a day for 7 days, ofloxacin 300 mg twice a day for 7 days, or levofloxacin 500 mg once daily for 7 days. Patients should be instructed to return for evaluation if symptoms persist or recur after completion of therapy (105).

The results of clinical trials indicate that azithromycin and doxycycline are equally efficacious for treatment of chlamydial infection (106,107). These investigations were conducted primarily in populations in which follow-up was encouraged and adherence to a 7-day regimen was good. Azithromycin should be used to treat patients for whom adherence is in question, and is more costeffective because a single dose and DOT can be used. Doxycycline costs less than azithromycin, and it has been used extensively for a longer period. Erythromycin is less efficacious than either azithromycin or doxycycline due to gastrointestinal side effects and lower adherence. Ofloxacin is similar in efficacy to doxycycline and azithromycin, but it is more expensive to use and offers no advantage with regard to the dosage regimen. Partner tracing and notification along with education regarding the use and efficacy of condoms remain a mainstay of prevention of gonorrheal and chlamydial infection.

Key Points:

- Single-dose SCAT regimens are efficacious in treating uncomplicated gonococcal and chlamydial infections.
- Testing for *Chlamydia* is encouraged in all cases of urethritis because the infection is often asymptomatic, highly sensitive and specific diagnostic assays are readily available, and a specific diagnosis may improve compliance and partner notification.

BLOODSTREAM INFECTIONS
Endocarditis
Classically, antibiotic therapy for infective endocarditis has been carried out for 4 to 6 weeks. Despite increasing frequency of antimicrobial resistance in the major

pathogens associated with this disease, primarily *S. aureus* and enterococci, antibiotic regimens of short duration are still possible for selected patients with susceptible isolates. Adjunctive diagnostic aids such as transesophageal echocardiography often permit earlier diagnosis of endocarditis, thereby increasing the possibility that short-course antibiotic therapy may be applied successfully. Two studies in viridans group streptococcal endocarditis demonstrated that, in selected patients, a 2-week regimen of either penicillin or ceftriaxone combined with an aminoglycoside yielded cure rates comparable to those seen when penicillin or ceftriaxone is given for 4 weeks (108,109). Additional studies of viridans streptococcal endocarditis showed that 2 weeks of therapy with once-daily ceftriaxone combined with either netilmicin or gentamicin given once daily was equivalent to 2 weeks of penicillin given with an aminoglycoside in divided doses (109,110). This 2-week regimen is appropriate for patients with uncomplicated endocarditis caused by highly penicillin-susceptible (MIC $\leq 0.1\,\mu g/mL$) viridans group streptococci or *Streptococcus bovis* who are also at low risk for gentamicin toxicity, but it is not recommended in the presence of known extracardiac infection or in patients with a creatinine clearance $< 20\,mL/min$ (111). Gentamicin has been shown to accelerate killing of methicillin-susceptible staphylococci (MSSA) in vitro. Several studies support the efficacy of a 2-week course of aminoglycoside–beta-lactam combination in injection drug users with right-sided staphylococcal endocarditis and no renal failure, extra-pulmonary metastatic infections, meningitis, or methicillin-resistant *S. aureus* (112–116). In one study of right-sided *S. aureus* endocarditis, 2-week monotherapy with cloxacillin was shown to be equivalent to cloxacillin plus gentamicin (115), while another study showed that regimens comprised of vancomycin plus gentamicin were less effective than regimens containing beta-lactams (114). Potential reasons for the decreased efficacy of glycopeptides include their limited bactericidal activity, poor penetration into vegetations, and increased drug clearance in injection drug users (117). In contrast to right-sided MSSA endocarditis, there are currently no evidence-based data that support treatment of left-sided MSSA endocarditis with courses shorter than 4 weeks duration (111). Standard 4- to 6-week antibiotic courses are recommended for prosthetic valve endocarditis; endocarditis caused by enterococci, fastidious organisms, or Gram-negative bacilli; and complicated endocarditis, including that caused by antibiotic resistant strains. Enterococci, by virtue of their relative resistance to beta-lactams and vancomycin, are inhibited but not killed by these antibiotics, requiring synergistic combinations with aminoglycosides to kill susceptible strains (111). Enterococci are also relatively impermeable to aminoglycosides, further complicating matters and making successful SCAT less likely for these pathogens. Investigations into the efficacy of short course therapy for organisms other than viridans group streptococci and MSSA remain to be conducted, but the complicating factor of antibiotic resistance in many of these isolates makes the success of SCAT less likely to be successful.

Key Points:

- Shorter course (2-week) regimens comprised of a beta-lactam with or without an aminoglycoside are effective for treatment of uncomplicated viridans streptococcal endocarditis and right-sided MSSA endocarditis.
- Evidence-based data are not yet available to support short-course regimens in other etiologies of endocarditis.

Catheter-Related Bloodstream Infections (CR-BSIs)

Each year in the United States, hospitals and clinics purchase more than 150 million intravascular devices to administer intravenous fluids, medications, blood products, and parenteral nutrition fluids to monitor hemodynamic status and to provide hemodialysis (118,119). The majority of these devices are peripheral venous catheters, but more than 5 million central venous devices are inserted each year. Over 80,000 cases of nosocomial bloodstream infections (BSIs) occur each year in the United States, most of which are related to the different types of the intravascular devices, especially the nontunneled central venous catheter (CVC).

Intravenous catheter device-related infection results in significantly increased hospital costs, length of stay, and morbidity and mortality. Mortality attributed to catheter-related *S. aureus* bacteremia significantly exceeded the rates for other pathogens, while mortality attributed to coagulase-negative staphylococcal catheter-related bacteremia is significantly lower than that for other pathogens (120). The pathogenesis of the nontunneled CVC infection is often related to extraluminal catheter colonization originating from the skin, whereas tunneled catheter or implantable catheters or devices may become infected by hematogenous seeding or intraluminal colonization (119,120).

Clinical findings for establishing the diagnosis of intravascular device-related infection are unreliable due to their poor specificity and sensitivity (120). Blood cultures positive for *S. aureus* or coagulase-negative staphylococci in the absence of any other identifiable source of infection should increase the suspicion for CR-BSI. Microorganisms most commonly associated with peripheral vascular and CVC infection are coagulase-negative staphylococci, *S. aureus*, and aerobic Gram-negative bacilli.

Laboratory techniques for clinical diagnosis of catheter-related infection employ a semiquantitative method, in which the catheter segment is rolled across the surface of an agar plate and colony-forming units (CFU) are assessed after overnight incubation. Growth of ≥ 15 CFU from a catheter by semiquantitative culture or growth of $\geq 10^2$ CFU from a catheter by quantitative culture, with accompanying signs of local or systemic inflammation, is indicative of a catheter-related infection.

Clinical Management

Antibiotic therapy for catheter-related infection is often initiated empirically. The initial choice of antibiotics depends on the severity of the patient's clinical disease, risk factors for infection, and likely pathogens associated with the specific intravascular device (Fig. 5) (120). Although there are no data supporting the use of specific empiric antibiotic therapy for device-related BSIs, vancomycin is usually recommended in those hospitals or countries with an increased incidence of methicillin-resistant staphylococci, because of its activity against coagulase-negative staphylococci and *S. aureus*. In the absence of MRSA, penicillinase-resistant penicillins, such as nafcillin or oxacillin, should be used. Additional empiric coverage for enteric Gram-negative bacilli and *P. aeruginosa*, with a third- or fourth-generation cephalosporin, such as ceftazidime or cefepime, may be indicated in severely ill or immunocompromised patients with suspected CR-BSI. Antimicrobial therapy should be given intravenously initially, but once the patient has stabilized and antibiotic sensitivities are known, an oral quinolone, such as ciprofloxacin, TMP-SMX, or linezolid could be administered, because of their excellent oral bioavailability and tissue penetration.

There are no compelling data to support specific recommendations for the duration of therapy for device-related infections. Patients with catheter-related bacteremia should be separated from those with complicated infections in which there is septic thrombosis, endocarditis, osteomyelitis, or possible metastatic seeding, and those with uncomplicated bacteremia in which there is no evidence of such complications (Fig. 5). If there is a prompt response to initial antibiotic therapy, most patients who are not immunocompromised, or lack underlying heart disease or a prosthetic device, should receive 10 to 14 days of antimicrobial therapy for pathogens other than coagulase-negative staphylococci. A more prolonged antibiotic course of 4 to 6 weeks should be considered for complicated infections due to *S. aureus*. Predictors of complicated *S. aureus* bacteremia include community acquisition, skin findings suggestive of acute systemic infection, persistent fever >72 hr and a positive follow-up blood culture at 48 to 96 hr (121). Also, if there is evidence of endocarditis, septic thrombosis, or osteomyelitis, a longer course of antibiotic therapy is recommended (120).

Surgically implantable vascular devices consist of either a surgically implantable catheter, such as tunneled silicone catheters (Hickman, Broviac, or Groshong), or implantable devices, such as Port-A-Cath (120). Because removal of a surgically-implantable vascular device is often a management challenge, it is important to be sure that one is dealing with a true CR-BSI rather than skin contamination, catheter colonization, or infection from another source. Patients with complicated device infections, such as tunnel infection or port abscess, require removal of the catheter and 7 to 10 days of antibiotic therapy. Septic thrombosis or endocarditis requires removal of the catheter or device and antibiotic treatment for 4 to 6 weeks. In cases complicated by osteomyelitis, the

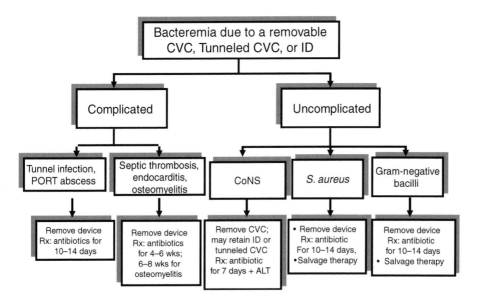

FIGURE 5 Summary of the duration of antibiotic therapy recommended for therapy of catheter-related bloodstream infections. Note the difference in duration of therapy for the different pathogens. *Abbreviations*: ALT, alanine aminotransferase test; CoNS, coagulase negative streptococci; CVC, central venous catheter; ID, implantable device. *Source*: From Ref. 120.

catheter should be removed and patients treated for 6 to 8 weeks. In the presence of uncomplicated infection due to coagulase-negative staphylococci, the tunneled CVC may be retained, if there is no evidence of persisting or relapsing bacteremia. Antibiotic lock therapy, using high concentrations of antibiotics locked into the catheter or implantable device, should be considered for salvage therapy in selected patients where there are compelling reasons why the catheter cannot be removed (120).

Key Points:

- There are no randomized clinical trials to support specific recommendations for the duration of therapy for device-related infections.
- Patients with catheter-related bacteremia should be separated into those with complicated infections in which there is septic thrombosis, endocarditis, osteomyelitis, or possible metastatic seeding that require longer courses of therapy versus those with uncomplicated bacteremia that can be treated for shorter periods (120).
- If there is a prompt response to initial antibiotic therapy, most patients with uncomplicated bacteremia who are not immunocompromised and without underlying heart disease or a prosthetic device should receive 10 to 14 days of antimicrobial therapy of Gram-negative bacilli and at least 14 days for *S. aureus*. Coagulase-negative staphylococci needs to be treated for only seven days, if the device is removed (120).
- Patients with tunnel infection or abscess require removal of the catheter and 7 to 10 days of antibiotic therapy.

SUMMARY

SCAT is an important strategy for decreasing selection pressure for the evolution and spread of MDR pathogens. SCAT is also valuable for improving patient outcomes and decreasing healthcare costs. Data presented in this chapter indicate that SCAT is effective for a spectrum of outpatient and inpatient infections. There is a need for more studies to better define the spectrum of infections and the more effective antibiotic regimens and to identify the most suitable patients for SCAT therapy. Recent guidelines for the management of pneumonia, UTIs, and BSIs have been published, but as we pointed out, there is often a lag period before these guidelines are implemented and evaluated in clinical practice.

SCAT has many advantages and potential disadvantages underscoring the need for rigorous study design and analysis. With the limited availability of new antimicrobial agents and the increased spread of MDR pathogens in our aging and more at-risk populations, it is imperative that we use our current resources wisely and continue to search for new anti-infective agents, as well as to explore better methods for the control and effective use of available antimicrobial agents. These initiatives must include the pharmaceutical industry, societies (IDSA, ATS, Society of Healthcare Epidemiologists of America, and the Association for Professionals in Infection Control), and state, federal, and international agencies. These groups could set an agenda to examine new ideas and work together to maximize our current knowledge and implement intervention strategies. Clearly, there is also a need for improved professional and public education, with more oversight by various regulatory agencies to emphasize and promulgate principles and practice for prevention of infections and quality improvement.

Hopefully, the data discussed in this chapter will be a catalyst for more interventions and use of methods to evaluate and monitor local and national antibiotic utilization and misuse. The key is to expand and continue a dialogue, coupled with specific goals and targets supported by more focused research support at multiple levels designed to improve current and future practices.

Although there has been progress in our understanding and practice of SCAT, there is still ample room for improvement. Our goals should be to push the envelope, think outside of the box, and to implement intervention strategies aimed at better infection control, risk reduction, education, and use of prophylaxis. There is clearly a need for change, but change will require leadership, a feasible strategic plan, incentives, appropriate resources, effective collaborations, and a commitment to developing new models.

REFERENCES

1. Naylor CD, Guyatt GH. Users' guides to the medical literature. X. How to use an article reporting variations in the outcomes of health services. The evidence-based medicine working group. J Am Med Assoc 1996; 275:554–8.
2. National Nosocomial Infections Surveillance (NNIS) System report, data summary from January 1990-May 1999, issued June 1999. Am J Infect Control 1999; 27:520–32.
3. Donskey CJ, Chowdhry TK, Hecker MT, et al. Effect of antibiotic therapy on the density of vancomycin-resistant enterococci in the stool of colonized patients. N Engl J Med 2000; 343:1925–32.
4. Guidelines for the management of adults with hospital-acquired, ventilator-associated, and healthcare-associated pneumonia. Am J Respir Crit Care Med 2005; 171:388–416.
5. Levy SB, Marshall B. Antibacterial resistance worldwide: causes, challenges and responses. Nat Med 2004; 10:S122–9.
6. David DR. In: Cohen JP, ed. Short-course antibiotic therapy. 2nd ed. New York: Mosby, 2004:1765–89.
7. Cohn DL. Treatment of latent tuberculosis infection. Semin Respir Infect 2003; 18:249
8. El-Sadr WM, Perlman DC, Denning E, Matts JP, Cohn DL. A review of efficacy studies of 6-month short-course therapy for tuberculosis among patients infected with human immunodeficiency virus: differences in study outcomes. Clin Infect Dis 2001; 32:623–32.
9. Guillemot D, Carbon C, Balkau B. Low dosage and long treatment duration of beta-lactam: risk factors for carriage of penicillin-resistant *Streptococcus pneumoniae*. J Am Med Assoc 1998; 279: 365–70.
10. Hecker MT, Aron DC, Patel NP, Lehmann MK, Donskey CJ. Unnecessary use of antimicrobials in hospitalized patients: current patterns of misuse with an emphasis on the antianaerobic spectrum of activity. Arch Intern Med 2003; 163:972–8.
11. Maki D, Schuna A. A study of antimicrobial misuse in a university hospital. Am J Med Sci 1987; 275:271–82.
12. Cosgrove SE, Carmeli Y. The impact of antimicrobial resistance on health and economic outcomes. Clin Infect Dis 2003; 36:1433–7.
13. McGowan JE Jr. Antimicrobial resistance in hospital organisms and its relation to antibiotic use. Rev Infect Dis 1983; 5:1033–48.
14. Duncan RA. Controlling use of antimicrobial agents. Infect Control Hosp Epidemiol 1997; 18:260–6.
15. Duncan RA. Antimicrobial Stewardship. In: Lautenbach EWK, ed. Practical Handbook for Hospital Epidmiologists. 2nd ed. Thorofare, New Jersey: Slack Inc., 2004:199–209.

16. Burke JP. Antibiotic resistance—squeezing the balloon? J Am Med Assoc 1998; 280:1270–1.
17. Burgess DS, Lewis JS. Effect of macrolides as part of initial empiric therapy on medical outcomes for hospitalized patients with community-acquired pneumonia. Clin Ther 2000; 22:872–8.
18. MacGowan AP. Role of pharmacokinetics and pharmacodynamics: does the dose matter? Clin Infect Dis 2001; 33(Suppl. 3):S238–9.
19. Richards MJ, Edwards JR, Culver DH, Gaynes RP. Nosocomial infections in medical intensive care units in the United States. National Nosocomial Infections Surveillance System. Crit Care Med 1999; 27:887–92.
20. Jacoby GA, Munoz-Price LS. The new beta-lactamases. N Engl J Med 2005; 352:380–91.
21. Francis JS, Doherty MC, Lopatin U, et al. Severe community-onset pneumonia in healthy adults caused by methicillin-resistant *Staphylococcus aureus* carrying the Panton-Valentine leukocidin genes. Clin Infect Dis 2005; 40:100–7.
22. Mongkolrattanothai K, Boyle S, Kahana MD, Daum RS. Severe *Staphylococcus aureus* infections caused by clonally related community-acquired methicillin-susceptible and methicillin-resistant isolates. Clin Infect Dis 2003; 37:1050–8.
23. Heffelfinger JD, Dowell SF, Jorgensen JH, et al. Management of community-acquired pneumonia in the era of pneumococcal resistance: a report from the Drug-Resistant *Streptococcus pneumoniae* Therapeutic Working Group. Arch Intern Med 2000; 160:1399–408.
24. Costerton JW, Stewart PS, Greenberg EP. Bacterial biofilms: a common cause of persistent infections. Science 1999; 284:1318–22.
25. Casey JR, Pichichero ME. Higher dosages of azithromycin are more effective in treatment of group A streptococcal tonsillopharyngitis. Clin Infect Dis 2005; 40:1748–55.
26. Bisno AL, Gerber MA, Gwaltney JM Jr, Kaplan EL, Schwartz RH. Diagnosis and management of group A streptococcal pharyngitis: a practice guideline. Infectious Diseases Society of America. Clin Infect Dis 1997; 25:574–83.
27. Pichichero ME, Cohen R. Shortened course of antibiotic therapy for acute otitis media, sinusitis and tonsillopharyngitis. Pediatr Infect Dis J 1997; 16:680–95.
28. Guay D. Short-course antimicrobial therapy of respiratory tract infections. Drugs 2003; 63:2169–84.
29. Wannamaker LW, Rammelkamp CH Jr, Denny FW, et al. Prophylaxis of acute rheumatic fever by treatment of the preceding streptococcal infection with various amounts of depot penicillin. Am J Med 1951; 10:673–95.
30. Wannamaker LW, Denny FW, Perry WD, et al. The effect of penicillin prophylaxis on streptococcal disease rates and the carrier state. N Engl J Med. 1953; 249:1–7.
31. Schwartz RH, Wientzen RL Jr, Pedreira F, Feroli EJ, Mella GW, Guandolo VL. Penicillin V for group A streptococcal pharyngotonsillitis. A randomized trial of seven vs ten days' therapy. J Am Med Assoc 1981; 246:1790–5.
32. Gerber MA, Randolph MF, Chanatry J, Wright LL, De MK, Kaplan EL. Five vs. ten days of penicillin V therapy for streptococcal pharyngitis. Am J Dis Child 1987; 141:224–7.
33. Pichichero ME. Short course antibiotic therapy for respiratory infections: a review of the evidence. Pediatr Infect Dis J 2000; 19:929–37.
34. Adam D, Scholz H, Helmerking M. Short-course antibiotic treatment of 4782 culture-proven cases of group A streptococcal tonsillopharyngitis and incidence of poststreptococcal sequelae. J Infect Dis 2000; 182:509–16.
35. McCarty JM. Clarithromycin in the management of community-acquired pneumonia. Clin Ther 2000; 22:281–94.
36. Williams JW Jr, Holleman DR Jr, Samsa GP, Simel DL. Randomized controlled trial of 3 vs. 10 s of trimethoprim/sulfamethoxazole for acute maxillary sinusitis. J Am Med Assoc 1995; 273:1015–21.
37. Casiano RR. Azithromycin and amoxicillin in the treatment of acute maxillary sinusitis. Am J Med 1991; 91:27S–30S.

38. Khong TK. Shortened therapies in acute sinusitis. Hosp Pract 1996; 31:11–3.
39. David DJ, Cooter RD. Craniofacial infection in 10 years of transcranial surgery. Plast Reconstr Surg 1987; 80:213–25.
40. Murphy TF, Kirkham C, Sethi S, Lesse AJ. Expression of a peroxiredoxin-glutaredoxin by *Haemophilus influenzae* in biofilms and during human respiratory tract infection. FEMS Immunol Med Microbiol 2005; 44:81–9.
41. Wilson R. Bacteria and airway inflammation in chronic obstructive pulmonary disease: more evidence. Am J Respir Crit Care Med 2005; 172:147–8.
42. Saint S, Bent S, Vittinghoff E, Grady D. Antibiotics in chronic obstructive pulmonary disease exacerbations. A meta-analysis. J Am Med Assoc 1995; 273:957–60.
43. Murphy TF, Brauer AL, Grant BJ, Sethi S. *Moraxella catarrhalis* in Chronic obstructive pulmonary disease: burden of disease and immune response. Am J Respir Crit Care Med 2005; 172:195–9.
44. Hoepelman IM, Mollers MJ, van Schie MH, et al. A short (3-day) course of azithromycin tablets versus a 10-day course of amoxycillin-clavulanic acid (co-amoxiclav) in the treatment of adults with lower respiratory tract infections and effects on long-term outcome. Int J Antimicrob Agents 1997; 9:141–6.
45. Lode H, Schaberg T. Azithromycin in lower respiratory tract infections. Scand J Infect Dis Suppl 1992; 83:26–33.
46. Gris P. Once-daily, 3-day azithromycin versus a three-times-daily, 10-day course of co-amoxiclav in the treatment of adults with lower respiratory tract infections: results of a randomized, double-blind comparative study. J Antimicrob Chemother. 1996; 37 (Suppl. C):93–101.
47. Mandell LA, Bartlett JG, Dowell SF, File TM, Jr, Musher DM, Whitney C. Update of practice guidelines for the management of community-acquired pneumonia in immunocompetent adults. Clin Infect Dis. 2003; 37:1405–33.
48. Mandell LA, Wunderink RG, Anzueto A, et al. Infectious Diseases Society of America/American Thoracic Society Consensus Guidelines on the Management of Community-Acquired Pneumonia in Adults. Clin Infect Dis 2007; 44:S27–S72.
49. Mandell LA, File TM, Jr. Short-course treatment of community-acquired pneumonia. Clin Infect Dis. 2003; 37:761–63.
50. Dunbar LM, Khashab MM, Kahn JB, Zadeikis N, Xiang JX, Tennenberg AM. Efficacy of 750-mg, 5-day levofloxacin in the treatment of community-acquired pneumonia caused by atypical pathogens. Curr Med Res Opin. 2004; 20:555–63.
51. Tellier G, Niederman MS, Nusrat R, Patel M, Lavin B. Clinical and bacteriological efficacy and safety of 5 and 7 regimens of telithromycin once daily compared with a 10 regimen of clarithromycin twice daily in patients with mild to moderate community-acquired pneumonia. J Antimicrob Chemother 2004; 54:515–23.
52. File TM Jr, Mandell LA, Leach T, Dostov K, Georgiev O. 5-day, short-course gemifloxacin Tehrapy to treat community-acquired pneumonia. Interscience Congress of Antimicrobial Therapy & Chemotherapy, New Orleans, LA. 9-22-2005. Ref Type: Abstract
53. O'Doherty B, Muller O. Randomized, multicentre study of the efficacy and tolerance of azithromycin versus clarithromycin in the treatment of adults with mild to moderate community-acquired pneumonia. Azithromycin Study Group. Eur J Clin Microbiol Infect Dis 1998; 17:828–33.
54. Drehobl MA. Use of a large, extended release 2 g dose of aziathromycin for treatment of community-acquired pneumonia. 44th Interscience Congress of Antimicrobial Agents and Chemotherapy (L660). 9-20-2004. Ref Type: Abstract.
55. Bartlett JG, Dowell SF, Mandell LA, File Jr TM, Musher DM, Fine MJ. Practice guidelines for the management of community-acquired pneumonia in adults. Infectious Diseases Society of America. Clin Infect Dis 2000; 31:347–82.
56. Mathers DL, Hassman J, Tellier G. Efficacy and tolerability of once-daily oral telithromycin compared with clarithromycin for the treatment of community-acquired pneumonia in adults. Clin Ther 2004; 26:48–62.
57. Chastre J, Fagon JY. Ventilator-associated pneumonia. Am J Respir Crit Care Med 2002; 165:867–903.

58. Dennesen PJ, Van DV, Kessels AG, Ramsay G, Bonten MJ. Resolution of infectious parameters after antimicrobial therapy in patients with ventilator-associated pneumonia. Am J Respir Crit Care Med 2001; 163:1371–5.
59. Luna CM, Blanzaco D, Niederman MS, et al. Resolution of ventilator-associated pneumonia: prospective evaluation of the clinical pulmonary infection score as an early predictor of outcome. Crit Care Med 2003; 31(3):676–82.
60. Micek ST, Ward S, Fraser VJ, Kollef MH. A randomized controlled trial of an antibiotic discontinuation policy for clinically suspected ventilator-associated pneumonia. Chest 2004; 125:1791–9.
61. Singh N, Rogers P, Atwood CW, Wagener MM, Yu VL. Short-course empiric antibiotic therapy for patients with pulmonary infiltrates in the intensive care unit. A proposed solution for indiscriminate antibiotic prescription. Am J Respir Crit Care Med 2000; 162:505–11.
62. Chastre J, Wolff M, Fagon JY, et al. Comparison of 8 vs. 15 days of antibiotic therapy for ventilator-associated pneumonia in adults: a randomized trial. J Am Med Assoc 2003; 290:2588–98.
63. Harbarth S, Holeckova K, Froidevaux C, et al. Diagnostic value of procalcitonin, interleukin-6, and interleukin-8 in critically ill patients admitted with suspected sepsis. Am J Respir Crit Care Med 2001; 164:396–402.
64. Duflo F, Debon R, Goudable J, Chassard D, Allaouchiche B. Alveolar and serum oxidative stress in ventilator-associated pneumonia. Br J Anaesth 2002; 89:231–6.
65. Luyt CE, Guerin V, Combes A, et al. Procalcitonin kinetics as a prognostic marker of ventilator-associated pneumonia. Am J Respir Crit Care Med 2005; 171:48–53.
66. Warren JW, Abrutyn E, Hebel JR, Johnson JR, Schaeffer AJ, Stamm WE. Guidelines for antimicrobial treatment of uncomplicated acute bacterial cystitis and acute pyelonephritis in women. Infectious Diseases Society of America (IDSA). Clin Infect Dis 1999; 29:745–58.
67. Gupta MN, Sturrock RD, Field M. A prospective 2-year study of 75 patients with adult-onset septic arthritis. Rheumatology (Oxford). 2001; 40:24–30.
68. Hooton TM, Scholes D, Gupta K, Stapleton AE, Roberts PL, Stamm WE. Amoxicillin-clavulanate vs ciprofloxacin for the treatment of uncomplicated cystitis in women: a randomized trial. J Am Med Assoc 2005; 293:949–55.
69. Naber KG. Treatment options for acute uncomplicated cystitis in adults. J Antimicrob Chemother 2000; 46(Suppl. A):23–7.
70. Lutters M, Vogt N. Antibiotic duration for treating uncomplicated, symptomatic lower urinary tract infections in elderly women. Cochrane Database Syst Rev 2002; CD001535.
71. Vogel T, Verreault R, Gourdeau M, Morin M, Grenier-Gosselin L, Rochette L. Optimal duration of antibiotic therapy for uncomplicated urinary tract infection in older women: a double-blind randomized controlled trial. CMAJ 2004; 170:469–73.
72. Stapleton A. Urinary tract infections in patients with diabetes. Am J Med 2002; 113 (Suppl. 1)A:80S–4S.
73. Hooton TM. The current management strategies for community-acquired urinary tract infection. Infect Dis Clin North Am 2003; 17:303–2.
74. Siroky MB. Pathogenesis of bacteriuria and infection in the spinal cord injured patient. Am J Med 2002; 113(Suppl. 1)A:67S–79S.
75. Dow G, Rao P, Harding G, et al. A prospective, randomized trial of 3 or 14 days of ciprofloxacin treatment for acute urinary tract infection in patients with spinal cord injury. Clin Infect Dis 2004; 39:658–64.
76. Kahan NR, Chinitz DP, Kahan E. Physician adherence to recommendations for duration of empiric antibiotic treatment for uncomplicated urinary tract infection in women: a national drug utilization analysis. Pharmacoepidemiol Drug Saf 2004; 13:239–42.
77. Wigton RS, Longenecker JC, Bryan TJ, Parenti C, Flach SD, Tape TG. Variation by specialty in the treatment of urinary tract infection in women. J Gen Intern Med 1999; 14:491–4.

78. Howden CW, Hunt RH. Guidelines for the management of *Helicobacter pylori* infection. Ad Hoc Committee on Practice Parameters of the American College of Gastroenterology. Am J Gastroenterol 1998; 93:2330–8.

79. Malfertheiner P, Megraud F, O'Morain C, et al. Current concepts in the management of *Helicobacter pylori* infection—the Maastricht 2-2000 Consensus Report. Aliment Pharmacol Ther 2002; 16:167–80.

80. Malfertheiner P, Megraud F, O'Morain C, et al. Current European concepts in the management of *Helicobacter pylori* infection—the Maastricht Consensus Report. The European *Helicobacter pylori* Study Group (EHPSG). Eur J Gastroenterol Hepatol 1997; 9:1–2.

81. Buckley MJ, Xia HX, Hyde DM, Keane CT, O'Morain CA. Metronidazole resistance reduces efficacy of triple therapy and leads to secondary clarithromycin resistance. Dig Dis Sci 1997; 42:2111–5.

82. Wong WM, Gu Q, Wang WH, et al. Effects of primary metronidazole and clarithromycin resistance to *Helicobacter pylori* on omeprazole, metronidazole, and clarithromycin triple-therapy regimen in a region with high rates of metronidazole resistance. Clin Infect Dis 2003; 37:882–9.

83. Osato MS, Reddy R, Reddy SG, Penland RL, Malaty HM, Graham DY. Pattern of primary resistance of *Helicobacter pylori* to metronidazole or clarithromycin in the United States. Arch Intern Med 2001; 161:1217–20.

84. Meyer JM, Silliman NP, Wang W, et al. Risk factors for *Helicobacter pylori* resistance in the United States: the surveillance of *H. pylori* antimicrobial resistance partnership (SHARP) study, 1993–1999. Ann Intern Med 2002; 136:13–24.

85. Calvet X, Ducons J, Guardiola J, et al. One-week triple versus quadruple therapy for *Helicobacter pylori* infection — a randomized trial. Aliment Pharmacol Ther 2002; 16:1261–7.

86. Prazeres MP, De Magalhaes Queiroz DM, Campos Barbosa DV, et al. *Helicobacter pylori* primary resistance to metronidazole and clarithromycin in Brazil. Antimicrob Agents Chemother 2002; 46:2021–3.

87. Xia HX, Fan XG, Talley NJ. Clarithromycin resistance in *Helicobacter pylori* and its clinical relevance. World J Gastroenterol 1999; 5:263–6.

88. McMahon BJ, Hennessy TW, Bensler JM, et al. The relationship among previous antimicrobial use, antimicrobial resistance, and treatment outcomes for *Helicobacter pylori* infections. Ann Intern Med 2003; 139:463–9.

89. Laine L, Estrada R, Trujillo M, Fukanaga K, Neil G. Randomized comparison of differing periods of twice-a-day triple therapy for the eradication of *Helicobacter pylori*. Aliment Pharmacol Ther 1996; 10:1029–33.

90. de Boer W, Driessen W, Jansz A, Tytgat G. Effect of acid suppression on efficacy of treatment for *Helicobacter pylori* infection. Lancet 1995; 345(8953):817–20.

91. Vakil N, Lanza F, Schwartz H, Barth J. Seven-day therapy for *Helicobacter pylori* in the United States. Aliment Pharmacol Ther 2004; 20:99–107.

92. Ford A, Delaney B, Forman D, Moayyedi P. Eradication therapy for peptic ulcer disease in *Helicobacter pylori* positive patients. Cochrane Database Syst Rev 2003; CD003840.

93. Treiber G, Wittig J, Ammon S, Walker S, van Doorn LJ, Klotz U. Clinical outcome and influencing factors of a new short-term quadruple therapy for *Helicobacter pylori* eradication: a randomized controlled trial (MACLOR study). Arch Intern Med 2002; 162:153–60.

94. de Boer WA, Driessen WM, Tytgat GN. Only four days of quadruple therapy can effectively cure *Helicobacter pylori* infection. Aliment Pharmacol Ther 1995; 9:633–38.

95. de Boer WA. How to achieve a near 100% cure rate for *Helicobacter pylori* infection in peptic ulcer patients. A personal viewpoint. J Clin Gastroenterol 1996; 22:313–6.

96. Treiber G, Ammon S, Schneider E, Klotz U. Amoxicillin/metronidazole/omeprazole/clarithromycin: a new, short quadruple therapy for *Helicobacter pylori* eradication. Helicobacter 1998; 3:54–8.

97. Mermin JH, Townes JM, Gerber M, Dolan N, Mintz ED, Tauxe RV. Typhoid fever in the United States, 1985–1994: changing risks of international travel and increasing antimicrobial resistance. Arch Intern Med 1998; 158:633–8.

98. Kubota K, Barrett TJ, Ackers ML, Brachman PS, Mintz ED. Analysis of *Salmonella enterica* serotype Typhi pulsed-field gel electrophoresis patterns associated with international travel. J Clin Microbiol 2005; 43:1205–9.

99. Nguyen TC, Solomon T, Mai XT, et al. Short courses of ofloxacin for the treatment of enteric fever. Trans R Soc Trop Med Hyg 1997; 91:347–9.

100. Wain J, Hoa NT, Chinh NT, et al. Quinolone-resistant Salmonella typhi in Viet Nam: molecular basis of resistance and clinical response to treatment. Clin Infect Dis 1997; 25:1404–10.

101. Chinh NT, Parry CM, Ly NT, et al. A randomized controlled comparison of azithromycin and ofloxacin for treatment of multidrug-resistant or nalidixic acid-resistant enteric fever. Antimicrob Agents Chemother 2000; 44:1855–9.

102. Islam A, Butler T, Kabir I, Alam NH. Treatment of typhoid fever with ceftriaxone for 5 days or chloramphenicol for 14 days: a randomized clinical trial. Antimicrob Agents Chemother 1993; 37:1572–5.

103. Moran JS, Levine WC. Drugs of choice for the treatment of uncomplicated gonococcal infections. Clin Infect Dis 1995; 20(Suppl. 1):S47–65.

104. Fenton KA, Ison C, Johnson AP, et al. Ciprofloxacin resistance in *Neisseria gonorrhoeae* in England and Wales in 2002. Lancet 2003; 361:1867–9.

105. Sexually transmitted disease treatment guidelines, 2006. Centers for Disease Control and Prevention. MMWR Recomm Rep 2006; 55:1–94.

106. Updates to CDC's Sexually Transmitted Diseases Treatment Guidelines, 2006: Fluoroquinolones no longer recommended for treatment of gonococcal infections. Centers for Disease Control and Prevention. MMWR 2007; 56:332–6.

107. Stamm WE, Hicks CB, Martin DH, et al. Azithromycin for empirical treatment of the nongonococcal urethritis syndrome in men. A randomized double-blind study. J Am Med Assoc 1995; 274:545–9.

108. Wilson WR. Ceftriaxone sodium therapy of penicillin G-susceptible streptococcal endocarditis. J Am Med Assoc 1992; 267:279–80.

109. Francioli P, Ruch W, Stamboulian D. Treatment of streptococcal endocarditis with a single daily dose of ceftriaxone and netilmicin for 14 days: a prospective multicenter study. Clin Infect Dis 1995; 21:1406–10.

110. Sexton DJ, Tenenbaum MJ, Wilson WR, et al. Ceftriaxone once daily for four weeks compared with ceftriaxone plus gentamicin once daily for two weeks for treatment of endocarditis due to penicillin-susceptible streptococci. Endocarditis Treatment Consortium Group. Clin Infect Dis 1998; 27:1470–4.

111. Baddour LM, Wilson WR, Bayer AS, et al. Infective endocarditis: diagnosis, antimicrobial therapy, and management of complications: a statement for healthcare professionals from the Committee on Rheumatic Fever, Endocarditis, and Kawasaki Disease, Council on Cardiovascular Disease in the Young, and the Councils on Clinical Cardiology, Stroke, and Cardiovascular Surgery and Anesthesia, American Heart Association: endorsed by the Infectious Diseases Society of America. Circulation 2005; 111:e394–434.

112. Chambers HF, Miller RT, Newman MD. Right-sided *Staphylococcus aureus* endocarditis in intravenous drug abusers: two-week combination therapy. Ann Intern Med 1988; 109:619–24.

113. DiNubile MJ. Short-course antibiotic therapy for right-sided endocarditis caused by *Staphylococcus aureus* in injection drug users. Ann Intern Med 1994; 121:873–6.

114. Fortun J, Navas E, Martinez-Beltran J, et al. Short-course therapy for right-side endocarditis due to *Staphylococcus aureus* in drug abusers: cloxacillin versus glycopeptides in combination with gentamicin. Clin Infect Dis 2001; 33:120–5.

115. Ribera E, Gomez-Jimenez J, Cortes E, et al. Effectiveness of cloxacillin with and without gentamicin in short-term therapy for right-sided *Staphylococcus aureus* endocarditis. A randomized, controlled trial. Ann Intern Med 1996; 125:969–74.

116. Torres-Tortosa M, de CM, Vergara A, Sanchez-Porto A, et al. Prospective evaluation of a two-week course of intravenous antibiotics in intravenous drug addicts with infective endocarditis. Grupo de Estudio de Enfermedades Infecciosas de la Provincia de Cadiz. Eur J Clin Microbiol Infect Dis 1994; 13:559–64.
117. Miro JM, del RA, Mestres CA. Infective endocarditis and cardiac surgery in intravenous drug abusers and HIV-1 infected patients. Cardiol Clin 2003; 21:167–vi.
118. O'Grady NP, Alexander M, Dellinger EP, et al. Guidelines for the prevention of intravascular catheter-related infections. Am J Infect Control 2002; 30:476–89.
119. O'Grady NP, Alexander M, Dellinger EP, et al. Guidelines for the prevention of intravascular catheter-related infections. Infect Control Hosp Epidemiol 2002; 23:759–69.
120. Mermel LA, Farr BM, Sherertz RJ, et al. Guidelines for the management of intravascular catheter-related infections. Clin Infect Dis 2001; 32:1249–72.
121. Fowler VG Jr, Olsen MK, Corey GR, et al. Clinical identifiers of complicated *Staphylococcus aureus* bacteremia. Arch Intern Med 2003; 163:2066–72.
122. Li JZ, Winston LG, Moore DH, Bent J. Efficacy of short-course antibiotic therapy regimens for community acquired pnuemonia: a meta-analysis. Am J Med 2007; 120 (9):783–90.
123. File TM Jr, Mandell LA, Tillotson G, Kostov K, Georgiev O. Gemifloxacin once daily for 5 days versus 7 days for the treatment of community-aquired pneumonia: a randomized, multicentre, double-blind study. J Antimicrob Chemother 2007; 60(1): 112–20.

19 Impact of Guidelines on Antimicrobial Treatment of Respiratory Tract Infections

Thomas M. File
Northeastern Ohio Universities College of Medicine, Rootstown, Ohio and Summa Health System, Akron, Ohio, U.S.A.

INTRODUCTION

Respiratory tract infections (RTIs) are the most common type of infection managed by healthcare providers and are of potentially great consequence (1). Overall, RTIs are the greatest single cause of death in children worldwide (4.3 million deaths in 1992), whereas lower RTIs are the most common cause of death caused by infectious disease in the United States. RTIs are also the source of most antibiotic use. Approximately three-quarters of all outpatient antimicrobial use are for respiratory infections (2). Although many RTIs require antimicrobial therapy for optimal management, respiratory viruses for which antibiotic use is not warranted cause most outpatient respiratory infections [i.e., acute bronchitis, nasal pharyngitis, colds, nonspecific upper respiratory tract infections (URIs)]. Use of antibiotics for these conditions is a source of great antibiotic abuse and increases the likelihood of further hindering the already high level of antibiotic resistance. Paradoxically, the progress previously made in dealing with the most common bacterial cause of respiratory infections, *Streptococcus pneumoniae*, is now associated with a global explosion of drug resistance that has made treatment decisions very difficult.

In order to address the appropriate use of antibiotics and to improve care of patients with RTIs who warrant antibiotics, various professional groups have developed numerous guidelines. The primary purposes of these guidelines are to standardize care and ultimately improve outcome of patients. Promoting the appropriate use of antibiotics through the development and application of such treatment guidelines and educational efforts aimed at clinicians as well as patients should not only optimize clinical outcomes, but also help curb inappropriate prescribing and misuse of antibiotics, decrease treatment costs, and increase patient satisfaction. It is important to understand that specific guidelines cannot always account for individual difference among patients. They are not intended to replace physician judgment with respect to particular patients or special clinical situations. The eventual determination regarding their application must be made by the physician in light of each patient's individual circumstances.

This chapter considers recommendations for judicious antibiotic use for RTIs, reviews guidelines for specific infections [with a greater emphasis on community-acquired pneumonia (CAP)], and reviews their impact on outcome.

PRINCIPLES OF JUDICIOUS USE OF ANTIBIOTICS TO TREAT RESPIRATORY TRACT INFECTIONS

The discovery of potent antimicrobial agents was one of the greatest contributions to medicine in the 20th century. Unfortunately, the emergence of antimicrobial-resistant pathogens now threatens these advances. The increase in resistance is a result of several factors, but a major factor driving resistance is the overall volume of antimicrobial prescribing—particularly for indications that do not warrant such therapy (3). It is vitally important that judicious use of antimicrobials be encouraged in order to curb this overuse, and, hopefully, minimize resistance emergence. One way to promote the appropriate use of antibiotics is through the development and application of treatment guidelines, which are based on sound scientific evidence.

Antimicrobial-Resistant S. pneumoniae

Antibiotic overuse and inappropriate antibiotic selection have been associated with increased drug resistance among several respiratory pathogens—most notably *S. pneumoniae*, the most common bacterial pathogen in RTI. However, the clinical significance of antimicrobial-resistant *S. pneumoniae* is not clear for the all RTIs. While there is adequate information to indicate penicillin-resistant *S. pneumoniae* is important when treating meningitis or otitis media, the relevance for lower RTIs, especially pneumonia, is unsettled (4). Presently the level of resistance of *S. pneumoniae* to beta-lactams and macrolides does not result in clinical treatment failures in most patients with pneumonia, but as a minimum inhibitory concentration (MIC) shift occurs (i.e., higher prevalence of *S. pneumoniae* with penicillin MIC $\geq 4\,\mu g/mL$), it is anticipated an adverse clinical impact of resistance among the pneumococci will become more apparent. Risk factors for penicillin-resistant *S. pneumoniae* have been identified (i.e., age < 2 years or > 65 years, beta-lactam therapy within 3 months, alcoholism, medical comorbidities, immunosuppressive illness or therapy, and exposure to a child in a day care center), although it is not clear these are specific enough for individual patients to be clinically reliable (5). In 2005, Vanderkooi and colleagues published results of a prospective cohort study of invasive pneumococcal infection that evaluated risk factors for antimicrobial resistances. The researchers concluded that the single most important risk factor for antimicrobial resistance was the previous use of an antibiotic from the same class of agents (6).

The clinical relevance of macrolide-resistant *S. pneumoniae* (MRSP) may be dependent on the type of resistance expressed by a particular strain. The most common mechanisms of resistance include methylation of a ribosomal target encoded by *erm* gene and efflux of the macrolides by cell membrane protein transporter, encoded by *mef* gene (7). *S. pneumoniae* strains with *mef* are resistant at a lower level (with MICs generally 1–$16\,\mu g/mL$) than *erm*-resistant strains, and it is possible that such strains (particularly with MIC $< 8\,\mu g/mL$) may be inhibited if sufficiently high levels of macrolide can be obtained within infected tissue (such as may occur with newer macrolides—clarithromycin or azithromycin) (8–11). However, there is recent evidence that the MICs of these strains are increasing and this may affect the efficacy of these macrolides (12). The *mef*-resistant strains are usually susceptible to clindamycin. Most *erm*-resistant isolates have a MIC $> 32\,\mu g/mL$ for erythromycin and are considered highly resistant for all macrolides and clindamycin. Until recently, reports of failure of CAP treated with macrolides have been rare, particularly for patients at low risk for drug-resistant strains. However, since 2000, anecdotal reports and one controlled study have documented failures due to MRSP in patients treated with an oral macrolide who have subsequently required admission to the hospital with *S. pneumoniae* bacteremia (13–16). Currently, *mef*-associated resistance predominates in North America. *erm*-associated resistance predominates in Europe and is common in Japan.

Although the worldwide prevalence of pneumococcal resistance to the newer fluoroquinolones (levofloxacin, moxifloxacin, gemifloxacin) remains low (less than 2%), in some countries resistance has increased markedly (17–19). The overall prevalence of fluoroquinolone resistance (levofloxacin >4 mcg/mL) in Hong Kong in 2000 had increased to 13.3% due to the dissemination of a fluoroquinolone-resistant clone (18). Treatment failures have already been reported, mostly in patients who have previously been treated with fluoroquinolones (20,21). Risk factors for levofloxacin resistance were identified as: prior exposure to a fluoroquinolone, nursing home residence, nosocomial infection, and chronic obstructive pulmonary disease (COPD) (22).

Principles of Judicious Antimicrobial Use

Because of the increase in resistance it is increasingly important that recommendations for judicious use of antibiotics for RTI be reviewed. Several organizations have published guidelines for appropriate antimicrobial usage (23–26). When recommendations from such guidelines are applied to select an appropriate empiric agent, the clinical outcome is hopefully optimized and the costs associated with incorrect prescribing and multiple courses of antibiotics can be avoided. Principles of optimized therapy should be promoted and utilized by prescribing clinicians in order to result in the best outcomes for our patients and reduce the emergence of antibiotic resistance. This is the conclusion of a consensus group on resistance and prescribing in RTI. This independent, multinational, interdisciplinary group was established to identify fundamental principles that should form the basis of prescribing in RTI and guideline formulation, with particular emphasis on countering bacterial resistance and maximizing beneficial patient outcomes (27).

The Consensus Group listed several core principles of antibiotic therapy that should provide optimal benefit for patients as well as minimize resistance; among these are:

1. Use antibacterial therapy only in those patients with bacterial infection.
2. Utilize diagnostic and other measures to reduce prescribing. Therapy should maximally reduce or eradicate the bacterial load.
3. Use antimicrobial agents with optimal pharmacodynamics to achieve eradication.
4. Use locally relevant resistance data in the decision process.
5. Understand that antimicrobial acquisition cost may be insignificant compared with therapeutic failure.

Reduction of Unnecessary Antimicrobials

The Consensus Group identified inappropriate prescribing to be the major influence on developing resistance and increasing costs, and called for antibiotic therapy to be limited to infections in which bacteria are the predominant cause. While this principle certainly seems self-evident, it is one to which adherence seems very difficult. The reasons for over-prescribing antibiotics are multifactorial. Patients may consult clinicians, expecting an antibiotic to be prescribed for an acute respiratory infection for which the etiology is most likely viral; as a result, clinicians may feel pressured to write antibiotic prescriptions to satisfy patients and to maintain good doctor–patient relationships. Receiving an antibiotic reinforces the patients' perception that antibiotics are warranted in similar situations. Thus, patients may continue to consult clinicians each time similar symptoms occur, expecting that antibiotics are again needed. Clinicians also may prescribe antibiotics as a rapid means of treating patients' symptoms rather than taking the time to educate patients that antibiotics are not always necessary, especially if a viral infection is suspected. However, clinicians should recognize that patient satisfaction is not compromised by the absence of an antibiotic prescription, provided patients understand the reasons. Hamm et al. demonstrated that patient satisfaction was influenced by patient perceptions that the clinician spent enough time discussing the illness and by patient knowledge about the treatment choice (28). Moreover, clinicians may prescribe antibiotics as part of a defensive approach to avoid the potential sequelae of not prescribing for patients with bacterial infection.

Unfortunately, most patients and many clinicians view "unnecessary" antibiotic prescribing as at worst a neutral intervention (i.e., cannot harm, but may help). It is imperative patients understand this is not the case. In fact, the unnecessary use of antibacterials has several possible harmful effects in addition to selection of resistance, such as increased cost and exposure to unnecessary adverse reactions. Decreasing excess antibiotic use is an important strategy for combating the increase in community-acquired antibiotic-resistant infections. Several studies have documented a benefit of combining physician intervention and patient education that has resulted in decreased use of antimicrobials and reduction of resistance (Table 1) (29–34).

Correct diagnosis to differentiate viral from bacterial infection is a key to limiting unnecessary antimicrobials. Unfortunately, there is a lack of rapidly available, cost-effective diagnostic tests, which reliably differentiate self-limiting, viral from bacterial infection. However, practice guidelines can offer pragmatic criteria for better antimicrobial usage. For example, restriction of antibiotic therapy in otitis media to those children with acute bacterial disease and avoidance in otitis media with effusion could reduce unnecessary use by two-thirds (35). The Consensus Group concluded that antibiotics that maximize bacterial eradication improve both short- and long-term clinical outcomes, reduce overall costs—particularly those relating to treatment failure and consequent hospital admission—and assist in the minimization of resistance emergence and dissemination. They believe that a radical re-evaluation of RTI therapy, incorporating these principles, is long overdue, to guide the decisions of both individuals and formulary and guideline committees more accurately.

In addition to reducing antimicrobial usage, more effective use of pneumococcal vaccines offers promise to decreasing the burden of this pathogen and resistance in both pediatric and adult populations. Preliminary data indicate significant reductions in hospitalization and mortality from use of these vaccines, suggesting an associated reduced necessity of prescribing (36). However, of primary importance is the continued promotion of principles of judicious antibiotic when they are warranted.

GUIDELINES FOR RTI
The Value of Guidelines
In general, clinical guidelines have been shown to improve medical practice (37). The use of clinical practice guidelines can be an effective means of changing

TABLE 1 Impact of Guideline Interventions on Antimicrobial Usage and Resistance

Study (reference)	Country	Intervention	Observations
Kristinsson et al. (29)	Iceland	Reduction in antibiotic use	Overall reduction in antibiotic use (penicillin from 20% to < 15%), associated with reduction of drug-resistant *Streptococcus pneumoniae*
Seppala et al. (30)	Finland	Reduction in macrolide use for certain infections	Resistance of *Streptococcus pyogenes* decreased from 19% to 9%
Pestonik et al. (31)	U.S.A.	Evaluation of antibiotic practice guidelines through computer-assisted decision support	Antibiotic use decreased by 22.8%, rate of antibiotic adverse events decreased by 30%, antibiotic resistance remained stable
Petersen et al. (32)	U.S.A.	Provider and community education for prescribing antibiotics for RTIs in Alaska	Education of healthcare providers and patients substantially decreased the number of visits and antimicrobial prescriptions for RTI, and the carriage of PRSP
Gonzales et al. (33)	U.S.A.	Use of household and/or office-based patient educational materials as well as clinician detailing compared to controls	Antibiotic prescription rates declined at sites implementing both use of office-based patient educational materials as well as clinician detailing
Guillenot et al. (34)	France	Educational interventions aimed at parents, physicians, and pharmacists designed to reduce antibiotic use for upper RTIs	Antibiotic sales fell 32–37% depending on the intervention. The rate of colonization with PRSP was seen in intervention groups

Abbreviations: RTI, respiratory tract infection; PRSP, penicillin-resistant *Streptococcus pneumoniae*.

behavior, such as promoting the appropriate use of antibiotics. Effective clinical guidelines should improve patient care while enhancing cost savings. However, cost savings should not be the primary motivating factor. A recent example reported by Beilby et al. described a government intervention in Australia intended to decrease costs by reducing the use of amoxicillin-clavulanate (38). As a result, costs increased through the occurrence of adverse outcomes in patients with acute otitis media (AOM), sinusitis, lower RTI, and acute exacerbations of chronic bronchitis (AECB).

To maximize effectiveness and applicability, antibiotic use guidelines should be evidence-based. The guidelines should also reflect data on resistance, recognizing that local patterns of resistance often differ across geographic regions. Hence, effective guidelines should be readily adaptable for implementation locally. Primary objectives of guidelines for treating RTIs should be to discourage antibiotic use to treat viral illness, to outline diagnostic criteria, and to avoid the use of ineffective antimicrobials.

Unfortunately, a meta-analysis of relevant studies has shown that there are numerous barriers to adherence to practice guidelines (Table 2) (39). For example,

TABLE 2   Barriers to Clinician Adherence to Clinical Practice Guidelines

Barrier	Explanation
Lack of awareness	Clinician unaware that the guidelines exist
Lack of familiarity	Clinician aware of guidelines but unfamiliar with specifics
Lack of agreement	Clinician does not agree with a specific recommendation made in guideline or is averse to the concept of guidelines in general
Lack of self-efficacy	Clinician doubts whether he/she can perform the behavior
Lack of outcome expectancy	Clinician believes the recommendations will be unsuccessful
Lack of motivation	Clinician is unable/unmotivated to change previous practices
Guideline-related barriers	Guidelines are not easy or convenient to use
Patient-related barriers	Clinician may be unable to reconcile guidelines with patient preferences
Environmental-related barriers	Clinician may not have control over some changes (e.g., time, resources, organizational constraints)

Source: Adapted from Ref. 39.

clinicians may not be aware of all of the available guidelines or may not be well versed in how to apply specific recommendations appropriately. In addition, clinicians may not agree with some or all of the recommendations made or, as a general principle, may resist the concept of guidelines. If clinicians are doubtful that they can perform the task called for in the guidelines or harbor a belief that the recommendations will be unsuccessful, they probably will not follow the guidelines. Time constraints or healthcare organization requirements may impose restrictions that hamper the clinician's ability to implement the guidelines. Furthermore, the clinician may not have control over some changes called for in guidelines, such as the acquisition of new resources to perform diagnostic tests. Patient preferences for alternatives not recommended in guidelines also may obstruct adherence to clinical practice guidelines. To be successful, educational efforts and interventions aimed at improving adherence to practice guidelines—such as use of checklists and reminder systems—should address all of the identified barriers.

Antimicrobial Recommendations in RTI Guidelines-General Approach

Guidelines are usually evidence-based as assessed by a panel of experts. Guidelines for the management of specific RTIs have been developed by numerous professional organizations. For their development, most groups have relied on information obtained from prospectively performed studies upon which to base recommendations. Thus, published data and expert opinion have served as major influences in the formulation of these documents.

The selections of specific antimicrobial agents in the guidelines are usually based on multiple factors that include: the most likely pathogens and pathogen susceptibility patterns, patient's age and comorbidities, ability to tolerate side effects, and cost. Dosing frequency and side effects play a significant role in promoting or deterring patient adherence to therapy. Selecting agents that have more favorable side-effect profiles and less-frequent dosing requirements can aid in achieving adherence. Epidemiological information that may indicate the likelihood of a particular pathogen (such as recent epidemics of influenza, recent travel, and recent exposure to animals or other patients with specific infections) and disease severity (i.e., outpatient vs. inpatient) also significantly influences therapeutic choices.

The following represents brief descriptions of the major guidelines published in North America concerning the most common RTIs.

The Use of Treatment Recommendations/Guidelines in RTIs Other Than Pneumonia

Acute Otitis Media

Treatment for bacterial AOM must take into account pathogens most commonly implicated in this condition (i.e., *S. pneumoniae, Haemophilus influenzae, Moraxella catarrhalis*) as well as their resistance patterns. AOM treatment recommendations have been developed in the context of increasing levels of drug-resistant bacteria and selecting the appropriate antibiotic agents. In 1999, guidelines were published from a multidisciplinary group coordinated by the Centers for Disease Control and Prevention (CDC) (40). After reviewing the data, the drug-resistant *S. pneumoniae* Therapeutic Working Group of the CDC recommended that amoxicillin (standard dose: 40–45 mg/kg/day or high-dose: 80–90 mg/kg/day) should be used as first-line therapy in AOM. If factors associated with the likelihood of resistance are present, the recommendations suggest using high-dose amoxicillin, high-dose amoxicillin-clavulanate, or cefuroxime axetil as first-line therapy. These factors include daycare attendance, age, and recent prior exposure to antibiotics (e.g., within 4–6 weeks). Amoxicillin-clavulanate, cefuroxime axetil, and intramuscular (IM) ceftriaxone are recommended for treatment if amoxicillin fails after 3 days of therapy. Although a single injection of IM ceftriaxone achieves high concentrations in middle ear fluid for several days, the clinical outcome is not improved compared with a 10-day course of amoxicillin-clavulanate (41). Furthermore, a series of daily injections given for 3 days may be needed to improve the effectiveness of ceftriaxone against penicillin-resistant *S. pneumoniae* (40). Other agents such as cefprozil, cefpodoxime, cefaclor, cefixime, ceftibuten, loracarbef, trimethoprim-sulfamethoxazole, and the macrolides are not included in the list of preferred antimicrobials for a variety of reasons, including inadequate pharmacokinetic properties and decreased activity against beta-lactamase enzymes and drug-resistant *S. pneumoniae* (DRSP).

Patients who are allergic to penicillin may be treated with a newer macrolide or trimethoprim-sulfamethoxazole. However, these agents have less activity against DRSP. Fluoroquinolones, although effective against common respiratory pathogens, are not approved for use in children.

More recently, the American Academy of Pediatrics and American Academy of Family Physicians published an evidenced-based clinical practice guideline for the diagnosis and management of AOM of children from 2 months through 12 years of age (42). The guideline provides a specific definition of AOM and addresses pain management, initial observation versus antibacterial treatment, and appropriate antibacterials. A diagnosis of AOM requires (*i*) a history of acute onset of signs and symptoms, (*ii*) the presence of middle ear effusion, and (*iii*) signs and symptoms of middle ear inflammation. Criteria for antibacterial-agent treatment and recommended antibacterial agents are listed in Tables 3 and 4.

Acute Bacterial Rhinosinusitis (ABRS)

Similar to the CDC's recommendations for AOM, the guidelines issued by the Sinus and Allergy Health Partnership recommends empiric choices for treating ABRS (43). As in AOM, *S. pneumoniae* and *H. influenzae* are frequently implicated in ABRS. However, *M. catarrhalis* is less likely to be the infectious cause of this

TABLE 3 Criteria for Initial Antibacterial Treatment or Observation in Children with Acute Otitis Media

Age	Certain diagnosis	Uncertain diagnosis
<6 mo	Antibacterial therapy	Antibacterial therapy
6 mo to 2 years	Antibacterial therapy	Antibacterial therapy if severe illness; observation option if non-severe illness when follow-up can be insured
≥2 years	Antibacterial therapy if severe illness; observation option if non-severe	Observation option

Source: Adapted from Ref. 42.

condition compared with its role in AOM (2% vs. 12%). The guidelines recognize that patients exposed to an antibiotic within 4 to 6 weeks of their current infection are likely to be infected with a resistant pathogen. In developing its antimicrobial guidelines, the panel employed the Poole Therapeutic Outcome Model to predict the therapeutic effectiveness of various antimicrobial agents. Recognizing that resistance rates may change over time and may vary from community to community, the Panel intends to revise the guidelines as resistance rates change and as new antibiotics are introduced. The model is available at the Sinus and Allergy website (76), where clinicians may input local resistance rates and develop their own optimal treatment recommendations.

Agents recommended for the treatment of ABRS are listed in Table 5. The antibiotic selections listed in the table are stratified by disease severity, age of the patient, and recent antibiotic exposure. The preferred agents are those that are active against the pathogens commonly implicated in acute sinusitis—*S. pneumoniae, H. influenzae,* and *M. catarrhalis.* Switching to a second agent is suggested if, after 72 hr, the patient's condition does not clinically improve or worsens. Selection of the appropriate antibiotic can help prevent the development of chronic sinusitis, decrease costs associated with multiple treatment failures, and curtail the development of resistance.

First-line therapy for adult patients with mild disease and no antibiotic therapy during the previous 4 to 6 weeks are limited to high-dose amoxicillin, amoxicillin-clavulanate, cefpodoxime proxetil, and cefuroxime axetil. The guidelines note that cefprozil may have a bacterial failure rate of up to 25%. Similarly, while clarithromycin, trimethoprim-sulfamethoxazole, doxycycline, azithromycin, or erythromycin may be considered for patients with beta-lactam allergies, they are generally less active for DRSP. The use of trimethoprim-sulfamethoxazole also has been associated with potentially fatal toxic epidermal necrolysis. For adults with mild disease who have had recent antibiotic therapy or for those with moderate disease with no recent antibiotic therapy, first-line treatment recommendations include amoxicillin-clavulanate, high-dose amoxicillin, cefpodoxime proxetil, and cefuroxime axetil. Appropriate agents for beta-lactam-allergic or -intolerant patients include gatifloxacin, levofloxacin, and moxifloxacin. In adult patients with moderate disease and recent antibiotic use, the indicated agents are amoxicillin-clavulanate, gatifloxacin, levofloxacin, moxifloxacin, or combination therapy—amoxicillin or clindamycin for Gram-positive coverage plus cefixime or cefpodoxime proxetil for Gram-negative coverage.

TABLE 4 Recommended Antibacterial Agents for Acute Otitis Media

>39°C or severe otalgia	At diagnosis for patients treated initially with antibacterials		Clinically defined treatment failure at 48–72 hr after initial observation		Clinically defined treatment failure 48–72 hr after initial treatment with antibacterials	
	Recommended	Alternative	Recommended	Alternative	Recommended	Alternative
No	Amoxicillin, 80–90 mg/kg/d	Non-type I: cefnidir, cefuroxime, cefpodoxime Type I: azithromycin, clarithromycin	Amoxicillin, 80–90 mg/kg/d	Non-type I: cefnidir, cefuroxime, cefpodoxime; Type I: azithromycin, clarithromycin	Amoxicillin-clavulanate, 90 mg/kd	Non-type I: ceftriaxone Type I: clindamycin
Yes	Amoxicillin-clavulanate, 90 mg/kd	Ceftriaxone	Amoxicillin-clavulanate, 90 mg/k/d	Ceftriaxone	Ceftriaxone	Tympanocentesis, clindamycin

Source: Adapted from Ref. 42.

TABLE 5 Agents Recommended for Treatment of Acute Bacterial Sinusitis

Population	Mild disease	Moderate disease

Adults (if no antibiotics in past 4–6 weeks)	Amoxicillin (high dose)[a]
	Amoxicillin-clavulanate
	Cefpodoxime proxetil
	Cefuroxime axetil
	Alternatives — limited effectiveness, bacterial failure rates 20%–25%
	  Cefprozil
	  Clarithromycin[b]
	  TMP/SMX[b]
	  Doxycycline[b]
	  Azithromycin[b]
	  Erythromycin[b]
		Amoxicillin (high dose)[a]
		Amoxicillin-clavulanate
		Cefpodoxime proxetil
		Cefuroxime axetil
		Alternatives
		  Gatifloxacin
		  Levofloxacin
		  Moxifloxacin

Adults (if antibiotics in past 4–6 weeks)	Amoxicillin (high dose)[a]
	Amoxicillin-clavulanate
	Cefpodoxime proxetil
	Cefuroxime axetil
	Alternatives:
	  Levofloxacin
	  Moxifloxacin
	  Gatifloxacin
		Amoxicillin-clavulanate
		Gatifloxacin
		Levofloxacin
		Moxifloxacin
		Combination therapy: Gram-positive coverage (amoxicillin or clindamycin) + Gram-negative coverage (cefixime or cefpodoxime proxetil)

Children (if no antibiotics in past 4–6 weeks)	Amoxicillin (high-dose)[a]
	Amoxicillin-clavulanate
	Cefpodoxime proxetil
	Cefuroxime axetil
	Alternatives — limited effectiveness, bacterial failure rates 20%–25%
	  TMP/SMX
	  Azithromycin
	  Clarithromycin
	  Erythromycin
		Amoxicillin (high-dose)[a]
		Amoxicillin-clavulanate
		Cefpodoxime proxetil
		Cefuroxime axetil

Children (if antibiotics in past 4–6 weeks)	Amoxicillin (high dose)[a] Amoxicillin-clavulanate Cefpodoxime proxetil Cefuroxime axetil	Amoxicillin-clavulanate Combination therapy: Gram-positive coverage (amoxicillin or clindamycin) + Gram-negative coverage (cefixime or cefpodoxime proxetil)

[a]High-dose amoxicillin (80–90 mg/kg/day).
[b]For penicillin allergy.
Abbreviations: ABRS, acute bacterial rhinosinusitis; TMP/SMX, trimethoprim-sulfamethoxazole.
Source: Adapted from Ref. 42.

In pediatric patients with mild disease and no antibiotic use in the previous 4 to 6 weeks, first-line therapy includes amoxicillin-clavulanate, high-dose amoxicillin, cefpodoxime proxetil, or cefuroxime axetil. In patients with a history of immediate type I hypersensitivity to beta-lactams, the use of trimethoprim-sulfamethoxazole, azithromycin, clarithromycin, or erythromycin is recommended, although bacterial failure rates of 20% to 25% are possible with these agents.

For children with moderate disease who have had no recent antibiotic therapy or for those with mild disease who have had recent antibiotic therapy, indicated treatment agents are high-dose amoxicillin, amoxicillin-clavulanate, cefpodoxime proxetil, and cefuroxime axetil. In children with moderate disease who have received recent antibiotic therapy, the recommended treatment is amoxicillin-clavulanate or combination therapy—amoxicillin or clindamycin for Gram-positive coverage plus cefixime or cefpodoxime proxetil for Gram-negative coverage.

Pharyngitis (Strep Throat)

The primary use of antibiotics in pharyngitis is to treat infection due to group A *Streptococcus* (GAS). GAS is the most common bacterial agent causing acute pharyngitis, and accounts for approximately 15% to 30% of cases in children and 5% to 10% of adults (44,45). However, streptococcal pharyngitis is difficult to differentiate from other causes (such as viral etiology) on clinical grounds (45).

Definitive diagnosis of streptococcal pharyngitis is based on the identification of GAS in the throat by culture, rapid antigen detection test, or by serologic means. Results of culture and serologic testing are not available at the time of clinical decision making and are therefore not timely. Rapid antigen detection test provides the result to the clinician within minutes. However, the sensitivity varies from 60% to 90%; thus, a false test does not rule out the diagnosis.

Intramuscular penicillin and oral penicillin V or oral amoxicillin continue to be the recommended first-line drugs by most guideline. Table 6 shows the most recent antimicrobial agents recommended for the treatment of streptococcal pharyngitis (46). GAS continues to be highly sensitive to penicillin and amoxicillin and these agents have been the first-line recommended therapy. In patients with penicillin allergy, an oral cephalosporin or a macrolide is recommended. An oral cephalosporin may be used in patients who do not have immediate-type hypersensitivity to beta-lactam agents. Macrolide antibiotic may be used in those patients who are allergic to penicillin regardless of the type of reaction. However, the increasing resistance of GAS to macrolides worldwide is of major concern (47). Macrolide resistance may reside in the *erm* gene or *mef* gene. Cross-resistance to all the macrolide antibiotics is the rule. Streptococci with low level of macrolide resistance are commonly associated with the *mef* gene that is responsible for the efflux of the antibiotic out of the bacterial cells. These bacteria are usually susceptible to clindamycin. Streptococci that are highly macrolide resistant are usually not susceptible to clindamycin as well, and the *erm* gene commonly mediates this resistance.

Acute Exacerbations of Chronic Bronchitis

Timely and accurate diagnosis and treatment of AECB remain challenges to clinicians because of the indefinite beginnings and uncertain treatment modalities of the condition. Because patients with AECB have chronic bronchitis as an underlying disease and because the definition of AECB is subjective, it is sometimes difficult to determine when an exacerbation has begun or ended.

The most common bacterial pathogens associated with AECB are *H. influenzae, M. catarrhalis,* and *S. pneumoniae* (48,49). Gram-negative pathogens, including *P. aeruginosa,* can be significant pathogens in patients with more severe underlying COPD. Because as many as 50% of AECB episodes may be nonbacterial in origin and because there is no reliable method of distinguishing bacterial episodes from nonbacterial episodes based on clinical criteria, the appropriateness of antimicrobial

TABLE 6 Recommendations for Antimicrobial Therapy for Group A Streptococcal Pharyngitis

Route	Antimicrobial agent, dosage	Duration
Oral	Children: 250 mg bid or tid	10 days
	Adolescents and adults: 250 mg tid or qid	10 days
	Adolescents and adults: 500 mg bid	10 days
Oral	Amoxicillin may be used in place of penicillin V using a 50 mg dose, or 750 mg dose	10 days
IM	Benzathine penicillin G 1.2 million units	1 dose
	Benzathine penicillin G 600,000 units (children < 27 kg)	1 dose
	Mixtures of benzathine and procaine penicillin (dose should be based on benzathine penicillin)	1 dose
Oral	Erythromycin (dose varies with formulation)	10 days
	Erythromycin stearate 1 g/day in 2 or 4 divided doses[a]	
Oral	First-generation cephalosporins (should not be used to treat patients with immediate-type hypersensitivity to beta-lactam antibiotics)	10 days
Oral	Cefadroxil	5 days
Oral	Cefixime	5 days
Oral	Cefdinir	5 days
Oral	Cefpodoxime	5 days
Oral	Azithromycin 500 mg first day followed by 250 mg daily for 4 more days	5 days
Oral	Clarithromycin 500 mg qid	5 days

[a]Data based on Ref. 44.
Source: Adapted from Ref. 46.
Abbreviations: bid, two times daily; IM, intramuscular; qid, daily; tid, three times daily.

therapy is controversial, particularly in light of current trends in resistance. However, since recurrent episodes of AECB can impair pulmonary function and can severely impact quality of life, many clinicians choose to treat the condition with antibiotics in order to address those cases that are bacterial in origin. To help decide whether antimicrobial therapy is warranted, clinicians may also stratify patients by the type of exacerbation and by the presence of risk factors associated with poor outcome. Several randomized, placebo-controlled trials have shown that antibiotic treatment is beneficial in selected patients with AECB. Specifically, studies show that patients with more severe exacerbation (type I) are more likely to experience benefit than those with less severe disease (50). Patients with type I exacerbation have all three cardinal symptoms: increased dyspnea, increased sputum volume, and increased sputum purulence; whereas patients with type II exacerbation have two symptoms and patients with type III have only one. In comparison, patients with moderate exacerbation (type II) experienced less benefit from antibiotics compared with those who received placebo, and patients with mild episodes (type III) did not appear to benefit from antibiotic treatment compared with the placebo group. In the Anthonisen study, patients with AECB who received antibiotic therapy had a more rapid return of peak flow, were more likely to achieve clinical success, and experienced clinical failure less frequently than patients given placebo (51). Other studies also have shown the benefit of antibiotic therapy in AECB (51). A clinical practice guideline for management of AECB formulated by the American College of Physicians, American Society of Internal Medicine, and the American College of Chest Physicians was recently published; this position paper recommends the use of antibiotics in patients with severe exacerbation (such as type I) of COPD (52).

In addition to stratification by type, high-risk patients for poor outcome of AECB have been identified: these include patients with a history of repeated infections (>4 per year), comorbid illnesses (such as diabetes, asthma, coronary heard disease), or marked airway obstruction (<50% FEV$_1$) (53).

In patients with AECB of bacterial origin, antibiotics may have a long-term benefit of decreasing the amount of bacteria chronically colonizing the airway once the patient is clinically stable, thus helping to prevent progression to parenchymal lung infection (48). Antibiotic treatment may also prevent progressive airway injury due to persistent infection and may prolong the duration between exacerbations.

Agents with activity against the most commonly encountered pathogens in AECB—*S. pneumoniae, H. influenzae,* and *M. catarrhalis*—should be selected for treatment. An appropriate agent also should be resistant to beta-lactamase destruction, should have good penetration into bronchial tissue and sputum, should promote patient adherence through convenient dosing, and should have a favorable side-effect profile. The specific choice of antibiotic for AECB remains controversial. Most previously published trials have demonstrated a benefit of narrow-spectrum antibiotics (i.e., amoxicillin, trimethoprim-sulfamethoxazole, and tetracycline) as initial treatment (52). However, most of these studies were done before the emergence of multidrug-resistant pathogens. Many experts recommend stratifying antibiotics on the basis of severity of disease and on the presence of risk factors of outcome.

The most recently North American guidelines for management of AECB were published by the Canadian Thoracic Society and the Canadian Infectious Disease Society (54). This guideline promotes patient stratification to identify patients at risk of failing standard antimicrobial therapy (because of the concern for resistant pathogens or of host factors), which may lead to improve clinical outcomes and overall lower costs if hospital admissions and respiratory failure can be prevented. The classification system divides patients into four groups, as listed in Table 7.

Guidelines for Community-Acquired Pneumonia

CAP is a common disorder that is potentially life threatening, especially in older adults and those with comorbid disease. Despite substantial progress in therapeutic options, CAP remains a significant cause of morbidity and death worldwide and continues to have major controversies concerning antimicrobial management. Guidelines from numerous international organizations have been developed over the past decade. For this chapter, however, only those from North American organizations are reviewed. Recent recommendations for empiric antimicrobial therapy are summarized in Table 8 (55–57). Although the different guidelines vary somewhat in their emphasis of the importance of defining the etiologic agents so that directed therapy can be implemented, it is acknowledged that the majority of patients will be treated empirically. This is particularly the case for outpatients where diagnostic testing is not cost efficient and is not emphasized. Moreover, even at tertiary level university centers where multiple diagnostic testing methods are used for patients who require hospitalization, an etiologic agent is found in only 50% (approximately) of cases.

While numerous pathogens have been associated as the etiology of CAP, a limited range of key pathogens causes the majority of CAP, with *S. pneumoniae* being the most common. Other common etiological agents to which empiric

TABLE 7 Classification and Therapy of Acute Bronchitis and Acute Exacerbations of Chronic Bronchitis

Group/clinical state	Symptoms/risk factors	Probable pathogens	Treatment
Acute tracheobronchitis	No underlying chronic inflammatory lung disease	Usually viral	None, unless symptoms >10–14 days
Chronic bronchitis without risk factors (simple)	Increased cough, increased sputum volume and purulence	*Haemophilus influenzae, Moraxella catarrhalis, Streptococcus pneumoniae*	Second-generation macrolide (azithromycin or clarithromycin), second- or third-generation cephalosporin, amoxicillin, doxycyline, trimethoprim-sulfamethoxazole
Chronic bronchitis with risk factors (complicated)	As for group I + any of: FEV_1 <50%; >4 exacerbations/year; cardiac disease; use of home oxygen; chronic oral steroid use; antibiotic use in the past 3 months	As in group I plus *Klebsiella* spp. + other Gram-negatives; increased probability of beta-lactam resistance	Quinolone, amoxicillin-clavulanate
Chronic bronchial infection	As in group II with constant purulent sputum, often with bronchiectasis, FEV_1 usually <35% predicted; multiple risk factors	As in group II + *Pseudomonas aeruginosa* and multiresistant enterobacteriaceae	Ciprofloxacin

Source: Modified from Ref. 54.

therapy is usually directed according to the North American guidelines include: *H. influenzae* (and *M. catarrhalis*) and the "atypical pathogens" (*M. pneumoniae, C. pneumoniae,* and *Legionella* spp.). Other pathogens considered important for empiric therapy under selected conditions include: *Staphylococcus aureus, Chlamydophila psittaci, Coxiella burnetii,* Gram-bacteria bacilli, fungi, *Mycobacterium* spp., anaerobes (aspiration pneumonia), and respiratory viruses.

The North American guidelines place a significant emphasis on the potential role of the "atypical" organisms (58). The rationale is that these organisms are becoming more commonly recognized in recent studies as the etiology of CAP; and in the several observational studies of therapy for patients who require hospitalization, antimicrobial regimens that have activity against the "atypicals" have been associated with better outcomes. In addition it is now well recognized that it is difficult in most cases to differentiate the etiology of CAP (i.e., atypical vs. *S. pneumoniae*) from the clinical and radiographic findings at presentation of the patient.

TABLE 8 Comparison of Recommendations of Recently Published North American Guidelines for Empiric Antimicrobial Therapy of Community-Acquired Pneumonia in Adults

Guideline (Ref.)	Outpatient	General ward	ICU/severe
Canadian Infectious Disease Society/ Canadian Thoracic Society (55)	*Without modifying factors* Macrolide Doxycycline *With modifying factors* COLD (no recent antibiotics or steroids) New macrolide[a] Doxycycline COLD (recent antibiotics or steroids) Antipseudomonal FQ[b] (amox-clav or 2G cephalosporin[c]) and macrolide	Antipseudomonal FQ[b] 2G, 3G, or 4G cephalosporin + macrolide	*Pseudomonas* not suspected IV antipseudomonal FQ + cefotaxime, ceftriaxone, or beta-lactam–beta-lactamase inhibitor or IV macrolide + cefotaxime, ceftriaxone, or beta-lactam–beta-lactamase inhibitor *Pseudomonas* suspected Antipseudomonal FQ (e.g., Cipro) + antipseudomonal beta-lactam or Aminoglycoside triple therapy with antipseudomonal beta-lactam + aminoglycoside + macrolide
IDSA (56)	*Previously healthy* No recent antibiotic therapy A macrolide or doxycycline Recent antibiotic therapy A respiratory FQ alone, or an advanced macrolide (azithromycin or clarithromycin) + high-dose amox (1 g tid or amox-clav XR 2 g bid) *Comorbidities (COPD, diabetes, renal or congestive heart failure, or malignancy)* No recent antibiotic therapy An advanced macrolide or a respiratory FQ Recent antibiotic therapy A respiratory FQ alone, or an advanced macrolide + a beta-lactam (high-dose amox or amox-clav, or cephalosporin[c])	Macrolide + [cefotaxime, ceftriaxone, or a beta-lactam–beta-lactamase inhibitor (ampicillin-sulbactam or piperacillin-tazobactam)] or Antipseudomonal FQ (regimen selected will depend on if recent antibiotic therapy; if recent antibiotic therapy, select the alternative)	IV antipseudomonal FQ or IV macrolide + [cefotaxime, ceftriaxone, or a beta-lactam–beta-lactamase inhibitor (ampicillin–sulbactam or piperacillin-tazobactam)]; if at risk for *Pseudomonas* (i.e., structural lung disease or recurrent antibiotic or steroid use): antipseudomonal agents with activity for *Streptococcus pneumoniae* (i.e., cefepime, imipenem, meropenem, piperacillin) + an FQ (including ciprofloxacin)

(Continued)

TABLE 8 Comparison of Recommendations of Recently Published North American Guidelines for Empiric Antimicrobial Therapy of Community-Acquired Pneumonia in Adults (*Continued*)

Guideline (Ref.)	Outpatient	General ward	ICU/severe
ATS (57)	*No cardiopulmonary disease, no modifying factors*[d] Azithromycin or clarithromycin (doxycycline if allergic or intolerant of macrolides) *Modifying factors*[d] Beta-lactam (cefpodoxime, cefuroxime, high-dose amox, amox-clav, or parenteral ceftriaxone, followed by PO cefpodoxime) + macrolide or doxycycline; or antipseudomonal FQ[b]	*No modifying factors*[d] IV azithromycin; doxycycline + a beta-lactam; or monotherapy with an antipseudomonal FQ[b] *Modifying factors*[d] IV beta-lactam (cefotaxime, ceftriaxone, ampicillin/sulbactam, high-dose ampicillin) + IV or PO macrolide or doxycycline; or IV antipseudomonal FQ	No risk for *Pseudomonas* IV beta-lactam (cefotaxime, ceftriaxone) + IV macrolide (azithromycin) or IV antipseudomonal FQ Risk for *Pseudomonas* IV antipseudomonal beta-lactam (cefepime, imipenem, meropenem, piperacillin-tazobactam) + IV antipseudomonal FQ (ciprofloxacin) or IV antipseudomonal beta-lactam + IV aminoglycoside + IV azithromycin or IV nonpseudomonal FQ
IDSA/ATS (76)	*Previously healthy and no recent antibiotic therapy* Macrolide or doxycycline *Presence of comorbidities or recent antibiotics*[e] Respiratory FQ (gemifloxacin, levofloxacin, moxifloxacin) or Beta-lactam + a macrolide	Respiratory FQ or Beta-lactam + a macrolide	Beta-lactam (cefotaxamine, ceftriaxone, ampicillin/sulbactam) + azithromycin or a respiratory FQ *Special Concerns* If *Pseudomonas* a concern, recommendations similar to IDSA and ATS above If community acquired MRSA a concern, add linezolid or vancomycin

[a]Clarithromycin, azithromycin.

[b]Levofloxacin, gatifloxacin, or moxifloxacin; trovafloxacin is restricted because of potential severe hepatotoxicity (for newest IDSA/ATS guidelines: gemifloxacin, levofloxacin, or moxifloxacin).

[c]Cefuroxime axetil, amoxicillin, amox-clav, cefpodoxime, cefprozil; does not cover atypical pathogens.

[d]Modifying factors: elderly, multiple comorbidities, risk factors for drug-resistance.

[e]In regions with a hight rate (>25%) of high-level macrolide-resistant pneumococci, these are preferred options even without comorbidities or recent antibiotics.

Abbreviations: Amox, amoxicillin; ATS, American Thoracic Society; bid, two times daily; Clav, clavulanate; COLD, chronic obstructive lung disease; COPD, chronic obstructive pulmonary disease; FQ, fluoroquinolone; IDSA, Infectious Diseases Society of America; IV, intravenous; PO, oral dosage; tid, three times daily.

Recommendations for Empiric Therapy of CAP—Outpatients

All of the new North American guidelines variably recommend macrolides, doxycycline, or an antipneumococcal fluoroquinolone (e.g., levofloxacin, gatifloxacin, and moxifloxacin) as treatment options for patients who are mildly ill and can be treated as outpatients. In general, the North American guidelines recommend a macrolide or doxycycline as first-line treatment for outpatients with no comorbidity or risk factors for DRSP. The rationale to position the macrolides as prominent first-line agents for mild CAP in otherwise healthy hosts is partly based on the fact that the rate of macrolide-resistant *S. Pneumoniae* is low for such patients who have not recently recieved antimicrobials. In addition, at the time of the development of the North American guidelines, cases of macrolide failure for outpatients, especially for cases not associated with risks for DRSP, had been infrequent.

In the North American guidelines, outpatients are generally stratified into those without modifying factors, for whom a macrolide or doxycycline may be used, and those with modifying factors (such as chronic obstructive lung disease or use of recent antibiotics or steroid—for which there may be a greater likelihood of DRSP), for whom fluoroquinolones are considered more appropriate as first-line empiric therapy.

Recommendations for Empiric Therapy of CAP—Inpatients

All of the NA guidelines recommend treatment with a beta-lactam plus a macrolide or monotherapy with a fluoroquinolone for patients admitted to the general ward. The rationale for recommending these regimens is based on studies showing these regimens were associated with a significant reduction in mortality, compared with that associated with administration of cephalosporin alone. For patients with severe CAP who require admission to an ICU all guidelines recommend comprehensive antimicrobial therapy to cover *S. pneumoniae* (including DRSP), *Legionella*, and the possibility of pseudomonas in selected cases. For this group of patients with severe disease, azithromycin is the preferred macrolide over erythromycin by the American Thoracic Society (ATS) because of difficulties in administration and tolerance with erythromycin (parenteral clarithromycin is not available in the United States).

New Recommendations by IDSA/ATS

In 2007, combined Infectious Diseases Society of America (IDSA)/ATS guidelines were published (59). The recommendations are listed in Table 8 and are similar to the prior guidelines. Two exceptions are that the standard dose recommended for levofloxacin is 750 mg daily, based on better pharmacodynamic target parameters than the 500 mg dose, and there are additional recommendations for the possible community-acquired MRSA for severe CAP. Finally, in this latest guideline, the more potent drugs are given preference because of their benefit in decreasing the risk of selection for antibiotic resistance.

IMPACT OF CAP GUIDELINES ON OUTCOMES

For guidelines to be of value they must be shown to be associated with an improvement of care of the patient. The efficacy of the management recommendations of guidelines can be evaluated by analyzing several parameters, which include: clinical outcomes, influence on antimicrobial prescribing, effect on bacterial resistance, and cost. Audits of practice guidelines and care pathways for patients with CAP have shown they can improve the quality of care and reduce cost (60–68). In a national evaluation of Medicare patients treated in hospitals from 1997 to 1999, Jencks et al. found that 79% of patients were treated with antimicrobial therapy consistent with current recommendations in the guidelines (69).

Several studies have attempted to evaluate the validity of the published treatment guidelines for CAP. Gleason et al. evaluated the therapies and outcomes of 864 outpatients with CAP from the Patients Outcomes Research Trial database (62). Most patients were treated with an oral macrolide, including older patients and those with comorbid conditions. Although monotherapy with a macrolide was not recommended by the guidelines for patients with more complex illness, they appeared to have good outcomes as well. However, the patients who were treated according to the guidelines were small and were more severely ill than those treated by nonguideline therapy. Gordon et al. evaluated more than 4000 patients admitted to the general wards of a hospital and found that therapy according to the ATS guidelines (1993 version) was associated with a lower mortality than if nonguideline therapy was used (63). In a more recent study, Menendez et al. studied 295 patients admitted to a hospital from February 1998 to March 1999 and compared the outcomes in relation to the initial antimicrobial therapy (64). In a multivariate analysis, adherence to the ATS guidelines was independently associated with decreased mortality.

Several observational studies have found that antimicrobial regimens as listed in the guidelines are associated with decreased mortality and shorter length of stay (LOS) for patients who require hospitalization. Stahl et al. evaluated 100 prospective patients hospitalized with CAP. Patients were stratified according to the antibiotic received. Patients who received macrolides (usually IV erythromycin or PO clarithromycin) within the first 24 hr of admission had a markedly shorter LOS (2.8 days) than those not so treated (65). The investigators speculate that the direct antimicrobial effect against "atypical" pathogens as well as a beneficial immunologic or anti-inflammatory effect may be responsible for the advantage of the macrolides. In a study of 12,945 Medicare patients (65 years of age), Gleason and colleagues found the addition of a macrolide to a second- or third-generation cephalosporin resulted in a significantly reduced 30-day mortality for elderly patients hospitalized with pneumonia (66). The authors suggest this finding of better outcome may be related to the better activity for the common "typical" and "atypical" bacterial pathogens. Dudas et al., in an observational study of 3035 patients hospitalized with pneumonia in one of 72 nonteaching hospitals with a national group purchasing organization, found the addition of a macrolide to either a second- or third-generation cephalosporin or a beta-lactam/beta-lactase inhibitor was associated with decreased mortality and reduced LOS (67). Houck et al. examined the risk for mortality during the 30 days after admission to the hospital of 10,069 Medicare patients in three time periods—1993, 1995, and 1997 (68). In 1993, therapy with a macrolide plus a beta-lactam was associated with significantly lower mortality than therapy with either a beta-lactam alone or other regimens that did not include a macrolide, beta-lactam, or fluoroquinolone. This association was not observed in 1995 or 1997. The authors speculate this may be a result of a temporal variation in the incidence of atypical pathogen pneumonia.

The impact of guidelines on a variety of outcomes of CAP are listed in Table 9. Many studies found a benefit in either mortality or cost (70–75). A retrospective cohort study in two Veterans' hospitals investigated the association between the use of IDSA or ATS guideline-concordant antimicrobial therapy and mortality among hospitalized patients with CAP (60). The 30-day survival was significantly greater for patients treated with guideline-concordant antibiotics (94% vs. 78% with nonconcordant therapy). The most common non-concordant regimen was a beta-lactam antibiotic used alone. A multicenter,

TABLE 9 Impact of Guideline Interventions on Outcome of Community-Acquired Pneumonia

Study (reference)	Country	Intervention	Outcome
Meehan et al. (60)	U.S.A.	Observational evaluation of timing of antimicrobials for older inpatients	30 day mortality less if first dose given within 8 hr of presentation
Bratzler et al. (61)	U.S.A.	Observational evaluation of timing of antimicrobials for older inpatients	30 day mortality less if first does given within 4 hr of presentation
Gordon et. al. (63)	U.S.A.	Examined initial choice of antimicrobial therapy of approx. 4,500 patients admitted to general ward	Therapy according to ATS guidelines was associated with lower mortality than if nonrecommended therapy was used
Menendez et al. (64)	Spain	Examined initial choice of antimicrobial therapy in 295 patients admitted to a hospital	Adherence to antibiotics of ATS guidelines was associated with decrease mortality when compared to nonadherent treatments
Gleason et al. (62)	U.S.A.	Evaluated 864 patients treated as outpatients	Recommended antimicrobials for younger, healthier patients in 1993 ATS guidelines were cost effective; for more complex outpatients, the recommendations were more costly without increased benefit
Gleason et al. (66)	U.S.A.	Observational study of 12,945 inpatients ($\geq$ 65 years of age)	Second- or third-generation cephalosporin plus a macrolide or fluoro-quinolone monotherapy reduced 30-day mortality
Dudas et al. (67)	U.S.A.	Observational study of 10,000 inpatients from 72 nonteaching hospitals	Beta-Lactam plus a macrolide or a fluoroquinolone; associated with decreased mortality and decreased length of stay
Stahl et al. (65)	U.S.A.	Prospective evaluation of 100 inpatients at single hospital	Patients receiving macrolides as part of initial therapy had shorter hospitalization stay
Houck et al. (68)	U.S.A.	Observational study of 10,000 Medicare patients admitted to hospital	Depending on the time period, beta-lactam plus a macrolide or fluoro-quinolone was associated with lower mortality

(Continued)

TABLE 9   Impact of Guideline Interventions on Outcome of Community-Acquired Pneumonia
(*Continued*)

Study (reference)	Country	Intervention	Outcome
Mortensen et al. (71)	U.S.A.	Retrospective, observational, 420 patients at 2 tertiary hospitals	30-day survival greater for patients treated according to IDSA or ATS guidelines
Menendez et al. (72)	Spain	Observational, multicenter, 1,288 patients	Adherence to recommended antibiotics in guideline was associated with reduced 30-day mortality and treatment failure
Bodi et al. (74)	Spain	Multicenter, 529 patients in ICU	
Yealy et al. (75)	U.S.A.	Randomized, controlled from 32 emergency departments, 3,219 patients	Guideline implementation increased performance of recommended processes of care, did not show significant difference in mortality

Abbreviations: ATS, American Thoracic Society; ICU, intensive care unit; IDSA, Infectious Diseases Society of America.

prospective, observational study of 1288 patients hospitalized with CAP in Spain found that after adjusting for severity of CAP, adherence to recommended antibiotics in guidelines was protective for 30-day mortality (OR, 0.55; 95% CI, 0.3–0.9) and for treatment failure (OR, 0.65; 95% CI, 0.4–0.9) (61). A prospective multicenter study of 529 patients with severe CAP admitted to the ICU found that age (OR, 1.7), APACHE II score (OR, 4.1), nonadherence to IDSA guidelines (OR, 1.6), and immunocompromise (OR, 1.9) were variables associated with death (63). The overall rate of adherence to IDSA guidelines was 58% and was the only modifiable prognostic factor for severe CAP. A randomized, controlled study demonstrated that increasing the intensity of guideline implementation increased the performance of recommended processes of care, although the authors did not observe any difference in mortality rates.

The validation of therapeutic recommendations as indicated by the findings of these studies suggests that CAP guidelines can be beneficial to doctors, patients, and healthcare organizations. Still, guidelines may be viewed by some clinicians as condescending, and the conscientious physician may consider them as promoting "cook book" medicine. However, the proliferation of newer antibiotics, diagnostic technologies, and therapeutic modalities exerts notable pressure on each physician to keep up with the new developments in order to provide optimal care to patients. Time constraints may leave a large percentage of healthcare professionals little opportunity to critically review the significance of newer information. Guidelines, which are evidenced-based and supported by expert review, can provide timely reviews of appropriate management, which can support the knowledge and judgment of the individual clinician. Thus, the intent of evidence-based guidelines is not to establish absolute rules, but rather to provide support to the clinician as to the standard of care, which is current and understandable. They have never been intended to supersede the clinical judgment of each physician, as they cannot cover all possible clinical situations; and ultimately the prescribing clinician is responsible for applying them as they seem appropriate.

Educational Strategies to Promote Rational Antibiotic Use

Issuing guidelines on appropriate antibiotic use for treatment of different types of infections is only the first step in ensuring that rational principles are adopted and followed in clinical practice. Educational strategies aimed at enhancing clinician awareness of guidelines and encouraging their implementation is necessary. Educational materials promoting the implementation of practice guidelines and emphasizing their benefits could be developed and provided to clinicians. Translation of guidelines into practice also must involve educational efforts geared toward patients. Patients need to understand that antibiotics are not appropriate for the treatment of viral infections. They also must be educated about the need to take antibiotics as directed and for the entire duration prescribed. Public health campaigns can help to spread the word and traditional print and audiovisual patient education materials also may be useful.

Educational efforts aimed at providers and patients already have proven successful in promoting the rational use of antibiotics in upper RTIs. In a study in rural Alaska, the education of healthcare workers and the community concerning appropriate antimicrobial use in children with upper RTIs was associated with a 22% reduction in the number of antibiotic prescriptions in children younger than 5 years and with a 28% decrease in penicillin-resistant pneumococcal nasopharyngeal isolates compared with the two control regions not provided with the educational intervention (36). In a National Ambulatory Medical Care Survey, McCraig et al. observed a decrease in antimicrobial prescribing for RTIs among children and adolescents from 838 per 1000 population in 1989 to 1990 to 503 in 1999 to 2000 (76). The authors of the study attributed this decrease in part to the educational efforts of various professionals and public health organizations to promote appropriate antimicrobial prescribing.

In addition to educational campaigns, there is no substitute for the few moments taken by the treating clinician to explain fully why antibiotics are not necessary or why they are being prescribed. This approach helps patients realize that their condition is being taken seriously. The investment in time and personal attention can increase patient satisfaction with the selected treatment and can help ensure that patients comply with therapy.

CONCLUSION

The widespread morbidity caused by RTIs is a serious problem for society in general and clinicians in particular. The appropriate management of RTIs poses multiple challenges for the clinician. Inappropriate prescribing practices (e.g., selecting agents with insufficient antimicrobial activity and treating viral infections with antibiotics) have contributed to the development of drug resistance among common respiratory pathogens (e.g., *S. pneumoniae, H. influenzae,* and *M. catarrhalis*). Factors contributing to inappropriate antimicrobial use include patient expectations, clinician time constraints, and the practice of defensive medicine. Antibiotic therapy with the appropriate agent shortens the course of the illness, lowers the risk of complications due to untreated disease, helps to prevent disease progression and airway impairment, and avoids the added cost of multiple courses of antibiotics.

Clinicians are now presented with several sets of guidelines for the care of RTIs. These guidelines are intended to provide clinicians with general principles of disease management, and it is envisaged that these will be adapted to suit regional circumstances, local healthcare practices, and individual patient characteristics. All of the guideline statements reflect thoughtful consideration by a panel of experts and should be viewed as recommendations for strategies of care and not definite stepwise rules of care. Indeed, clinicians must interpret such statements in the context that these recommendations cannot apply to all hypothetical settings. Rather, these statements represent general state-of-the-art documents, which require continuing change because of the changes in our understanding of these important infections. Educational efforts targeted toward clinicians as well as patients are necessary to encourage the implementation of guidelines, to avoid misuse of antibiotics for viral infections, and to prevent the prescription of antibiotics that are ineffective for treating the most likely respiratory pathogens. The judicious and rational use of appropriate antibiotic agents in the treatment of RTIs can help to improve the care of patients, and reduce the complexities, costs, and disease complications that currently burden the management of these common conditions.

REFERENCES

1. File TF Jr. The epidemiology of respiratory tract infections. Semin Respir Infect 2000; 15:184–94.
2. Armstrong GL, Pinner RW. Outpatient visits for infectious diseases in the United States, 1980 through 1996. Arch Intern Med 1999; 159:2531–6.
3. Wenzel RP, Edmond MB. Managing antibiotic resistance. N Engl J Med 2001; 343:1961–2.
4. File TM Jr. Appropriate use of antimicrobials for drug-resistant pneumonia: focus on the significance of Beta-lactam-resistant *Streptococcus pneumoniae*. Clin Infect Dis 2002; 34(Suppl. 1):S17–26.
5. Campbell GD Jr, Silberman R. Drug-resistant *Streptococcus pneumoniae*. Clin Infect Dis 1998; 26:1188–95.
6. Vanderkooi OG, Low DE, Green K, et al. Toronto invasive bacterial disease network: predicting antimicrobial resistance in invasive pneumococcal infections. Clin Infect Dis 2005; 40:1288–97.
7. Leclercq R, Courvalin P. Resistance to macrolides and related antibiotics in *Streptococcus pneumoniae*. Antimicrob Agents Chemother 2002; 46:2727–34.
8. Amsden GW. Pneumococcal macrolide resistance—myth or reality? J Antimicrob Chemother 1999; 44:1–6.
9. Bishai W. The in vivo–in vitro paradox in pneumococcal respiratory tract infections. J Antimicrob Chemother 2002; 49:433–6.
10. Lynch JP III, Martinez FJ. Clinical relevance of macrolide-resistant *Streptococcus pneumoniae* for community-acquired pneumonia. Clin Infect Dis 2002; 34(Suppl. 1):S27–46.
11. Siegel RE. The significance of serum vs tissue levels of antibiotics in the treatment of penicillin-resistant *Streptococcus pneumoniae* and community-acquired pneumonia. Are we looking in the wrong place? Chest 1999; 116:535–8.
12. Hyde TB, Gay K, Stephens DS, et al. Macrolide resistance among invasive *Streptococcus pneumoniae* isolates. J Am Med Assoc 2001; 286:1857–62.
13. Fogarty C, Goldschmidt R, Bush K. Bacteremic pneumonia due to multidrug-resistant pneumococci in 3 patients treated unsuccessfully with azithromycin and successfully with levofloxacin. Clin Infect Dis 2000; 31:613–5.
14. Kelley MA, Weber DJ, Gilligan P, et al. Breakthrough pneumococcal bacteremia in patients being treated with azithromycin and clarithromycin. Clin Infect Dis 2000; 31:1008–11.
15. Musher DM, Dowell ME, Shortridge VD, et al. Emergence of macrolide resistance during treatment of pneumococcal pneumonia. N Engl J Med 2002; 346:630–1.

16. Lonks JR, Garau J, Gomez L, et al. Failure of macrolide antibiotic treatment in patients with bacteremia due to erythromycin-resistant *Streptococcus pneumoniae*. Clin Infect Dis 2002; 35:556–9.
17. Chen D, McGeer A, deAzavedo JC, Low DE. The Canadian Bacterial Surveillance Network. Decreased susceptibility of *Streptococcus pneumoniae* to fluoroquinolones in Canada. N Engl J Med 1999; 341:233–9.
18. Ho PL, Yung RWH, Tsang DNC, et al. Increasing resistance of *Streptococcus pneumoniae* to fluoroquinolones: results of a Hong Kong multicentre study in 2000. J Antimicrob Chemother 2002; 49:173–6.
19. McGee L, Goldsmith CE, Klugman KP. Fluoroquinolone resistance among clinical isolates of *Streptococcus pneumoniae* belonging to international multi-resistant clones. J Antimicrob Chemother 2002; 49:173–6.
20. Davidson R, Cavalcanti R, Brunton JL, et al. Levofloxacin treatment failures of pneumococcal pneumonia in association with resistance. N Engl J Med 2002; 346:747–50.
21. Kays NB, Smith DW. Levofloxacin treatment failure in a patient with fluoroquinolone resistant *Streptococcus pneumoniae* pneumonia. Pharmacotherapy 2002; 22:395–9.
22. Ho PL, Tse WS, Tsang KW, et al. Risk factors for acquisition of levofloxacin-resistant *Streptococcus pneumoniae*: a case-control study. Clin Infect Dis 2001; 32:701–7.
23. Interagency Task Force on antimicrobial resistance. Public Health Action Plan to Combat Antimicrobial Resistance. Atlanta: Centers for Disease Control and Prevention, 2001 (www.cdc.gov/drugresistance/actionplan/).
24. Alliance for the Prudent Use of Antibiotics (www.apua.org).
25. World Health Organization. Global Strategy for the Containment of Antimicrobial Resistance. Geneva: World Health Organization, 2001 (www.who.International).
26. The European Commission. Communication from the Commission on a Community Strategy Against Antimicrobial Resistance, Comm, Vol. 1. Brussels: Commission of the European Communities, 2001, 201, 333 (www.europa.eu.int).
27. Ball P, Baquero F, Cars O, et al. Antibiotic therapy of community respiratory tract infection: strategies for optimal outcomes and minimized resistance emergence. J Antimicrob Chemother 2002; 49:31–40.
28. Hamm RM, Hicks RJ, Bemben DA. Antibiotics and respiratory infections: are patients more satisfied when expectations are met? J Fam Pract 1996; 43:56–62.
29. Kristinsson KG, Hjalmarsdottir MA, Gudnason T. Continued decline in the incidence of penicillin non-susceptible pneumococci in Iceland. In: 38th Interscience Conference of Antimicrobial Agents and Chemotherapy. San Diego: American Society for Microbiology, September, 1998.
30. Seppala H, Klanda T, Vuopio-Varkila J, et al. The effects of changes in the consumption of macrolide antibiotics on erythromycin resistance in group A Streptococcus in Finland. N Engl J Med 1997; 337:441–6.
31. Pestonik SL, Classen DC, Evans S, Burke JP. Implementing antibiotic practice guidelines through computer-assisted decision support: clinical and financial outcomes. Ann Intern Med 1996; 124:884–90.
32. Petersen KL, Hennessy TW, Parkinson AJ, et al. Provider and community education decreases antimicrobial use and carriages of penicillin-resistant *S. pneumoniae* in rural Alaska communities. In: 37th Annual meeting of Infectious Diseases Society of America, Philadelphia, 18–21 November, 1999.
33. Gonzales R, Steiner JF, Lum A, Barrett PH Jr. Decreasing antibiotic use in ambulatory practice: impact of a multidimensional intervention on the treatment of uncomplicated acute bronchitis in adults. J Am Med Assoc 1999; 281:1512–9.
34. Guillenot D, Henriet L, Lecoeur H, Weber P, Carbon C. Optimization of antibiotic rapidly decreases penicillin resistant *Streptococcus pneumoniae* carriage: the Aubeppin Study. In: 41st Interscience Congress on Antimicrobial Agents and Chemotherapy, Chicago, Illinois, December, 2001.
35. Dowell SF, Marcy SM, Phillips WR, et al. Otitis media—principles of judicious use of antimicrobial agents. Pediatrics 1998; 101:165–71.

36. Christenson B, Lunberg P, Hedlund J, Ortqvist A. Effects of a large-scale intervention with influenza and 23-pneumococcal vaccines in adults aged 65 years or older: a prospective study. Lancet 2001; 357:1008–11.
37. Grimshaw JM, Russell IT. Effect of clinical guidelines on medical practice: A systematic review of rigorous evaluations. Lancet 1993; 342:1317–22.
38. Beilby J, Marley J, Walder D, et al. The impact of changing antibiotic prescribing on patient outcomes in a community setting: a natural experiment in Australia. In: 37th Annual Meeting of the Infectious Diseases Society of America, Philadelphia, 18–21 November, 1999.
39. Cabana MD, Rand CS, Powe NR, et al. Why don't physicians follow clinical practice guidelines? A framework for improvement. J Am Med Assoc 1999; 282:1458–65.
40. Dowell SF, Butler JC, Giebink GS, et al. Acute otitis media: management and surveillance in an era of pneumococcal resistance. A report from the drug-resistant *Streptococcus pneumoniae* therapeutic working group. Pediatr Infect Dis J 1999; 18:1–9.
41. Varsano I, Volovitz B, Horev Z, et al. Intramuscular ceftriaxone compared with oral amoxicillin-clavulanate for treatment of acute otitis media in children. Eur J Pediatr 1997; 156:858–63.
42. American Academy of Pediatrics and American Academy of Family Physicians. Clinical Practice Guideline: Diagnosis and Management of Acute Otitis Media. Pediatrics 2004; 113:1451–65.
43. Sinus and Allergy Heath Partnership. Antimicrobial treatment guidelines for acute bacterial rhinosinusitis. Otlolaryngol Heal Neck Surg 2000; 123(Suppl.):S1–32.
44. Bisno AL. Acute pharyngitis. N Engl J Med 2001; 344:205–11.
45. Snow V, Mottur-Pilson C, Cooper RJ, Hoffman JR. Principles of appropriate antibiotic use for acute pharyngitis in adults. Ann Intern Med 2001; 134:506–8.
46. Bisno AL, Gerber MA, Gwaltney JM Jr, Kaplan EL, Schwartz RH. Practice guideline for the diagnosis and management of group A streptococcal pharyngitis. Clin Infect Dis 2002; 35:113–25.
47. Martin JM, Green M, Barbadora KA, Wald ER. Erythromycin-resistant group A streptococci in schoolchildren in Pittsburgh. N Engl J Med 2002; 346:1200–6.
48. Niederman MS. Acute exacerbations of chronic bronchitis: the role of infection and the selection of appropriate therapy. Pulmonary Crit Care Update 1996; 27:1–8.
49. Bach PB, Brown C, Gelfand SE, McGory DC. Management of acute exacerbations of chronic obstructive pulmonary disease: a summary and appraisal of published evidence. Ann Intern Med 2001; 134:600–20.
50. Anthonisen NR, Manfreda J, Warren CPW, Hershfield ES, Harding GKM, Nelson NA. Antibiotic therapy in exacerbations of chronic obstructive pulmonary disease. Ann Intern Med 1987; 106:196–204.
51. Saint S, Bent S, Vittinghoff E, Grady D. Antibiotics in chronic obstructive pulmonary disease exacerbations: a meta-analysis. J Am Med Assoc 1995; 273:957–60.
52. Snow V, Lascher S, Mottur-Pilson C. For the joint expert panel on chronic obstructive pulmonary disease of the American College of chest physicians and the American College of Physicians-American Society of Internal Medicine. Ann Intern Med 2001; 134:595–9.
53. Adams SG, Anzueto A. Antibiotic therapy in acute exacerbations of chronic bronchitis. Semin Respir Infect 2000; 15:234–47.
54. Balter MS, La Forge J, Low DE, et al. Canadian guidelines for the management of acute exacerbations of chronic bronchitis. Can Respir J 2003; 10(Suppl. B):3B–32.
55. Mandell LA, Marrie TJ, Grossman RE, et al. Canadian guidelines for the initial management of community-acquired pneumonia: an evidence-based update by the Canadian infectious diseases society and the Canadian thoracic society. Clin Infect Dis 2000; 31:383–421.
56. Mandell LA, Bartlett JG, Dowell SF, File TM Jr, Musher DM, Whitney C. Update of Practice Guidelines for the Management of adults with Community-Acquired Pneumonia in Adults. Clin Infect Dis 2003; 37:1405–33.
57. Niederman MS, Mandell LA, Anzueto A, et al. Guidelines for the Management of adults with Community-Acquired Pneumonia (American Thoracic Society). Am J Respir Crit Care Med 2001; 163:1730–54.

58. File TM Jr, Garau J, Blasi F, et al. Guidelines for empiric antimicrobial prescribing in community-acquired pneumonia. Chest 2004; 125:1888–901.
59. Mandell LA, Wunderink RG, Anzueto A, et al. Infectious Diseases Society of America-American Thoracic Society Concensus Guidelines on the Management of Community-Acquired Pneunomia in Adults. Clin Infect Dis 2007; 44:S27–S72.
60. Meehan TP, Fine MJ, Krumholz HM, et al. Quality of care, process, and outcomes in elderly patients with pneumonia. J Am Med Assoc 1997; 278:2080–4.
61. Bratzler DW, Houck PM, Nsa W, et al. Initial processes of care and outcomes in elderly patients with pneumonia. Ann Emerg Med 2001; 38(Suppl.):S36.
62. Gleason PP, Kapoor WN, Stone RA, et al. Medical outcomes and antimicrobial costs with the use of the American Thoracic Society guidelines for outpatients with community-acquired pneumonia. J Am Med Assoc 1997; 278:32–9.
63. Gordon GS, Throop D, Berberian L, et al. Validation of the therapeutic recommendations of the American Thoracic Society (ATS) guidelines for community-acquired pneumonia in hospitalized patients. Chest 1996; 110:55S.
64. Menendez R, Ferrando D, Valles JM, Vallterra J. Influence of deviation from guidelines on the outcome of community-acquired pneumonia. Chest 2002; 122:612–7.
65. Stahl JE, Barza M, DesJardin J, et al. Effect of macrolides as part of initial empiric therapy on length of stay in patients hospitalized with community-acquired pneumonia. Arch Intern Med 1999; 159:2576–80.
66. Gleason PP, Meehan TP, Fine JM, et al. Association between initial antimicrobial therapy and medical outcomes for hospitalized elderly patients with pneumonia. Arch Intern Med 1999; 159:2562–72.
67. Dudas V, Hopefl A, Jacobs R, et al. Antimicrobial selection for hospitalized patients with presumed community-acquired pneumonia: a survey of non-teaching US community hospitals. Ann Pharmacother 2000; 34:446–52.
68. Houck PM, MacLehose RF, Niederman MS, et al. Empiric antibiotic therapy and mortality among Medicare pneumonia inpatients in 10 western states: 1993, 1995, and 1997. Chest 2001; 119:1420–6.
69. Jencks SF, Cuerdon T, Burwen DR, et al. Quality of medical care delivered to Medicare beneficiaries. J Am Med Assoc 2000; 284:1670–6.
70. Marrie TJ, Lau CY, Wheeler SL, et al. A controlled trial of a critical pathway for treatment of community-acquired pneumonia. CAPITAL Study Investigators. Community-Acquired Pneumonia Intervention Trial Assessing Levofloxacin. J Am Med Assoc 2000; 283:749.
71. Mortensen EM, Restrepo M, Anzueto A, Pugh J. Effects of guideline-concordant antimicrobial therapy on mortality among patients with community-acquired pneumonia. Am J Med 2004; 117:726.
72. Menendez R, Torres A, Zalacain R, et al. Guidelines for the treatment of community-acquired pneumonia: predictors of adherence and outcome. Am J Respir Crit Care Med 2005; 172:757.
73. Menendez R, Ferrando D, Valles JM, Vallterra J. Influence of deviation from guidelines on the outcome of community-acquired pneumonia. Chest 2002; 122:612.
74. Bodi M, Rodriguez A, Sole-Violan J, et al. Antibiotic prescription for community-acquired pneumonia in the intensive care unit: impact of adherence to Infectious Diseases Society of America guidelines on survival. Clin Infect Dis 2005; 41:1709.
75. Yealy DM, Auble TE, Stone RA, et al. Effect of increasing the intensity of implementing pneumonia guidelines. Ann Intern Med 2005; 143:881–94.
76. McCaig LF, Besser RF, Hughes JM. Treads in antimicrobial prescribing rates for children and adolescents. J Am Med Assoc 2002; 287:3133–5.

20 The Impact of Hospital Epidemiology on the Management and Control of Antimicrobial Resistance: Issues and Controversies

August J. Valenti
Department of Hospital Epidemiology and Infection Prevention, Division of Infectious Diseases, Maine Medical Center, Portland, Maine and Department of Medicine, College of Medicine, University of Vermont, Burlington, Vermont, U.S.A.

INTRODUCTION

The ever-escalating human and global economic significance of antimicrobial resistance makes the proper selection, dosing, and duration of antimicrobial agents the subjects of initiatives from a number of interest groups (1,2). But, while antimicrobial optimization is an important component in a comprehensive program for combating resistance, the services of a competent microbiology laboratory and a vigorous infection control program are essential elements as well. Infections, real or suspected (and occasionally imagined), drive antimicrobial use, which, in turn, drives resistance. Interventions designed to interrupt or modify this antimicrobial use-resistance pathway (Fig. 1) are among the chief concerns of infection control programs. Prevention should be the highest priority in infection control. Accordingly, the primary prevention of infections, their transmission, and the development and spread of resistance remain among the chief preoccupations for the hospital epidemiologist.

Once they establish a beachhead, drug-resistant organisms (DROs) survive and are spread in a variety of ways throughout the continuum of healthcare. The degree to which a resistant organism will spread within a hospital—and, for that matter, a healthcare system or region—is analogous to the degree to which a pathogen's ability to cause disease depends on host-factors and largely depends on the type of organism, the populations at risk, the nature of a hospital's activities, and the efficacy of its policies to prevent infection. It is also true that, while excellent, evidence-based policies and procedures may be in place, the willingness and ability of healthcare workers to follow them are a function of how well they understand the policies, accept the evidence supporting them, and the adequacy of the resources and systems dedicated to encourage good practice. Hence, there are today complex interactions inside and outside healthcare institutions, which have a collective impact on the spread of resistance. Hospital epidemiology continually strives to identify and understand the processes that lead to healthcare-associated infections (HAIs) in order to develop and evaluate interventional strategies directed at preventing and controlling them.

Interest in antimicrobial resistance and preventing the spread of resistant organisms has literally erupted in the last two decades among providers, consumers, and regulators (3,4). Proposed mandates on healthcare institutions coming from the public, politicians, and third party payers to monitor appropriate antimicrobial use, DROs, and infection control policies are not always guided by

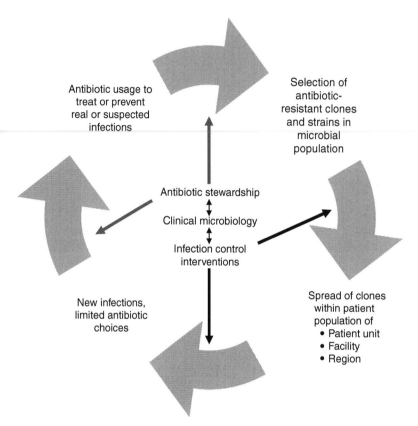

FIGURE 1 Antibiotic use-resistance pathway and opportunities for interventions in a healthcare facility or system.

sound epidemiologic principles. The intended aims of improving healthcare by providing transparency, information for healthcare consumers, and incentives for monitoring and improving outcomes, are sometimes undermined by emotional arguments and poorly conceived programs that reflect a lack of understanding of epidemiological methodology and the difficulties in developing valid comparative data. Furthermore, in some states, concern over the repercussions of resistant organisms in hospitals has precipitated consideration of legislative mandates requiring hospitals to control resistant organisms utilizing designated approaches such as actively screening patients and isolating patients colonized or infected with certain organisms (5).

There is reason for optimism, however. The fear and furor surrounding patient safety and DROs is spawning a renewed interest in infection control. Healthcare quality improvement is maturing, and a number of new and fruitful initiatives, which include infection prevention, are boasting dramatic results (6). Several initiatives incorporating evidence-based interventions, including several based on years of science done by healthcare epidemiologists, have been adopted by hospitals or healthcare systems around the country. Participants are seeing significant reductions in HAIs such as catheter-associated blood stream infections, ventilator-associated pneumonias (VAPs), and surgical site infections (SSIs) (6).

Moreover, where successes are occurring, they can be attributed, in large part, to administrative support and collaborative, multidisciplinary efforts to implement these interventions. The infection control professional should play a central role in translating science into practice through education, surveillance, identification of process breakdowns, development of sound policies and procedures, monitoring outcomes, and providing feedback to staff—their traditional responsibilities.

IMPACT OF HAIs

Increasingly, HAIs are framed within the context of preventable adverse events and patient safety. Nosocomial infections are the leading adverse events affecting patients in hospitals (7). Five to ten percent of all patients admitted to acute care hospitals can be expected to develop one or more infections during their stay; approximately 2 million patients are affected annually (8). With nearly 90,000 deaths a year, at an annual cost in the billions of dollars, HAIs are coming under increased public scrutiny (9). At least a third of HAIs have been shown to be preventable through effective infection control programs (10).

The major HAIs are bloodstream infections (BSIs); pneumonias, especially VAP; urinary tract infections (UTIs); and SSIs. In many healthcare facilities, *Clostridium difficile*-infection (CDI) is also a significant problem, especially those where the epidemic, more virulent (BI/NAP1/027) strain is prevalent. There are cost and safety issues surrounding these infections, especially those involving DROs: increased morbidity and mortality, more expensive and limited treatment options, longer hospital stays, patient dissatisfaction, the cost and inconvenience of precautions, litigation, and adverse publicity for healthcare facilities (particularly where drug resistance is publicly reported and/or considered a measure of quality)—an increasing reality in today's consumer-driven patient safety movement (11–15). It follows that interventions that successfully reduce HAIs should have an impact on DROs.

EPIDEMIOLOGY OF DRUG RESISTANCE IN HEALTHCARE INSTITUTIONS

Some DROs of epidemiologic importance in hospitals are listed in Table 1. The prevalence of DROs depends on the location, size, type of facility, and level of services offered by a healthcare institution, especially if intensive care units (ICUs) are included (16–20). The burden of colonization and severity of infection may differ among pediatric, adult, elderly, and ICU hospital populations (21,22). Methicillin-resistant *Staphylococcus aureus* (MRSA) and vancomycin-resistant enterococci (VRE) prevalence rates have been climbing over the last twenty to thirty years (23,24). Similarly, rates of multi-drug resistant (MDR) Gram-negative rods have been rising (25,26).

Since the first case of vancomycin-intermediate *Staphylococcus aureus* (VISA) or glycopeptide-intermediate *Staphylococcus aureus* was identified in Japan in 1996, these strains are being isolated from around the world and outbreaks have been described (27,28). Of even greater concern is the discovery of vancomycin-resistant strains (VRSA), first reported in the United States in 2002. Both VISA and VRSA strains can cause severe disease. With so few cases of VRSA reported to date, the epidemiology of these organisms is uncertain, but co-colonization with VRE and MRSA has preceded VRSA colonization or infection to date (29). The importance of a good clinical laboratory is underscored by the fact that VISA strains are not

TABLE 1 Drug-Resistant Organisms of Epidemiologic Importance to Hospitals

Organisms	Antimicrobial resistance to these drugs/drug classes
Bacteria	
Staphylococcus aureus	Methicillin/oxacillin
	Vancomycin
	Aminoglycosides
	Linezolid
	Daptomycin
Enterococci	Ampicillin
	Vancomycin
	Linezolid
	Aminoglycosides
	Daptomycin
	Tigecycline
Enterobacteriaceae	3rd generation cephalosporins
	4th generation cephalosporins
	Monobactams
	Aminoglycosides
	Fluoroquinolones
Pseudomonas aeruginosa	Extended-spectrum penicillins
	3rd and 4th generation cephalosporins
	Fluoroquinolones
	Carbapenems
	Aminoglycosides
Acinetobacter sp.	All classes of antibiotics
	Carbapenems
	Tigecycline
Stenotrophomonas sp.	Trimethoprim/sulfamethoxazole
	Fluoroquinolones
	Ticarcillin/clavulanate
Mycobacteria	
Mycobacterium tuberculosis	Isoniazid
	Rifampin
	Ethambutol
	Pyrazinamide
	Streptomycin
	Fluoroquinolones
Fungi	
Candida species	Azoles
	Amphotericin B
	Echinocandins
Viruses	
Cytomegalovirus	Foscarnet
	Gancylclovir
	Cidofovir

readily detected by routine disc diffusion; broth dilution, agar dilution, or E-tests (AB Biodisk) are more reliable (30–32).

In recent years, an increase in community-acquired strains of MRSA colonizing and infecting patients is contributing to hospital rates of MRSA and complicating the epidemiology of MRSA in healthcare settings. These strains can produce mild to severe disease in patients and are now clearly part of the MRSA population in outpatient and inpatient settings in the United States (33). It has been speculated that antimicrobial usage trends in hospitals and the community (e.g., fluoroquinolone usage) and poor compliance with infection control interventions, including proper hand hygiene procedures, are contributing to these trends (34–38).

Transmission of infection within a hospital requires a source, a susceptible population, and a means of transmission (39). Factors that contribute to the survival and spread of organisms within a healthcare facility include the vulnerability of the patient population, colonization pressure (the point prevalence; i.e., number of patients colonized or infected at any given time on a ward can potentially facilitate transmission), patient proximity, staffing levels, and antimicrobial usage (which exerts selective pressure on intestinal microbiota) (38,40–43).

The major route of transmission of DROs in healthcare settings is person-to-person, either by direct contact or indirect spread (38,43). Besides their presence on and within colonized or infected patients, resistant organisms can be found on environmental surfaces in patient areas and on equipment (stationary or portable) (44). Patients may acquire resistant organisms from contact with such sources. Healthcare workers' hands, portable equipment (e.g., stethoscopes), and clothing can become contaminated with DROs from contact with colonized or infected patients or contaminated surfaces (45). Healthcare workers themselves may become colonized with DROs, contributing to the survival and spread of these organisms within the facility (46–49). An important point is that patients carrying DROs are more likely to develop nosocomial infection with these organisms (50).

Organisms may be transmitted as a result of the commerce among various healthcare facilities where there is ample opportunity for patients—and even shared staff—to carry DROs among treatment centers (Fig. 2). These are obvious "trade routes" along which resistance can spread beyond a single institution. A study by Evans et al. described a system-wide surveillance system that allowed them to trace the movements of patients colonized or infected with MRSA and VRE within a healthcare system. These patients had encounters at 62 different facilities up to 304 miles away over a 5 year period (51). As we will discuss below, this has implications for regional approaches to combating resistance.

IMPORTANT HAIs—OVERVIEW OF INFECTION CONTROL AND PREVENTION STRATEGIES
General Strategies for Preventing HAIs
Precautions

The containment of certain pathogens by isolating patients, placing patients and staff into cohorts, and using barrier precautions (hand hygiene, gloves, gowns, masks, and protective equipment) has been traditionally associated with infection control. Over the past thirty or more years there has been a marked evolution in isolation policies recommended by the Centers for Disease Control and Prevention (CDC) (39). These guidelines, originally published in 1996, have been recently revised (see Ref. 216).

As with other communicable diseases, HAIs are transmitted by contact, the airborne route, through a common source, droplet spread, or via a vector (39). Standard Precautions are applied to all hospitalized patients to reduce the spread of pathogenic organisms. Transmission-Based Precautions (airborne, droplet, contact) and empiric use of Transmission-based Precautions supplement Standard

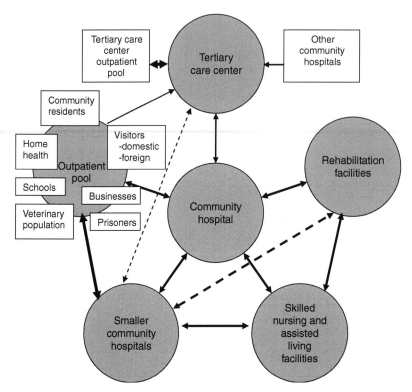

FIGURE 2 Relationships among diverse healthcare facilities in a region—external "trade routes" along which drug-resistant organisms may disseminate. *Source*: Adapted from Ref. 213.

Precautions in those situations where patients are known or suspected to be colonized or infected with pathogens of epidemiologic significance. Since recommendations may not anticipate every contingency, it remains the prerogative of the infection control professional to modify precautions to fit institutional needs and special situations.

Contact precautions (CP), which utilize barriers (e.g., gowns, gloves, and masks) worn by healthcare workers (HCWs), are intended to prevent transmission of certain pathogens—DROs among them—spread by direct or indirect contact with the patient or the patient's environment. It is recommended that the patient be in a private room when possible, but cohorting patients and staff may be necessary when private rooms are not available. Personnel and others, when appropriate, don gowns and gloves prior to entering the patient's room, which they remove and place into specified containers before exiting the room and performing hand hygiene (39).

Hand Hygiene
Although hand washing is nearly universally regarded as the single most important thing a healthcare worker can do to prevent the acquisition and transmission of infections, studies have consistently demonstrated a significant lack of adherence to good practice (52). A host of reasons can be cited for this discordance and

need to be considered in campaigns to increase compliance with hand hygiene policies (Fig. 3) (53). Boyce and Pittet prepared a comprehensive review of hand hygiene for the Healthcare Infection Control Practices Advisory Committee (HICPAC), the Society for Healthcare Epidemiology of America (SHEA), the Association for Professionals in Infection Control and Epidemiology (APIC), and the Infectious Diseases Society of America (IDSA) Hand Hygiene Task Force (53). Based on studies of the efficacy of alcohol-based hand rubs, the task force strongly recommended the use of these products for routine decontamination of the hands, unless the hands are visibly soiled. Hand washing is recommended "when hands are visibly dirty or contaminated with proteinaceous material or are visibly soiled with blood or other body fluids." Alcohol-based hand rubs decrease the time needed for hand hygiene, are less irritating, and are better accepted by healthcare personnel (54). In addition, they can be conveniently placed in areas where it is difficult to provide sinks; although, there are problems in some areas surrounding the use and placement of gel dispensers due to rules promulgated by local fire marshals. In addition, alcohol hand hygiene products are ineffective against *C. difficile* spores, so when caring for patients with CDI, HCWs should revert to the first-line use of hand washing with soap and running water. The wearing of artificial fingernails for those whose responsibilities include direct contact with high-risk patients, such as those in surgery and ICUs, is discouraged. Adherence to hand hygiene should be monitored, and information regarding their performance be given to personnel.

Improved compliance with hand hygiene may easily reduce transmission in settings where the number of infected or colonized patients is low. However, in settings where the average daily point prevalence is high, only a few lapses in hand hygiene may be all that is needed to sustain cross-transmission (40,52). The efficacy of efforts to improve hand hygiene requires further investigation, but institutions should make hand hygiene a priority. This requires education,

---

Self-reported reasons for poor adherence to hand hygiene

- Irritation and dryness of the skin
- Inconveniently placed sinks or shortage of sinks
- Lack of soap or paper towels
- Too busy or insufficient time
- Understaffing or overcrowding
- Patient needs take priority
- Hand hygiene interferes with healthcare worker-patient relationship
- Low risk of acquiring infection from patient
- Wearing gloves or the belief that gloves obviate the need for hand hygiene
- Lack of knowledge of guidelines
- Forgetfulness or not thinking about it
- No role model from colleagues or superiors
- Doubts about the value of hand hygiene
- Disagreement with the recommendations
- Lack of scientific information on the impact of improved hand hygiene on healthcare-associated infections

FIGURE 3 Reasons cited by healthcare workers for poor adherence to hand hygiene. *Source:* Adapted from Ref. 53.

Hand Hygiene: Motivating and Educating Healthcare Workers

- Healthcare worker educational training and motivational programs should focus specifically on factors currently found to significantly influence behavior, and not solely on the type of hand hygiene products.
- The strategy must be multifaceted, multimodal, and include education and senior executive support for implementation.
- Educate healthcare workers about the type of patient-care activities that can result in hand contamination and about the advantages and disadvantages of various methods used to clean hands.
- Monitor adherence to recommended hand hygiene practices and provide performance feedback to healthcare workers.
- Encourage partnerships between patients, their families, and healthcare workers to promote hand hygiene.

FIGURE 4   Hand hygiene health guidelines. *Source*: Adapted from Ref. 212.

motivation, and overcoming the systems problems that impede compliance (53). Systems problems that lead to poor adherence include lack of available sinks or alcohol-based hand rubs, products that irritate the skin, overcrowding, and excessive workload. Improving compliance with evidence-based hand-hygiene practices must be a multimodal and multidisciplinary effort—part of a broader strategy to enhance the culture of patient safety within hospitals (Fig. 4).

Gloves
The hand hygiene guideline addresses glove use as well. Proper use of gloves requires that they be changed—not washed—after each patient or if moving from a contaminated body site to a clean site on the same patient. Glove use does not eliminate the need for proper hand hygiene, and, after removing gloves, hands should be properly washed or decontaminated by applying an alcohol-based rub. Universal gloving—i.e., using disposable examination gloves during contact with high-risk patients or their environment—has been proposed by Weinstein and others. It has been shown to reduce the spread of CDI and transmission of VRE (55–57). In a study by Tenorio et al., gloving reduced the risk of acquisition of VRE on healthcare workers' hands by 71% (58). The ease and convenience of this approach has a certain appeal over the gowning and gloving required by traditional CP (59). In some studies, gowning offered no demonstrable advantage over universal gloving in the control of VRE, MRSA, ceftazidime-resistant *Escherichia coli*, and *Klebsiella pneumoniae* (52,59,60). However, gowns have been shown to be of benefit in other studies (see discussion of the control of resistant organisms below) and remain a recommendation for CP.

    Universal glove use is directed at the reservoir of colonized patients in hospitals who are unrecognized and have the potential to transmit pathogens. Others advocate active surveillance cultures (ASC) on all patients or those at high risk for colonization so that CP (gloves and gowns) can be applied. In one institution where screening cultures and full CP for infected or colonized patients were already in place, universal gloving on high-risk units for patients whose colonization status was unknown was associated with significant reductions in the acquisition of VRE (61).

Specific Strategies for Preventing HAIs
The prevention and control of HAIs should, in general, serve to reduce antimicrobial resistance by decreasing opportunities for infection and the accompanying use of antimicrobials. Putting aside the occasional exposure of a hospital population to highly contagious diseases, such as varicella, measles, and pertussis, most health-care epidemiologists in developed countries are daily preoccupied with four categories of infections: UTIs; catheter-related BSIs; pneumonias, primarily VAPs; and SSIs. A fifth, CDI, due to a disturbing increase in the incidence and severity of this disease, is discussed in Chapter 11. Some appreciation of the issues surrounding these categories of infections is necessary background for understanding interventions directed against DROs.

Catheter-Associated UTIs
UTIs account for about 40% of all HAIs (62). Instrumentation, particularly indwelling catheterization, is responsible for the majority of nosocomial UTIs (63). Therefore, using these catheters only when indicated, inserting and maintaining them properly, and removing them when they are no longer needed is important.

Urinary catheters are frequently overused and are left in for longer than needed; catheters should never be used for convenience (64). Personnel who insert and maintain catheters should be trained in aseptic technique. Strict adherence to the sterile, continuously closed system of urinary drainage is the standard and has been shown to be superior to open drainage (63). The use of prophylactic antimicrobials in the prevention of catheter-related UTIs is not currently recommended and has been shown to increase resistance in some studies (65,66). Most episodes of catheter-associated UTI appear to be caused by the migration of bacteria from the urethral meatus along the external surface of the catheter into the bladder rather than intraluminally (67). Studies of the efficacy of catheters coated with antimicrobials or silver alloy in reducing bacteriuria and UTIs have had mixed results, but silver alloy/hydrogel-coated catheters have shown promise and may be cost-effective (68). A recent prospective trial of a silicone-based, silver-coated Foley catheter did not demonstrate a reduction in nosocomial UTIs, although there were differences in the study groups (69). The use of antimicrobial coatings may encourage resistance. Newer approaches include the use of catheters impregnated with synergistic combinations of antiseptics or coated with an avirulent strain of *E. coli* (70,71).

Nosocomial Pneumonia and VAP
The attributable mortality of nosocomial pneumonias is about 30%, and they are the leading cause of death from nosocomial infection in this country (72). Several experts have published reviews of the concepts of diagnosis, management, and prevention of nosocomial pneumonia (73–75). Guidelines published by the CDC present a comprehensive strategy for the prevention of this important HAI (76).

Pneumonia is the third most common cause of infection in U.S. medical-surgical ICUs, and mechanical ventilation is the most significant risk factor for the development of pneumonia (75,77). The diagnosis, antimicrobial therapy, length of therapy, and nonpharmacologic interventions directed against VAPs are areas of intense research. Unfortunately, this widely studied area has often produced disappointing results in terms of elucidating effective preventive measures. In addition, there are definitional problems that make this a difficult area to study.

Pneumonia in the ICU contributes significantly to antimicrobial resistance, in large part, for two reasons: (*i*) because the diagnosis of pneumonia is not solidified with objective data in many institutions resulting in the unnecessary antimicrobial use in patients that do not actually have pneumonia and (*ii*) therapy is extended for too long (clinicians failing to use shorter course therapy for 7 to 8 days of therapy; discussed further in Chapter 18). It has been shown that the initial choice of antimicrobials is important in determining patient outcomes, that local antibiograms should be used to guide therapy, and clinicians frequently select an inadequate initial therapeutic regimen (78–80). Better antimicrobial choices may be aided by real-time susceptibility testing such as a rapid E-test (AB Biodisk) (81) or having knowledge of unit-specific antibiograms to guide empiric therapy. Shortening the length of therapy for pneumonia is one strategy for decreasing colonization pressures in a unit. Chastre et al. demonstrated that an 8-day course of therapy was as effective as 15 days for treating VAPs in adults (82). Finally, rotating antimicrobials in the ICU—antibiotic cycling—has been studied as a deterrent to resistance, without any demonstrable success, and is discussed in Chapter 14.

Nonpharmacologic strategies such as reducing the number of ventilated patients and reducing the length of time on mechanical ventilation are obvious strategies. In this regard, studies of positive-pressure ventilation methods that do not require intubation are encouraging (83,84). In some studies, continuous suctioning of secretions that pool in the subglottic space over the tracheal cuff has been shown to be an effective strategy once patients are intubated and ventilated (85–87). However, not all studies have clearly shown benefit (88). Simply placing patients in a semi-recumbent rather than supine position, aimed at reducing the aspiration of gastric contents, can be helpful (89,90). As with other recommended practices, there is inconsistent application of evidence-based guidelines in U.S. ICUs (91). As a result, there are quality campaigns that require participating institutions to use multiple, evidence-based interventions "bundled" into guidelines, which are monitored for compliance and impact on outcomes.

The use of systemic or nonabsorbable antimicrobials to selectively decontaminate the digestive tract (selective digestive decontamination) has been proposed, but is controversial, especially since increased antimicrobial use has been associated with the development of resistance (92). While this strategy can decrease VAPs in select populations of ventilated patients, it has not been shown to significantly affect mortality (93). Previous studies reported reductions in ventilator-associated pneumonias when antimicrobials were rotated on a regular basis (94–96). However, uncertainties as to the efficacy of this strategy remain (97).

Addressing VAP (as well as hospital- and healthcare-associated pneumonias) from an institutional perspective exemplifies the complimentary nature of infection control programs and antimicrobial stewardship programs. A variety of preventative strategies for pneumonia as well as tracking rates of pneumonia for feedback to clinicians and administrators are managed typically by the infection conrol practitioners under the guidance of the hospital epidemiologist. Antimicrobial stewardship programs may focus on developing treatment algorithms in concert with intensivists, surgeons, infectious diseases specialists, the hospital epidemiologist, respiratory therapists, and the clinical microbiology loboratory. Importantly, because most do not respond to paper guidelines, active intervention is necessary (rounding in the ICU; helping clinicians to calculate diagnostic scoring systems, which are part of many algorithms; deciphering and compiling data from, in some cases, off-site microbiology laboratories to construct unit-specific antibiograms, which in turn can be used to guide empiric therapy; and serving to remind clinicians that 7 to 8 days of therapy has been administered and the patient has responded by objective criteria; thus treatment can be stopped). In this example, the complimentary roles for infection control and antimicrobial stewardship are illustrated by "dividing and conquering."

Bloodstream Infection

Among hospitals submitting data to NNIS, BSIs are the third most common HAI in medical and surgical ICUs (77). These infections contribute to increased costs, lengths of stay, mortality, and excess antimicrobial use. Most healthcare-acquired BSIs are related to intravascular catheterization. When the integrity of a vascular catheter system is broken for the purpose of introducing medications or fluids into a line or withdrawing blood from a line, bacteria may contaminate the lumen and enter the bloodstream. Bacteria also track along the outer surface of the catheter and penetrate the mechanical barrier to infection provided by the integument.

Mermel has published a concise overview of this area (98). Education of staff on proper insertion and care of catheters, the designation of special intravenous teams responsible for the insertion and maintenance of peripheral lines, and feedback of infection rates to personnel should be part of an overall strategy for the prevention of catheter-related infections. Institutional policies should focus on appropriate use of catheters, proper insertion and maintenance, minimizing interruptions in the integrity of intravascular access systems, and removing them when they are no longer necessary or when they become infected. Designating specially trained teams of personnel for the insertion and maintenance of vascular catheters and providing feedback to personnel appear to be effective strategies in reducing BSIs (99,100).

Insertion under sterile conditions using full barrier technique including large drapes, sterile gowns, and surgical masks for all in attendance has been shown to be a highly cost-effective measure (101). Additional measures such as tunneling catheters and avoiding the femoral area for intravenous catheterization have also proven effective (102,103). Skin preparation with chlorhexidine has been shown to be superior to povidone-iodine; covering catheter insertion sites with chlorhexidine dressings may reduce line-associated bacteremias (98).

Technological strategies have included the development of catheters impregnated with antiseptics or antimicrobials, catheter hubs that contain antimicrobials, and contamination shields on pulmonary artery catheters. Catheters treated with antiseptics and antimicrobials have been associated with reductions in BSIs in many studies, but these catheters are costly. A review of eleven randomized, controlled trials of antimicrobial-impregnated central venous catheters pointed out methodological and statistical flaws in many of these studies and concluded that no significant clinical advantage to antimicrobial-impregnated central lines could be demonstrated (104). While antimicrobial- and antiseptic-impregnated catheters can be shown to reduce catheter-related BSIs, it is unclear that employing these expensive catheters is more effective than following proper insertion and post-insertion care guidelines (105).

As with VAPs, the adoption of bundled, evidence-based preventative guidelines, such as those developed by HICPAC in 1996, have been shown to be effective institutional strategies for reducing BSIs, but, again, adherence, is variable (106–109). A number of studies, including one large multicenter study by Warren et al., have shown that education-based interventions using evidence-based guidelines reduce catheter-associated BSIs (105). The Institute for Healthcare Improvement has initiated a highly visible program for preventing catheter-related BSIs as part of their 100,000 Lives and 5 Million Lives campaigns' quality improvement initiatives focusing on a number of preventable adverse events in healthcare (110). The group of interventions, described in more detail in documents readily available on the worldwide web (214) include the following components: proper hand hygiene; maximal barrier precautions; chlorhexidine skin antisepsis; optimal catheter site selection, with subclavian vein as the preferred site for nontunneled catheters; and daily review of line necessity, with prompt removal of unnecessary lines. All of these components are considered necessary for appropriate, safe central line insertion to have been performed. It is clear from good studies that substantial, sustained reductions in catheter-related BSIs can be gained by promoting evidence-based guidelines for their insertion, and, if widely implemented, can result in significant reduction in morbidity, mortality, and costs (105,111).

Surgical Site Infections
Nosocomial infections related to surgery, especially SSIs, are among the most common nosocomial infections, occurring in 9% to 30% of post-surgical patients (112). They are the second most common HAI in the United States (7). Herwaldt et al. have carefully analyzed the complexities of determining the true impact of postoperative nosocomial infections on costs, length of stay, and mortality in a recently published prospective study of postoperative nosocomial infections in patients undergoing general, cardiothoracic, and neurosurgical operations in a tertiary care medical center (113). It is clear that, along with the sometimes devastating consequences to patients, these infections increase costs and consume medical resources.

In 1999, HICPAC published guidelines that provide detailed information on the prevention of SSIs (114). While the most important factors in the prevention of SSIs are the skill of the surgeon, proper technique, and the health of the patient, infection control has an important role in the reduction of SSIs (115–117). Surveillance of SSIs with feedback of surgeon-specific infection rates has been shown to be an effective intervention, reducing overall SSI rates by up to 56% (10,118–121). Despite methodological difficulties (e.g., with definitions and capturing infections that occur after discharge), surveillance and feedback of SSIs are among the most important responsibilities of infection control professionals.

The practice of administering perioperative antimicrobials for the prevention of surgical infections has evolved since Burke's landmark study in 1961, which showed the relationship between the timing of antimicrobial administration and efficacy in preventing experimental skin infection (122). Recommendations for antimicrobial prophylaxis emphasize that the appropriate antimicrobial must have adequate levels in the target tissue before or at the time of expected contamination. An appropriate preoperative antimicrobial should be chosen in procedures where the evidence supports its use and given at a time that ensures bactericidal serum and tissue levels are present when the incision is made (preferably within 30 minutes of the incision). It is not necessary to maintain therapeutic levels for more than a few hours after closure; therefore, additional doses should be given only when indicated in published guidelines (114). If antimicrobials are not discontinued in a timely manner, cost, resistance, and CDI risks are adversely affected. Appropriate use and timing of preoperative antimicrobials is emerging as an important quality indicator. Poor compliance with established guidelines is a problem for many hospitals. Studies have demonstrated that the use of a computer-based reminder system to prompt appropriate timing of antimicrobials can be an effective technological solution (123,124). With the concept of pay-for-performance at the doorstep, the government is no longer willing to reimburse hospitals that are "poor performers," and surgical prophylaxis is one of the areas being scrutinized by regulators.

The application of mupirocin to the nares to eliminate intranasal carriage of *S. aureus* prior to surgery has been the subject of much recent study and has been reviewed within the larger context of decolonization before surgery by Napolitano (125). A recent double-blind, randomized, placebo-controlled trial in 263 patients undergoing cardiovascular surgery did not demonstrate a reduction in the rates of overall SSIs by *S. aureus* (126). A meta-analysis of 60 articles published by Kallen et al. in 2005 suggests that perioperative intranasal mupirocin appears to be effective in reducing SSIs in general and nongeneral surgery, and, given its safety, should be considered in clean surgeries that carry a risk of staphylococcal infection (127). However, decolonization requires further study, and, at present, this strategy cannot be routinely recommended.

As with other HAIs, multifaceted and multidisciplinary approaches to improve compliance with evidence-based guidelines are being promoted by quality improvement organizations hoping to reduce surgical complications. One such effort is the Surgical Care Improvement Project (SCIP), a project sponsored by a national quality partnership of organizations, which hopes to reduce surgical complications by 25% by 2010 (128,129). Among their process and outcome measures for preventing SSIs are: prophylactic antibiotic timing (within one hour of surgical incision), selection, and discontinuation (within 24 hr after surgery or 48 hr after cardiovascular procedures); diagnosis of wound infection during index hospitalization; appropriate hair removal; and immediate postoperative normothermia in colorectal surgery patients (129).

INTERVENTIONS DIRECTED AT DROs

The importance of good practice and consistent application of evidence-based guidelines, as discussed above, cannot be overemphasized when discussing the prevention and control of DROs. In 2003, the CDC launched its Campaign to Prevent Antimicrobial Resistance in Healthcare Settings. General principles were presented in the form of a "twelve step" program to prevent infections and diminish opportunities for development of resistance in the hospitalized adult population (Fig. 5). This ambitious program includes guidance and resources for preventing resistance in dialysis patients, long-term care residents, hospitalized children, and surgical patients.

Two important guidelines for managing DROs in healthcare settings, one from SHEA and the other from HICPAC, have appeared in recent years (38,43). These guidelines reflect differences in interpretation of the evidence derived from extensive examination and analysis of the literature. The debate that ensued over these guidelines began in their pre-publication phase and is likely to persist for some time. And, while the differences between the two recommendations seem small, the controversy has prompted parties from each viewpoint to publish their separate "tales" of the evolution of these guidelines (130,131).

The major difference between the two guidelines is the screen and isolate or, as some refer to it, the "search and destroy" practice (130). The SHEA guidelines recommend aggressive use of active surveillance to identify patients

Prevent Infection
- Step 1. Vaccinate
  - Give influenza/pneumococcal vaccine to at-risk patients before discharge
  - Get influenza vaccine annually

- Step 2. Get the catheters out
  - Use catheters only when essential
  - Use the correct catheter
  - Use proper insertion and catheter-care protocols
  - Remove catheters when they are no longer essential

Diagnose and Treat Infection Effectively
- Step 3. Target the pathogen
  - Culture the patient
  - Target empiric therapy to likely pathogens and local antibiogram
  - Target definitive therapy to known pathogens and antimicrobial susceptibility test results

- Step 4. Access the experts
  - Consult infectious diseases experts for patients with serious infections

Use Antimicrobials Wisely
- Step 5. Practice antimicrobial control
  - Engage in local antimicrobial control efforts

- Step 6. Use local data
  - Know your antibiogram
  - Know your patient population

- Step 7. Treat infection, not contamination
  - Use proper antisepsis for blood and other cultures
  - Culture the blood, not the skin or catheter hub
  - Use proper methods to obtain and process all cultures

- Step 8. Treat infection, not colonization
  - Treat pneumonia, not the tracheal aspirate
  - Treat bacteremia, not the catheter tip or hub
  - Treat urinary tract infection, not the indwelling catheter

- Step 9. Know when to say "no" to vanco
  - Treat infection, not contaminants or colonization
  - Fever in a patient with an intravenous catheter is not a routine indication for vancomycin

- Step 10. Stop antimicrobial treatment:
  - When infection is cured
  - When cultures are negative and infection is unlikely
  - When infection is not diagnosed

Prevent Transmission
- Step 11. Isolate the pathogen
  - Use standard infection control precautions.
  - Contain infectious body fluids (follow airborne, droplet, and contact precautions)
  - When in doubt, consult infection control experts

- Step 12. Break the chain of contagion
  - Stay home when you are sick
  - Keep your hands clean
  - Set an example

FIGURE 5 The Centers for Disease Control and Prevention's Campaign to Prevent Antimicrobial Resistance. *Source*: Adapted from Ref. 211.

colonized with these organisms. These patients are then placed on CP to decrease further transmission. The HICPAC guideline favors a graduated approach with greater intensity of control activities in settings where baseline measures fail to decrease transmission rates. Until some of the more contentious issues are resolved, most hospitals will be faced with deciding what they will take from each of the guidelines to develop strategies for preventing the dissemination of resistance. In this section we briefly examine some of the evidence behind the controversy.

GRAM-POSITIVE RESISTANT ORGANISMS (MRSA AND VRE)

MRSA. The acquisition of the staphylococcal cassette chromosome *mec* by a sensitive strain confers resistance to methicillin (and all beta-lactams currently marketed) (132). Exceptions to this include certain beta-lactams that target penicillin-binding protein 2a such as 2 cephalosporins in development (ceftaroline and ceftobiprole) and an early investigational carbapenem. Epidemiologic evidence suggests that the spread of MRSA has been due to a few clonal types, introduced into a population by infected or colonized patients, rather than the frequent de novo development of new MRSA clones (132–138). Interrupting transmission is an appropriate strategy in controlling this type of spread (43).

VRE (See Also Chapter 6). The majority of vancomycin resistance in enterococci is the result of *vanA* and *vanB* gene clusters (139). Most, if not all, VRE infection and colonization is due to the transmission of VRE or from the transfer of these gene clusters; vancomycin-resistance does not appear to arise spontaneously in patients exposed to vancomycin (140–142). VRE is almost always associated with healthcare in the United States, as opposed to Europe where *vanA* or *vanB* VRE isolates have been found in healthy people, farm animals, and food products (43). In general, a single clonal strain is usually responsible for an initial outbreak of VRE in a healthcare setting. However, where the organism has persisted, multiple clones may be found—possibly due to the transfer of resistance genes to multiple strains of sensitive enterococci, the introduction of new strains, or both (43,143,144).

Antimicrobials exert selective pressure that favors the growth of acquired VRE strains in the stool, making transmission more likely (42). The colonization pressure of VRE in a given unit is a strong predictor of VRE acquisition, and the effect of selective pressure exerted by antimicrobials may be less of a factor in transmission when colonization pressure is high (40). Muto et al. concluded that only modest reductions in VRE transmission can be achieved through antimicrobial controls, and, as with MRSA, infection control interventions are more likely to be successful (43). Nonetheless, under most circumstances, antimicrobial exposure is an important risk factor for VRE acquisition, especially in patients who have been given multiple antibiotics, antimicrobials with anaerobic activity, and third-generation cephalosporins (42). This has implications for a broad-based strategy for control that includes limiting contact transmission as well as antibiotic stewardship.

Interventions for the Control of MRSA and VRE

Hand Hygiene. Both VRE and MRSA can survive on the hands of healthcare workers, and persistence on environmental surfaces can be a source of contamination of healthcare workers' hands and gloves (44,45,145). Proximity to patients with VRE, shared caregivers, and colonization pressure within a unit are predictors of VRE acquisition (40,44,61,146). One stochastic mathematical model predicted that even a moderate increase in hand hygiene during periods of understaffing or overcrowding—conditions that are likely to favor poor hand hygiene—in an ICU could decrease transmission as effectively as placing patients in cohorts (147).

Barriers (Gloves, Gowns, and Masks). As previously noted, universal gloving has been associated with reduction in the transmission of VRE. While studies support the role of gloves in reducing hand contamination, changing gloves between patients (VRE can be recovered from gloves following routine examination of a patient) and hand hygiene are still strongly advocated (44,45). One large outbreak of severe disease secondary to VISA in a French ICU could not be controlled with barrier precautions alone. Only after restricting admissions to the unit, enhanced environmental disinfection, and hand hygiene with a hydroalcoholic preparation was the outbreak brought under control.

Some transmission of DROs is probably the result of contamination of healthcare workers' clothing. While the efficacy of gowns is not entirely clear, they have been shown to reduce transmission of VRE and MRSA, and most studies appear to support their utility (43). Slaughter et al. could not demonstrate that gowns added additional benefit over gloving, whereas Puzniak and colleagues demonstrated a beneficial effect of gowns in reducing VRE transmission in a medical ICU when colonization pressure was high (60,146).

The utility of masks has not been established for preventing the transmission of MRSA. Because of potential airborne transmission of staphylococci, nasal colonization, and shedding of staphylococci by patients and healthcare workers, there is, at least, a theoretical rationale for the use of masks in CP for MRSA, VISA, and VRSA (148).

Equipment and Environmental Disinfection. Portable equipment that is used on more than one patient can transport pathogens either directly or by contaminating hands and gloves (41,149–151). Using dedicated or disposable equipment and cleaning equipment between patients is recommended (38,43,152). The cleaning and disinfection of equipment and environmental surfaces to inactivate DROs, particularly in areas that come into frequent contact with the hands of healthcare workers, should be carried out as outlined in the current CDC guidelines for environmental infection control (152). Routine cultures of the environment add to the expense of controlling outbreaks and are not recommended, but may be useful in verifying that adequate environmental cleaning is taking place, especially in settings where VRE transmission is continuing despite control measures (152).

Active Surveillance Cultures and Contact Precautions. In response to the rising incidence of VRE infections in the United States, HICPAC issued guidelines in 1994 that raised the possibility that periodic screening cultures of stool or rectal swabs might facilitate the control of VRE by identifying colonized patients, especially among high-risk populations. Yet, even after publication of the 1995 HICPAC guidelines, the incidence of VRE infections continued to rise (23). However, screening cultures were not widely used. Subsequently, studies that applied the CDC guidelines more rigorously, incorporating ASC/CP, demonstrated that VRE could be controlled effectively.

The obvious intent of ASC/CP is to identify patients colonized—a hidden reservoir of resistance—or infected with a resistant pathogen in order to interrupt person-to-person transmission by placing them on precautions. Vriens et al.

reported a higher frequency of transmission of MRSA from unidentified carriers than from identified patients who were isolated in an ICU (153). In one outbreak, proximity to colonized, nonisolated patients with VRE was a risk factor for acquisition of VRE; however, proximity to isolated patients who were VRE positive was not (61). Indeed, the proportion of colonized patients who are undetected in the absence of ASC can be significant (154). In addition, patients colonized with VRE or MRSA are at greater risk for developing infections with these organisms, especially in more vulnerable populations (21).

Ostrowsky et al. demonstrated that control of VRE could be accomplished in a healthcare system through surveillance cultures to detect colonization in high-risk patients, isolation of colonized patients, and the use of barrier precautions—interestingly, without an active attempt to reduce antimicrobial use (155). A large number of studies in a variety of settings report control of VRE and MRSA when ASC/CP are part of control measures (38,43,156,157).

Among the more controversial recommendations in the SHEA guideline is a call for widespread application of ASC/CP in addition to standard control measures. Yet, ASC in conjunction with CP for colonized or infected patients may be better than Standard Precautions alone and is associated with reductions in rates of colonization and infection with MRSA and VRE in many studies (43,157,158). Calfee et al. reported sustained control of VRE at the University of Virginia Hospital over a 5-year period, which they largely attributed to the use of surveillance cultures to identify asymptomatic, colonized patients (159). In fact, most published reports of successful control of these two organisms have included ASC/CP among their interventions (38,160).

Supporters of the SHEA guideline find the correlation of these measures with control of MRSA and VRE in so many studies compelling enough to urge broad adoption of ASC/CP. The potential for transfer of genetic resistance factors from VRE to staphylococci—which has been demonstrated to occur in vitro—and the possibility of creating a highly resistant staphylococcus, lends urgency to the argument for aggressive control of these organisms (161). So what, then, are the barriers to recommending greater utilization of ASC/CP, and why the debate?

Most critics of the SHEA approach take issue with its analysis of the literature on several fronts. For one, most of the evidence up to that time came from studies of outbreaks, many in ICUs or among more vulnerable, special populations of patients (5). Opponents are not satisfied with the evidence that the results of such studies are applicable to all hospitals or patient populations—especially where transmission risks are not as great. Secondly, there are methodological problems in many of the studies cited. To be sure, evaluating infection control interventions in hospital settings is fraught with potentially confounding variables. An excellent discussion by Nijssen and colleagues explores the uncertainty of attributing significance to interventions designed to control resistance that are introduced into a system where multiple, continuously interacting processes are occurring (e.g., changing prevalence of resistance, infection control interventions, antimicrobial use) (162).

Nearly all of the studies employed multiple, concurrent interventions, which also makes it difficult to determine the proportionate contribution of each intervention. However, Huang et al. have evaluated the impact of routine ASC/CP in ICUs on BSIs caused by MRSA. They achieved a 75% reduction in the incidence density of MRSA BSI in the ICU and a 40% reduction in non-ICU cases. This amounted to a 67% reduction hospital-wide over a sixteen-month period. Their study design was an interrupted time series in which they analyzed nine years of data. They concluded that the statistically significant factor in bringing about these reductions was ASC/CP in the ICU. A number of usual interventions, added one at a time over the study period, such as the introduction of alcohol gels, a handwashing campaign, and maximal sterile barrier precautions for insertion of central lines, did not have significant impact on the rates.

Unfortunately, many of the studies are of quasi-experimental design rather than prospective, randomized controlled trials (163). There is an ongoing multi-center, randomized trial sponsored by the National Institutes of Health to evaluate the efficacy of control measures including ASC/CP in 19 adult ICUs (215). However, Muto et al. have expressed reservations regarding this study's design and whether it is adequately evaluating ASC/CP (164).

Other criticisms of ASC/CP have centered around the burden on healthcare resources (personnel, labor, and costs) and adverse effects of isolation on patients. There are studies supporting the cost benefit of ASC/CP, although more are needed, especially in nonoutbreak situations (5,157,165–167). Part of the cost and burden include the labor associated with screening, culturing, and CP. Technological advances in PCR are making it possible to identify resistant organisms in screening cultures in a more timely fashion, which could reduce the time patients must spend on CP (168,169). This is an important point, because concerns over the care patients receive while on precautions have been raised by several authors (170–172).

Supporters of the SHEA guidelines point to the success of northern European countries and Western Australia, where aggressive approaches to ASC/CP have controlled these infections (164). They contrast this with the failure of Standard Precautions and failure to control these organisms in other areas of Europe and Australia, where a less aggressive approach is used (164,173). In the United States, MRSA is responsible for nearly 60% of staphylococcal infections in some ICUs; however, the occurrence of MRSA among staphylococcal isolates is much smaller in the Netherlands, Belgium, and Scandinavia, where such reductions have been seen (38,174). The differences among medical delivery systems in these countries and in the United States, for whom these guidelines are intended, may be a factor as well. Finally, it is unclear whether standard precautions are truly ineffective when used properly, especially given the widely reported variability in HCWs' adherence to recommended practices.

The extent to which control measures should be adopted universally, particularly in regions with low prevalence rates of resistance, is one of the issues surrounding the debate. Most studies of the epidemiology and control of resistant organisms have come from large, academic centers. The question of whether ASC/CP is an appropriate strategy for community hospitals or small rural hospitals has underscored a need for more study of resistance rates in the community healthcare setting. Diekema et al. in a survey of over 400 hospitals in the United States found that antimicrobial resistance rates were strongly associated with the size, geographic location, and academic affiliation of hospitals (17). Data comparing percentages of nosocomial *Staphylococcus aureus* infections with MRSA in NNIS hospitals with less than 200 beds with those with greater than 200 beds between 1992 and 2002 demonstrates that smaller hospitals have caught up with larger hospitals in their percentage of HAI due to MRSA (23). A study by West et al. has demonstrated benefits of ASC/CP in a community setting (175).

The implications of these guidelines for hospitals are significant. As Strausbaugh et al. point out, neither the SHEA nor the HICPAC guideline addresses, in a more comprehensive sense, the goal of these control efforts (130). The problem of how resources should be allocated for control programs—an important issue for poorer community and rural hospitals—was not addressed in these documents. While the control of antimicrobial resistance is of undeniable import, there are other programs seeking to improve patient safety competing for resources. High "front-end" costs, such as would be required for widespread adoption of ASC/CP, as recommended in the SHEA guidelines, remain an issue for those who support the two-tiered protocol recommended by HICPAC.

Control of MDR Gram-Negative Bacteria

Extended-spectrum and AmpC beta-lactamase-producing bacteria are important causes of HAIs. Organisms known to harbor these potent beta-lactamases as well as other resistance determinants in some cases include: *Pseudomonas aeruginosa* that are resistant to quinolones, carbapenems, and third-generation cephalosporins; MDR *Enterobacter* spp.; and MDR *Acinetobacter* spp. *E. coli* and *Klebsiella* spp. are on the rise worldwide (176). Infections caused by MDR Gram-negative organisms are associated with higher morbidity and mortality than infections caused by less resistant bacteria for a number of reasons, including their propensity for delaying appropriate therapy (177). In addition, it has been demonstrated that MDR Gram-negative bacteria consume more healthcare resources than matched infections due to susceptible strains of the same bacterium (171,178–181) Another pressing issue is that treatment options for MDR Gram-negative organisms are rapidly diminishing, as there is little ongoing development of antibiotics with activity against these organisms. Therefore, limiting the spread of these organisms is imperative. Unfortunately, there has been less attention paid to these organisms than to Gram-positive organisms in recent studies, and information comes largely from outbreaks reported in the literature (176). Recommendations for the control of these organisms are reviewed and presented in the HICPAC guidelines (38).

Understanding the epidemiology, clinical management, and control of these organisms depends on the capacity to identify them and their reservoirs. Yet, despite current recommendations, not all clinical microbiology laboratories routinely identify extended-spectrum beta-lactamase (ESBL)-producing organisms. Surveys looking at the ability of clinical laboratories to detect ESBLs identified a serious gap in this regard (182,183). Laboratory identification and access to molecular typing technology is essential for preventing and controlling outbreaks.

The environment is an important source of these organisms. Outbreaks have been associated with hospital water supplies, bronchoscopes, portable equipment, artificial nails, ultrasound gel, contaminated intravenous solutions, and other environmental sources (184). As with Gram-positive DROs, Gram-negative DROs can be spread by person-to-person transmission, as they are carried on the hands of HCWs (184–187). Colonized patients and, rarely, colonized HCWs are another reservoir, which has led to the obvious question as to whether ASC/CP over an above CP should be part of control efforts (47,176). As a survey conducted by the IDSA Emerging Infections Network determined, such interventions are used in U.S. hospitals (176,188), although infectious diseases experts surveyed are less certain about the role of ASC.

Risk factors for acquiring these organisms are similar to those for the acquisition of other nosocomial Gram-negative organisms: indwelling catheters, increased severity of illness, urgent abdominal surgery, ventilator use, and prolonged hospital stay. Lautenbach et al. found patients infected with ESBLs had a greater cumulative antimicrobial exposure than did controls; total antimicrobial exposure was the only independent predictor of infections with these organisms (189). Their study suggested that curbing the use of all classes of antimicrobials used against Gram-negative organisms may be important. However, studies have documented clonal spread of these organisms (187,190–193). Patterson has recently discussed current knowledge about the control of MDR Gram-negative organisms (194). Control measures should be broader than antibiotic management alone and should include limiting contact transmission of resistant isolates. Determining local patterns and mechanisms of resistance is essential for choosing antimicrobial interventions in a healthcare facility (194).

An excellent discussion and analysis of the data on active surveillance to identify colonized patients and whether they should be placed on CP has been published by Harris et al. (176). Their paper provides a framework for decision making and recommendations for future investigations of ASC/CP in the control of MDR Gram-negative organisms. It is too early to recommend the routine use of ASC/CP for these organisims. In outbreak situations where there is failure to control spread, this seems reasonable. As with Gram-positive DROs, the HICPAC guidelines favor a graduated approach to control (38). Hospital epidemiologists must determine what is best in their institution. The following recommendations are modifications of suggestions originally published in 1999 by Paterson and Yu for ESBLs and could also be applied to other highly resistant Gram-negative organisms of epidemiologic importance, but further study is needed (195):

- Laboratories should follow the Clinical Laboratory Standards Institute (CLSI) guidelines for detecting ESBLs among all isolates of *Klebsiella pneumoniae* and *E. coli* and should report these to clinicians and infection control.
- Proper hand hygiene, gloves, and gowns should be employed when caring for infected or colonized patients.
- Educate clinical and laboratory staff, patients, and their visitors about these organisms.
- Affected patients should be grouped in cohorts, and staffing assignments should minimize the potential for cross-transmission.
- Antimicrobial controls, based on local antibiograms and mechanisms of resistance, should be instituted.
- Consider periodic rectal swabs and urine cultures of patients in ICUs to identify carriers. In some institutions, active surveillance is only used in outbreak situations.
- Inform receiving units or other facilities of infected or colonized patients.
- Carriage can persist for months. Previously colonized or infected patients should be regarded as colonized until proven otherwise and medical records should be flagged to indicate status at readmission.
- Colonized or infected patients may be admitted to nursing homes, where they should be placed in single rooms with private bathrooms. The use of common areas by colonized patients should be considered on an individual basis.

INFECTION CONTROL AND FORMULARY CONTROL IN MANAGING RESISTANCE IN HEALTHCARE SETTINGS

There is a sizeable body of evidence supporting the role of infection control in limiting the dissemination of resistant organisms. However, effective control of resistant organisms requires the services of a competent microbiology laboratory and a program for overseeing and optimizing antimicrobial use. But, antimicrobial optimization should not focus simply on proscribing the use of antimicrobials; the underutilization of antimicrobials can have undesirable effects on outcomes and resistance as well as over-utilization. The favorable impact of antimicrobial stewardship on antimicrobial use, healthcare expenditures, and antimicrobial resistance has been reported in a number of studies in large as well as small hospitals (196). Depending on how a hospital's various quality improvement programs are configured, hospital epidemiologists either administer or are closely allied with antibiotic stewardship programs at their institutions.

Antibiotic stewardship is reviewed in detail in Chapter 15. The proportionate influence of infection control interventions compared with antibiotic optimization on reducing resistance may depend, to some extent, on the organism and the mode of transmission: horizontally transmitted resistant organisms such as MRSA seem more susceptible to infection control interventions, whereas resistant organisms arising from the endogenous flora of patients undergoing antibiotic therapy may be more influenced by antimicrobial stewardship (197). However, this cannot be too strictly interpreted in light of studies demonstrating clonal spread of certain Gram-negative DROs (184).

Hospital epidemiologists have long understood that surveillance without feedback to providers, education, and the implementation of evidence-based guidelines is ineffectual. Similarly, a number of studies have confirmed the importance of surveillance, education, feedback, and prescribing controls on inappropriate antimicrobial use (198–201) as well as resistance (202,203). Providing resources for surveillance (especially if surveillance is done using administrative data—a methodology fraught with problems) without support for education and implementing best practices will not reduce inappropriate antimicrobial use or antimicrobial resistance (3). Rather than competing, antimicrobial stewardship programs and infection control professionals should be well-integrated with a good clinical microbiology laboratory and have administrative as well as information services support. They should communicate frequently, share data, and look for opportunities in the "antimicrobial usage-resistance" cycle (Fig. 1) to effectively identify process breakdowns, educate clinicians at the point of care, and effect the "cultural" changes necessary to reduce situations that favor the development and spread of resistant microbes.

THE IMPORTANCE OF A REGIONAL VIEW

As we have pointed out, and Evans et al. has demonstrated, populations of patients (and HCWs) move along trade routes, potentially affecting the resistance patterns within regions (Fig. 2) (51). Polgreen and colleagues looked at patient and institutional risk factors for the acquisition of MRSA and VRE among hospitals in Iowa (ranging from ~86 to >858 beds in diverse geographic regions of the state) between 1998 and 2001. Their study revealed differences in the epidemiology of these two organisms (16). They found that VRE and MRSA shared some risk factors for acquisition, but there were also some significant differences in that MRSA was endemic in rural hospitals (rural location and hospital size of <200 beds were significant risk factors for MRSA infection), while hospitalization at a smaller hospital had a negative correlation with VRE infection. This has important implications for control of these organisms. Understanding the regional epidemiology of resistance and identifying reservoirs of these organisms are essential elements in developing intelligent control strategies.

Combating resistance regionally has been of benefit in controlling VRE and MRSA within a geographic area. The landmark investigation reported by Ostrowsky et al. in 32 healthcare facilities in the Siouxland region demonstrated that control of VRE could be accomplished in a regional healthcare system by implementing a standard set of guidelines in all participating facilities (155). The Veterans Affairs Pittsburgh Health System and participating hospitals in the region reported dramatic reductions in HAIs with MRSA after implementing a systems engineering approach, intense educational campaign, and bundled, evidence-based interventions (6,204). Kaye et al. recently reported on the work of the Duke Infection Control Outreach Network, a consortium of hospitals in North Carolina and Virginia (205). They achieved a reduction in BSIs, nosocomial MRSA infections, VAP, and blood-borne pathogen exposures in 12 participating hospitals by using uniform approaches to surveillance, frequent analysis and feedback, and interventions based on CDC recommendations. They estimated significant economic benefits to this approach, and their 32 hospital consortium continues to report reductions in these infections as well as in Foley-associated UTIs on their website (http://dicon.mc.duke.edu/). There is a growing number of examples of successful regional approaches to DROs (206).

CAN MANDATORY PUBLIC REPORTING OF HAIs AND LEGISLATIVE MANDATES HELP COMBAT DROs?
Public Reporting

Publicity surrounding HAIs and public impatience, spurred by the media and consumer groups, about lack of information regarding infections in hospitals has culminated in legislative actions designed to inform the public and motivate healthcare institutions to do better. As of this writing, 16 states have legislation requiring hospitals to report infections publicly, and nearly all others are considering such laws, but have not yet passed legislation. While many in healthcare favor greater transparency, there are legitimate concerns that such data can be flawed, abused, or misleading. In addition, the collection, reporting, and validation will increase labor and costs associated with healthcare.

These concerns induced SHEA and HICPAC to produce documents describing potential methodological problems and providing guidance for valid measures (207,208). Both documents consider process measures easier to use and validate. While some legislation has asked for hospital-wide infection rates, total hospital surveillance has been largely abandoned by healthcare epidemiologists because low HAI rates for some services or units diminishes the usefulness of routine surveillance, house-wide surveillance is labor-intensive and diverts resources from more important infection prevention activities, and risk adjustment is not possible for all patient populations in a hospital (208). A major concern of healthcare epidemiologists is the temptation to utilize administrative data for reporting. Such data are convenient and available, but studies have shown administrative data to be inferior (207). Public reporting systems must employ standardized methods for case-finding, have a system for external validation of data, and consider the resources and infrastructure (personnel, training, technological support) necessary for developing this data. Risk adjustment is necessary for valid comparisons.

Both the SHEA and HICPAC documents confront some of the unintended consequences of mandatory reporting. It is unlikely that most laypersons will come easily to an understanding of the inherent complexities of collecting and interpreting comparative data. Unless reports are presented in a way that allows most people to understand the information and its potential limitations, they can be misleading and potentially counterproductive. Hospitals or HCWs, concerned about keeping rates of HAIs low, may be less inclined to treat patients at high risk for HAI. The re-engineering of current surveillance practices that will be required for public reporting will place additional burdens on busy infection control professionals. As with any intervention, scientific validation will be required to see whether mandatory reporting is a cost-effective way to prevent HAIs and DROs.

Legislating Control Measures

At least two states have launched legislative initiatives mandating the use of ASC/CP to control MRSA or VRE. Even proponents of aggressive control are troubled by legislative attempts to mandate potentially costly interventions that were intended as guidelines—guidelines based on evidence that is still being analyzed and debated among healthcare epidemiologists. Ill-conceived initiatives can increase the burden on hospitals and providers and may not result in improved outcomes. A joint task force of SHEA and APIC has addressed this issue. They recently published a review of the evidence supporting ASC/CP and the legislation making it mandatory for healthcare facilities to implement these measures (5). They included a discussion of the effect of such legislation on infection control programs; its requirements for data management, validation, and compliance monitoring; enforcement; and the practical problems with implementation. While they emphasize a need for more research in this area and improved collaboration among public health authorities and institutional infection control professionals, they do not support legislation mandating ASC/CP for control. It is unclear how the opinion of experts will resonate with the public and legislators.

Many epidemiologists—including this author—feel that, when dealing with a serious threat such as resistance, which may outstrip our ability to contain it, the most aggressive tactics should be employed initially until scientific analysis can discern which of the tactics can be peeled away. This is why ASC/CP has the support it does; it is nearly always associated with interventions that work. The question is one of how to best allocate resources along with a will to control antimicrobial resistance. Many feel it will take a *national* will to manage this problem, as it has in Northern Europe.

CONCLUSIONS

This chapter might just as easily have been titled "The Impact of Antimicrobial Resistance on the Management of Infection Control." There is no doubt among infection control professionals that reducing DROs is among their most important priorities; reaching a sound scientific consensus on how to achieve this is proving difficult. What is clear is that, more than ever before, the infection control professional must be fully cognizant of the external (community relations, medical advances, accrediting and regulatory forces) and internal forces (people, processes, and technology) operating on and within healthcare if they are to effect the cultural changes, implement the necessary policies to prevent HAIs, and reduce antimicrobial resistance (Fig. 6). Infection control professionals, previously preoccupied with the internal forces operating in their healthcare facility, must now see and act beyond their units and wards. Communities expect that medical advances will be translated into local action. However, worry over biological disasters such as biological terrorism, highly resistant microbes, pandemic influenza, newly emerging infections, and adverse events in hospitals can drive both rational and irrational solutions. In addition, publicity surrounding programs with improved outcomes and motivational catch-phrases such as "getting to zero" can create unrealistic expectations and costly unintended consequences (e.g., reluctance to report adverse events, unwarranted patient dissatisfaction, and increased litigation). This must be considered along with the serious need for improved patient safety and a reduction in antimicrobial resistance.

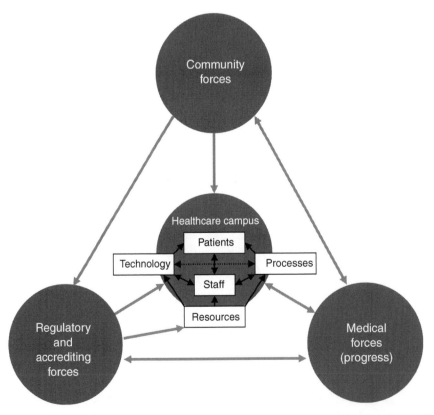

FIGURE 6 Interplay of forces in healthcare that affect responses to problems such as antibiotic resistance.

Understanding human behavior aids programs that aim to educate and motivate HCWs' adherence to good practice, such as in hand hygiene (53,209). It is time for healthcare epidemiologists to redouble their efforts toward educating the populations that they study and serve both within their hospitals and outside of them. They must be involved in the public debate over antimicrobial resistance and reporting of HAIs. Ideally, they will help inform any legislative processes at all stages of development and remain involved in monitoring the outcomes.

Resources and commitment must back programs to combat antimicrobial resistance; unfunded mandates only serve to discourage those attempting to translate science into practice. It is fortunate that in recent years some regulatory and accrediting agencies are verbalizing expectations that hospital leaders will commit resources to infection control commensurate with the work at hand. Infection control professionals must be prepared to defend the impact of measures directed at preventing HAIs on resources as well. This is not so difficult when interventions reduce costs and increase benefits; however, more careful analysis is needed when interventions that prevent infections also increase costs (210).

Infection control, antimicrobial stewardship, and the clinical microbiology laboratory remain central for the effective prevention and management of DROs. Unfortunately, there are still indications that infection control professionals face increasing responsibilities, an uncertain future, and inadequate support. If antimicrobial resistance is to be controlled or defeated, this must certainly change.

ACKNOWLEDGMENT

The author wishes to thank Rob Owens, PharmD, for his review and many helpful comments.

REFERENCES

1. Shlaes DM, Gerding DN, John JF Jr, et al. Society for Healthcare Epidemiology of America and Infectious Diseases Society of America Joint Committee on the Prevention of Antimicrobial Resistance: guidelines for the prevention of antimicrobial resistance in hospitals. Clin Infect Dis 1997; 25(3):584–99.
2. Bell D. Development of the *Public Health Action Plan to Combat Antimicrobial Resistance*, In: Knobler SL, Lemon SM, Najafi M, Burroughs T, eds. The Resistance Phenomenon in Microbes and Infectious Disease Vectors: Implications for Human Health and Strategies for Containment—Workshop Summary. Forum On Emerging Infections. Washington, DC: National Academy Press, 2003.
3. Nouwen JL. Controlling antibiotic use and resistance. Clin Infect Dis 2006; 42(6):776–7.
4. Livermore DM. Minimising antibiotic resistance. Lancet Infect Dis 2005; 5(7):450–9.
5. Weber SG, Huang SS, Oriola S, et al. Legislative mandates for use of active surveillance cultures to screen for methicillin-resistant *Staphylococcus aureus* and vancomycin-resistant enterococci: position statement from the Joint SHEA and APIC Task Force. Infect Control Hosp Epidemiol 2007; 28(3):249–60.
6. Zell BL, Goldmann DA. Healthcare-associated infection and antimicrobial resistance: moving beyond description to prevention. Infect Control Hosp Epidemiol 2007; 28(3):261–4.
7. Burke JP. Infection control—a problem for patient safety. N Engl J Med 2003; 348(7):651–6.
8. Public health focus: surveillance, prevention, and control of nosocomial infections. MMWR Morb Mortal Wkly Rep 1992; 41(42):783–7.
9. Weinstein RA. Nosocomial infection update. Emerg Infect Dis 1998; 4(3):416–20.

10. Haley RW, Culver DH, White JW, et al. The efficacy of infection surveillance and control programs in preventing nosocomial infections in US hospitals. Am J Epidemiol 1985; 121(2):182–205.
11. Cosgrove SE, Sakoulas G, Perencevich EN, Schwaber MJ, Karchmer AW, Carmeli Y. Comparison of mortality associated with methicillin-resistant and methicillin-susceptible *Staphylococcus aureus* bacteremia: a meta-analysis. Clin Infect Dis 2003; 36(1):53–9.
12. Cosgrove SE, Qi Y, Kaye KS, Harbarth S, Karchmer AW, Carmeli Y. The impact of methicillin resistance in *Staphylococcus aureus* bacteremia on patient outcomes: mortality, length of stay, and hospital charges. Infect Control Hosp Epidemiol 2005; 26(2):166–74.
13. Abramson MA, Sexton DJ. Nosocomial methicillin-resistant and methicillin-susceptible *Staphylococcus aureus* primary bacteremia: at what costs? Infect Control Hosp Epidemiol 1999; 20(6):408–11.
14. Engemann JJ, Carmeli Y, Cosgrove SE, et al. Adverse clinical and economic outcomes attributable to methicillin resistance among patients with *Staphylococcus aureus* surgical site infection. Clin Infect Dis 2003; 36(5):592–8.
15. Shorr AF, Combes A, Kollef MH, Chastre J. Methicillin-resistant *Staphylococcus aureus* prolongs intensive care unit stay in ventilator-associated pneumonia, despite initially appropriate antibiotic therapy. Crit Care Med 2006 Mar; 34(3):700–6.
16. Polgreen PM, Beekmann SE, Chen YY, et al. Epidemiology of methicillin-resistant *Staphylococcus aureus* and vancomycin-resistant *Enterococcus* in a rural state. Infect Control Hosp Epidemiol 2006; 27(3):252–6.
17. Diekema DJ, BootsMiller BJ, Vaughn TE, et al. Antimicrobial resistance trends and outbreak frequency in United States hospitals. Clin Infect Dis 2004; 38(1):78–85.
18. Harbarth S, Albrich W, Goldmann DA, Huebner J. Control of multiply resistant cocci: do international comparisons help? Lancet Infect Dis 2001; 1(4):251–61.
19. Zinn CS, Westh H, Rosdahl VT. An international multicenter study of antimicrobial resistance and typing of hospital *Staphylococcus aureus* isolates from 21 laboratories in 19 countries or states. Microb Drug Resist 2004; 10(2):160–8.
20. Kollef MH, Fraser VJ. Antibiotic resistance in the intensive care unit. Ann Intern Med 2001; 134(4):298–314.
21. Bradley SF, Terpenning MS, Ramsey MA, et al. Methicillin-resistant *Staphylococcus aureus*: colonization and infection in a long-term care facility. Ann Intern Med 1991; 115(6):417–22.
22. Saiman L, Cronquist A, Wu F, et al. An outbreak of methicillin-resistant *Staphylococcus aureus* in a neonatal intensive care unit. Infect Control Hosp Epidemiol 2003; 24(5): 317–21.
23. National Nosocomial Infections Surveillance (NNIS) System Report, data summary from January 1992 through June 2003, issued August 2003. Am J Infect Control 2003; 31(8):481–98.
24. Fridkin SK, Edwards JR, Courval JM, et al. The effect of vancomycin and third-generation cephalosporins on prevalence of vancomycin-resistant enterococci in 126 U.S. adult intensive care units. Ann Intern Med 2001; 135(3):175–83.
25. Neuhauser MM, Weinstein RA, Rydman R, Danziger LH, Karam G, Quinn JP. Antibiotic resistance among gram-negative bacilli in US intensive care units: implications for fluoroquinolone use. JAMA 2003; 289(7):885–8.
26. Fridkin SK. Increasing prevalence of antimicrobial resistance in intensive care units. Crit Care Med 2001; 29(4 Suppl.):N64–N68.
27. Centers for Disease Control and Prevention. *Staphylococcus aureus* resistant to vancomycin–United States, 2002. MMWR Morb Mortal Wkly Rep 2002; 51(26):565–7.
28. de Lassence A, Hidri N, Timsit JF, et al. Control and outcome of a large outbreak of colonization and infection with glycopeptide-intermediate *Staphylococcus aureus* in an intensive care unit. Clin Infect Dis 2006; 42(2):170–8.
29. Furuno JP, Perencevich EN, Johnson JA, et al. Methicillin-resistant *Staphylococcus aureus* and vancomycin-resistant *Enterococci* co-colonization. Emerg Infect Dis 2005; 11(10):1539–44.

30. Tenover FC, Lancaster MV, Hill BC, et al. Characterization of staphylococci with reduced susceptibilities to vancomycin and other glycopeptides. J Clin Microbiol 1998; 36(4):1020–7.
31. Tenover FC, Biddle JW, Lancaster MV. Increasing resistance to vancomycin and other glycopeptides in *Staphylococcus aureus*. Emerg Infect Dis 2001; 7(2):327–32.
32. Cosgrove SE, Carroll KC, Perl TM. *Staphylococcus aureus* with reduced susceptibility to vancomycin. Clin Infect Dis 2004; 39(4):539–45.
33. Seybold U, Kourbatova EV, Johnson JG, et al. Emergence of community-associated methicillin-resistant *Staphylococcus aureus* USA300 genotype as a major cause of health care-associated blood stream infections. Clin Infect Dis 2006; 42(5):647–56.
34. Fridkin SK, Hill HA, Volkova NV, et al. Temporal changes in prevalence of antimicrobial resistance in 23 US hospitals. Emerg Infect Dis 2002; 8(7):697–701.
35. Madaras-Kelly KJ, Remington RE, Lewis PG, Stevens DL. Evaluation of an intervention designed to decrease the rate of nosocomial methicillin-resistant *Staphylococcus aureus* infection by encouraging decreased fluoroquinolone use. Infect Control Hosp Epidemiol 2006; 27(2):155–69.
36. Fridkin SK, Hageman JC, Morrison M, et al. Methicillin-resistant *Staphylococcus aureus* disease in three communities. N Engl J Med 2005; 352(14):1436–44.
37. Kuehnert MJ, Kruszon–Moran D, Hill HA, et al. Prevalence of *Staphylococcus aureus* nasal colonization in the United States, 2001–2002. J Infect Dis 2006; 193(2):172–9.
38. Jane D. Siegel, MD; Emily Rhinehart, RN MPH CIC; Marguerite Jackson, PhD; Linda Chiarello, RN MS; the Healthcare Infection Control Practices Advisory Committee, Centers for Disease Control and Prevention. Management of multidrug-resistant organisms in healthcare settings, 2006. http://www.cdc.gov/ncidod/dhqp/pdf/ar/mdroGuideline2006.pdf Accessed October 26, 2006, 2007
39. Garner JS. Guideline for isolation precautions in hospitals. The Hospital Infection Control Practices Advisory Committee. Infect Control Hosp Epidemiol 1996; 17(1):53–80.
40. Bonten MJ, Slaughter S, Ambergen AW, et al. The role of "colonization pressure" in the spread of vancomycin-resistant enterococci: an important infection control variable. Arch Intern Med 1998; 158(10):1127–32.
41. Bhalla A, Pultz NJ, Gries DM, et al. Acquisition of nosocomial pathogens on hands after contact with environmental surfaces near hospitalized patients. Infect Control Hosp Epidemiol 2004; 25(2):164–7.
42. Donskey CJ, Chowdhry TK, Hecker MT, et al. Effect of antibiotic therapy on the density of vancomycin-resistant enterococci in the stool of colonized patients. N Engl J Med 2000; 343(26):1925–32.
43. Muto CA, Jernigan JA, Ostrowsky BE, et al. SHEA guideline for preventing nosocomial transmission of multidrug-resistant strains of *Staphylococcus aureus* and *Enterococcus*. Infect Control Hosp Epidemiol 2003; 24(5):362–86.
44. Boyce JM, Potter-Bynoe G, Chenevert C, King T. Environmental contamination due to methicillin-resistant *Staphylococcus aureus*: possible infection control implications. Infect Control Hosp Epidemiol 1997; 18(9):622–7.
45. Zachary KC, Bayne PS, Morrison VJ, Ford DS, Silver LC, Hooper DC. Contamination of gowns, gloves, and stethoscopes with vancomycin-resistant enterococci. Infect Control Hosp Epidemiol 2001; 22(9):560–4.
46. Boyce JM, Opal SM, Potter-Bynoe G, Medeiros AA. Spread of methicillin-resistant *Staphylococcus aureus* in a hospital after exposure to a health care worker with chronic sinusitis. Clin Infect Dis 1993; 17(3):496–504.
47. Zawacki A, O'Rourke E, Potter-Bynoe G, Macone A, Harbarth S, Goldmann D. An outbreak of *Pseudomonas aeruginosa* pneumonia and bloodstream infection associated with intermittent otitis externa in a healthcare worker. Infect Control Hosp Epidemiol 2004; 25(12):1083–9.
48. Faibis F, Laporte C, Fiacre A, et al. An outbreak of methicillin-resistant *Staphylococcus aureus* surgical-site infections initiated by a healthcare worker with chronic sinusitis. Infect Control Hosp Epidemiol 2005; 26(2):213–5.
49. Sheretz RJ, Reagan DR, Hampton KD, et al. A cloud adult: the *Staphylococcus aureus*-virus interaction revisited. Ann Intern Med 1996; 124(6):539–47.

50. Galoisy-Guibal L, Soubirou JL, Desjeux G, et al. Screening for multidrug-resistant bacteria as a predictive test for subsequent onset of nosocomial infection. Infect Control Hosp Epidemiol 2006; 27(11):1233–41.
51. Evans RS, Lloyd JF, Abouzelof RH, Taylor CW, Anderson VR, Samore MH. System-wide surveillance for clinical encounters by patients previously identified with MRSA and VRE. Medinfo 2004; 11(Pt 1):212–6.
52. Weinstein RA. Controlling antimicrobial resistance in hospitals: infection control and use of antibiotics. Emerg Infect Dis 2001; 7(2):188–92.
53. Boyce JM, Pittet D. Guideline for Hand Hygiene in Health-Care Settings. Recommen-dations of the Healthcare Infection Control Practices Advisory Committee and the HICPAC/SHEA/APIC/IDSA Hand Hygiene Task Force. Am J Infect Control 2002; 30(8):S1–46.
54. Boyce JM, Kelliher S, Vallande N. Skin irritation and dryness associated with two hand-hygiene regimens: soap-and-water hand washing versus hand antisepsis with an alcoholic hand gel. Infect Control Hosp Epidemiol 2000; 21(7):442–8.
55. Weinstein RA, Kabins SA. Strategies for prevention and control of multiple drug-resistant nosocomial infection. Am J Med 1981; 70(2):449–54.
56. Johnson S, Gerding DN, Olson MM, et al. Prospective, controlled study of vinyl glove use to interrupt *Clostridium difficile* nosocomial transmission. Am J Med 1990; 88(2):137–40.
57. Hartstein AI, Denny MA, Morthland VH, LeMonte AM, Pfaller MA. Control of methicillin-resistant *Staphylococcus aureus* in a hospital and an intensive care unit. Infect Control Hosp Epidemiol 1995; 16(7):405–11.
58. Tenorio AR, Badri SM, Sahgal NB, et al. Effectiveness of gloves in the prevention of hand carriage of vancomycin-resistant *Enterococcus* species by health care workers after patient care. Clin Infect Dis 2001; 32(5):826–9.
59. Trick WE, Weinstein RA, DeMarais PL, et al. Comparison of routine glove use and contact-isolation precautions to prevent transmission of multidrug-resistant bacteria in a long-term care facility. J Am Geriatr Soc 2004; 52(12):2003–9.
60. Slaughter S, Hayden MK, Nathan C, et al. A comparison of the effect of universal use of gloves and gowns with that of glove use alone on acquisition of vancomycin-resistant enterococci in a medical intensive care unit. Ann Intern Med 1996; 125(6):448–56.
61. Byers KE, Anglim AM, Anneski CJ, et al. A hospital epidemic of vancomycin-resistant *Enterococcus*: risk factors and control. Infect Control Hosp Epidemiol 2001; 22(3):140–7.
62. Centers for Disease Control. National Nosocomial Infections Study Report. Atlanta: Centers for Disease Control, 1979:2–14.
63. Wong ES, Hooton TM. Guidelines for Prevention of Catheter Associated Urinary Tract Infections. Atlanta: U.S. Department of Commerce, National Technical Information Service. 1982:1–5.
64. Jain P, Parada JP, David A, Smith LG. Overuse of the indwelling urinary tract catheter in hospitalized medical patients. Arch Intern Med 1995; 155(13):1425–9.
65. Gribble MJ, Puterman ML. Prophylaxis of urinary tract infection in persons with recent spinal cord injury: a prospective, randomized, double-blind, placebo–controlled study of trimethoprim-sulfamethoxazole. Am J Med 1993; 95(2):141–52.
66. Saint S, Lipsky BA. Preventing catheter-related bacteriuria: should we? Can we? How? Arch Intern Med 1999; 159(8):800–8.
67. Tambyah PA, Halvorson KT, Maki DG. A prospective study of pathogenesis of catheter-associated urinary tract infections. Mayo Clin Proc 1999; 74(2):131–6.
68. Salgado CD, Karchmer TB, Farr BM. Prevention of catheter associated urinary tract infections. In: Wenzel RP, ed. Prevention and Control of Nosocomial Infections. Philadelphia: Lippincott Williams & Wilkins, 2003:297–311.
69. Srinivasan A, Karchmer T, Richards A, Song X, Perl TM. A prospective trial of a novel, silicone-based, silver-coated foley catheter for the prevention of nosocomial urinary tract infections. Infect Control Hosp Epidemiol 2006; 27(1):38–43.
70. Gaonkar TA, Sampath LA, Modak SM. Evaluation of the antimicrobial efficacy of urinary catheters impregnated with antiseptics in an in vitro urinary tract model. Infect Control Hosp Epidemiol 2003; 24(7):506–13.

71. Trautner BW, Hull RA, Thornby JI, Darouiche RO. Coating urinary catheters with an avirulent strain of *Escherichia coli* as a means to establish asymptomatic colonization. Infect Control Hosp Epidemiol 2007; 28(1):92–4.

72. Steger KA, Tablan OC, Mir J, Craven DE. Preventing nosocomial pneumonia: guidelines for health care workers. In: Abrutyn E, Goldmann DA, Scheckler WE, eds. Saunders Infection Control Reference Service: the Experts' Guide to the Guidelines. 2nd Ed. Philadelphia, PA: W.B. Saunders Company, 2001:269–79.

73. Mayhall CG. Nosocomial pneumonia. Diagnosis and prevention. Infect Dis Clin North Am 1997; 11(2):427–57.

74. Craven DE, De Rosa FG, Thornton D. Nosocomial pneumonia: emerging concepts in diagnosis, management, and prophylaxis. Curr Opin Crit Care 2002; 8(5):421–9.

75. Shorr AF, Kollef MH. Ventilator-associated pneumonia: insights from recent clinical trials. Chest 2005; 128(5 Suppl. 2):583S–91S.

76. Centers for Disease Control and Prevention. Guidelines for the prevention of nosocomial pneumonia. *MMWR* 1997; 46:1–79.

77. Richards MJ, Edwards JR, Culver DH, Gaynes RP. Nosocomial infections in combined medical-surgical intensive care units in the United States. Infect Control Hosp Epidemiol 2000; 21(8):510–5.

78. Kolleff MH. Appropriate antibiotic therapy for ventilator-associated pneumonia and sepsis: a necessity, not an issue for debate. Intensive Care Med 2003; 29(2):147–9.

79. Iregui M, Ward S, Sherman G, Fraser VJ, Kollef MH. Clinical importance of delays in the initiation of appropriate antibiotic treatment for ventilator-associated pneumonia. Chest 2002; 122(1):262–8.

80. Beardsley JR, Williamson JC, Johnson JW, Ohl CA, Karchmer TB, Bowton DL. Using local microbiologic data to develop institution-specific guidelines for the treatment of hospital-acquired pneumonia. Chest 2006; 130(3):787–93.

81. Bouza E, Torres MV, Radice C, et al. Direct E-test (AB Biodisk) of respiratory samples improves antimicrobial use in ventilator-associated pneumonia. Clin Infect Dis 2007; 44(3):382–7.

82. Chastre J, Wolff M, Fagon JY, et al. Comparison of 8 vs 15 days of antibiotic therapy for ventilator-associated pneumonia in adults: a randomized trial. JAMA 2003; 290(19):2588–98.

83. Brochard L. Mechanical ventilation: invasive versus noninvasive. Eur Respir J Suppl 2003; 47:31s–7s.

84. Burns KE, Adhikari NK, Meade MO. Noninvasive positive pressure ventilation as a weaning strategy for intubated adults with respiratory failure. Cochrane Database Syst Rev 2003; (4):CD004127.

85. Valles J, Artigas A, Rello J, et al. Continuous aspiration of subglottic secretions in preventing ventilator-associated pneumonia. Ann Intern Med 1995; 122(3):179–86.

86. Kollef MH, Skubas NJ, Sundt TM. A randomized clinical trial of continuous aspiration of subglottic secretions in cardiac surgery patients. Chest 1999; 116(5):1339–46.

87. Shorr AF, O'Malley PG. Continuous subglottic suctioning for the prevention of ventilator-associated pneumonia: potential economic implications. Chest 2001; 119(1):228–35.

88. Girou E, Buu-Hoi A, Stephan F, et al. Airway colonisation in long-term mechanically ventilated patients. Effect of semi-recumbent position and continuous subglottic suctioning. Intensive Care Med 2004; 30(2):225–33.

89. Torres A, Serra-Batlles J, Ros E, et al. Pulmonary aspiration of gastric contents in patients receiving mechanical ventilation: the effect of body position. Ann Intern Med 1992; 116(7):540–3.

90. Drakulovic MB, Torres A, Bauer TT, Nicolas JM, Nogue S, Ferrer M. Supine body position as a risk factor for nosocomial pneumonia in mechanically ventilated patients: a randomised trial. Lancet 1999; 354(9193):1851–8.

91. Cook DJ, Meade MO, Hand LE, McMullin JP. Toward understanding evidence uptake: semirecumbency for pneumonia prevention. Crit Care Med 2002; 30(7):1472–7.

92. Kollef MH. Selective digestive decontamination should not be routinely employed. Chest 2003; 123(5Suppl.):464S–8S.

93. Eggimann P, Pittet D. Infection control in the ICU. Chest 2001; 120(6):2059–93.
94. Kollef MH, Vlasnik J, Sharpless L, Pasque C, Murphy D, Fraser V. Scheduled change of antibiotic classes: a strategy to decrease the incidence of ventilator-associated pneumonia. Am J Respir Crit Care Med 1997; 156(4 Pt. 1):1040–8.
95. Gruson D, Hilbert G, Vargas F, et al. Rotation and restricted use of antibiotics in a medical intensive care unit. Impact on the incidence of ventilator-associated pneumonia caused by antibiotic-resistant gram-negative bacteria. Am J Respir Crit Care Med 2000; 162(3 Pt. 1):837–43.
96. Gruson D, Hilbert G, Vargas F, et al. Strategy of antibiotic rotation: long-term effect on incidence and susceptibilities of Gram-negative bacilli responsible for ventilator-associated pneumonia. Crit Care Med 2003; 31(7):1908–14.
97. Kollef MH. Is antibiotic cycling the answer to preventing the emergence of bacterial resistance in the intensive care unit? Clin Infect Dis 2006; 43(Suppl. 2):S82–8.
98. Mermel LA. New technologies to prevent intravascular catheter-related bloodstream infections. Emerg Infect Dis 2001; 7(2):197–9.
99. Soifer NE, Borzak S, Edlin BR, Weinstein RA. Prevention of peripheral venous catheter complications with an intravenous therapy team: a randomized controlled trial. Arch Intern Med 1998; 158(5):473–7.
100. Curran ET, Coia JE, Gilmour H, McNamee S, Hood J. Multi-centre research surveillance project to reduce infections/phlebitis associated with peripheral vascular catheters. J Hosp Infect 2000; 46(3):194–202.
101. Raad II, Hohn DC, Gilbreath BJ, et al. Prevention of central venous catheter-related infections by using maximal sterile barrier precautions during insertion. Infect Control Hosp Epidemiol 1994; 15(4 Pt. 1):231–8.
102. Timsit JF, Bruneel F, Cheval C, et al. Use of tunneled femoral catheters to prevent catheter-related infection. A randomized, controlled trial. Ann Intern Med 1999; 130(9):729–35.
103. Merrer J, De JB, Golliot F, et al. Complications of femoral and subclavian venous catheterization in critically ill patients: a randomized controlled trial. JAMA 2001; 286(6):700–7.
104. McConnell SA, Gubbins PO, Anaissie EJ. Do antimicrobial-impregnated central venous catheters prevent catheter-related bloodstream infection? Clin Infect Dis 2003; 37(1):65–72.
105. Warren DK, Cosgrove SE, Diekema DJ, et al. A multicenter intervention to prevent catheter-associated bloodstream infections. Infect Control Hosp Epidemiol 2006; 27(7):662–9.
106. Reduction in central line-associated bloodstream infections among patients in intensive care units–Pennsylvania, April 2001-March 2005. MMWR Morb Mortal Wkly Rep 2005; 54(40):1013–6.
107. Sherertz RJ, Ely EW, Westbrook DM, et al. Education of physicians-in-training can decrease the risk for vascular catheter infection. Ann Intern Med 2000; 132(8):641–8.
108. Berenholtz SM, Pronovost PJ, Lipsett PA, et al. Eliminating catheter-related bloodstream infections in the intensive care unit. Crit Care Med 2004; 32(10):2014–20.
109. Pearson ML. Guideline for prevention of intravascular device-related infections. Part I. Intravascular device-related infections: an overview. The Hospital Infection Control Practices Advisory Committee. Am J Infect Control 1996; 24(4):262–77.
110. Berwick DM, Calkins DR, McCannon CJ, Hackbarth AD. The 100,000 lives campaign: setting a goal and a deadline for improving health care quality. JAMA 2006; 295(3):324–7.
111. Pronovost P, Needham D, Berenholtz S, et al. An intervention to decrease catheter-related bloodstream infections in the ICU. N Engl J Med 2006; 355(26):2725–32.
112. Horan TC, Culver DH, Gaynes RP, Jarvis WR, Edwards JR, Reid CR. Nosocomial infections in surgical patients in the United States, January 1986-June 1992. National Nosocomial Infections Surveillance (NNIS) System. Infect Control Hosp Epidemiol 1993; 14(2):73–80.
113. Herwaldt LA, Cullen JJ, Scholz D, et al. A prospective study of outcomes, healthcare resource utilization, and costs associated with postoperative nosocomial infections. Infect Control Hosp Epidemiol 2006; 27(12):1291–8.

114. Mangram AJ, Horan TC, Pearson ML, Silver LC, Jarvis WR. Guideline for prevention of surgical site infection, 1999. Hospital Infection Control Practices Advisory Committee. Infect Control Hosp Epidemiol 1999; 20(4):250–78.
115. Nichols RL. Postoperative wound infection. N Engl J Med 1982; 307(27):1701–2.
116. Nichols RL. Surgical wound infection. Am J Med 1991; 91(3B):54S–64S.
117. Nichols RL. Preventing surgical site infections: a surgeon's perspective. Emerg Infect Dis 2001; 7(2):220–4.
118. Condon RE, Schulte WJ, Malangoni MA, Anderson-Teschendorf MJ. Effectiveness of a surgical wound surveillance program. Arch Surg 1983; 118(3):303–7.
119. Mead PB, Pories SE, Hall P, Vacek PM, Davis JH Jr, Gamelli RL. Decreasing the incidence of surgical wound infections. Validation of a surveillance-notification program. Arch Surg 1986; 121(4):458–61.
120. McConkey SJ, L'Ecuyer PB, Murphy DM, Leet TL, Sundt TM, Fraser VJ. Results of a comprehensive infection control program for reducing surgical-site infections in coronary artery bypass surgery. Infect Control Hosp Epidemiol 1999; 20(8):533–8.
121. Olson MM, Lee JT Jr. Continuous, 10-year wound infection surveillance. Results, advantages, and unanswered questions. Arch Surg 1990; 125(6):794–803.
122. Burke JF. The effective period of preventive antibiotic action in experimental incisions and dermal lesions. Surgery 1961; 50:161–8.
123. Larsen RA, Evans RS, Burke JP, Pestotnik SL, Gardner RM, Classen DC. Improved perioperative antibiotic use and reduced surgical wound infections through use of computer decision analysis. Infect Control Hosp Epidemiol 1989; 10(7):316–20.
124. Burke JP. Maximizing appropriate antibiotic prophylaxis for surgical patients: an update from LDS Hospital, Salt Lake City. Clin Infect Dis 2001 1; 33(Suppl. 2):S78–83.
125. Napolitano LM. Decolonization of the skin of the patient and surgeon. Surg Infect (Larchmt) 2006; 7(Suppl. 3):s3–15.
126. Konvalinka A, Errett L, Fong IW. Impact of treating *Staphylococcus aureus* nasal carriers on wound infections in cardiac surgery. J Hosp Infect 2006; 64(2):162–8.
127. Kallen AJ, Wilson CT, Larson RJ. Perioperative intranasal mupirocin for the prevention of surgical-site infections: systematic review of the literature and meta-analysis. Infect Control Hosp Epidemiol 2005; 26(12):916–22.
128. Bratzler DW. The Surgical Infection Prevention and Surgical Care Improvement Projects: promises and pitfalls. Am Surg 2006; 72(11):1010–6.
129. SCIP Project Information. (Accessed May 11, 2007, at http://www.medqic.org/dcs/ ContentServer?cid = 1122904930422 & pagename =Medqic%2FContent%2FParentShell Template&parentName&Topic&c=MQParents)
130. Strausbaugh LJ, Siegel JD, Weinstein RA. Preventing transmission of multidrug-resistant bacteria in health care settings: a tale of 2 guidelines. Clin Infect Dis 2006; 42(6):828–35.
131. Muto CA, Jarvis WR, Farr BM. Another tale of two guidelines. Clin Infect Dis 2006; 43(6):796–7.
132. Hiramatsu K, Cui L, Kuroda M, Ito T. The emergence and evolution of methicillin-resistant *Staphylococcus aureus*. Trends Microbiol 2001; 9(10):486–93.
133. Kreiswirth B, Kornblum J, Arbeit RD, et al. Evidence for a clonal origin of methicillin resistance in *Staphylococcus aureus*. Science 1993; 259(5092):227–30.
134. Oliveira DC, Tomasz A, de LH. The evolution of pandemic clones of methicillin-resistant *Staphylococcus aureus*: identification of two ancestral genetic backgrounds and the associated mec elements. Microb Drug Resist 2001; 7(4):349–61.
135. Musser JM, Kapur V. Clonal analysis of methicillin-resistant *Staphylococcus aureus* strains from intercontinental sources: association of the mec gene with divergent phylogenetic lineages implies dissemination by horizontal transfer and recombination. J Clin Microbiol 1992; 30(8):2058–63.
136. Givney R, Vickery A, Holliday A, Pegler M, Benn R. Evolution of an endemic methicillin-resistant *Staphylococcus aureus* population in an Australian hospital from 1967 to 1996. J Clin Microbiol 1998; 36(2):552–6.
137. Crisostomo MI, Westh H, Tomasz A, Chung M, Oliveira DC, de LH. The evolution of methicillin resistance in *Staphylococcus aureus*: similarity of genetic backgrounds in

historically early methicillin-susceptible and -resistant isolates and contemporary epidemic clones. Proc Natl Acad Sci USA 2001; 98(17):9865–70.

138. Enright MC, Robinson DA, Randle G, Feil EJ, Grundmann H, Spratt BG. The evolutionary history of methicillin-resistant *Staphylococcus aureus* (MRSA). Proc Natl Acad Sci USA 2002; 99(11):7687–92.

139. Gold HS. Vancomycin-resistant enterococci: mechanisms and clinical observations. Clin Infect Dis 2001; 33(2):210–9.

140. Murray BE. What can we do about vancomycin-resistant enterococci? Clin Infect Dis 1995; 20(5):1134–6.

141. Martone WJ. Spread of vancomycin-resistant enterococci: why did it happen in the United States? Infect Control Hosp Epidemiol 1998; 19(8):539–45.

142. Bonten MJ, Willems R, Weinstein RA. Vancomycin-resistant enterococci: why are they here, and where do they come from? Lancet Infect Dis 2001; 1(5):314–25.

143. Morris JG Jr, Shay DK, Hebden JN, et al. Enterococci resistant to multiple antimicrobial agents, including vancomycin. Establishment of endemicity in a university medical center. Ann Intern Med 1995; 123(4):250–9.

144. Kim WJ, Weinstein RA, Hayden MK. The changing molecular epidemiology and establishment of endemicity of vancomycin resistance in enterococci at one hospital over a 6-year period. J Infect Dis 1999; 179(1):163–71.

145. Smith TL, Iwen PC, Olson SB, Rupp ME. Environmental contamination with vancomycin-resistant enterococci in an outpatient setting. Infect Control Hosp Epidemiol 1998; 19(7):515–8.

146. Puzniak LA, Leet T, Mayfield J, Kollef M, Mundy LM. To gown or not to gown: the effect on acquisition of vancomycin-resistant enterococci. Clin Infect Dis 2002; 35(1):18–25.

147. Grundmann H, Hori S, Winter B, Tami A, Austin DJ. Risk factors for the transmission of methicillin-resistant *Staphylococcus aureus* in an adult intensive care unit: fitting a model to the data. J Infect Dis 2002; 185(4):481–8.

148. Karchmer TB, Giannetta ET, Muto CA, Strain BA, Farr BM. A randomized crossover study of silver-coated urinary catheters in hospitalized patients. Arch Intern Med 2000; 160(21):3294–8.

149. Livornese LL Jr, Dias S, Samel C, et al. Hospital-acquired infection with vancomycin-resistant Enterococcus faecium transmitted by electronic thermometers. Ann Intern Med 1992; 117(2):112–6.

150. Smith MA, Mathewson JJ, Ulert IA, Scerpella EG, Ericsson CD. Contaminated stethoscopes revisited. Arch Intern Med 1996; 156(1):82–4.

151. Duckro AN, Blom DW, Lyle EA, Weinstein RA, Hayden MK. Transfer of vancomycin-resistant enterococci via health care worker hands. Arch Intern Med 2005; 165(3):302–7.

152. Sehulster L, Chinn RY. Guidelines for environmental infection control in health-care facilities. Recommendations of CDC and the Healthcare Infection Control Practices Advisory Committee (HICPAC). MMWR Recomm Rep 2003 6; 52 (RR-10):1–42.

153. Vriens MR, Fluit AC, Troelstra A, Verhoef J, van der WC. Is methicillin-resistant *Staphylococcus aureus* more contagious than methicillin-susceptible *S. aureus* in a surgical intensive care unit? Infect Control Hosp Epidemiol 2002; 23(9):491–4.

154. Calfee DP, Giannetta ET, Durbin LJ, Germanson TP, Farr BM. Control of endemic vancomycin-resistant Enterococcus among inpatients at a university hospital. Clin Infect Dis 2003; 37(3):326–32.

155. Ostrowsky BE, Trick WE, Sohn AH, et al. Control of vancomycin-resistant enterococcus in health care facilities in a region. N Engl J Med 2001; 344(19):1427–33.

156. Calfee DP, Giannetta ET, Durbin LJ, Germanson TP, Farr BM. Control of endemic vancomycin-resistant Enterococcus among inpatients at a university hospital. Clin Infect Dis 2003; 37(3):326–32.

157. Farr BM. Prevention and control of methicillin-resistant *Staphylococcus aureus* infections. Curr Opin Infect Dis 2004; 17(4):317–22.

158. Farr BM, Jarvis WR. Would active surveillance cultures help control healthcare-related methicillin-resistant *Staphylococcus aureus* infections? Infect Control Hosp Epidemiol 2002; 23(2):65–8.

159. Calfee DP, Giannetta ET, Durbin LJ, Germanson TP, Farr BM. Control of endemic vancomycin-resistant Enterococcus among inpatients at a university hospital. Clin Infect Dis 2003; 37(3):326–32.
160. Harbarth S, Pittet D. Control of nosocomial methicillin-resistant *Staphylococcus aureus*: where shall we send our hospital director next time? Infect Control Hosp Epidemiol 2003; 24(5):314–6.
161. Noble WC, Virani Z, Cree RG. Co-transfer of vancomycin and other resistance genes from *Enterococcus faecalis* NCTC 12201 to *Staphylococcus aureus*. FEMS Microbiol Lett 1992; 72(2):195–8.
162. Nijssen S, Bootsma M, Bonten M. Potential confounding in evaluating infection-control interventions in hospital settings: changing antibiotic prescription. Clin Infect Dis 2006; 43(5):616–23.
163. Harris AD, Bradham DD, Baumgarten M, Zuckerman IH, Fink JC, Perencevich EN. The use and interpretation of quasi-experimental studies in infectious diseases. Clin Infect Dis 2004; 38(11):1586–91.
164. Muto CA, Jarvis WR, Farr BM. Another tale of two guidelines. Clin Infect Dis 2006; 43(6):796–7.
165. Montecalvo MA, Jarvis WR, Uman J, et al. Costs and savings associated with infection control measures that reduced transmission of vancomycin-resistant enterococci in an endemic setting. Infect Control Hosp Epidemiol 2001; 22(7):437–42.
166. Chaix C, Durand-Zaleski I, Alberti C, Brun-Buisson C. Control of endemic methicillin-resistant *Staphylococcus aureus*: a cost-benefit analysis in an intensive care unit. JAMA 1999; 282(18):1745–51.
167. Karchmer TB, Durbin LJ, Simonton BM, Farr BM. Cost-effectiveness of active surveillance cultures and contact/droplet precautions for control of methicillin-resistant *Staphylococcus aureus*. J Hosp Infect 2002; 51(2):126–32.
168. de SN, Denis O, Gasasira MF, De MR, Nonhoff C, Struelens MJ. Controlled evaluation of the IDI-MRSA assay for detection of colonization by methicillin-resistant *Staphylococcus aureus* in diverse mucocutaneous specimens. J Clin Microbiol 2007; 45(4):1098–101.
169. Drews SJ, Johnson G, Gharabaghi F, et al. A 24-hr screening protocol for identification of vancomycin-resistant *Enterococcus faecium*. J Clin Microbiol 2006; 44(4):1578–80.
170. Stelfox HT, Bates DW, Redelmeier DA. Safety of patients isolated for infection control. JAMA 2003; 290(14):1899–905.
171. Evans HL, Shaffer MM, Hughes MG, et al. Contact isolation in surgical patients: a barrier to care? Surgery 2003; 134(2):180–8.
172. Saint S, Higgins LA, Nallamothu BK, Chenoweth C. Do physicians examine patients in contact isolation less frequently? A brief report. Am J Infect Control 2003; 31(6):354–6.
173. Farr BM. Doing the right thing (and figuring out what that is). Infect Control Hosp Epidemiol 2006; 27(10):999–1003.
174. National Nosocomial Infections Surveillance (NNIS) System Report, data summary from January 1992 through June 2004, issued October 2004. Am J Infect Control 2004; 32(8):470–85.
175. West TE, Guerry C, Hiott M, Morrow N, Ward K, Salgado CD. Effect of targeted surveillance for control of methicillin-resistant *Staphylococcus aureus* in a community hospital system. Infect Control Hosp Epidemiol 2006; 27(3):233–8.
176. Harris AD, McGregor JC, Furuno JP. What infection control interventions should be undertaken to control multidrug-resistant Gram-negative bacteria? Clin Infect Dis 2006; 43(Suppl. 2):S57–61.
177. Ibrahim EH, Sherman G, Ward S, Fraser VJ, Kollef MH. The influence of inadequate antimicrobial treatment of bloodstream infections on patient outcomes in the ICU setting. Chest 2000; 118(1):146–55.
178. Cosgrove SE, Kaye KS, Eliopoulous GM, Carmeli Y. Health and economic outcomes of the emergence of third-generation cephalosporin resistance in *Enterobacter* species. Arch Intern Med 2002; 162(2):185–90.
179. Carmeli Y, Troillet N, Karchmer AW, Samore MH. Health and economic outcomes of antibiotic resistance in *Pseudomonas aeruginosa*. Arch Intern Med 1999; 159(10):1127–32.

180. Schwaber MJ, Navon-Venezia S, Kaye KS, Ben-Ami R, Schwartz D, Carmeli Y. Clinical and economic impact of bacteremia with extended-spectrum-beta-lactamase-producing *Enterobacteriaceae*. Antimicrob Agents Chemother 2006; 50(4):1257–62.
181. Lautenbach E, Weiner MG, Nachamkin I, Bilker WB, Sheridan A, Fishman NO. Imipenem resistance among *Pseudomonas aeruginosa* isolates: risk factors for infection and impact of resistance on clinical and economic outcomes. Infect Control Hosp Epidemiol 2006; 27(9):893–900.
182. Steward CD, Wallace D, Hubert SK, et al. Ability of laboratories to detect emerging antimicrobial resistance in nosocomial pathogens: a survey of project ICARE laboratories. Diagn Microbiol Infect Dis 2000; 38(1):59–67.
183. Tenover FC, Mohammed MJ, Gorton TS, Dembek ZF. Detection and reporting of organisms producing extended-spectrum beta-lactamases: survey of laboratories in Connecticut. J Clin Microbiol 1999; 37(12):4065–70.
184. Paterson DL, Yilmaz M. Antibiotic-resistant Gram-negative infections. In: Lautenbach E, Woeltje K, eds. Practical Handbook for Healthcare Epidemiologists. SLACK Incorporated, 2004:189–98.
185. Royle J, Halasz S, Eagles G, et al. Outbreak of extended spectrum beta lactamase producing *Klebsiella pneumoniae* in a neonatal unit. Arch Dis Child Fetal Neonatal Ed 1999 Jan; 80 (1):F64-F68.
186. Eisen D, Russell EG, Tymms M, Roper EJ, Grayson ML, Turnidge J. Random amplified polymorphic DNA and plasmid analyses used in investigation of an outbreak of multiresistant *Klebsiella pneumoniae*. J Clin Microbiol 1995; 33(3):713–7.
187. Gunale A, von BH, Wendt C. Survival of cephalosporin-resistant enterobacteriaceae on fingers. Infect Control Hosp Epidemiol 2006; 27(9):974–7.
188. Sunenshine RH, Liedtke LA, Fridkin SK, Strausbaugh LJ. Management of inpatients colonized or infected with antimicrobial-resistant bacteria in hospitals in the United States. Infect Control Hosp Epidemiol 2005; 26(2):138–43.
189. Lautenbach E, Patel JB, Bilker WB, Edelstein PH, Fishman NO. Extended-spectrum beta-lactamase-producing *Escherichia coli* and *Klebsiella pneumoniae*: risk factors for infection and impact of resistance on outcomes. Clin Infect Dis 2001; 32(8):1162–71.
190. Cornaglia G, Mazzariol A, Lauretti L, Rossolini GM, Fontana R. Hospital outbreak of carbapenem-resistant *Pseudomonas aeruginosa* producing VIM-1, a novel transferable metallo-beta-lactamase. Clin Infect Dis 2000; 31(5):1119–25.
191. Yan JJ, Ko WC, Tsai SH, Wu HM, Wu JJ. Outbreak of infection with multidrug-resistant *Klebsiella pneumoniae* carrying bla(IMP-8) in a university medical center in Taiwan. J Clin Microbiol 2001; 39(12):4433–9.
192. Giakkoupi P, Xanthaki A, Kanelopoulou M, et al. VIM-1 Metallo-beta-lactamase-producing *Klebsiella pneumoniae* strains in Greek hospitals. J Clin Microbiol 2003; 41(8):3893–6.
193. Jones RN, Kehrberg EN, Erwin ME, Anderson SC. Prevalence of important pathogens and antimicrobial activity of parenteral drugs at numerous medical centers in the United States, I. Study on the threat of emerging resistances: real or perceived? Fluoroquinolone Resistance Surveillance Group. Diagn Microbiol Infect Dis 1994; 19(4):203–15.
194. Patterson JE. Multidrug-resistant Gram-negative pathogens: multiple approaches and measures for prevention. Infect Control Hosp Epidemiol 2006; 27(9):889–92.
195. Paterson DL, Yu VL. Extended-spectrum beta-lactamases: a call for improved detection and control. Clin Infect Dis 1999; 29(6):1419–22.
196. Fraser G, Stogsdill P, Owens RC Antimicrobial stewardship initiatives: A programmatic approach to optimizing antimicrobial use In: Owens RC, Ambrose PG, Nightingale CH, Eds. Antibiotic Optimization: Concepts and Strategies in Clinical Practice. New York, NY: Marcel Dekker, 2005:261–326.
197. Rice LB. Controlling antibiotic resistance in the ICU: different bacteria, different strategies. Cleve Clin J Med 2003; 70(9):793–800.
198. Apisarnthanarak A, Danchaivijitr S, Khawcharoenporn T, et al. Effectiveness of education and an antibiotic-control program in a tertiary care hospital in Thailand. Clin Infect Dis 2006 15; 42(6):768–75.

199. Thuong M, Shortgen F, Zazempa V, Girou E, Soussy CJ, Brun-Buisson C. Appropriate use of restricted antimicrobial agents in hospitals: the importance of empirical therapy and assisted re-evaluation. J Antimicrob Chemother 2000; 46(3):501–8.

200. van Kasteren ME, Mannien J, Kullberg BJ, et al. Quality improvement of surgical prophylaxis in Dutch hospitals: evaluation of a multi-site intervention by time series analysis. J Antimicrob Chemother 2005; 56(6):1094–102.

201. Thamlikitkul V, Danchaivijitr S, Kongpattanakul S, Ckokloikaew S. Impact of an educational program on antibiotic use in a tertiary care hospital in a developing country. J Clin Epidemiol 1998; 51(9):773–8.

202. Bantar C, Sartori B, Vesco E, et al. A hospitalwide intervention program to optimize the quality of antibiotic use: impact on prescribing practice, antibiotic consumption, cost savings, and bacterial resistance. Clin Infect Dis 2003; 37(2):180–6.

203. White AC Jr, Atmar RL, Wilson J, Cate TR, Stager CE, Greenberg SB. Effects of requiring prior authorization for selected antimicrobials: expenditures, susceptibilities, and clinical outcomes. Clin Infect Dis 1997; 25(2):230–9.

204. Muder R, McCray, E Cunnigham C. Sustained reduction in methicillin-resistant *Staphylococcus aureus* (MRSA) infection following implementation of a systems engineering approach. In: Program and abstracts of the 16th annual meeting of the Society of Healthcare Epidemiology of America; March 18–21 2006; Chicago, Illinois. Abstract 66.

205. Kaye KS, Engemann JJ, Fulmer EM, Clark CC, Noga EM, Sexton DJ. Favorable impact of an infection control network on nosocomial infection rates in community hospitals. Infect Control Hosp Epidemiol 2006; 27(3):228–32.

206. Nicolle LE, Dyck B, Thompson G, et al. Regional dissemination and control of epidemic methicillin-resistant *Staphylococcus aureus*. Manitoba Chapter of CHICA-Canada. Infect Control Hosp Epidemiol 1999; 20(3):202–5.

207. Wong ES, Rupp ME, Mermel L, et al. Public disclosure of healthcare-associated infections: the role of the Society for Healthcare Epidemiology of America. Infect Control Hosp Epidemiol 2005; 26(2):210–12.

208. McKibben L, Horan T, Tokars JI, et al. Guidance on public reporting of healthcare-associated infections: recommendations of the Healthcare Infection Control Practices Advisory Committee. Am J Infect Control 2005; 33(4):217–26.

209. Grol R, Grimshaw J. From best evidence to best practice: effective implementation of change in patients' care. Lancet 2003; 362(9391):1225–30.

210. Graves N, Halton K, Lairson D. Economics and preventing hospital-acquired infection: broadening the perspective. Infect Control Hosp Epidemiol 2007; 28(2):178–84.

211. Centers for Disease Control and Prevention, Campaign to Prevent Antimicrobial Resistance in Healthcare Settings. http://www.cdc.gov/drugresistance/healthcare/default.htm (Accessed May 6, 2007).

212. WHO Guidelines on Hand Hygiene in Health Care (Advanced Draft): A Summary. http://www.who.int/patientsafety/events/05/HH_en.pdf (Accessed May 6, 2007).

213. Scheckler WE, Valenti AJ. The practice of epidemiology in community hospitals. In: Jarvis W, ed. Bennett and Brachman's Hospital Infections, 5th ed. Philadelphia: Lippincott Williams & Wilkins, 2008.

214. Implement the central line bundle. Institute for Healthcare Improvement. http://www.ihi.org/IHI/Topics/Critical Care/Intensive Care/Changes/Implement the Central Line Bundle. htm (Accessed May 6, 2007).

215. Hand hygiene to reduce bacteria in ICUs. National Institute of Allergy and Infectious Diseases. http://clinicaltrials.gov/ct/show/nct00100386?order=1 (Accessed May 13, 2007).

216. Centers for Disease Control and Prevention. Guideline for isolation precautions: preventing transmission of infections agents in healthcare settings, 2007. http://www.cdc.gov/ncidod/dhqp/gl_isolation.html (Accessed October 31, 2007).

21 Combination Antimicrobial Therapy for Gram-Negative Infections: What Is the Evidence?

Nasia Safdar and Cybele L. Abad
Department of Medicine, University of Wisconsin Medical School, Madison, Wisconsin, U.S.A.

INTRODUCTION

The late 20th century witnessed a rapidly growing crisis in antimicrobial resistance, especially among microorganisms that cause nosocomial infections (1–4). In particular, multidrug-resistant Gram-negative bacteria are re emerging as a major threat, especially in patients who are immune compromised, or admitted to the intensive care unit (ICU) (5,6). Infections with resistant strains of Gram-negative bacilli are associated with prolonged hospitalization, higher costs, and increased mortality compared with infection by an antimicrobial-susceptible organism (7–11). Effective treatment is essential to reduce the considerable morbidity and mortality associated with these serious infections. Combination therapy with two or more antimicrobials for treatment of Gram-negative infections has been used widely for decades, with the perception that it improves clinical outcomes and reduces the emergence of resistance. However, rising rates of resistance, driven in large part by overuse of antimicrobials, have made it necessary to scrutinize antimicrobial treatment strategies to ensure appropriate therapy and optimize clinical outcomes while promoting judicious antimicrobial use. This chapter examines the evidence for, and against, the use of combination therapy in comparison with monotherapy for the treatment of infections caused by Gram-negative bacilli.

ANTIMICROBIAL RESISTANCE AMONG GRAM-NEGATIVE BACILLI

Many species of Gram-negative bacilli that cause serious infections associated with high mortality in the healthcare setting are intrinsically resistant and/or easily acquire resistance to antimicrobials (12–14). Data from the National Nosocomial Infection Surveillance System at the U.S. Centers for Disease Control and Prevention showed that by December 2003, nosocomial infections in ICU patients caused by Gram-negative bacilli resistant to third-generation cephalosporins accounted for 31% of all *Enterobacter* infections, 32% of all *Pseudomonas* infections, and 20% of all Klebsiella spp. infections. Thirty percent of *Pseudomonas aeruginosa* isolates were resistant to fluoroquinolones and 21% were resistant to carbapenems. These rates represent 20% to 47% increases compared with isolates from 1998 to 2002 (15). Many species of commonly encountered nosocomially acquired Gram-negative bacteria, such as *Klebsiella pneumoniae*, produce extended-spectrum beta-lactamases (ESBLs), rendering the organisms multidrug resistant. Paterson et al. reported a multicenter multinational study of *K. pneumoniae* bacteremia, where the isolates were examined for ESBL production. Overall, 30.8% (78 of 253) of episodes of nosocomial bacteremia and 43.5% (30 of 69) of episodes acquired in ICUs were due to ESBL-producing organisms (16). ESBL-producing Gram-negative bacilli are also more likely to be resistant to fluoroquinolones, further limiting treatment options (17,18). The rising rates of multidrug resistance in Gram-negative bacilli (Table 1) (19) have major implications for the selection of anti-infective therapy.

TREATMENT OF INFECTIONS CAUSED BY GRAM-NEGATIVE BACILLI: THE RATIONALE FOR COMBINATION ANTI-INFECTIVE THERAPY

An ongoing debate has centered on the issue of whether or not use of two or more antimicrobials, rather than a single antimicrobial agent, may be more advantageous for treatment of serious infections caused by Gram-negative bacilli, either as empiric therapy before susceptibilities are available, or as definitive therapy (20–23). In theory, there are three major potential advantages to using combination anti-infective therapy for Gram-negative infections: (*i*) an increased likelihood that the infecting pathogen will be susceptible to at least one of the components of the regimen, thereby allowing initial appropriate anti-infective therapy; (*ii*) preventing of emergence of resistance during therapy; and (*iii*) additive or synergistic effect of the antimicrobials (24–26), translating into improved patient outcomes, such as reduction in mortality, regardless of whether the strains of organisms are susceptible or multidrug resistant. The disadvantages in using combination therapy include a greater likelihood of adverse effects, increased cost, possible antagonism between specific drug combinations (27) and the societal implications of antibiotic overuse, propagating antimicrobial resistance (28,29).

Although a number of studies have been undertaken to address this key question, they all suffer from several limitations. In general, randomized controlled trials (RCTs) do not have sufficient numbers of a particular type of microorganism to allow robust subgroup analyses, and as such, synergy and emergence of resistance is not rigorously assessed. Of the number of observational studies that exist, the great majority suffer from selection bias. Factors beyond the choice of treatment may (and do) impact the outcome. These factors include underlying comorbidities, severity of illness, and other unmeasured confounding variables, which may differ in the combination and monotherapy groups. Inadequate adjustment for many of these factors may compromise the internal validity of these studies.

TABLE 1 Rates of Antimicrobial Resistance Among Gram-Negative Organisms Most Frequently Isolated from Patients with Nosocomial Bloodstream Infection From 1995 to 2002

Antimicrobial	No. of isolates (% resistance)			
	Escherichia coli	*Enterobacter* spp.	*Klebsiella* spp.	*Pseudomonas aeruginosa*
Ampicillin	1126 (44)	—	894 (98)	—
Ampicillin/sulbactam	711 (41)	—	667 (40)	—
Piperacillin	630 (39)	467 (34)	562 (34)	554 (11)
Ceftazidime	793 (2)	658 (39)	777 (13)	825 (16)
Imipenem	682 (0.4)	643 (0.6)	636 (0.8)	700 (14)
Ciprofloxacin	754 (5)	468 (8)	646 (9)	732 (20)
Tobramycin	600 (4)	469 (13)	579 (17)	643 (10)

Source: Adapted from Ref. 19.

Meta-analyses that have combined the results of these studies allow for critical assessment of the literature, identification of important gaps and limitations, and generation of hypotheses for future trials, but cannot be considered definitive, given the heterogeneity and limitations of included studies (Table 2). Major reasons to consider use of combination therapy, such as reducing emergence of resistance and promoting synergy, have not been adequately assessed in either clinical trials or observational studies.

Combination Therapy to Increase the Likelihood of Providing Early Appropriate Anti-Infective Therapy

Several studies have shown that, in general, appropriate antimicrobial therapy, defined as the use of at least one antibiotic subsequently found to be active in vitro against the causative organism, leads to lower mortality rates in bacteremia (30–33). A landmark study by McCabe and Jackson in the early 1960s reported a reduction in mortality associated with Gram-negative bacteremia in 173 patients from 48% to 22% with the use of early appropriate anti-infective therapy (34).

More recent studies have confirmed these results, which seem to be most pronounced for critically ill patients (35,36). Although resistance rates vary across regions and institutions, based on overall resistance rates prevalent among Gram-negative bacilli, the likelihood that a single antimicrobial agent will provide appropriate anti-infective therapy when given empirically for Gram-negative infection is increasingly small (37). This happens particularly in ICU settings where intrinsically resistant organisms such as *Acinetobacter* species, *Stenotrophomonas maltophilia*, *Citrobacter*, and *P. aeruginosa* are major pathogens. Local patterns of the microbiology and antimicrobial susceptibility of infecting organisms should guide the choice of initial anti-infective therapy. Importantly, Binkley et al. in their analysis of 9970 bacterial isolates over a 3-year period, showed that unit-specific antibiograms may be more useful in making decisions regarding initial empiric therapy than hospital-wide antibiograms (38). Very broad-spectrum agents, such as carbapenems, may provide initial appropriate therapy as monotherapy; however, carbapenem-resistant Gram-negative bacilli are increasingly being reported (39–42).

Combination Therapy to Reduce Emergence of Resistance

The emergence of resistance during antimicrobial therapy is well documented, especially with use of third-generation cephalosporins against infections caused by members of the family *Enterobacteriaceae* (43,44). The resistant organisms are generally thought to be naturally occurring mutants selected by drug exposure. With mutation frequencies varying from 10^{-4} to 10^{-8}, it is not surprising that emergence of resistant organisms occurs primarily at sites of high organism density, such as the lower respiratory tract (45).

Combination therapy has been studied as a means of reducing the emergence of resistance, with the underlying premise that two drugs with differing mechanisms of action may thwart the capacity of the organism to become resistant (46,47). A plethora of in vitro and animal studies support the hypothesis that combination therapy reduces the emergence of resistance (48–52). Michea-Hamzehpour et al. evaluated the ability of antibiotic combinations to limit the emergence of resistance during therapy in a murine model of peritonitis (50).

TABLE 2 Meta-Analyses Comparing Combination Therapy with Monotherapy for Sepsis, Neutropenic Fever, and Gram-Negative Bacteremia

Study, year (ref.)	Description	Study population	Predominant organisms or syndromes	Number of patients	Resistance point estimate (95°7. CI)	All cause mortality point estimate	Treatment failure point estimate	Treatment failure due to emergence of resistance	Treatment failure due to super-infection	Comments
Bliziotis et al. 2005 (55)	Meta-analysis of 8 RCTs comparing combination beta-lactam and aminoglycoside treatment for infections to beta-lactam monotherapy	Children, neutropenia, cystic fibrosis, languages other than english excluded	*Escherichia coli, Pseudomonas aeruginosa, Klebsiella pneumoniae*	1394	0.90 (0.56–1.47)	0.70 (0.40–1.25)	0.62 (0.38–1.01)	3.09 (0.75–12.82)	0.60 (0.33–1.10)	Only 8 of 65 relevant studies met criteria for inclusion
Safdar et al. 2004 (22)	Meta-analysis of 17 observational studies and trials comparing combination treatment with monotherapy	Languages other than english and outcomes other than mortality excluded	*Escherichia coli, Pseudomonas aeruginosa, Klebsiella pneumoniae*	3077	NR	0.96 (0.70–1.32)	NR	NR	NR	Only studies of bacteremia were included
Paul et al. 2006 (169)	Meta-analysis of 64 RCTs comparing combination beta-lactam and aminoglycoside treatment for infections to beta-lactam monotherapy	Trials in cystic fibrosis patients excluded	*Escherichia coli, Pseudomonas aeruginosa, Klebsiella pneumoniae,* urinary tract infection, biliary tract infection, pneumonia, endocarditis	7586	NR	1.10 (0.75–1.35)	1.11 (0.95–1.29)	0.88 (0.54–1.45)	0.76 (0.57–1.01)	
Paul et al. 2003 (72)	Meta-analysis of 47 RCTs comparing combination beta-lactam and aminoglycoside treatment for infections to beta-lactam monotherapy	Only patients with fever and neutropenia included	Multiple Gram-positive and Gram-negative organisms; bacteremia in 24% of patients	7807	NR	0.85 (0.72–1.02)	0.92 (0.85–0.00)[a]	NR	0.97 (0.82–1.14)	<2% of patients had pseudomonas infection
Elphick and Tan 2005 (170)	Meta-analysis of 8 RCTs comparing combination beta-lactam and aminoglycoside treatment to beta-lactam alone or aminoglycoside alone	Only patients with cystic fibrosis included	NR	356	NR	NR	NR	NR	NR	Important outcomes could not be calculated because of heterogeneity and poor methodologic quality of the studies

[a]treatment success favoring monotherapy.

Abbreviations: CI, confidence interval; NR, not reported; RCT, randomized controlled trial.

Resistance was defined as at least a fourfold increase in minimum inhibitory concentrations (MICs). Following a single dose of antibiotic, resistance to ceftriaxone and pefloxacin emerged, respectively, in 15% and 83% of animals infected with *K. pneumoniae,* 71% and 54% with *Enterobacter cloacae,* 0% and 83% with *Serratia marcescens,* 25% and 100% with *P. aeruginosa,* and 0% with both *Escherichia coli* and *Staphylococcus aureus.* Any dual combination of amikacin, pefloxacin, and ceftriaxone was associated with less acquired resistance than monotherapy in mice with *K. pneumoniae* and *E. cloacae.* Lister et al. studied the combination of levofloxacin and imipenem and the use of each drug alone against *P. aeruginosa* strains in vitro. They found that the use of combination therapy eradicated all three clinical isolates and failed to produce any resistant subpopulations. In contrast, exposure to a single agent at a time showed initial killing followed by emergence of a resistant subpopulation 24 hr after drug exposure (48).

Whether combination therapy will prevent emergence of resistance in infections in humans in the current era, where the promise of more potent antibiotics is tempered by the increasing crisis in antimicrobial resistance, is less clear (20,53). Paul et al. reported a meta-analysis of 64 randomized trials comparing beta-lactam monotherapy with beta-lactam plus aminoglycoside combination therapy for patients with sepsis. They found no difference in the rate of development of resistance in the two groups (Fig. 1), which they determined by comparing pre- and post-treatment isolates (54). Another meta-analysis of eight RCTs, comparing beta-lactam monotherapy to beta-lactam plus aminoglycoside combination therapy that considered emergence of resistance as a primary outcome found that monotherapy was not associated with a greater emergence of resistance than combination (OR, 0.90, 95% CI 0.56–1.47) (55). Heterogeneity in study design, type of beta-lactam used, and lack of rigorous methodology in assessing the emergence of resistance in the studies should be acknowledged as important limitations of these meta-analyses.

A number of reports using mathematical models to predict the impact of antimicrobial therapy on the emergence of resistance have been published. Bonhoeffer et al. found that combination antimicrobial therapy was more effective in preventing resistance than monotherapy for the treatment of infections that did

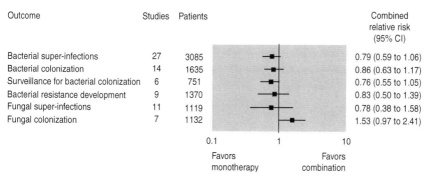

Outcome	Studies	Patients		Combined relative risk (95% CI)
Bacterial super-infections	27	3085		0.79 (0.59 to 1.06)
Bacterial colonization	14	1635		0.86 (0.63 to 1.17)
Surveillance for bacterial colonization	6	751		0.76 (0.55 to 1.05)
Bacterial resistance development	9	1370		0.83 (0.50 to 1.39)
Fungal super-infections	11	1119		0.78 (0.38 to 1.58)
Fungal colonization	7	1132		1.53 (0.97 to 2.41)

0.1   1   10

Favors monotherapy   Favors combination

FIGURE 1 Summary of relative risks for outcome relating to resistance development in comparison of beta-lactam monotherapy versus beta-lactam-aminoglycoside combination therapy for treatment of sepsis. Log scale of relative risks [95% confidence intervals (CI)], random effect model. Studies are ordered by weight. *Source*: From Ref. 54.

not result in prolonged carriage of the infecting organism, a scenario that is more in keeping with community infections than healthcare-associated infection (56). Drug dosing and achievable high concentrations were shown to be important factors in predicting the development of resistance by Jumbe et al. who used a mouse-thigh infection model and mathematical modeling to characterize the relationship between varying doses of levofloxacin and drug-susceptible and resistant populations of *P. aeruginosa* (57).

In summary, although the bulk of the currently available evidence from clinical studies does not support the contention that combination therapy with beta-lactam and aminoglycoside for treatment of infections caused by Gram-negative bacilli such as *E. coli, P. aeruginosa,* and *K. pneumoniae* reduces the emergence of resistance in these organisms, these findings are in contrast to animal studies and mathematical models and further research is needed in this area.

Combination Therapy to Provide Synergistic Killing of Gram-Negative Bacilli

Demonstration of clinical benefit from synergy has been studied in neutropenic patients with fever (58). Since the early 1990s, synergy was considered as an important factor in overcoming impaired host defenses. However, this was recently re-examined; in one randomized trial, piperacillin monotherapy was compared with ceftriaxone and gentamicin in 212 neutropenic febrile patients with hematologic malignancy. The authors found that 89.8% of patients receiving piperacillin-tazobactam had responded at 21 days compared with 71.8% in the combination therapy group ($p = 0.005$). The mean total antibiotic drug cost in the monotherapy group was 39.4% of that in group B ($p = 0.010$). Several patients in both groups required modifications of their antimicrobial regimen with the addition of teicoplanin and/or meropenem, which may also have impacted the study results (59).

In general, in vitro studies use four methods to assess synergistic activity: checkerboard, Etest, time-kill, and in vitro pharmacodynamic models. Unfortunately, there is discordance between the results of checkerboard titration and time-kill curve methods. Burgess and Hastings compared the activity of piperacillin/tazobactam in combination with amikacin, ciprofloxacin, or trovafloxacin at different concentrations against *P. aeruginosa* using time-kill methodology. MICs were determined for four clinical isolates of *P. aeruginosa*. Time-kill studies were conducted over 24 hr. Each drug was tested alone and in combination, which was classified as synergistic, indifferent, or antagonistic. Synergy was defined as $\geq 2 - \log(10)$ decrease in CFU/mL at 24 hr with the combination when compared to the most active single agent. In addition, the number of surviving organisms for the antimicrobial combination must be $\geq 2 - \log(10)$ less than the initial inoculum. Overall, synergy was most frequently (42%) noted with the piperacillin/tazobactam and amikacin combinations, followed by 33% and 8% of the piperacillin/tazobactam and trovafloxacin and ciprofloxacin combinations. No combination demonstrated antagonism.

In summary, a number of different methodologies have been used to measure in vitro synergy, none of which has correlated well, either with each other or with clinical outcomes. It is unclear whether the presence of in vitro synergy should determine selection of antibiotic treatment of Gram-negative infections (60). Focusing on optimizing therapy using pharmacodynamic principles is likely to produce more benefit than combination therapy for the purpose of achieving synergy.

Combination Therapy for Infections Caused by Completely Resistant Gram-Negative Bacilli

In the last decade, a new rationale for combination therapy has emerged, namely the use of combination anti-infective therapy for strains of bacteria that have become resistant to all, or nearly all, available antibacterial agents. This is a particular challenge with *P. aeruginosa* and *Acinetobacter* species. In this instance, the goal is merely to find any clinical activity of an antibiotic combination that may result in either additive or "subadditive" activity of the combination, or enhancement of a single active agent by an otherwise inactive agent (5).

In vitro and animal studies assessing the utility of combination antimicrobial therapy against *P. aeruginosa*, despite resistance to individual drugs, have yielded results showing better outcomes with combination therapy (Table 3) (61–64). Rifampin in combination with either polymyxin B or azithromycin has increased activity in vitro against multidrug-resistant *P. aeruginosa*. Other combinations with greater activity against *P. aeruginosa* than the individual components of the combination include ceftazidime or cefepime with a fluoroquinolone; ceftazidime plus colistin; clarithromycin plus tobramycin; and azithromycin plus tobramycin, doxycycline, or trimethoprim (62). Not all studies, however, show in vitro synergy with combination therapy. Wareham et al. found that rifampin in combination with polymyxin, imipenem, or azithromycin was not synergistic in vitro against *Acinetobacter* spp. (65).

Data in humans showing the efficacy of this approach is extremely scant, but increasing. Isolated case reports and case series of favorable outcomes with combinations of colistin, imipenem, and rifampin for multidrug-resistant *P. aeruginosa* infections have been described (66).

MAJOR INFECTIOUS SYNDROMES WITH GRAM-NEGATIVE BACILLI
Neutropenic Fever

Infection remains the most frequent life-threatening complication in patients with hematologic malignancies or solid tumors. It is the underlying cause of death of 50% of patients with solid tumors and lymphomas, and 75% of patients with leukemia (67,68). The epidemiology and microbiology of infections in patients

TABLE 3 Selected Antibiotic Combinations Showing Activity against Multidrug-Resistant Strains of Gram-Negative Bacilli

Pathogen	Combinations	Type of evidence	References
Pseudomonas aeruginosa	Colistin and rifampin	In vitro and in patients	64,66,171
	Colistin and doxycyline	In vitro	64
	Ticarcillin, tobramycin, rifampin	In vitro and mouse model	172,173
	Colistin and ceftazidime	In vitro	174
	Colistin and rifampin	In vitro	64,175
Acinetobacter baumannii	Colistin and meropenem	In vitro	64
	Colistin and azithromycin	In vitro	64
	Polymyxin B, rifampin, ampicillin/sulbactam	In vitro	171
	Polymyxin B, rifampin, imipenem	In vitro	176

Source: Adapted from Ref. 62.

with granulocytopenia and malignancy has undergone a shift from predominantly Gram-negative bacilli in the 1960s and 1970s, to a preponderance of Gram-positive organisms in more recent years (69). Between 30% and 50% of febrile episodes in granulocytopenic patients can be confirmed microbiologically, and of these, most represent bacteremia (70).

Empiric antimicrobial therapy should be instituted without delay in all granulocytopenic patients with fever, ideally within 2 hr of the clinical evaluation. Afebrile patients who are granulocytopenic but who have signs or symptoms suggestive of infection should also receive empiric antimicrobial therapy, begun in the same manner as for febrile patients (70). The choice of initial antimicrobial regimens should be based on knowledge of most common infecting pathogens in that center or patient population, and the antibiotic susceptibilities at that institution. Because of the ever-present risk of life-threatening infection by *P. aeruginosa*, all initial antimicrobial regimens must include at least one drug with antipseudomonal activity.

Despite many randomized trials, no single empiric regimen can be recommended for treatment of all patients with granulocytopenic fever. Comparing numerous studies is difficult because of differing definitions of disease, and varied criteria used to assess response to treatment.

Multiple studies have shown no differences in outcome between monotherapy and multidrug combinations for empiric treatment of uncomplicated fever in granulocytopenic patients, i.e., those without clinical evidence of local infection or sepsis at the outset. Two recent meta-analyses encompassing more than 4000 patients found that patients with uncomplicated granulocytopenic fever treated with a beta-lactam alone, in contrast with a beta-lactam plus an aminoglycoside regimen, found no significant difference in all-cause mortality (relative risk 0.85–0.87, $p = 0.057$) (71,72). While rates of super-infection in both groups were similar, the frequency of adverse events was higher in patients receiving combination therapy. Another meta-analysis, which used clinical failure of antimicrobial therapy as the outcome measure, also found beta-lactam monotherapy to be comparable to aminoglycoside-containing combinations in uncomplicated granulocytopenic fever (73).

The antimicrobial agents that have been best studied for monotherapy include a third- (ceftazidime) or fourth-generation cephalosporin (cefepime) or a carbapenem (imipenem-cilastatin or meropenem). The emergence of ESBLs in *Enterobacteriaceae* has reduced the utility of ceftazidime for monotherapy (74). Imipenem-cilastatin, meropenem, and cefepime, unlike ceftazidime, are active against ESBL-producing *Enterobacteriaceae* and have excellent activity against viridans streptococci and pneumococci. A prospective double-blind study of 411 patients with cancer showed that the rate of clinical response was higher in febrile granulocytopenic patients treated with meropenem than in those treated with ceftazidime (75).

Two-drug combination therapy most often comprises an aminoglycoside (gentamicin, tobramycin, or amikacin) plus an antipseudomonal penicillin (ticarcillin-clavulanate or piperacillin-tazobactam), an antipseudomonal cephalosporin (cefepime or ceftazidime), or a carbapenem (imipenem-cilastatin or meropenem). These regimens have been shown to have comparable efficacy in numerous trials (72). Because of intrinsic and growing acquired resistance in many species of Gram-negative bacteria causing serious infections (13), and the high mortality associated with these, combination antimicrobial therapy is intuitively appealing. However, as previously discussed, the studies to date have not shown combination therapy to be superior (72). Although widely used, the combination of antipseudomonal penicillin with a fluoroquinolone has not yet been adequately studied. In one multicenter randomized trial of 471 clinically evaluable febrile episodes, piperacillin plus tobramycin was compared with piperacillin with cipro-floxacin (234 episodes in the ciprofloxacin-piperacillin group and 237 in the tobramycin-piperacillin group). Success rates in the ciprofloxacin-piperacillin group (63 of 234 febrile episodes) and tobramycin-piperacillin group (52 of 237 episodes) were similar [27% vs. 22%, respectively; difference, 5.0% points (95% CI, −2.3 to 12.8% points)]. Survival was also similar in these groups [96.2% of patients receiving ciprofloxacin-piperacillin vs. 94.1% of patients receiving tobra-mycin-piperacillin; difference, 2.1% points (CI, −2.2 to 6.4% points)]. No significant differences in adverse events or toxicity were noted ($p = 0.083$) (76). In our opinion, fluoroquinolones in initial empiric regimens should not be used if the patient has had heavy exposure to this class of drugs in the past, such as for prophylaxis, or treatment of a recent infection. In summary, institutional trends in resistance profiles should guide empiric therapy for neutropenic fever. In general, combination therapy offers no advantage over monotherapy.

Healthcare-Associated Pneumonia

The majority of healthcare-associated pneumonia is ventilator-associated pneumonia (VAP), which is the most frequent nosocomial infection in the ICU (77); between 10% and 20% of mechanically ventilated patients develop VAP (78). The published literature suggests that the impact of VAP on outcomes in ICU patients is considerable. Several studies report that patients with VAP have an increased length of stay and hospital costs (79,80); some studies have also found mortality attributable to VAP (81–83). An increasing proportion of VAP episodes, particularly those occurring 5 or more days after admission, are caused by multidrug-resistant microorganisms such as *P. aeruginosa*, *Enterobacter* spp., *Acinetobacter* spp., and methicillin-resistant *S. aureus* (84,85).

Early appropriate anti-infective therapy has been clearly shown to result in more favorable outcomes with VAP (Table 4) (86–97), and most treatment failures have been related to inappropriate initial antibiotic treatment with insufficient coverage of these pathogens. Therefore, initial empiric combination therapy has been advocated to provide a broad spectrum of antimicrobial coverage until culture and susceptibility results become available. A recent guideline from the American Thoracic Society and the Infectious Diseases Society of America recommends that patients at risk for infection with multidrug-resistant organisms, which includes almost all patients in the ICU, should initially receive a combination of agents that can provide a broad spectrum of coverage to minimize the potential for inappropriate antibiotic treatment. To ensure pseudomonal coverage, therapy should involve an antipseudomonal beta-lactam plus either an antipseudomonal quinolone or an aminoglycoside. The choice of agents should be based on local patterns of antimicrobial susceptibility, and anticipated side effects, and should also take into account which therapies patients have recently received (i.e., within the past 2 weeks), avoiding use of agents from those same antimicrobial classes (98).

Combination therapy as definitive treatment of VAP is commonly used, presumably to promote synergy and improve clinical outcomes. However,

TABLE 4 Selected Studies of the Effect of Adequate Therapy on Mortality from Ventilator-Associated Pneumonia

Author (Ref.)	Number of patients	Adequate treatment Death/patients (%)	Inadequate treatment Death/patients (%)	p-value
Celis et al. (86)	118	33/118 (28)	11/12 (92)	<0.001
Alvarez-Lerma (87)	430	46/284 (16)	36/146 (25)	0.003
Luna et al. (88)	50	6/16 (38)	31/34 (91)	<0.01
Sanchez-Nieto et al. (89)	38	6/24 (25)	6/14 (43)	NS
Kollef et al. (90)	411	48/106 (45)	51/305 (17)	<0.01
Bercault and Boulain (91)	135	37/92 (40)	18/34 (53)	NS
Dupont et al. (92)	111	21/55 (38)	27/57 (47)	NS
Iregui et al. (93)	107	21/74 (28)	23/33 (70)	<0.01
Hanes et al. (94)	163	9/79 (11)	21/84 (25)	0.02
Dupont et al. (95)	322	37/220 (17)	21/92 (23)	NS
Leroy et al. (96)	132	42/106 (40)	16/26 (62)	0.04
Mueller et al. (97)	82	1/28 (4)	12/54 (22)	<0.01

Abbreviation: NS, not significant.
Source: Adapted from Ref. 177.

the relationship of in vitro synergy with clinical outcomes is far from clear, as mentioned earlier. Combination therapy has been proposed as a means of preventing emergence of resistance during treatment of VAP. Although emergence of resistance during therapy is especially well documented for *Enterobacter* infections and for *P. aeruginosa* infections, the utility of combination therapy in minimizing emergence of resistance has not been shown convincingly (99).

In a meta-analysis by Paul et al., which included 7586 patients from prospective randomized trials of beta-lactam monotherapy compared with beta-lactam–aminoglycoside combination regimens in patients with sepsis, approximately 1000 had pneumonia, and combination therapy was not superior to monotherapy in achieving clinical cure. Furthermore, there was greater nephrotoxicity in the combination therapy group (54).

Thus it appears the only reason to use combination therapy that is currently supported by evidence is to increase the likelihood of initiating appropriate antimicrobial therapy. Once the organism is identified, monotherapy should be used, if permitted by the antibiogram. Agents that have been shown to be effective as monotherapy in patients with moderately severe healthcare-associated pneumonia not due to multidrug-resistant pathogens include ciprofloxacin, levofloxacin, imipenem, meropenem, cefepime, and piperacillin–tazobactam (100–105).

SPECIFIC PATHOGENS
Enterobacter Spp.

Enterobacter species are becoming increasingly important nosocomial pathogens, especially in the ICU setting (15,44,106,107). In the Surveillance and Control of Pathogens of Epidemiologic (SCOPE) importance project, nosocomial bloodstream infections from 1995 to 2002 were analyzed. *Enterobacter* species were among the most common Gram-negative organisms following *P. aeruginosa*; both bacteria were more common in the ICU setting than in the wards, each representing 4.7% of bloodstream infections. *Enterobacter* species also accounted for 3.1% of bloodstream infections in non-ICU wards (107). Data from the

National Nosocomial Infections Surveillance (NNIS) system demonstrated that *Enterobacter* species caused 11.2% of pneumonia cases in all types of ICUs, ranking third after *S. aureus* (18.1%) and *P. aeruginosa* (17%). *Enterobacter* were also among the most frequent pathogens for surgical site infections, as reported in the NNIS from October 1986 to April 1997. The isolation rate was 9.5% after enterococci (15.3), coagulase-negative staphylococci (12.6), *S. aureus* (11.2), and *P. aeruginosa* (10.3).

Enterobacter species cause a wide variety of infections, principally hospital-acquired pneumonia and bacteremia; common reservoirs for the organism include the urinary, respiratory, and gastrointestinal tracts, as well as surgical and burn wounds (108,109). Comorbidities, critical illness, immunocompromised states, prolonged ICU stay, invasive devices, antimicrobial use, and surgical procedures, all predispose patients to infection with *Enterobacter* species (110–113). *Enterobacter* bacteremia is associated with a 20% to 70% mortality, in part because of the severe underlying conditions in the host population (114).

An important feature of *Enterobacter* organisms is their predilection to develop resistance to antimicrobials during therapy (108). This is especially true for the third-generation cephalosporins. *Enterobacter* species possess, as do many other Gram-negative bacilli, the chromosomal gene *AmpC* that encodes for the ampC beta-lactamase that hydrolyzes penicillins and cephalosporins. In most cases, small amounts of the enzyme are produced that do not have significant impact on treatment outcomes. However, in response to antimicrobial pressure, *Enterobacter* species are able to produce large amounts of this enzyme. This is mediated by a mutation in *AmpD* gene, which normally inhibits ampC expression. This results in permanent, constitutive, hyperproduction of ampC beta-lactamase; the result is resistance to all penicillins, cephalosporins, and monobactams (4,7,22–30). The mutation occurs at a frequency of 10^{-5} to 10^{-7} (115) and the multidrug resistance that results is associated with adverse clinical outcomes from failure of therapy (116).

Several reports have documented the emergence of resistance to cephalosporins in *Enterobacter* infections (117,118). Resistance emerged as early as 2 days and as late as 20 days after initiation of antibiotic therapy. Resistance to oxyimino-cephalosporins has emerged during therapy in 19% of patients treated for *Enterobacter* bacteremia in academic medical centers in the United States (108). Rates are highest for patients with high-density infections such as deep-seated abscesses and pneumonia, and lower among patients with urinary tract infections, where beta-lactams reach very high concentrations (119). Risk factors for resistance to cephalosporins in *Enterobacter* spp. include prior use of cephalosporins. Against this backdrop, the selection of therapy for *Enterobacter* infections becomes difficult.

In particular, the use of newer cephalosporins has been associated with increased prevalence of resistance to beta-lactam antibiotics (120). Other factors that have been shown to influence the emergence of resistant strains include previous receipt of aminoglycosides, care in the ICU, presence of intravascular or urinary catheters, or invasive procedures (114). The size and complexity of the hospital, and the kind or type of hospital unit, may also influence this (18–21).

Third-generation cephalosporins are commonly used as initial empiric therapy for bacteremias. However, since studies have shown that resistance and poor outcomes are associated with previous use of third-generation cephalosporins (7,10,46), it is suggested that use of these drugs be avoided where *Enterobacter* is a suspected pathogen. In the study by Chow et al. emergence of resistance to third-generation cephalosporins occurred with the same frequency regardless of whether the patient received the cephalosporin alone, or in combination with an aminoglycoside.

Instead of third-generation cephalosporins, monotherapy with a carbapenem can be instituted (47–51). In one study, for example, the use of ertapenem proved as effective as a beta-lactam/beta-lactamase-inhibitor combination in the treatment of serious infections (121).

Kim et al. reported data on 249 patients with bacteremia due to third-generation cephalosporin-resistant *Citrobacter freundii*, *E. aerogenes*, *E. cloacae*, and *S. marcescens*. Of 152 patients given appropriate therapy, most received monotherapy (128) and 11% died. Twenty-four patients received combination therapy and 25% of these patients died. There was no statistically significant difference in mortality between the two groups. In those given monotherapy, no differences in mortality were seen comparing imipenem, aminoglycoside, and ciprofloxacin (122).

Klebsiella Spp.

As early as the 1960s, *Klebsiella* spp. have been a prominent cause of Gram-negative infections in hospitalized patients. They are the second most frequent cause of Gram-negative bacteremia after *E. coli*, accounting for 3% to 7% of all nosocomial bacterial infections. They are frequently implicated in healthcare-associated pneumonia, intra-abdominal infections and urinary tract infections (123). Infection due to this organism has historically been felt to be difficult to treat, with bacteremia associated with high mortality rates (124). As with many other organisms, initial appropriate antimicrobial therapy has been shown to improve clinical outcomes including mortality (124). However, with multidrug resistance now increasingly common, the choice of anti-infective for initial empiric therapy is more limited and multidrug resistance is an independent risk factor for initial inadequate therapy (125). Inappropriate antimicrobial therapy is an important predictor of mortality in *Klebsiella* bacteremia (126–128). Whether to use a single broad-spectrum antibiotic versus combination therapy as empiric treatment, or as definitive treatment once susceptibility results are available, is a key issue.

A major concern regarding infections with *Klebsiella* spp. is the expanding presence of ESBL-producing strains (16). Infections caused by ESBL-producing strains of *Enterobacteriaceae* are associated with greater morbidity, and in some studies, mortality, when compared to bacteremia caused by non-ESBL producing *K. pneumoniae* (31,129–131).

A number of risk factors for colonization and eventual infection with ESBL *K. pneumoniae* (ESBL-KP) have been identified and include prior antibiotic use, especially with extended-spectrum cephalosporins, placement of an indwelling catheter, intravascular catheter, feeding tube, or prior invasive procedure (132–136).

Of five major studies that have assessed the utility of combination antimicrobial therapy for *Klebsiella* bacteremia (Table 5) for reducing mortality (31,131,137–139), only one found a statistically significant result favoring combination therapy (139). Feldman et al. reported a retrospective study of 47 patients with *K. pneumoniae* bacteremia (139). Severe comorbidities were present in most of the patients and the most common source of bacteremia was pneumonia. None of the patients who received combination therapy with a beta-lactam and an aminoglycoside, died compared with 83% of those who received monotherapy with an appropriate beta-lactam, aminoglycoside, or ciprofloxacin. No formal adjustment for severity of illness was performed and this represents a major confounding factor in observational studies addressing the issue of antimicrobial treatment for infection.

Korvick et al. reported a prospective, observational, multicenter study to evaluate the efficacy of antibiotic combination therapy versus that of monotherapy in 230 consecutive patients with *Klebsiella* bacteremia (137). The major species was *K. pneumoniae* and half of the infections were nosocomially acquired. The most common source of bacteremia was urinary tract followed by the biliary tract, lung, and abdomen. Overall, there was no difference in 14-day mortality in the group that received beta-lactam and aminoglycoside combination therapy compared with monotherapy alone (20% and 18%, respectively). However, in a subgroup analysis limited to patients with hypotension related to sepsis, the investigators found that fewer patients who received combination therapy died (24%) than those who received monotherapy (50%). In this study, monotherapy was defined as treatment with a single antibiotic active in vitro against the *Klebsiella* strain isolated from the blood. Combination therapy was defined as treatment with two antibiotics, both of which were active in vitro against the *Klebsiella* strain. In both groups, treatment was given for a minimum of 2 days but data on the total duration of therapy and changes in the treatment regimen following susceptibility results of the isolates was not reported, both of which might be expected to influence outcomes of bacteremia. In another study of 100 cases of *Klebsiella* bacteremia, most of which were nosocomial, inadequate antimicrobial treatment was a risk factor for mortality; no differences were observed in mortality with combination and monotherapy (138). Kang et al. compared 91 patients who received a carbapenem or ciprofloxacin as definitive treatment, and found no mortality difference between those who received the combination of these two antibiotics and those that received mono-therapy (31).

Combination therapy in so far as it provides adequate initial antimicrobial therapy, may be used for empiric treatment of *Klebsiella* bacteremia. Alternatively, a carbapenem may be effective as monotherapy in institutions where carbapenem resistance is not widespread. The site of treatment is also important to take into account when selecting anti-infective therapy; outcomes are worse with nonurin-ary sites of infection. No convincing advantage to using combination therapy for the entire course of treatment has been demonstrated.

Pseudomonas aeruginosa

P. aeruginosa is a major nosocomial pathogen, especially in neutropenic patients, and those with compromised immunity (30,32,140–142). A frequent cause of bacteremia and pneumonia in hospitalized patients, *P. aeruginosa* infections are associated with a 20% to 60% mortality rate, despite potent antimicrobial therapy (30). A number of factors have been found to be associated with poor prognosis following *Pseudomonas* bacteremia, including severe underlying disease (i.e., malignancy) (143), pneumonia as the source for bacteremia, septic shock (142), and neutropenia (144).

P. aeruginosa is intrinsically resistant to many antibiotics at concentrations achievable in vivo. Moreover, under selective antibiotic pressure, *P. aeruginosa* has been shown to rapidly acquire antibiotic resistance, by a number of different mechanisms (145). Beta-lactam resistance is mediated by production of beta-lactamases, permeability alterations, and penicillin-binding protein modifications. *P. aeruginosa* also contains inducible chromosomal beta-lactamases that confer resistance to cephalosporins. Resistance to fluoroquinolones continues to increase; both mutations in DNA gyrase and efflux pumps have been described.

The relationship of antibiotic therapy to outcome has been the subject of several observational studies, most of which have concluded that inappropriate antibiotic therapy is associated with adverse outcomes (30,31). *Pseudomonas* infection is clinically indistinguishable from other forms of Gram-negative bacterial infection. For this reason, patients with *Pseudomonas* infection might receive empiric antibiotics that are inactive against the pathogen, especially before antibiotic susceptibility results become available. Combination therapy is more likely to encompass appropriate therapy (37). In an analysis of 136 cases of *P. aeruginosa* bacteremia in Korea, Kang et al. found that patients who received delayed effective antimicrobial therapy, defined as the administration of empiric antibiotics ineffective against the *P. aeruginosa* isolate pending results of antibiotic susceptibility testing, with a delay of more than 24 hr after blood culture samples were obtained, had a 43% (33 of 76) 30-day mortality. In comparison, patients who did not receive delayed effective empiric treatment had a 28% (13 of 47) mortality ($p = 0.079$). Other studies have found similar results; Vidal et al. noted that when appropriateness of initial antimicrobial therapy was redefined using results of in vitro testing, only half of their cohort with *P. aeruginosa* bacteremia received appropriate therapy (146).

However, the importance of monotherapy versus combination therapy for *P. aeruginosa* infections is controversial, whether for empiric therapy, or definitive treatment. RCTs of Gram-negative infections have too few cases of *P. aeruginosa* to allow a statistically robust analysis of the relative value of combination versus monotherapy. This was shown in a review of 10 randomized trials of antimicrobial therapy in patients with cancer and neutropenia. In this analysis, only 90 of a total of 909 episodes of bacteremia were caused by *Pseudomonas* species. Therefore, observational studies are important. Many have problems with selection bias, such as differences in severity of illness and comorbidities among patients receiving one or the other type of therapy. Other major shortcomings include lack of assessment of objective endpoints such as mortality. In addition, some do not account for the results of in vitro susceptibility testing in the definition of adequate therapy. Given these limitations, definitive conclusions regarding whether empiric or definitive combination therapy are superior to adequate monotherapy are difficult to make.

Eight major studies compared combination therapy with monotherapy for *P. aeruginosa* bacteremia (Table 6) (30,32,141,142,147–150). All were observational. Patient populations in these studies included those with malignancy, neutropenia, or critical illness. The sources of bacteremia were the respiratory and urinary tract. With a few exceptions, monotherapy referred to treatment with an antipseudomonal beta-lactam, and combinations were generally a beta-lactam plus an aminoglycoside (Table 2). One of these eight studies reported clinical cure as the primary outcome and did not provide data on mortality. In this study by Chatzinikolaou et al. (30), records of 245 patients with consecutive episodes of *P. aeruginosa* bacteremia from 1991 to 1995 at the MD Anderson Cancer Center were reviewed. The overall cure rate was 80% and there were no differences in cure rates observed between initial monotherapy with a beta-lactam and initial combination therapy (i.e., two beta-lactams or a beta-lactam and an aminoglycoside). The presence or absence of shock or pneumonia did not influence cure rates. Importantly, seven

TABLE 5 Studies Comparing Combination with Monotherapy for *Klebsiella* Bacteremia

Study, year (Ref.)	Study description	Number of patients	Portal of entry	Nosocomial cases (%)	Patient population	Mortality in monotherapy	Mortality in combination therapy group	OR or RR comparing combination with monotherapy (95% CI)
Garcia de la Torre et al. 1985 (138)	Retrospective cohort study	100	Urinary tract	77 (77)	General inpatients	9/41	9/45	0.89 (0.27–2.88)
Feldman et al. 1990 (139)	Prospective cohort study	47	Respiratory tract	25 (53)	General inpatients	12/16	0/9	0.00 (0.00–0.29)
Korvick et al. 1992 (137)	Prospective cohort	230	Urinary tract, biliary tract	122 (53)	General inpatients	20/113	23/117	1.14 (0.56–2.34)
Kim et al. 2002 (131)	Retrospective cohort	125	Biliary tract	65 (52)	General inpatients	13/66	11/42	1.45 (0.52–3.98)
Kang et al. 2004 (31)	Retrospective cohort	133	Biliary tract	105/133 (79)	General inpatients	5/67	6/24	4.13 (0.91–18.9)

Abbreviations: CI, confidence interval; OR, odds ratio; RR, relative risk.

patients received aminoglycosides alone and none responded. Antipseudomonal cephalosporins and carbapenems were associated with better cure rates compared with antipseudomonal penicillins.

Of the remaining seven studies that reported mortality rates, no statistically significant mortality differences were seen between the combination and mono-therapy group in six studies; however, all of these studies lacked adequate statistical power. Hilf et al. in a prospective study of 200 patients found that in vitro synergy did not correlate with clinical outcomes; however, combination therapy with a beta-lactam and aminoglycoside had better outcomes (27% mortality) versus 47% with monotherapy (141). Some patients in the monotherapy arm received aminoglycoside alone, which is not considered optimal therapy for *P. aeruginosa* infection.

Recently, much attention has focused on the appropriate application of pharmacodynamic principles in dosing treatment regimens for Pseudomonas infection. Zelenitsky et al. undertook a retrospective study of antibiotic pharmaco-dynamics in the treatment of *P. aeruginosa* bacteremia. Among the 38 cases they included in their analysis, 87% of patients received an aminoglycoside or cipro-floxacin, and 79% received piperacillin or ceftazidime. Most patients received combination therapy. Peak/MIC ratio was associated independently with treat-ment outcome, with a predicted probability of cure $\geq 90\%$ when peak/MIC was at least eight (143).

Given the rapid rise in multidrug-resistant *P. aeruginosa* and the clear link between appropriate initial antibiotic therapy and clinical outcomes, we recom-mend that empiric combination antibiotic therapy be initiated for suspected severe infection, such as respiratory tract infection or bacteremia. Therapy should be de-escalated immediately when susceptibility results become available. Definitive therapy should be monotherapy with an agent active in vitro, with the caveat that aminoglycosides alone should not be used.

With regards to the risk of development of resistance, in vitro animal studies and mathematical models suggest that combination therapy may reduce the risk of emergence of resistance. However, there is scant data in humans to support this contention. Moreover, the adverse consequences of prolonged com-bination therapy, such as super-infection, toxicity, and cost, must be taken into consideration. Current literature has focused on beta-lactam and aminoglycoside combination, but the use of beta-lactam with a fluoroquinolone is increasingly utilized in clinical settings and should be formally studied for its efficacy in *Pseudomonas* infections.

Other Gram-Negative Bacilli

Citrobacter species are increasingly being recognized as an important, although still relatively infrequent cause of bacteremia in hospitalized patients (151). *Citrobacter* species have been implicated in various infections including surgical wound infections (152,153), cellulitis (154–156), urinary tract infections (153,157), and bacteremias (158). Most patients who develop these infections have underlying risk factors such as prolonged hospital stays, immunosuppression, malignancy, hepatobiliary disease, and invasive devices (159–161). Frequently associated with polymicrobial bacteremia, studies have found mortality associated with this pathogen ranging from 22% to 56% (158,160,162–164), probably a reflection of the critically ill state of the host.

TABLE 6 Studies Assessing Mortality from *Pseudomonas* Infections Comparing Combination with Monotherapy

Author, year (Ref.)	Study description	Number of patients	Common sources of bacteremia	Use of combination therapy	Mortality with empiric therapy		Mortality with definitive therapy	
					Monotherapy	Combination therapy	Monotherapy	Combination therapy
Chamot et al. 2003 (150)	Retrospective cohort study	115	Respiratory tract, urinary tract	Empiric and definitive	15/49	5/36	9/33	10/46
Vidal et al. 1996 (32)[a]	Retrospective cohort study	189	Respiratory tract, IV catheter-related	Definitive	NR	NR	NR	NR
Hilf et al. 1989 (141)	Prospective cohort study	200	Respiratory tract, urinary tract	Empiric	20/43	38/143	NR	NR
Kuikka and Valtonen 1998 (142)	Retrospective cohort study	132	Respiratory tract	Definitive	NR	NR	28/70	11/41
Tapper and Armstrong 1974 (148)	Retrospective cohort study	50	Respiratory tract, urinary tract	Empiric	27/34	30/44	NR	NR
Mendelson et al. 1994 (149)	Retrospective cohort study	21	Respiratory tract	Empiric	4/9	4/15	NR	NR
Siegman-Igra et al. 1998 (147)	Retrospective cohort study	57	Urinary tract	Empiric	6/42	2/15	NR	NR

[a]No differences in mortality between definitive combination and monotherapy noted; numbers provided not statistically significant.
Abbreviations: NR, not reported.

Citrobacter species are frequently resistant to one or more antimicrobials (151) and recent use of antimicrobial agents, especially extended-spectrum cephalosporins, has been found to be a risk factor for infection with resistant *Citrobacter* (164). Resistance rates to cephalosporins, fluoroquinolones, and aminoglycosides have increased over the last few years, probably due to multiple factors including widespread antimicrobial use, an increasingly elderly and immunocompromised population, and greater use of procedures and invasive devices (165). In a series of 48 cases of *Citrobacter* bacteremia in India, Gupta et al. found that 79% of their isolates were resistant to three or more antimicrobials (162). Similar findings were reported by Chen et al. from Taiwan, where rates of resistance to third-generation cephalosporins and extended-spectrum penicillins were high both in nosocomial and community acquired isolates (158). The mechanisms of resistance included production of both inducible ampC cephalosporinases, as with other members of *Enterobacteriaceae*, and ESBL production.

Scant data exist on combination therapy for *Citrobacter* bacteremia. In the series by Chen and colleagues, 18 patients received empiric combination therapy with an aminoglycoside and a beta-lactam, and one of these patients died (5%). In comparison, 11 patients received monotherapy with a third-generation cephalosporin, five of whom died (45%) (OR 0.07, 0.01–0.73, $p = 0.018$); the investigators found that while both empiric and definitive combination therapy were associated with improved outcomes, another major predictor of response was the appropriateness of antimicrobial therapy (164). Given the paucity of data, evidence-based recommendations regarding treatment are not possible; however, if data from other members of the family *Enterobacteriaceae* is extrapolated to *Citrobacter*, combination therapy may need to be used initially pending susceptibility results, but may subsequently be de-escalated to appropriate monotherapy.

Acinetobacter baumannii has emerged as a significant nosocomial pathogen in hospitalized patients worldwide. The rising incidence of infections caused by *Acinetobacter* spp. is of particular concern because of the high rates of multidrug resistance (166). Data from the SCOPE study showed that, over a 7-year period from 1995 to 2002, 25% of nosocomial bacteremias (24,179 total isolates) were caused by Gram-negative bacilli (19). *Acinetobacter* species accounted for 1.6% of nosocomial bacteremia and were the 10th leading cause of bacteremia. At present, more than 85% of isolates are susceptible to carbapenems, but resistance is increasing due to either IMP-type metalloenzymes or carbapenemases of the OXA type (167,168).

Given the high rates of multidrug resistance among *Acinetobacter* species, combination therapy for the purpose of providing initial appropriate empiric treatment may be necessary and is especially recommended for hospital-acquired pneumonia where *Acinetobacter* poses a major threat. Combination therapy for the purposes of reducing resistance during therapy and improving clinical outcomes is commonly used but has not been studied.

CONCLUSION

Infections caused by Gram-negative bacilli pose a serious dilemma for the treating clinician, because of a high propensity for drug resistance. Empiric antimicrobial therapy, whether with a single drug, or a combination of two or more drugs, should be initiated without delay. The choice of anti-infectives should be guided by local institutional prevalence of specific organisms and their antibiograms. For most Gram-negative bacilli in the hospital setting, it is reasonable to initiate therapy with combination antimicrobials with the goal of providing early effective therapy, since it is clear that inappropriate therapy and delayed therapy are associated with a high mortality. The continuing use of combination therapy as definitive treatment once susceptibility results become available is not supported by current evidence.

Combination therapy for synergy and for reducing emergence of resistance has been studied best in in vitro animal models and mathematical models, but there is little clinical data to support its use in humans. Clinical outcomes and mortality do not appear to be reduced by combination therapy, provided that the monotherapy chosen has activity against the infecting organism, is an appropriate choice for the site of infection, and pharmacodynamic principles are followed for dosing to ensure optimal efficacy. For patients with granulocytopenia and fever, and those with sepsis, combination therapy offers no clinical advantage and appears to have a greater risk of adverse events and super-infections. In this era of an inexorable rise in antimicrobial resistance worldwide, more research on the optimal treatment of serious Gram-negative infections is urgently needed.

REFERENCES

1. Maki DG. Risk factors for nosocomial infection in intensive care. Devices vs nature and goals for the next decade. Arch Intern Med 1989; 149:30–5.
2. Kollef MH, Fraser VJ. Antibiotic resistance in the intensive care unit. Ann Intern Med 2001; 134:298–314.
3. Helfand MS, Bonomo RA. Current challenges in antimicrobial chemotherapy: the impact of extended-spectrum beta-lactamases and metallo-beta-lactamases on the treatment of resistant Gram-negative pathogens. Curr Opin Pharmacol 2005; 5:452–8.
4. Kaye KS, Engemann JJ, Fraimow HS, et al. Pathogens resistant to antimicrobial agents: epidemiology, molecular mechanisms, and clinical management. Infect Dis Clin North Am 2004; 18:467–511, viii.
5. Obritsch MD, Fish DN, MacLaren R, et al. Nosocomial infections due to multidrug-resistant *Pseudomonas aeruginosa*: epidemiology and treatment options. Pharmacotherapy 2005; 25:1353–64.
6. Waterer GW, Wunderink RG. Increasing threat of Gram-negative bacteria. Crit Care Med 2001; 29:N75–81.
7. Aloush V, Navon-Venezia S, Seigman-Igra Y, et al. Multidrug-resistant *Pseudomonas aeruginosa*: risk factors and clinical impact. Antimicrob Agents Chemother 2006; 50:43–8.
8. Kang CI, Kim SH, Park WB, et al. Risk factors for antimicrobial resistance and influence of resistance on mortality in patients with bloodstream infection caused by *Pseudomonas aeruginosa*. Microb Drug Resist 2005; 11:68–74.
9. Lautenbach E, Weiner MG, Nachamkin I, et al. Imipenem resistance among *Pseudomonas aeruginosa* isolates: risk factors for infection and impact of resistance on clinical and economic outcomes. Infect Control Hosp Epidemiol 2006; 27:893–900.
10. Hsu DI, Okamoto MP, Murthy R, et al. Fluoroquinolone-resistant *Pseudomonas aeruginosa*: risk factors for acquisition and impact on outcomes. J Antimicrob Chemother 2005; 55:535–41.
11. Carmeli Y, Troillet N, Karchmer AW, et al. Health and economic outcomes of antibiotic resistance in *Pseudomonas aeruginosa*. Arch Intern Med 1999; 159:1127–32.
12. Kollef MH. Gram-negative bacterial resistance: evolving patterns and treatment paradigms. Clin Infect Dis 2005; 40(Suppl. 2):S85–8.
13. Livermore DM. Multiple mechanisms of antimicrobial resistance in *Pseudomonas aeruginosa*: our worst nightmare? Clin Infect Dis 2002; 34:634–40.
14. Sanders CC, Sanders WE Jr. Clinical importance of inducible beta-lactamases in Gram-negative bacteria. Eur J Clin Microbiol 1987; 6:435–8.

15. National Nosocomial Infections Surveillance (NNIS) System Report, data summary from January 1992 through June 2004, issued October 2004. Am J Infect Control 2004; 32:470–85.
16. Paterson DL, Ko WC, Von Gottberg A, et al. International prospective study of *Klebsiella pneumoniae* bacteremia: implications of extended-spectrum beta-lactamase production in nosocomial Infections. Ann Intern Med 2004; 140:26–32.
17. Paterson DL, Mulazimoglu L, Casellas JM, et al. Epidemiology of ciprofloxacin resistance and its relationship to extended-spectrum beta-lactamase production in *Klebsiella pneumoniae* isolates causing bacteremia. Clin Infect Dis 2000; 30:473–8.
18. Lautenbach E, Strom BL, Bilker WB, et al. Epidemiological investigation of fluoroquinolone resistance in infections due to extended-spectrum beta-lactamase-producing *Escherichia coli* and *Klebsiella pneumoniae*. Clin Infect Dis 2001; 33:1288–94.
19. Wisplinghoff H, Bischoff T, Tallent SM, et al. Nosocomial bloodstream infections in US hospitals: analysis of 24,179 cases from a prospective nationwide surveillance study. Clin Infect Dis 2004; 39:309–17.
20. Chow JW, Yu VL. Combination antibiotic therapy versus monotherapy for Gram-negative bacteraemia: a commentary. Int J Antimicrob Agents 1999; 11:7–12.
21. Klibanov OM, Raasch RH, Rublein JC. Single versus combined antibiotic therapy for Gram-negative infections. Ann Pharmacother 2004; 38:332–7.
22. Safdar N, Handelsman J, Maki DG. Does combination antimicrobial therapy reduce mortality in Gram-negative bacteraemia? A meta-analysis. Lancet Infect Dis 2004; 4:519–27.
23. Calandra T, Cometta A. Antibiotic therapy for Gram-negative bacteremia. Infect Dis Clin North Am 1991; 5:817–34.
24. Giamarellou H. Aminoglycosides plus beta-lactams against Gram-negative organisms. Evaluation of in vitro synergy and chemical interactions. Am J Med 1986; 80:126–37.
25. Giamarellou H, Zissis NP, Tagari G, et al. In vitro synergistic activities of aminoglycosides and new beta-lactams against multiresistant *Pseudomonas aeruginosa*. Antimicrob Agents Chemother 1984; 25:534–6.
26. Klastersky J, Zinner SH. Synergistic combinations of antibiotics in Gram-negative bacillary infections. Rev Infect Dis 1982; 4:294–301.
27. Moellering RC Jr, Eliopoulos GM, Allan JD. Beta-lactam/aminoglycoside combinations: interactions and their mechanisms. Am J Med 1986; 80:30–4.
28. Manian FA, Meyer L, Jenne J, et al. Loss of antimicrobial susceptibility in aerobic Gram-negative bacilli repeatedly isolated from patients in intensive-care units. Infect Control Hosp Epidemiol 1996; 17:222–6.
29. Weinstein RA. Occurrence of cefotaxime-resistant *Enterobacter* during therapy of cardiac surgery patients. Chemioterapia 1985; 4:110–2.
30. Chatzinikolaou I, Abi-Said D, Bodey GP, et al. Recent experience with *Pseudomonas aeruginosa* bacteremia in patients with cancer: retrospective analysis of 245 episodes. Arch Intern Med 2000; 160:501–9.
31. Kang CI, Kim SH, Park WB, et al. Bloodstream infections caused by antibiotic-resistant Gram-negative bacilli: risk factors for mortality and impact of inappropriate initial antimicrobial therapy on outcome. Antimicrob Agents Chemother 2005; 49:760–6.
32. Vidal F, Mensa J, Almela M, et al. Epidemiology and outcome of *Pseudomonas aeruginosa* bacteremia, with special emphasis on the influence of antibiotic treatment. Analysis of 189 episodes. Arch Intern Med 1996; 156:2121–6.
33. Osmon S, Ward S, Fraser VJ, et al. Hospital mortality for patients with bacteremia due to *Staphylococcus aureus* or *Pseudomonas aeruginosa*. Chest 2004; 125:607–16.
34. McCabe WR, Jackson GG. Gram-negative bacteremia. I. Etiology and ecology. Arch Intern Med 1962; 110:847–55.
35. Kreger BE, Craven DE, McCabe WR. Gram-negative bacteremia. IV. Re-evaluation of clinical features and treatment in 612 patients. Am J Med 1980; 68:344–55.
36. Harbarth S, Nobre V, Pittet D. Does antibiotic selection impact patient outcome? Clin Infect Dis 2007; 44:87–93.
37. Micek ST, Lloyd AE, Ritchie DJ, et al. *Pseudomonas aeruginosa* bloodstream infection: importance of appropriate initial antimicrobial treatment. Antimicrob Agents Chemother 2005; 49:1306–11.

38. Binkley S, Fishman NO, LaRosa LA, et al. Comparison of unit-specific and hospital-wide antibiograms: potential implications for selection of empirical antimicrobial therapy. Infect Control Hosp Epidemiol 2006; 27:682–7.
39. Mena A, Plasencia V, Garcia L, et al. Characterization of a large outbreak by CTX-M-1-producing *Klebsiella pneumoniae* and mechanisms leading to in vivo carbapenem resistance development. J Clin Microbiol 2006; 44:2831–7.
40. Coelho J, Woodford N, Turton J, et al. Multiresistant Acinetobacter in the UK: how big a threat? J Hosp Infect 2004; 58:167–9.
41. Crespo MP, Woodford N, Sinclair A, et al. Outbreak of carbapenem-resistant *Pseudomonas aeruginosa* producing VIM-8, a novel metallo-beta-lactamase, in a tertiary care center in Cali, Colombia. J Clin Microbiol 2004; 42:5094–101.
42. Woodford N, Tierno PM Jr, Young K, et al. Outbreak of *Klebsiella pneumoniae* producing a new carbapenem-hydrolyzing class A beta-lactamase, KPC-3, in a New York Medical Center. Antimicrob Agents Chemother 2004; 48:4793–9.
43. Siebert JD, Thomson RB Jr, Tan JS, et al. Emergence of antimicrobial resistance in Gram-negative bacilli causing bacteremia during therapy. Am J Clin Pathol 1993; 100:47–51.
44. Paterson DL. Resistance in Gram-negative bacteria: Enterobacteriaceae. Am J Infect Control 2006; 34:S20–8; discussion S64–73.
45. Kosmidis J, Koratzanis G. Emergence of resistant bacterial strains during treatment of infections in the respiratory tract. Scand J Infect Dis. (Suppl.) 1986; 49:135–9.
46. Barriere SL. Bacterial resistance to beta-lactams, and its prevention with combination antimicrobial therapy. Pharmacotherapy 1992; 12:397–402.
47. Mouton JW. Combination therapy as a tool to prevent emergence of bacterial resistance. Infection 1999; 27(Suppl. 2):S24–8.
48. Lister PD, Wolter DJ. Levofloxacin-imipenem combination prevents the emergence of resistance among clinical isolates of *Pseudomonas aeruginosa*. Clin Infect Dis 2005; 40(Suppl. 2):S105–14.
49. Michea-Hamzehpour M, Auckenthaler R, Regamey P, et al. Resistance occurring after fluoroquinolone therapy of experimental *Pseudomonas aeruginosa* peritonitis. Antimicrob Agents Chemother 1987; 31:1803–8.
50. Michea-Hamzehpour M, Pechere JC, Marchou B, et al. Combination therapy: a way to limit emergence of resistance? Am J Med 1986; 80:138–42.
51. Pechere JC. Emergence of resistance during beta-lactam therapy of Gram-negative infections. Bacterial mechanisms and medical responses. Drugs 1988; 35(Suppl. 2):22–8.
52. Pechere JC, Marchou B, Michea-Hamzehpour M, et al. Emergence of resistance after therapy with antibiotics used alone or combined in a murine model. J Antimicrob Chemother 1986; 17(Suppl A):11–8.
53. Craig WA, Salamone FR. Do antibiotic combinations prevent the emergence of resistant organisms? Infect Control Hosp Epidemiol 1988; 9:417–9.
54. Paul M, Benuri-Silbiger I, Soares-Weiser K, et al. Beta lactam monotherapy versus beta lactam-aminoglycoside combination therapy for sepsis in immunocompetent patients: systematic review and meta-analysis of randomised trials. BMJ 2004; 328:668.
55. Bliziotis IA, Samonis G, Vardakas KZ, et al. Effect of aminoglycoside and beta-lactam combination therapy versus beta-lactam monotherapy on the emergence of antimicrobial resistance: a meta-analysis of randomized, controlled trials. Clin Infect Dis 2005; 41:149–58.
56. Bonhoeffer S, Lipsitch M, Levin BR. Evaluating treatment protocols to prevent antibiotic resistance. Proc Natl Acad Sci USA 1997; 94:12106–11.
57. Jumbe N, Louie A, Leary R, et al. Application of a mathematical model to prevent in vivo amplification of antibiotic-resistant bacterial populations during therapy. J Clin Invest 2003; 112:275–85.
58. Young LS. Review of clinical significance of synergy in Gram-negative infections at the University of California Los Angeles hospital. Infection 1978; 6(Suppl. 1):S47–52.
59. Gorschluter M, Hahn C, Fixson A, et al. Piperacillin-tazobactam is more effective than ceftriaxone plus gentamicin in febrile neutropenic patients with hematological malignancies: a randomized comparison. Support Care Cancer 2003; 11:362–70.

60. Bodey GP. Synergy. Should it determine antibiotic selection in neutropenic patients? Arch Intern Med 1985; 145:1964–6.
61. Sader HS, Jones RN. Comprehensive in vitro evaluation of cefepime combined with aztreonam or ampicillin/sulbactam against multi-drug resistant *Pseudomonas aeruginosa* and *Acinetobacter* spp. Int J Antimicrob Agents 2005; 25:380–4.
62. Rahal JJ. Novel antibiotic combinations against infections with almost completely resistant *Pseudomonas aeruginosa* and *Acinetobacter* species. Clin Infect Dis 2006; 43(Suppl. 2):S95–9.
63. Tatman-Otkun M, Gurcan S, Ozer B, et al. Annual trends in antibiotic resistance of nosocomial *Acinetobacter baumannii* strains and the effect of synergistic antibiotic combinations. New Microbiol 2004; 27:21–8.
64. Timurkaynak F, Can F, Azap OK, et al. In vitro activities of non-traditional antimicrobials alone or in combination against multidrug-resistant strains of *Pseudomonas aeruginosa* and *Acinetobacter baumannii* isolated from intensive care units. Int J Antimicrob Agents 2006; 27:224–8.
65. Wareham DW, Bean DC. In-vitro activity of polymyxin B in combination with imipenem, rifampicin and azithromycin versus multidrug resistant strains of *Acinetobacter baumannii* producing OXA-23 carbapenemases. Ann Clin Microbiol Antimicrob 2006; 5:10.
66. Tascini C, Menichetti F, Gemignani G, et al. Clinical and microbiological efficacy of colistin therapy in combination with rifampin and imipenem in multidrug-resistant *Pseudomonas aeruginosa* diabetic foot infection with osteomyelitis. Int J Low Extreme Wounds 2006; 5:213–6.
67. Chang HY, Rodriguez V, Narboni G, et al. Causes of death in adults with acute leukemia. Medicine (Baltimore) 1976; 55:259–68.
68. Feld R, Bodey GP, Rodriguez V, et al. Causes of death in patients with malignant lymphoma. Am J Med Sci 1974; 268:97–106.
69. Zinner SH. Changing epidemiology of infections in patients with neutropenia and cancer: emphasis on Gram-positive and resistant bacteria. Clin Infect Dis 1999; 29:490–4.
70. Hughes WT, Armstrong D, Bodey GP, et al. 2002 guidelines for the use of antimicrobial agents in neutropenic patients with cancer. Clin Infect Dis 2002; 34:730–51.
71. Furno P, Bucaneve G, Del Favero A. Monotherapy or aminoglycoside-containing combinations for empirical antibiotic treatment of febrile neutropenic patients: a meta-analysis. Lancet Infect Dis 2002; 2:231–42.
72. Paul M, Soares-Weiser K, Leibovici L. Beta lactam monotherapy versus beta lactam-aminoglycoside combination therapy for fever with neutropenia: systematic review and meta-analysis. BMJ 2003; 326:1111.
73. Paul M, Soares-Weiser K, Grozinsky S, et al. Beta-lactam versus beta-lactam-aminoglycoside combination therapy in cancer patients with neutropaenia. Cochrane Database Syst Rev 2003: CD003038.
74. Smith CE, Tillman BS, Howell AW, et al. Failure of ceftazidime-amikacin therapy for bacteremia and meningitis due to *Klebsiella pneumoniae* producing an extended-spectrum beta-lactamase. Antimicrob Agents Chemother 1990; 34:1290–3.
75. Fleischhack G, Hartmann C, Simon A, et al. Meropenem versus ceftazidime as empirical monotherapy in febrile neutropenia of paediatric patients with cancer. J Antimicrob Chemother 2001; 47:841–53.
76. Peacock JE, Herrington DA, Wade JC, et al. Ciprofloxacin plus piperacillin compared with tobramycin plus piperacillin as empirical therapy in febrile neutropenic patients. A randomized, double-blind trial. Ann Intern Med 2002; 137:77–87.
77. Chastre J, Fagon JY. Ventilator-associated pneumonia. Am J Respir Crit Care Med 2002; 165:867–903.
78. Safdar N, Dezfulian C, Collard HR, et al. Clinical and economic consequences of ventilator-associated pneumonia: a systematic review. Crit Care Med 2005; 33:2184–93.
79. Papazian L, Bregeon F, Thirion X, et al. Effect of ventilator-associated pneumonia on mortality and morbidity. Am J Respir Crit Care Med 1996; 154:91–7.

80. Rello J, Ollendorf DA, Oster G, et al. Epidemiology and outcomes of ventilator-associated pneumonia in a large US database. Chest 2002; 122:2115–21.
81. Cunnion KM, Weber DJ, Broadhead WE, et al. Risk factors for nosocomial pneumonia: comparing adult critical-care populations. Am J Respir Crit Care Med 1996; 153:158–62.
82. Craig CP, Connelly S. Effect of intensive care unit nosocomial pneumonia on duration of stay and mortality. Am J Infect Control 1984; 12:233–8.
83. Fagon JY, Chastre J, Hance AJ, et al. Nosocomial pneumonia in ventilated patients: a cohort study evaluating attributable mortality and hospital stay. Am J Med 1993; 94:281–8.
84. Trouillet JL, Chastre J, Vuagnat A, et al. Ventilator-associated pneumonia caused by potentially drug-resistant bacteria. Am J Respir Crit Care Med 1998; 157:531–9.
85. Richards MJ, Edwards JR, Culver DH, et al. Nosocomial infections in medical intensive care units in the United States. National Nosocomial Infections Surveillance System. Crit Care Med 1999; 27:887–92.
86. Celis R, Torres A, Gatell JM, et al. Nosocomial pneumonia. A multivariate analysis of risk and prognosis. Chest 1988; 93:318–24.
87. Alvarez-Lerma F. Modification of empiric antibiotic treatment in patients with pneumonia acquired in the intensive care unit. ICU-Acquired Pneumonia Study Group. Intensive Care Med 1996; 22:387–94.
88. Luna CM, Vujacich P, Niederman MS, et al. Impact of BAL data on the therapy and outcome of ventilator-associated pneumonia. Chest 1997; 111:676–85.
89. Sanchez-Nieto JM, Torres A, Garcia-Cordoba F, et al. Impact of invasive and non-invasive quantitative culture sampling on outcome of ventilator-associated pneumonia: a pilot study. Am J Respir Crit Care Med 1998; 157:371–6.
90. Kollef MH, Sherman G, Ward S, et al. Inadequate antimicrobial treatment of infections: a risk factor for hospital mortality among critically ill patients. Chest 1999; 115:462–74.
91. Bercault N, Boulain T. Mortality rate attributable to ventilator-associated nosocomial pneumonia in an adult intensive care unit: a prospective case-control study. Crit Care Med 2001; 29:2303–9.
92. Dupont H, Mentec H, Sollet JP, et al. Impact of appropriateness of initial antibiotic therapy on the outcome of ventilator-associated pneumonia. Intensive Care Med 2001; 27:355–62.
93. Iregui M, Ward S, Sherman G, et al. Clinical importance of delays in the initiation of appropriate antibiotic treatment for ventilator-associated pneumonia. Chest 2002; 122:262–8.
94. Hanes SD, Demirkan K, Tolley E, et al. Risk factors for late-onset nosocomial pneumonia caused by *Stenotrophomonas maltophilia* in critically ill trauma patients. Clin Infect Dis 2002; 35:228–35.
95. Dupont H, Montravers P, Gauzit R, et al. Outcome of postoperative pneumonia in the Eole study. Intensive Care Med 2003; 29:179–88.
96. Leroy O, Meybeck A, d'Escrivan T, et al. Impact of adequacy of initial antimicrobial therapy on the prognosis of patients with ventilator-associated pneumonia. Intensive Care Med 2003; 29:2170–3.
97. Mueller EW, Hanes SD, Croce MA, et al. Effect from multiple episodes of inadequate empiric antibiotic therapy for ventilator-associated pneumonia on morbidity and mortality among critically ill trauma patients. J Trauma 2005; 58:94–101.
98. American Thoracic Society/Infectious Diseases Society of America. Guidelines for the management of adults with hospital-acquired, ventilator-associated, and healthcare-associated pneumonia. Am J Respir Crit Care Med 2005; 171:388–416.
99. Cometta A, Baumgartner JD, Lew D, et al. Prospective randomized comparison of imipenem monotherapy with imipenem plus netilmicin for treatment of severe infections in nonneutropenic patients. Antimicrob Agents Chemother 1994; 38:1309–13.
100. Chapman TM, Perry CM. Cefepime: a review of its use in the management of hospitalized patients with pneumonia. Am J Respir Med 2003; 2:75–107.
101. Jaccard C, Troillet N, Harbarth S, et al. Prospective randomized comparison of imipenem-cilastatin and piperacillin-tazobactam in nosocomial pneumonia or peritonitis. Antimicrob Agents Chemother 1998; 42:2966–72.

102. West M, Boulanger BR, Fogarty C, et al. Levofloxacin compared with imipenem/cilastatin followed by ciprofloxacin in adult patients with nosocomial pneumonia: a multicenter, prospective, randomized, open-label study. Clin Ther 2003; 25:485–506.
103. Sieger B, Berman SJ, Geckler RW, et al. Empiric treatment of hospital-acquired lower respiratory tract infections with meropenem or ceftazidime with tobramycin: a randomized study. Meropenem Lower Respiratory Infection Group. Crit Care Med 1997; 25:1663–70.
104. Rubinstein E, Lode H, Grassi C. Ceftazidime monotherapy vs. ceftriaxone/tobramycin for serious hospital-acquired Gram-negative infections. Antibiotic Study Group. Clin Infect Dis 1995; 20:1217–28.
105. Nicolau DP, McNabb J, Lacy MK, et al. Continuous versus intermittent administration of ceftazidime in intensive care unit patients with nosocomial pneumonia. Int J Antimicrob Agents 2001; 17:497–504.
106. Paterson DL. Serious infections caused by enteric Gram-negative bacilli—mechanisms of antibiotic resistance and implications for therapy of Gram-negative sepsis in the transplanted patient. Semin Respir Infect 2002; 17:260–4.
107. Wisplinghoff H, Bischoff T, Tallent SM, et al. Nosocomial bloodstream infections in US hospitals: analysis of 24,179 cases from a prospective nationwide surveillance study. Clin Infect Dis 2004; 39:309–17.
108. Chow JW, Fine MJ, Shlaes DM, et al. Enterobacter bacteremia: clinical features and emergence of antibiotic resistance during therapy. Ann Intern Med 1991; 115:585–90.
109. Chow JW, Yu VL, Shlaes DM. Epidemiologic perspectives on Enterobacter for the infection control professional. Am J Infect Control 1994; 22:195–201.
110. Bouza E, Garcia de la Torre M, Erice A, et al. Enterobacter bacteremia. An analysis of 50 episodes. Arch Intern Med 1985; 145:1024–7.
111. Watanakunakorn C, Weber J. Enterobacter bacteremia: a review of 58 episodes. Scand J Infect Dis 1989; 21:1–8.
112. Burchard KW, Barrall DT, Reed M, et al. Enterobacter bacteremia in surgical patients. Surgery 1986; 100:857–62.
113. Gallagher PG. Enterobacter bacteremia in pediatric patients. Rev Infect Dis 1990; 12:808–12.
114. Kang CI, Kim SH, Park WB, et al. Bloodstream infections caused by Enterobacter species: predictors of 30-day mortality rate and impact of broad-spectrum cephalosporin resistance on outcome. Clin Infect Dis 2004; 39:812–8.
115. Medeiros AA. Relapsing infection due to Enterobacter species: lessons of heterogeneity. Clin Infect Dis 1997; 25:341–2.
116. Cosgrove SE, Kaye KS, Eliopoulous GM, et al. Health and economic outcomes of the emergence of third-generation cephalosporin resistance in Enterobacter species. Arch Intern Med 2002; 162:185–90.
117. Murray PR, Granich GG, Krogstad DJ, et al. In vivo selection of resistance to multiple cephalosporins by Enterobacter cloacae. J Infect Dis 1983; 147:590.
118. Black AS, Cohen J. Multiple beta-lactam resistance in Enterobacter cloacae following ceftazidime monotherapy. Lancet 1985; 2:331–2.
119. Sanders WE Jr, Tenney JH, Kessler RE. Efficacy of cefepime in the treatment of infections due to multiply resistant Enterobacter species. Clin Infect Dis 1996; 23:454–61.
120. Kaye KS, Cosgrove S, Harris A, et al. Risk factors for emergence of resistance to broad-spectrum cephalosporins among Enterobacter spp. Antimicrob Agents Chemother 2001; 45:2628–30.
121. Gesser RM, McCarroll K, Teppler H, et al. Efficacy of ertapenem in the treatment of serious infections caused by Enterobacteriaceae: analysis of pooled clinical trial data. J Antimicrob Chemother 2003; 51:1253–60.
122. Kim BN, Lee SO, Choi SH, et al. Outcome of antibiotic therapy for third-generation cephalosporin-resistant Gram-negative bacteraemia: an analysis of 249 cases caused by Citrobacter, Enterobacter and Serratia species. Int J Antimicrob Agents 2003; 22:106–11.
123. Stein GE. Antimicrobial resistance in the hospital setting: impact, trends, and infection control measures. Pharmacotherapy 2005; 25:44S–54.

124. Anderson DJ, Engemann JJ, Harrell LJ, et al. Predictors of mortality in patients with bloodstream infection due to ceftazidime-resistant *Klebsiella pneumoniae*. Antimicrob Agents Chemother 2006; 50:1715–20.
125. Hyle EP, Lipworth AD, Zaoutis TE, et al. Impact of inadequate initial antimicrobial therapy on mortality in infections due to extended-spectrum beta-lactamase-producing Enterobacteriaceae: variability by site of infection. Arch Intern Med 2005; 165:1375–80.
126. Tsay RW, Siu LK, Fung CP, et al. Characteristics of bacteremia between community-acquired and nosocomial *Klebsiella pneumoniae* infection: risk factor for mortality and the impact of capsular serotypes as a herald for community-acquired infection. Arch Intern Med 2002; 162:1021–7.
127. Du B, Long Y, Liu H, et al. Extended-spectrum beta-lactamase-producing *Escherichia coli* and *Klebsiella pneumoniae* bloodstream infection: risk factors and clinical outcome. Intensive Care Med 2002; 28:1718–23.
128. Lautenbach E, Metlay JP, Bilker WB, et al. Association between fluoroquinolone resistance and mortality in *Escherichia coli* and *Klebsiella pneumoniae* infections: the role of inadequate empirical antimicrobial therapy. Clin Infect Dis 2005; 41:923–9.
129. Schwaber MJ, Navon-Venezia S, Kaye KS, et al. Clinical and economic impact of bacteremia with extended-spectrum-beta-lactamase-producing Enterobacteriaceae. Antimicrob Agents Chemother 2006; 50:1257–62.
130. Tumbarello M, Spanu T, Sanguinetti M, et al. Bloodstream infections caused by extended-spectrum-beta-lactamase-producing *Klebsiella pneumoniae*: risk factors, molecular epidemiology, and clinical outcome. Antimicrob Agents Chemother 2006; 50:498–504.
131. Kim YK, Pai H, Lee HJ, et al. Bloodstream infections by extended-spectrum beta-lactamase-producing *Escherichia coli* and *Klebsiella pneumoniae* in children: epidemiology and clinical outcome. Antimicrob Agents Chemother 2002; 46:1481–91.
132. Zaoutis TE, Goyal M, Chu JH, et al. Risk factors for and outcomes of bloodstream infection caused by extended-spectrum beta-lactamase-producing *Escherichia coli* and Klebsiella species in children. Pediatrics 2005; 115:942–9.
133. Safdar N, Maki DG. The commonality of risk factors for nosocomial colonization and infection with antimicrobial-resistant *Staphylococcus aureus*, enterococcus, Gram-negative bacilli, *Clostridium difficile*, and *Candida*. Ann Intern Med 2002; 136:834–44.
134. Skippen I, Shemko M, Turton J, et al. Epidemiology of infections caused by extended-spectrum beta-lactamase-producing *Escherichia coli* and Klebsiella spp.: a nested case-control study from a tertiary hospital in London. J Hosp Infect 2006; 64:115–23.
135. Lautenbach E, Patel JB, Bilker WB, et al. Extended-spectrum beta-lactamase-producing *Escherichia coli* and *Klebsiella pneumoniae*: risk factors for infection and impact of resistance on outcomes. Clin Infect Dis 2001; 32:1162–71.
136. Panhotra BR, Saxena AK, Al-Ghamdi AM. Extended-spectrum beta-lactamase-producing *Klebsiella pneumoniae* hospital acquired bacteremia. Risk factors and clinical outcome. Saudi Med J 2004; 25:1871–6.
137. Korvick JA, Bryan CS, Farber B, et al. Prospective observational study of Klebsiella bacteremia in 230 patients: outcome for antibiotic combinations versus monotherapy. Antimicrob Agents Chemother 1992; 36:2639–44.
138. Garcia de la Torre M, Romero-Vivas J, Martinez-Beltran J, et al. Klebsiella bacteremia: an analysis of 100 episodes. Rev Infect Dis 1985; 7:143–50.
139. Feldman C, Smith C, Levy H, et al. *Klebsiella pneumoniae* bacteraemia at an urban general hospital. J Infect 1990; 20:21–31.
140. Baltch AL, Griffin PE. *Pseudomonas aeruginosa* bacteremia: a clinical study of 75 patients. Am J Med Sci 1977; 274:119–29.
141. Hilf M, Yu VL, Sharp J, et al. Antibiotic therapy for *Pseudomonas aeruginosa* bacteremia: outcome correlations in a prospective study of 200 patients. Am J Med 1989; 87:540–6.
142. Kuikka A, Valtonen VV. Factors associated with improved outcome of *Pseudomonas aeruginosa* bacteremia in a Finnish university hospital. Eur J Clin Microbiol Infect Dis 1998; 17:701–8.

143. Zelenitsky SA, Harding GK, Sun S, et al. Treatment and outcome of *Pseudomonas aeruginosa* bacteraemia: an antibiotic pharmacodynamic analysis. J Antimicrob Chemother 2003; 52:668–74.
144. Mathews WC, Caperna J, Toerner JG, et al. Neutropenia is a risk factor for Gram-negative bacillus bacteremia in human immunodeficiency virus-infected patients: results of a nested case-control study. Am J Epidemiol 1998; 148: 1175–83.
145. Philippe E, Weiss M, Shultz JM, et al. Emergence of highly antibiotic-resistant *Pseudomonas aeruginosa* in relation to duration of empirical antipseudomonal antibiotic treatment. Clin Perform Qual Health Care 1999; 7:83–7.
146. Vidal F, Mensa J, Martinez JA, et al. *Pseudomonas aeruginosa* bacteremia in patients infected with human immunodeficiency virus type 1. Eur J Clin Microbiol Infect Dis 1999; 18:473–7.
147. Siegman-Igra Y, Ravona R, Primerman H, et al. *Pseudomonas aeruginosa* bacteremia: an analysis of 123 episodes, with particular emphasis on the effect of antibiotic therapy. Int J Infect Dis 1998; 2:211–5.
148. Tapper ML, Armstrong D. Bacteremia due to *Pseudomonas aeruginosa* complicating neoplastic disease: a progress report. J Infect Dis 1974; 130(Suppl.):S14–23.
149. Mendelson MH, Gurtman A, Szabo S, et al. *Pseudomonas aeruginosa* bacteremia in patients with AIDS. Clin Infect Dis 1994; 18:886–95.
150. Chamot E, Boffi El Amari E, et al. Effectiveness of combination antimicrobial therapy for *Pseudomonas aeruginosa* bacteremia. Antimicrob Agents Chemother 2003; 47:2756–64.
151. Pfaller MA, Jones RN, Marshall SA, et al. Inducible amp C beta-lactamase producing Gram-negative bacilli from blood stream infections: frequency, antimicrobial susceptibility, and molecular epidemiology in a national surveillance program (SCOPE). Diagn Microbiol Infect Dis 1997; 28:211–9.
152. Stone AM, Tucci VJ, Isenberg HD, et al. Wound infection: a prospective study of 7519 operations. Am Surg 1976; 42:849–52.
153. Lipsky BA, Hook EW III, Smith AA, et al. Citrobacter infections in humans: experience at the Seattle Veterans Administration Medical Center and a review of the literature. Rev Infect Dis 1980; 2:746–60.
154. Bishara J, Gabay B, Samra Z, et al. Cellulitis caused by *Citrobacter diversus* in a patient with multiple myeloma. Cutis 1998; 61:158–9.
155. Shukla PC. Plantar cellulitis. Pediatr Emerg Care 1994; 10:23–5.
156. Hicks CB, Chulay JD. Bacteremic *Citrobacter freundii* cellulitis associated with tub immersion in a patient with the nephrotic syndrome. Mil Med 1988; 153:400–1.
157. Jones SR, Ragsdale AR, Kutscher E, et al. Clinical and bacteriologic observations on a recently recognized species of Enterobacteriaceae, *Citrobacter diversus.* J Infect Dis 1973; 128:563–5.
158. Chen YS, Wong WW, Fung CP, et al. Clinical features and antimicrobial susceptibility trends in *Citrobacter freundii* bacteremia. J Microbiol Immunol Infect 2002; 35:109–14.
159. Samonis G, Anaissie E, Elting L, et al. Review of Citrobacter bacteremia in cancer patients over a sixteen-year period. Eur J Clin Microbiol Infect Dis 1991; 10:479–85.
160. Drelichman V, Band JD. Bacteremias due to *Citrobacter diversus* and *Citrobacter freundii.* Incidence, risk factors, and clinical outcome. Arch Intern Med 1985; 145:1808–10.
161. Hodges GR, Degener CE, Barnes WG. Clinical significance of Citrobacter isolates. Am J Clin Pathol 1978; 70:37–40.
162. Gupta N, Yadav A, Choudhary U, et al. Citrobacter bacteremia in a tertiary care hospital. Scand J Infect Dis 2003; 35:765–8.
163. Jacobson KL, Cohen SH, Inciardi JF, et al. The relationship between antecedent antibiotic use and resistance to extended-spectrum cephalosporins in group I beta-lactamase-producing organisms. Clin Infect Dis 1995; 21:1107–13.
164. Shih CC, Chen YC, Chang SC, et al. Bacteremia due to Citrobacter species: significance of primary intraabdominal infection. Clin Infect Dis 1996; 23:543–9.
165. Wang JT, Chang SC, Chen YC, et al. Comparison of antimicrobial susceptibility of *Citrobacter freundii* isolates in two different time periods. J Microbiol Immunol Infect 2000; 33:258–62.

166. Wisplinghoff H, Edmond MB, Pfaller MA, et al. Nosocomial bloodstream infections caused by Acinetobacter species in United States hospitals: clinical features, molecular epidemiology, and antimicrobial susceptibility. Clin Infect Dis 2000; 31:690–7.
167. Corbella X, Montero A, Pujol M, et al. Emergence and rapid spread of carbapenem resistance during a large and sustained hospital outbreak of multiresistant *Acinetobacter baumannii*. J Clin Microbiol 2000; 38:4086–95.
168. Nordmann P, Poirel L. Emerging carbapenemases in Gram-negative aerobes. Clin Microbiol Infect 2002; 8:321–31.
169. Paul M, Silbiger I, Grozinsky S, et al. Beta lactam antibiotic monotherapy versus beta lactam-aminoglycoside antibiotic combination therapy for sepsis. Cochrane Database Syst Rev 2006: CD003344.
170. Elphick HE, Tan A. Single versus combination intravenous antibiotic therapy for people with cystic fibrosis. Cochrane Database Syst Rev 2005; CD002007.
171. Tascini C, Gemignani G, Ferranti S, et al. Microbiological activity and clinical efficacy of a colistin and rifampin combination in multidrug-resistant *Pseudomonas aeruginosa* infections. J Chemother 2004; 16:282–7.
172. Zuravleff JJ, Chervenick P, Yu VL, et al. Addition of rifampin to ticarcillin-tobramycin combination for the treatment of *Pseudomonas aeruginosa* infections: assessment in a neutropenic mouse model. J Lab Clin Med 1984; 103:878–85.
173. Zuravleff JJ, Yu VL, Yee RB. Ticarcillin-tobramycin-rifampin: in vitro synergy of the triplet combination against *Pseudomonas aeruginosa*. J Lab Clin Med 1983; 101:896–902.
174. Gunderson BW, Ibrahim KH, Hovde LB, et al. Synergistic activity of colistin and ceftazidime against multiantibiotic-resistant *Pseudomonas aeruginosa* in an in vitro pharmacodynamic model. Antimicrob Agents Chemother 2003; 47:905–9.
175. Hogg GM, Barr JG, Webb CH. In-vitro activity of the combination of colistin and rifampicin against multidrug-resistant strains of *Acinetobacter baumannii*. J Antimicrob Chemother 1998; 41:494–5.
176. Yoon J, Urban C, Terzian C, et al. In vitro double and triple synergistic activities of Polymyxin B, imipenem, and rifampin against multidrug-resistant *Acinetobacter baumannii*. Antimicrob Agents Chemother 2004; 48:753–7.
177. Eggimann P, Revelly JP. Should antibiotic combinations be used to treat ventilator-associated pneumonia? Semin Respir Crit Care Med 2006; 27:68–81.

Antibiotic Resistance: Modern Principles and Management Strategies to Optimize Outpatient Use of Antibiotics

Sharon B. Meropol
Center for Clinical Epidemiology and Biostatistics, Penn Center for Education and Research on Therapeutics, and Department of Biostatistics and Epidemiology, University of Pennsylvania School of Medicine, Philadelphia, Pennsylvania, U.S.A.

Joshua P. Metlay
Center for Clinical Epidemiology and Biostatistics, Penn Center for Education and Research on Therapeutics, Department of Biostatistics and Epidemiology, and Division of General Internal Medicine, Department of Medicine, University of Pennsylvania School of Medicine, and Veterans Administration Medical Center, Philadelphia, Pennsylvania, U.S.A.

"The epidemic increase in antibiotic-resistant Streptococcus pneumoniae *is an ambulatory care problem."* (1)

INTRODUCTION

Antimicrobial use is the key risk factor for emerging antimicrobial resistance among both community-acquired and hospital-acquired pathogens. However, while much attention has been focused on programs to reduce antimicrobial resistance in hospital settings, strategies developed to improve the quality of inpatient antibiotic use may not translate to the outpatient setting. There are numerous differences between the inpatient and outpatient settings, particularly in terms of the opportunities for regulating patterns of drug prescribing and the availability of microbiological data to guide decision making.

We begin this chapter discussing why decreasing unnecessary antimicrobial use in the outpatient setting is of such key importance. We then examine some factors associated with outpatient antimicrobial use, and present a conceptual framework for decreasing unnecessary use. Next, we provide some examples of successful programs for decreasing unnecessary antimicrobial use. Last, we consider potential directions for future strategies to optimize the effectiveness of our available antimicrobial therapies.

IMPORTANCE OF ADULT AND, ESPECIALLY, PEDIATRIC OUTPATIENT ANTIBIOTIC USE

In 2000, the U.S. population-based rate of antimicrobial drug use in ambulatory care settings was 461 antimicrobial drug prescriptions per 1000 persons per year, and the office visit-based rate was 125 antimicrobial drug prescriptions per 1000 visits. The age-based rate of antimicrobial use ranged from a low of approximately 75 antimicrobial drug prescriptions per 1000 office visits per year for individuals greater than or equal to age 45 years to a high of approximately 230 antimicrobial drug prescriptions per 1000 office care visits per year for children under age 15 years (2).

Importance for Resistance at the Individual Level

This enormous level of antimicrobial drug use in the community has implications at the individual level, especially for *Streptococcus pneumoniae*, the leading cause of community-acquired bacterial pneumonia, meningitis, sinusitis, and otitis media in the United States (3–5). Prior antibiotic use is a risk factor for carriage of, and infection with, antimicrobial-resistant *S. pneumoniae* (1,6–9). The very high rate of pediatric antibiotic use is especially important, particularly for individuals in childcare. As young children are the age group most likely to be pneumococcal carriers and most likely to be exposed to antimicrobial drugs, they are not surprisingly major carriers of resistant organisms (1,10) and at high risk of resistant infections (8). Colonized individuals in close quarters with symptoms of upper respiratory infection are at increased risk of spreading resistant organisms to other individuals (1). The transmission of drug-resistant pneumococci is of clinical importance, as shown by studies of inpatients with community-acquired pneumonia, infection with antimicrobial-resistant organisms demonstrating an increased risk of treatment failure, complications, and mortality (11–14).

Importance for Resistance at the Community Level

Antimicrobial resistance is influenced by selective forces related to the community volume of antimicrobial use (15,16). Many correlational studies have demonstrated that countries with higher antimicrobial consumption have higher rates of antimicrobial resistance (17–19). Consumption of beta-lactams is correlated with community levels of erythromycin and penicillin resistance, and macrolides can be strong drivers for local differences in erythromycin and penicillin resistance (17). Although these ecologic studies are not definitive proof of causality, the biologic plausibility and consistency of their findings are striking, and more ideal human experimental conditions are unlikely to be met (17).

A pair of natural experiments has shown that it is possible to reverse the trend toward increasing antimicrobial resistance. For example, in Finland during the 1980s, erythromycin consumption nearly tripled, and streptococcal erythromycin resistance increased from 5% to 13% between 1988 and 1990. Widely publicized recommendations were directed at physicians and the public to decrease outpatient macrolide use. The subsequent 43% decrease in macrolide consumption in Finland was followed by a fall in the prevalence of macrolide-resistant streptococci from a peak of 19.0% in 1993 to 15.6% by 1994, and 8.6% by 1996 (20).

In Iceland, the first penicillin-resistant *S. pneumoniae* (PRSP) was isolated in 1988. By 1993, PRSP accounted for nearly 20% of pneumococcal infections. PRSP surveillance among healthy day care children was instituted, and children found to be carrying PRSP were asked not to attend day care while they had symptoms of upper respiratory infection. Educational messages regarding appropriate antibiotic use were targeted to the public through the media, and the medical community through professional meetings and journals. The focus was on more selective diagnosis and antimicrobial treatment of otitis media, the most frequent reason for pediatric antimicrobial treatment. Propitiously, government outpatient antibiotic subsidies ended in 1991, making families responsible for the full cost of outpatient antimicrobial prescriptions. Antibiotic sales in Iceland declined (although not shown to be statistically significant), and PRSP infection declined from a peak of nearly 20% in 1993 to 16.9% in 1994. In 1992, 47% of healthy day care children were pneumococcal carriers and 20% of these organisms were PRSP. By 1995, 52% of children carried pneumococcus, of which 15% were PRSP (21).

SCOPE OF INAPPROPRIATE ANTIBIOTIC USE

Many descriptive studies show that, while recent efforts to curtail unnecessary antibiotic use have met with some success, there is evidence that there is still a long-standing and continuing problem with unnecessary antibiotic use in the United States for both adults and children, and that use of broad-spectrum antibiotics has been increasing. During the 1990s, adult antibiotic use fell by 23% for upper respiratory infections, and by 22% for bronchitis, but broad-spectrum antibiotic use doubled. By 2001–2002, 49% of adult outpatient visits for "respiratory tract infections" (acute bronchitis, cough, upper respiratory tract infection, and laryngitis, all conditions for which an antibiotic is rarely indicated) still received an antibiotic prescription, and 77% of these were for a broad-spectrum antibiotic, an increase of 87% over 6 years (22). Among children during the 1990s, antibiotic use decreased by 49% for upper respiratory tract infections, and by 13% for bronchitis, but broad-spectrum antibiotic use increased by 74%. By 1999–2000, when pediatric upper respiratory tract infection was diagnosed, antibiotics were still prescribed at 26% to 33% of visits (23), and 40% of pediatric antibiotic prescriptions were for broad-spectrum antibiotics (24).

These data demonstrate that inappropriate patterns of antimicrobial drug use remain a problem in the United States and additional interventions are needed. Promoting improved outpatient antibiotic use involves reducing overall antibiotic use for inappropriate indications, and targeting broad-spectrum antibiotics for those appropriate uses for which they are most likely to be of benefit.

FACTORS ASSOCIATED WITH INCREASED UNNECESSARY ANTIBIOTIC USE

As described by Avorn and Solomon, many elements are associated with "(mis)shaping antibiotic use" (25). Any decision to prescribe antibiotics results from the interaction of three factors, based on an adaptation of Kleinman and colleagues' model for clinician decision-making: medical provider factors, patient factors, and organizational factors (26).

Medical Provider Factors

Providers' perceptions of patients' and parents' expectations can often influence antibiotic prescribing decisions (27–31), although there is some evidence that prescribing behavior is not always associated with actual expectations (31). Other medical provider factors include knowledge regarding optimal diagnostic and treatment strategies, influence of provider-directed marketing campaigns (32), diagnostic uncertainty (33–35), time management strategies, provider sociodemographics (36), training/specialty (37,38), previous experience, clinical judgment, and heuristics, or "rule-of-thumb" (39,40).

Patient Factors

It is commonly stated that a key driver of antibiotic overprescribing is patient expectation or demand for antibiotics when they are sick. However, several studies (28,31,41,42), but not all (27), show that a decreased rate of antibiotic prescribing for patients with acute respiratory infection is not accompanied by decreased patient satisfaction and that satisfaction does not necessarily depend on antibiotic prescribing, as long as patients or parents are satisfied with the time spent on explaining the management plan (28,31). Parents who were offered a contingency plan for antibiotics in the future if the child did not improve were more satisfied with the encounter (43). Other patient factors include particular symptoms experienced and reported, illness severity, demographic, socioeconomic and cultural factors (36,38,44), knowledge about the nature of infectious conditions and the benefits expected from antibiotics (45,46), and past experiences (47,48).

Organizational Factors

Organizational factors include practice setting, provider visit and pharmacy co-payments (49), restrictive formularies including over-the-counter prescribing restrictions (50), availability of acute appointments and telephone advice (51), continuity of care, pharmaceutical sample availability, urban versus rural setting (36), patient volumes (35), patient-centered system navigational features, pressure for high patient volumes (52), and processes involved in obtaining diagnostic testing and results, such as those from radiological studies and rapid viral diagnostic testing. Different care delivery systems may influence decisions to prescribe antimicrobials, apart from a patient's clinical presentation. For example, an antibiotic treatment decision made for a patient in an urgent care clinic might be different than the decision made for the same patient if he/she were seen in a tertiary care hospital emergency department experiencing a broader array of patient illnesses and severity (53).

FRAMEWORK FOR DECREASING UNNECESSARY ANTIBIOTIC USE
Models for Successful Behavior Change

Many different types of strategies can be used to improve patterns of antibiotic prescribing by clinicians and antibiotic use by patients. Interventions that aim to change behavior are more likely to be successful than those that simply provide information to clinicians or patients (10,54–56). Strategies can be aimed at changing physician prescribing behavior, changing patient expectations about the need for an antibiotic, or changing organizational factors to support improved antibiotic utilization. Although strategies are discussed individually here, in practice it is often more effective to simultaneously use a combination of approaches, for example, employing a variety of communication methods targeting multiple relevant groups including patients, parents, children, day care staff, and healthcare professionals, and directed at their specific expectations. However, these complex interventions can be difficult to evaluate; effects are likely to be small to modest, the effect of confounders is difficult to assess, and false results can be costly (57–59).

Conceptual models of behavior change support the finding that successful change is often best accomplished with multifaceted interventions addressing the problem on multiple levels. For instance, the Predisposing, Reinforcing, and Enabling Constructs in Educational-Environmental Diagnosis and Evaluation (PRECEDE) model for health promotion goes beyond individual-level factors to address the social and environmental context in which behaviors occur (60–62). The model includes three types of influences on health behaviors: predisposing, reinforcing, and enabling factors. Predisposing factors include the knowledge, attitudes, beliefs, values, and perceptions that provide the rationale or motivation for behavior. Reinforcing factors are those that provide reward, incentive, or punishment for behavior to be perpetuated or terminated. Enabling factors either block or promote behavior and can make it possible to transform aspiration for behavior into reality.

The Stages of Change model, also known as the Transtheoretical Model, supposes that people must progress, or cycle back and forth, through successive specific stages of readiness-to-change (63,64). The stages are Precontemplation (the person is not motivated to consider change), Contemplation (the subject is considering making a change, is open to new information), Preparation (the person has a strong intention or concrete plan to change), Action (the person is changing behavior), and Maintenance (the person is routinely employing the changed behavior). Particularly effective interventions would target the stage transition pertinent to the specific personal, social, and environmental situation.

Intervention Examples

Some tools that can improve antibiotic treatment are listed in Table 1 and discussed below.

Medical Provider Interventions

Physicians need to balance their obligations toward society with their obligations toward their individual patients (4). The public health concern of antibiotic resistance does not always exert a compelling impact on physicians' antibiotic prescribing. For this reason, guideline recommendations and educational programs alone are unlikely to achieve ideal prescribing unless physician interventions highlight the problem of antimicrobial resistance from the standpoint of how

TABLE 1 Tools to Improve Antibiotic Treatment

Method	References
Professional-directed	
Academic detailing	7, 39, 65–70, 88, 95, 112
Practice guidelines	3, 68, 69, 71–79, 88, 113, 114
Practice profiling	68, 80–82, 113, 114
Public/patient/family-directed	
Home mailings	39, 68, 69, 83–85, 95, 113, 114
Posters, pamphlets	39, 55, 68, 69, 88, 95, 112–114
Videotapes	55, 86, 87
Video kiosks, computer module	90, 112
Viral prescription pads, "cold kits"	88, 89
Media (television, newspaper, radio)	7, 10, 69, 95
System-directed	
Delayed prescriptions	43, 91, 92
Restrictive formularies	50, 93, 94
Telephone advice/access to primary care	51, 84
Decision-support tools	95
Increased diagnostic specificity	96–102

it affects their patients. Physicians must be reassured regarding the safety of withholding antibiotics for patients with certain conditions, and given tools to distinguish between bacterial and viral infections and facilitate effective patient and family communication regarding antimicrobial use (10). Some tools that are available for changing physician behavior include:

1. Academic detailing: Education outreach using local "peer leader" experts to conduct one-on-one or small-group sessions with physicians is an effective approach (7,65–70).
2. Practice guidelines: The U.S. Centers for Disease Control and Prevention (CDC) has recently completed a series of practice guidelines regarding appropriate antibiotic use for adult acute respiratory infection, including: bronchitis (71), exacerbations of chronic obstructive pulmonary disease (72), pharyngitis (73), sinusitis (74), and nonspecific upper respiratory tract infections (75), and publishes regular guideline updates for influenza (76). The Infectious Diseases Society of America (3) and the American Thoracic Society (77) published recommendations for the management of adult community-acquired pneumonia. The American Academy of Pediatrics published guidelines for the diagnosis and antibiotic treatment of pediatric acute otitis media, the most common outpatient diagnosis for which an antibiotic is prescribed for children (78,79), and pediatric sinusitis (79).
3. Practice profiling: Information and feedback to physicians regarding their individual and practice group's prescribing patterns is another intervention that can be effective for certain outcomes (68,80–82).

Patient/Public Interventions

Similarly, a variety of methods have been developed for providing educational messages to patients and their parents. While limited information is available on the individual impact of each method, most successful interventions have used combinations of the following educational tools:

1. Home mailings: Household mailings of brochures to patients, parents, and the public can increase knowledge regarding appropriate antibiotic use and antibiotic resistance, and reduce office visits for minor illnesses (83–85).
2. In-office posters, pamphlets, videotapes: Office waiting room videotapes have also been used to deliver information to parents. Wheeler et al. found videotapes to be preferred by families to waiting room pamphlets and effective in reducing antibiotic-seeking for viral infections (86), but Bauchner et al. showed no significant effect of a videotape on parent attitudes or behaviors (87). Taylor et al. could demonstrate no decreased antibiotic prescriptions after a parent intervention involving a pamphlet and videotape promoting judicious antibiotic use for children (55). Posters and pamphlets have been most often evaluated as part of multifaceted interventions.
3. Viral prescription pads and "cold kits": Imitation "prescription pads" and "cold kits" have been used to deliver written information regarding symptomatic management of viral upper respiratory infections, usually as part of a larger multifaceted intervention (88,89).
4. Public media: Dissemination of information via newspapers, magazines, and radio, and dissemination of brochures using public mailings and at hospitals, clinics, pharmacies, day cares, schools, dental offices, and community

centers have also been used successfully (7,69). Strong branding of these materials by public health and government endorsements may enhance their effectiveness (10). Evidence suggests that television is likely to be the most effective public medium, especially during January when airtime is cheapest and respiratory tract infections (at least in the Northern Hemisphere) are most common (10).

5. Video kiosks: Video kiosks have been used to deliver interactive personalized information to patients in urgent care waiting rooms (90). The computer provided audio- and text-based educational information in English or Spanish, based upon the patient's most bothersome symptom. An English or Spanish printout to facilitate communication with the physician was provided at the end of the encounter.

Healthcare System Interventions

Organizational-level interventions provide an interface between providers and patients. While the feasibility of specific types of interventions is strongly dependent on characteristics of the healthcare environment, a list of potential interventions includes:

1. Delayed prescriptions: Delayed prescription for antibiotics have been evaluated in terms of antibiotic use and patient/parent satisfaction. Siegel et al. evaluated watchful waiting in 194 children (mean age 5 years) with nonsevere acute otitis media. Parents were given a "safety net" antibiotic prescription to fill if symptoms either worsened or did not improve in 48 hr. All subjects received comfort measures and analgesics. Thirty-one percent of the 175 contacted for follow-up had filled the antibiotic prescription. Sixty-three percent of parents reported they would be willing to follow a watchful waiting strategy for acute otitis media in the future (91). McCormick et al. evaluated watchful waiting without antibiotics for children aged 6 months to 12 years with nonsevere otitis media. All unimproved untreated subjects received antibiotic. Over all age groups combined, 5% and 21% of subjects in the immediate-antibiotic group and watchful waiting group, respectively, failed treatment, defined as a return office visit within 0 to 12 days with worsening acute ear symptoms and an abnormal tympanic membrane on physical examination. Sixty-six percent of subjects in the watchful waiting group did not receive antibiotics. Parent satisfaction did not differ between treatment groups (92). As discussed above, Mangione-Smith et al. have shown that parent satisfaction with watchful waiting is improved if the physician communicates a contingency plan to follow if their child does not improve (43).

2. Restrictive formularies: There is evidence that outpatient utilization of specific antimicrobials can be influenced by formulary inclusion (50,93). A recent study demonstrated that hospital formularies that restrict access to fluoroquinolones have reduced rates of fluoroquinolone prescriptions for outpatients evaluated in the ambulatory care and emergency department settings (94).

3. Decision support tools: Decision support tools can help with guideline adherence and include paper forms, computerized entry, electronic medical records, and personal digital assistants (PDAs) (95). In particular, the ability to connect PDAs to laboratory data, decision support software, and prescription-writing software provides a significant opportunity for implementing antibiotic quality improvement interventions into ambulatory care settings.

4. Increase diagnostic specificity: Rapid diagnostic testing for specific bacterial and viral organisms is increasingly available, and may eventually help clinicians distinguish between bacterial and viral conditions and choose the most appropriate therapy. For example, testing for streptococcal pharyngitis has become routine in office practice. Newer molecular diagnostic techniques facilitate rapid testing for pertussis, influenza, parainfluenza, respiratory syncytial virus, herpesviruses, parvovirus, adenovirus, rotavirus, gonorrhea, chlamydia, and orthopedic infection (96,97), although their sensitivity is not always ideal (98–102). As these methods improve, and as their costs come down, they may have wider usefulness in the acute outpatient setting (96,100).

Office-based rapid testing for serologic inflammatory markers may eventually help guide our management. For instance, serum C-reactive protein (CRP) is an acute-phase response protein with 100- to 1000-fold increased levels (11mg/L to >200 mg/L) during acute infections and inflammatory states. CRP has been shown to be elevated in patients with community-acquired pneumonia compared with viral respiratory illnesses (103,104). Flanders et al. studied 168 patients seeking care for an acute cough illness (105). Twenty (12%) of the 168 patients had radiographic evidence of pneumonia, and 17 (85%) of those twenty had elevated CRP >11 mg/L. Although the lower specificity of CRP creates limitations, if this result is replicated in larger studies, a low CRP level could provide reassurance to refrain from using antibiotics for acute respiratory illnesses. Procalcitonin is another systemic marker of inflammation, and has been shown to be higher in adults and children with community-acquired bacterial pneumonia compared with nonbacterial respiratory disease (106,107), and in children with pyelonephritis compared with those with lower renal tract infection (108). Christ-Crain et al. randomized 243 patients admitted with suspected pneumonia to either standard care or procalcitonin-guided treatment, where antibiotics were discouraged for those with lower procalcitonin levels. Relative risk of antibiotic use in the procalcitonin group was 0.49 compared with the standard care group. Clinical outcome was similar in both groups (109). The triggering receptor expressed on myeloid cells-1 (TREM-1) may be more specific than CRP and procalcitonin for distinguishing bacterial from nonbacterial inflammatory disorders (110). In 76 adults admitted to an intensive care unit with suspected bacterial infection, TREM-1 had a sensitivity of 96% and a specificity of 89% for identifying patients with bacterial infection (111).

EXAMPLES OF SUCCESSFUL INTERVENTIONS TO REDUCE INAPPROPRIATE ANTIBIOTIC USE

Several successful interventions to reduce inappropriate antibiotic use have been described in the literature. All used multiple simultaneous interventions targeting relevant groups to affect change among provider, patient, and organizational factors. Some included interventions specifically targeted at antibiotic use, and some focused on other utilization issues, such as self-care, symptom treatment, or day care policies.

Gonzales et al. published the results of their multidimensional intervention on the treatment of adult acute bronchitis in 1999 (39). This was a nonrandomized quasi-experimental study involving four primary care practices in Denver, Colorado that were part of a nonprofit group-model health maintenance organization.

The full intervention site received household- and office-based patient educational materials. Household materials were mailed to families and included magnets outlining preventive and self-care issues, what to expect for a visit for respiratory illness, a CDC pamphlet entitled "Your Child and Antibiotics," an industry-sponsored pamphlet regarding handwashing, and a letter from their practice's medical director about the importance of reducing unnecessary antibiotic use. Office-based materials, directed at patients and family medicine and internal medicine clinicians, included posters regarding: (*i*) the lack of effect of antibiotic treatment on duration of illness for "bronchitis or chest colds," (*ii*) a graphic showing the increased prevalence of invasive antibiotic-resistant *S. pneumoniae* in Colorado, and (*iii*) a graph showing risk of carriage of PRSP stratified by prior antibiotic use. The clinician intervention consisted of a 30-min education session about how to reduce unnecessary antibiotic use for bronchitis, and site-specific practice profiling about bronchitis treatment the previous winter season. The limited intervention site received only office-based educational materials, and two control sites provided usual care without added interventions. All outcomes were compared to baseline values. During the study period, there was a decrease in antibiotic prescription rates for bronchitis at the full intervention site (from 74% to 48%) but not at the control and limited intervention sites. There were no differences in changes in nonantibiotic prescription rates, and return visits did not differ between sites. This group has published several other quasi-experimental trials of similar interventions used for different patient groups in different settings (112–114).

Finkelstein et al. tested the impact of a family and physician educational outreach intervention on pediatric antibiotic use in Massachusetts and Washington State managed care practices. They randomized 12 practices to either intervention or control groups. The physician intervention consisted of two small-group practice meetings with a physician peer leader. At the first meeting, leaders reviewed six one-page CDC-endorsed summaries of prescribing guidelines, focusing on differentiating pediatric bacterial acute otitis media from chronic otitis with effusion, which does not require antibiotics. Four months later, leaders at the second meeting reinforced the recommendations, and presented practitioner- and practice-level feedback regarding antibiotic prescribing rates for the previous year. Parents in intervention practices were mailed the CDC pamphlet: "Your Child and Antibiotics," with a cover letter signed by their own pediatricians. CDC waiting room posters and pamphlets reinforced the same key messages. Antibiotic dispensing for children 3 to 36 months of age decreased by 18.6% in intervention practices compared with 11.5% in control practices. Among children 36 to <72 months of age, antibiotic dispensing decreased by 15% in intervention practices and 9.8% in control practices. The intervention had an overall adjusted effect of 16% in the younger and 12% in the older age group (68).

Belongia et al. reported their Wisconsin nonrandomized controlled before-and-after intervention trial of parent and clinician education on pediatric antibiotic prescribing and PRSP carriage by children using child care facilities. The intervention region consisted of three adjacent countries in northern Wisconsin and their two adjacent cities. The control region was a geographically distinct area surrounding the city of Marshfield, Wisconsin. Children in licensed child care facilities were screened for nasopharyngeal carriage of PRSP. Intervention region clinicians received grand rounds presentations by a peer leader, followed by practice-based small-group meetings with peer educators, presenting five key educational messages regarding antibiotic use for pediatric respiratory illnesses. Clinicians received written practice guidelines for five types of pediatric upper respiratory illnesses developed by a local physician working group, CDC fact sheets for physicians on judicious antibiotic use for common respiratory illnesses and bacterial resistance, samples of parent education pamphlets and information sheets, a sample letter allowing a child to return to childcare with an acute upper respiratory infection, and an imitation "prescription pad" providing written recommendations for symptomatic treatment of upper respiratory infections. Intervention region community procedures included: presentations for child care providers, local public health agencies, parent groups, and community organizations; CDC pamphlets and posters distributed to clinics, pharmacies, child care facilities, and schools; and presentations by project nurses to primary care clinic medical assistants and office staff regarding appropriate antibiotic use. "Cold kits" were provided to intervention region offices for distribution to adolescents and adults. The solid antibiotic prescription rate per clinician declined by 19% in the intervention region compared with 8% in the control region. The liquid antibiotic prescribing rates declined by 11% in the intervention region and increased by 12% in the control region. Retail antibiotic sales declined in the intervention but not in the control region. For participating children attending child care facilities, neither antibiotic use nor nasopharyngeal PRSP carriage rates differed between the intervention and control regions (88).

Perz et al. used data from Tennessee's Medicaid Managed Care Program to study the impact of the Knox County Health Department multifaceted yearlong campaign to decrease pediatric unnecessary antibiotic use. Tennessee's three other large urban counties did not receive the intervention and served as controls. Knox County's intervention was directed at three audiences: the 250 key primary care providers in the county, parents of young children, and the general public. Physician education consisted of peer leader lectures by a CDC physician to 150 key providers, presentations at hospital staff meetings, grand rounds, continuing medical education and resident conferences, distribution of treatment guidelines for pediatric respiratory infections to all 250 providers, and published articles in the Knox County Health Department newsletter mailed to all 1500 Knox County physicians. Most parent education materials were developed by and available from the CDC and consisted of pamphlets mailed to 40,000 households with children in day care and grades K-3, patient education materials distributed to the 250 key providers, and pamphlets distributed to the parents of every newborn. Public education consisted of; 30,000 pamphlets distributed to hospitals, clinics, and dental offices; television, radio, and newspaper announcements; 38,000 pamphlets distributed to families receiving influenza vaccine; and 53,000 pamphlets distributed at pharmacies. Antibiotic prescription rates declined in both intervention and control counties, with an intervention-attributable decline of 11% (69).

Hennessy et al. surveyed 13 rural Alaskan villages annually for 2 years for *S. pneumoniae* carriage and resistance, and collected population-based data on outpatient antibiotic use. Antibiotic use and pneumococcal carriage were both followed after a medical provider and community education campaign was introduced in four villages and then expanded the following year to include the remaining nine villages. The intervention included workshops for community health aides and physicians and follow-up visits to community health aides to reinforce the issues. Community residents received information regarding appropriate antibiotic use and antibiotic resistance in village meetings, at community fairs, through health newsletters, and in high school classrooms. Antibiotic use decreased by 31% in the initial intervention villages and by 35% in the remaining villages when they were included. No decrease in carriage of penicillin-resistant pneumococci was demonstrated after the intervention (7).

Samore et al. reported their cluster randomized trial in 12 rural Idaho and Utah communities, testing the impact of a community intervention with and without a clinical decision support system (CDSS) on reducing inappropriate primary care and emergency department antibiotic prescribing for respiratory infections. The community intervention was introduced in two waves. The first wave included meetings with community leaders, print news releases, distribution of bilingual examination room posters and brochures about appropriate antibiotic use in physician offices and pharmacies, and a mailing of a "do not treat viral infections with antibiotics" information card and refrigerator magnet to parents of children under 6 years of age. The second community intervention wave centered on self-care for respiratory illnesses. A spiral bound self-care guide for respiratory tract infections was distributed at clinics, health fairs, special events, and through one-to-one interactions with community residents. Articles regarding self-care were sent to community newspapers. Decision support tools distributed to clinicians covered guidelines for the treatment of pharyngitis, otitis media, bronchitis, upper respiratory tract infection, sinusitis, pneumonia, croup, and influenza. Three different support tools were offered to clinicians. In one version, a paper form was filled out by the patient, answering questions about specific symptoms. The paper form served as an information resource for the provider. The second tool was a paper-based flowchart designed to lead the clinician to the most appropriate diagnosis and treatment decision. The third tool was a PDA that generated patient-specific diagnostic and treatment recommendations based on clinical data entered by the clinician. Clinician education regarding antibiotic resistance, appropriate antibiotic use, and the decision support tools were provided to clinicians through lectures, small-group meetings, and one-on-one interactions with the study team. The antibiotic prescribing rate decreased by 10% from baseline in the clinical decision support arm, and increased by 1% and 6%, respectively, in the community intervention alone and nonstudy communities. Antibiotic use for "never-indicated" indications and macrolide use decreased more in the clinical decision support arm compared with the other communities (95).

FUTURE DIRECTIONS

Future advances to help us slow or reverse the trend of antibiotic resistance by improving the quality of antibiotic use will need to be multifaceted and would benefit from improvements in behavior change methodologies. Further elucidation of setting- and system-specific factors that influence intervention effectiveness is needed and can help us to understand how to translate and successfully implement promising interventions across clinical and organizational settings (10).

In addition, electronic medical records and decision support software offer key opportunities for integrating appropriate antibiotic use guidelines into ambulatory care decision making. Increasingly sophisticated and realigned electronic medical records, collection methods, and surveillance systems could improve collection and analysis of individual-level data and help define more precisely the relationship between prescribing, colonization, resistance, and disease at the individual and community levels. Improved ability to define and monitor diverse patient outcomes would help ensure that any reductions achieved in antibiotic use do not have adverse effects, and could explore the cost-effectiveness of specific intervention strategies (10).

Finally, improved rapid diagnostic testing options, with capability for real-time pathogen identification informing diagnosis strategies and treatment decisions, would improve targeting antibiotic use to patients who are most likely to benefit (3,115).

CONCLUSIONS

The optimal use of antibiotics in the outpatient setting is vital to maximizing the utility of our available antimicrobial therapies. Considerable evidence supports the combination of specific tools to help us educate medical caregivers and the public, and change antibiotic prescribing behaviors. Application of these methods can decrease unnecessary antibiotic use and improve the overall quality of antibiotic prescribing decisions. Future research will need to determine the cost-effectiveness of these strategies and seek ever more efficient methods for delivering decision support to the point of care. In addition, ongoing surveillance for patterns of drug resistance among community-acquired pathogens is critically important to help gauge the public health impact of these interventions.

LIST OF WEB RESOURCES

Resource (Ref.)	Web site
U.S. Centers for Disease Control and Prevention, Get Smart (89)	http://www.cdc.gov/getsmart/ http://www.cdc.gov/drugresistance/community/
Capital Health, Canada, Do Bugs Need Drugs® (116)	http://www.dobugsneeddrugs.org
Australian National Prescribing Service, Antibiotics in Primary Care (117)	http://www.nps.org.au/site.php?page=2&content=/ resources/ccncs/index.htm
Belgian National Campaign for more appropriate use of antibiotics (118)	http://www.antibiotiques.org/english/index.html
American College of Physicians Principles of Judicious Antibiotic use for Adult Acute Respiratory Tract Infections	http://www.acponline.org/ear/vas2000/principles.htm
Rosenfeld, RM, New York Regional Otitis Project (119), Observation option toolkit	http://www.health.state.ny.us/nysdoh/antibiotic/toolkt.pdf http://www.health.state.ny.us/nysdoh/antibiotic/tktintro.htm

REFERENCES

1. Gonzales R, Bartlett JG, Besser RE, et al. Principles of appropriate antibiotic use for treatment of uncomplicated acute bronchitis: background. Ann Intern Med 2001; 134(6):521–9.
2. McCaig LF, Besser RE, Hughes JM. Antimicrobial drug prescription in ambulatory care settings, United States, 1992–2000. Emerg Infect Dis 2003; 9(4):432–7.
3. Bartlett JG, Dowell SF, Mandell LA, File TM Jr, Musher DM, Fine MJ. Practice guidelines for the management of community-acquired pneumonia in adults. Infectious Diseases Society of America. Clin Infect Dis 2000; 31(2):347–82.

4. Metlay JP, Shea JA, Crossette LB, Asch DA. Tensions in antibiotic prescribing: pitting social concerns against the interests of individual patients. J Gen Intern Med 2002; 17(2):87–94.
5. Mandell G, Bennett BJ, Dolin R. Principles and practice of infectious diseases. 6th ed. Philadelphia: Churchill Livingstone, 2005.
6. Kwan-Gett TS, Davis RL, Shay DK, Black S, Shinefield H, Koepsell T. Is household antibiotic use a risk factor for antibiotic-resistant pneumococcal infection? Epidemiol Infect 2002; 129(3):499–505.
7. Hennessy TW, Petersen KM, Bruden D, et al. Changes in antibiotic-prescribing practices and carriage of penicillin-resistant *Streptococcus pneumoniae*: a controlled intervention trial in rural Alaska. Clin Infect Dis 2002; 34(12):1543–50.
8. Klugman KP. Pneumococcal resistance to antibiotics. Clin Microbiol Rev 1990; 3(2):171–96.
9. Nasrin D, Collignon PJ, Roberts L, Wilson EJ, Pilotto LS, Douglas RM. Effect of beta lactam antibiotic use in children on pneumococcal resistance to penicillin: prospective cohort study. BMJ 2002; 324(7328):28–30.
10. Finch RG, Metlay JP, Davey PG, Baker LJ. Educational interventions to improve antibiotic use in the community: report from the International Forum on Antibiotic Resistance (IFAR) colloquium, 2002. Lancet Infect Dis 2004; 4(1):44–53.
11. Feikin DR, Schuchat A, Kolczak M, et al. Mortality from invasive pneumococcal pneumonia in the era of antibiotic resistance, 1995–97. Am J Public Health 2000; 90(2):223–9.
12. Kelley MA, Weber DJ, Gilligan P, Cohen MS. Breakthrough pneumococcal bacteremia in patients being treated with azithromycin and clarithromycin. Clin Infect Dis 2000; 31(4):1008–11.
13. Metlay JP, Hofmann J, Cetron MS, et al. Impact of penicillin susceptibility on medical outcomes for adult patients with bacteremic pneumococcal pneumonia. Clin Infect Dis 2000; 30(3):520–8.
14. Metlay JP. Update on community-acquired pneumonia: impact of antibiotic resistance on clinical outcomes. Curr Opin Infect Dis 2002; 15(2):163–7.
15. Lipsitch M. The rise and fall of antimicrobial resistance. Trends Microbiol 2001; 9(9):438–44.
16. Lipsitch M, Samore MH. Antimicrobial use and antimicrobial resistance: a population perspective. Emerg Infect Dis 2002; 8(4):347–54.
17. Garcia-Rey C, Aguilar L, Baquero F, Casal J, Dal-Re R. Importance of local variations in antibiotic consumption and geographical differences of erythromycin and penicillin resistance in *Streptococcus pneumoniae*. J Clin Microbiol 2002; 40(1):159–64.
18. Bronzwaer SL, Cars O, Buchholz U, et al. A European study on the relationship between antimicrobial use and antimicrobial resistance. Emerg Infect Dis 2002; 8(3):278–82.
19. Goossens H, Ferech M, Vander Stichele R, Elseviers M. Outpatient antibiotic use in Europe and association with resistance: a cross-national database study. Lancet 2005; 365(9459):579–87.
20. Seppala H, Klaukka T, Vuopio-Varkila J, et al. The effect of changes in the consumption of macrolide antibiotics on erythromycin resistance in group A streptococci in Finland. Finnish Study Group for Antimicrobial Resistance. N Engl J Med 1997; 337(7):441–6.
21. Stephenson J. Icelandic researchers are showing the way to bring down rates of antibiotic-resistant bacteria. JAMA 1996; 275(3):175.
22. Roumie CL, Halasa NB, Grijalva CG, et al. Trends in antibiotic prescribing for adults in the United States-1995 to 2002. J Gen Intern Med 2005; 20(8):697–702.
23. Halasa NB, Griffin MR, Zhu Y, Edwards KM. Differences in antibiotic prescribing patterns for children younger than five years in the three major outpatient settings. J Pediatr 2004; 144(2):200–5.
24. Steinman MA, Gonzales R, Linder JA, Landefeld CS. Changing use of antibiotics in community-based outpatient practice, 1991–1999. Ann Intern Med 2003; 138(7):525–33.

25. Avorn J, Solomon DH. Cultural and economic factors that (mis)shape antibiotic use: the nonpharmacologic basis of therapeutics. Ann Intern Med 2000; 133(2):128–35.
26. Kleinman A, Eisenberg L, Good B. Culture, illness, and care: clinical lessons from anthropologic and cross-cultural research. Ann Intern Med 1978; 88(2):251–8.
27. Macfarlane J, Holmes W, Macfarlane R, Britten N. Influence of patients' expectations on antibiotic management of acute lower respiratory tract illness in general practice: questionnaire study. BMJ 1997; 315(7117):1211–4.
28. Hamm RM, Hicks RJ, Bemben DA. Antibiotics and respiratory infections: are patients more satisfied when expectations are met? J Fam Pract 1996; 43(1):56–62.
29. Cockburn J, Pit S. Prescribing behaviour in clinical practice: patients' expectations and doctors' perceptions of patients' expectations—a questionnaire study. BMJ 1997; 315(7107):520–3.
30. Bauchner H, Pelton SI, Klein JO. Parents, physicians, and antibiotic use. Pediatrics 1999; 103(2):395–401.
31. Mangione-Smith R, McGlynn EA, Elliott MN, Krogstad P, Brook RH. The relationship between perceived parental expectations and pediatrician antimicrobial prescribing behavior. Pediatrics 1999; 103(4 Pt. 1):711–8.
32. Dieperink ME, Drogemuller L. Industry-sponsored grand rounds and prescribing behavior. JAMA 2001; 285(11):1443–4.
33. Gonzalez-Vallejo C, Sorum PC, Stewart TR, Chessare JB, Mumpower JL. Physicians' diagnostic judgments and treatment decisions for acute otitis media in children. Med Decis Making 1998; 18(2):149–62.
34. Froom J, Culpepper L, Grob P, et al. Diagnosis and antibiotic treatment of acute otitis media: report from International Primary Care Network. BMJ 1990; 300(6724):582–6.
35. Arnold SR, Allen UD, Al-Zahrani M, Tan DH, Wang EE. Antibiotic prescribing by pediatricians for respiratory tract infection in children. Clin Infect Dis 1999; 29(2):312–7.
36. Gonzales R, Steiner JF, Sande MA. Antibiotic prescribing for adults with colds, upper respiratory tract infections, and bronchitis by ambulatory care physicians. JAMA 1997; 278(11):901–4.
37. Mainous AG III, Hueston WJ, Love MM. Antibiotics for colds in children: who are the high prescribers? Arch Pediatr Adolesc Med 1998; 152(4):349–52.
38. Nyquist AC, Gonzales R, Steiner JF, Sande MA. Antibiotic prescribing for children with colds, upper respiratory tract infections, and bronchitis. JAMA 1998; 279(11):875–7.
39. Gonzales R, Steiner JF, Lum A, Barrett PH Jr. Decreasing antibiotic use in ambulatory practice: impact of a multidimensional intervention on the treatment of uncomplicated acute bronchitis in adults. JAMA 1999; 281(16):1512–9.
40. Stone S, Gonzales R, Maselli J, Lowenstein SR. Antibiotic prescribing for patients with colds, upper respiratory tract infections, and bronchitis: a national study of hospital-based emergency departments. Ann Emerg Med 2000; 36(4):320–7.
41. Gonzales R, Steiner JF, Maselli J, Lum A, Barrett PH Jr. Impact of reducing antibiotic prescribing for acute bronchitis on patient satisfaction. Eff Clin Pract 2001; 4(3):105–11.
42. Gonzales R, Camargo CA, MacKenzie TD, et al. Patient satisfaction with emergency department care is not associated with antibiotic treatment for acute respiratory tract infections [abstract]. J Gen Intern Med 2006; 21(s4):97.
43. Mangione-Smith R, McGlynn EA, Elliott MN, McDonald L, Franz CE, Kravitz RL. Parent expectations for antibiotics, physician-parent communication, and satisfaction. Arch Pediatr Adolesc Med 2001; 155(7):800–6.
44. Melnick SL, Sprafka JM, Laitinen DL, Bostick RM, Flack JM, Burke GL. Antibiotic use in urban whites and blacks: the Minnesota Heart Survey. Ann Pharmacother 1992; 26(10):1292–5.
45. Gonzales R, Wilson A, Crane LA, Barrett PH Jr. What's in a name? Public knowledge, attitudes, and experiences with antibiotic use for acute bronchitis. Am J Med 2000; 108(1):83–5.
46. Wilson AA, Crane LA, Barrett PH, Gonzales R. Public beliefs and use of antibiotics for acute respiratory illness. J Gen Intern Med 1999; 14(11):658–62.

47. Ray DA, Rohren CH. Characteristics of patients with upper respiratory tract infection presenting to a walk-in clinic. Mayo Clin Proc 2001; 76(2):169–73.
48. Shlomo V, Adi R, Eliezer K. The knowledge and expectations of parents about the role of antibiotic treatment in upper respiratory tract infection—a survey among parents attending the primary physician with their sick child. BMC Fam Pract 2003; 4:20.
49. Shapiro MF, Ware JE Jr, Sherbourne CD. Effects of cost sharing on seeking care for serious and minor symptoms. Results of a randomized controlled trial. Ann Intern Med 1986; 104(2):246–51.
50. Carlson JA. Antimicrobial formulary management: meeting the challenge in a health maintenance organization. Pharmacotherapy 1991; 11(1) (Pt. 2):32S–5.
51. Stirewalt CF, Linn MW, Godoy G, Knopka F, Linn BS. Effectiveness of an ambulatory care telephone service in reducing drop-in visits and improving satisfaction with care. Med Care 1982; 20(7):739–48.
52. Aspinall SL, Berlin JA, Zhang Y, Metlay JP. Facility-level variation in antibiotic prescriptions for veterans with upper respiratory infections. Clin Ther 2005; 27(2):258–62.
53. Gonzales R, Camargo CA Jr, MacKenzie T, et al. Antibiotic treatment of acute respiratory infections in acute care settings. Acad Emerg Med 2006; 13(3):288–94.
54. Little P, Rumsby K, Kelly J, et al. Information leaflet and antibiotic prescribing strategies for acute lower respiratory tract infection: a randomized controlled trial. JAMA 2005; 293(24):3029–35.
55. Taylor JA, Kwan-Gett TS, McMahon EM Jr. Effectiveness of a parental educational intervention in reducing antibiotic use in children: a randomized controlled trial. Pediatr Infect Dis J 2005; 24(6):489–93.
56. Oxman AD, Thomson MA, Davis DA, Haynes RB. No magic bullets: a systematic review of 102 trials of interventions to improve professional practice. CMAJ 1995; 153(10):1423–31.
57. Shojania KG, Grimshaw JM. Still no magic bullets: pursuing more rigorous research in quality improvement. Am J Med 2004; 116(11):778–80.
58. Schunemann HJ, Cook D, Grimshaw J, et al. Antithrombotic and thrombolytic therapy: from evidence to application: the Seventh ACCP Conference on Antithrombotic and Thrombolytic Therapy. Chest 2004; 126(Suppl. 3):688S–96.
59. Grimshaw JM, Thomas RE, MacLennan G, et al. Effectiveness and efficiency of guideline dissemination and implementation strategies. Health Technol Assess 2004; 8(6): iii–iv, 1–72.
60. Hendrickson SG, Becker H. Reducing one source of pediatric head injuries. Pediatr Nurs 2000; 26(2):159–62.
61. Goodson P, Gottlieb NH, Smith MM. Put prevention into practice. Evaluation of program initiation in nine Texas clinical sites. Am J Prev Med 1999; 17(1):73–8.
62. DeJoy DM, Searcy CA, Murphy LR, Gershon RR. Behavioral-diagnostic analysis of compliance with universal precautions among nurses. J Occup Health Psychol 2000; 5(1):127–41.
63. Dijkstra A. The validity of the stages of change model in the adoption of the self-management approach in chronic pain. Clin J Pain 2005; 21(1):27–37; discussion 69–72.
64. Wagner TH, Goldstein MK. Behavioral interventions and cost-effectiveness analysis. Prev Med 2004; 39(6):1208–14.
65. Avorn J, Soumerai SB. Improving drug-therapy decisions through educational outreach. A randomized controlled trial of academically based detailing. N Engl J Med 1983; 308(24):1457–63.
66. Schaffner W, Ray WA, Federspiel CF, Miller WO. Improving antibiotic prescribing in office practice. A controlled trial of three educational methods. JAMA 1983; 250(13):1728–32.
67. Ray WA, Schaffner W, Federspiel CF. Persistence of improvement in antibiotic prescribing in office practice. JAMA 1985; 253(12):1774–6.
68. Finkelstein JA, Davis RL, Dowell SF, et al. Reducing antibiotic use in children: a randomized trial in 12 practices. Pediatrics 2001; 108(1):1–7.

69. Perz JF, Craig AS, Coffey CS, et al. Changes in antibiotic prescribing for children after a community-wide campaign. JAMA 2002; 287(23):3103–9.
70. Thomson O'Brien MA, Oxman AD, Davis DA, Haynes RB, Freemantle N, Harvey EL. Educational outreach visits: effects on professional practice and healthcare outcomes. Cochrane Database Syst Rev 2000(2):CD000409.
71. Snow V, Mottur-Pilson C, Gonzales R. Principles of appropriate antibiotic use for treatment of acute bronchitis in adults. Ann Intern Med 2001; 134(6):518–20.
72. Snow V, Lascher S, Mottur-Pilson C. Evidence base for management of acute exacerbations of chronic obstructive pulmonary disease. Ann Intern Med 2001; 134(7):595–9.
73. Snow V, Mottur-Pilson C, Cooper RJ, Hoffman JR. Principles of appropriate antibiotic use for acute pharyngitis in adults. Ann Intern Med 2001; 134(6):506–8.
74. Snow V, Mottur-Pilson C, Hickner JM. Principles of appropriate antibiotic use for acute sinusitis in adults. Ann Intern Med 2001; 134(6):495–7.
75. Snow V, Mottur-Pilson C, Gonzales R. Principles of appropriate antibiotic use for treatment of nonspecific upper respiratory tract infections in adults. Ann Intern Med 2001; 134(6):487–9.
76. Harper SA, Fukuda K, Uyeki TM, Cox NJ, Bridges CB. Prevention and control of influenza. Recommendations of the Advisory Committee on Immunization Practices (ACIP). MMWR Recomm Rep 2005; 54(RR-8):1–40.
77. Niederman MS, Mandell LA, Anzueto A, et al. Guidelines for the management of adults with community-acquired pneumonia. Diagnosis, assessment of severity, antimicrobial therapy, and prevention. Am J Respir Crit Care Med 2001; 163(7):1730–54.
78. Subcommittee on Management of Acute Otitis Media. Diagnosis and management of acute otitis media. Pediatrics 2004; 113(5):1451–65.
79. Subcommittee on Management of Sinusitis and Committee on Quality Improvement. Clinical practice guideline: management of sinusitis. Pediatrics 2001; 108(3):798–808.
80. Hux JE, Melady MP, DeBoer D. Confidential prescriber feedback and education to improve antibiotic use in primary care: a controlled trial. CMAJ 1999; 161(4):388–92.
81. Pimlott NJ, Hux JE, Wilson LM, Kahan M, Li C, Rosser WW. Educating physicians to reduce benzodiazepine use by elderly patients: a randomized controlled trial. CMAJ 2003; 168(7):835–9.
82. Herbert CP, Wright JM, Maclure M, et al. Better prescribing project: a randomized controlled trial of the impact of case-based educational modules and personal prescribing feedback on prescribing for hypertension in primary care. Fam Pract 2004; 21(5):575–81.
83. Roberts CR, Imrey PB, Turner JD, Hosokawa MC, Alster JM. Reducing physician visits for colds through consumer education. JAMA 1983; 250(15):1986–9.
84. Vickery DM, Kalmer H, Lowry D, Constantine M, Wright E, Loren W. Effect of a self-care education program on medical visits. JAMA 1983; 250(21):2952–6.
85. Trepka MJ, Belongia EA, Chyou PH, Davis JP, Schwartz B. The effect of a community intervention trial on parental knowledge and awareness of antibiotic resistance and appropriate antibiotic use in children. Pediatrics 2001; 107(1):E6.
86. Wheeler JG, Fair M, Simpson PM, Rowlands LA, Aitken ME, Jacobs RF. Impact of a waiting room videotape message on parent attitudes toward pediatric antibiotic use. Pediatrics 2001; 108(3):591–6.
87. Bauchner H, Osganian S, Smith K, Triant R. Improving parent knowledge about antibiotics: a video intervention. Pediatrics 2001; 108(4):845–50.
88. Belongia EA, Sullivan BJ, Chyou PH, Madagame E, Reed KD, Schwartz B. A community intervention trial to promote judicious antibiotic use and reduce penicillin-resistant *Streptococcus pneumoniae* carriage in children. Pediatrics 2001; 108(3):575–83.
89. Get SMART: Know When Antibiotics Work, US Centers for Disease Control and Prevention, US Department of Human Services. US Centers for Disease Control and Prevention, US Department of Human Services, 1995 (accessed at http://www.cdc.gov/getsmart/)
90. MacKenzie TD, Gonzales GR, Levin SK, et al. Patterns of use and acceptability of a bilingual interactive computer kiosk designed to teach patients about appropriate antibiotic use for acute respiratory tract infections [abstract]. J Gen Intern Med 2006; 21(s4):98.

91. Siegel RM, Kiely M, Bien JP, et al. Treatment of otitis media with observation and a safety-net antibiotic prescription. Pediatrics 2003; 112(3 Pt. 1):527–31.
92. McCormick DP, Chonmaitree T, Pittman C, et al. Nonsevere acute otitis media: a clinical trial comparing outcomes of watchful waiting versus immediate antibiotic treatment. Pediatrics 2005; 115(6):1455–65.
93. Marra F, Patrick DM, White R, Ng H, Bowie WR, Hutchinson JM. Effect of formulary policy decisions on antimicrobial drug utilization in British Columbia. J Antimicrob Chemother 2005; 55(1):95–101.
94. Aspinall SM, Metlay JP, Maselli JH, Gonzales R. Hospital formulary status affects outpatient fluoroquinolone prescribing in the emergency department. Presentation at the Annual Meeting of the Infectious Diseases Society of America, San Francisco, CA, 2005 October.
95. Samore MH, Bateman K, Alder SC, et al. Clinical decision support and appropriateness of antimicrobial prescribing: a randomized trial. JAMA 2005; 294(18):2305–14.
96. Tarkin IS, Dunman PM, Garvin KL. Improving the treatment of musculoskeletal infections with molecular diagnostics. Clin Orthop Relat Res 2005; (437):83–8.
97. Leichhardt H, Grunert HP. Enteroviruses: polioviruses, coxsackieviruses, echoviruses and enteroviruses. In: Cohen J, Powderly WG, eds. Infectious Disease. 2nd ed. St. Louis, MO: Mosby, 2004.
98. Prevention and Control of Influenza: recommendations of the Advisory Committee on Immunization Practices (ACIP). MMWR 2005; 54[RR08]:1–40.
99. Stein J, Louie J, Flanders S, et al. Performance characteristics of clinical diagnosis, a clinical decision rule, and a rapid influenza test in the detection of influenza infection in a community sample of adults. Ann Emerg Med 2005; 46(5):412–9.
100. Vega R. Rapid viral testing in the evaluation of the febrile infant and child. Curr Opin Pediatr 2005; 17(3):363–7.
101. Grondahl B, Puppe W, Weigl J, Schmitt HJ. Comparison of the BD Directigen Flu A+B Kit and the Abbott TestPack RSV with a multiplex RT-PCR ELISA for rapid detection of influenza viruses and respiratory syncytial virus. Clin Microbiol Infect 2005; 11(10):848–50.
102. Rothberg MB, Fisher D, Kelly B, Rose DN. Management of influenza symptoms in healthy children: cost-effectiveness of rapid testing and antiviral therapy. Arch Pediatr Adolesc Med 2005; 159(11):1055–62.
103. Melbye H, Straume B, Aasebo U, Brox J. The diagnosis of adult pneumonia in general practice. The diagnostic value of history, physical examination and some blood tests. Scand J Prim Healthcare 1988; 6(2):111–7.
104. Macfarlane J, Holmes W, Gard P, et al. Prospective study of the incidence, aetiology and outcome of adult lower respiratory tract illness in the community. Thorax 2001; 56(2):109–14.
105. Flanders SA, Stein J, Shochat G, et al. Performance of a bedside C-reactive protein test in the diagnosis of community-acquired pneumonia in adults with acute cough. Am J Med 2004; 116(8):529–35.
106. Moulin F, Raymond J, Lorrot M, et al. Procalcitonin in children admitted to hospital with community acquired pneumonia. Arch Dis Child 2001; 84(4):332–6.
107. Masia M, Gutierrez F, Shum C, et al. Usefulness of procalcitonin levels in community-acquired pneumonia according to the patients outcome research team pneumonia severity index. Chest 2005; 128(4):2223–9.
108. Pecile P, Miorin E, Romanello C, et al. Procalcitonin: a marker of severity of acute pyelonephritis among children. Pediatrics 2004; 114(2):e249–54.
109. Christ-Crain M, Jaccard-Stolz D, Bingisser R, et al. Effect of procalcitonin-guided treatment on antibiotic use and outcome in lower respiratory tract infections: cluster-randomised, single-blinded intervention trial. Lancet 2004; 363(9409):600–7.
110. Bouchon A, Facchetti F, Weigand MA, Colonna M. TREM-1 amplifies inflammation and is a crucial mediator of septic shock. Nature 2001; 410(6832):1103–7.
111. Gibot S, Kolopp-Sarda MN, Bene MC, et al. Plasma level of a triggering receptor expressed on myeloid cells-1: its diagnostic accuracy in patients with suspected sepsis. Ann Intern Med 2004; 141(1):9–15.

112. Harris RH, MacKenzie TD, Leeman-Castillo B, et al. Optimizing antibiotic prescribing for acute respiratory tract infections in an urban urgent care clinic. J Gen Intern Med 2003; 18(5):326–34.
113. Gonzales R, Sauaia A, Corbett KK, et al. Antibiotic treatment of acute respiratory tract infections in the elderly: effect of a multidimensional educational intervention. J Am Geriatr Soc 2004; 52(1):39–45.
114. Gonzales R, Corbett KK, Leeman-Castillo BA, et al. The minimizing antibiotic resistance in Colorado project: impact of patient education in improving antibiotic use in private office practices. Health Serv Res 2005; 40(1):101–16.
115. Walsh C. Contexts and challenges for the use of new antibiotics, Chapter 17. In: Walsh C, ed. Antibiotics: Actions, Origins, Resistance. Washington, D.C.: ASM Press, 2003.
116. Do Bugs Need Drugs: A Community Project for Wise use of Antibiotics. In: Capital Health, 2000. http://www.dobugsmeeddrugs.org (Accessed September 26, 2007).
117. Antibiotics in Primary Care. National Prescribing Service Limited, Australian Government Department of Health and Ageing, 2005 (accessed February 1, 2006, at http://www.nps.org.au/site.php?page=2&content=/resources/ccncs/index.htm.)
118. Belgian National Campaign for more appropriate use of antibiotics. 2004.
119. Rosenfeld RM. Observation option toolkit for acute otitis media. Int J Pediatr Otorhinolaryngol 2001; 58(1):1–8.

Index

Printed and bound by CPI Group (UK) Ltd, Croydon, CR0 4YY

23/10/2024

01778239-0005